The International Libra Psychology

PRINCIPLES OF GESTALT PSYCHOLOGY

Founded by C. K. Ogden

The International Library of Psychology

COGNITIVE PSYCHOLOGY
In 21 Volumes

I	The Psycho-Analysis of Artistic Vision and Hearing	*Ehrenzweig*
II	A Source Book of Gestalt Psychology	*Ellis*
III	Common Sense and its Cultivation	*Hankin*
IV	The Nature of Learning	*Humphrey*
V	Eidetic Imagery and Typological Methods of Investigation	*Jaensch*
VI	The World of Colour	*Katz*
VII	Principles of Gestalt Psychology	*Koffka*
VIII	Colour and Colour Theories	*Ladd-Franklin*
IX	Sense-Perception and Matter	*Lean*
X	Invention and the Unconscious	*Montmasson*
XI	Psychology and Education	*Ogden*
XII	Human Speech	*Paget*
XIII	The Gestalt Theory and the Problem of Configuration	*Petermann*
XIV	Surprise and the Psycho-Analyst	*Reik*
XV	The Psychology of a Musical Prodigy	*Révész*
XVI	Biological Memory	*Rignano*
XVII	The Psychology of Reasoning	*Rignano*
XVIII	The Effects of Music	*Schoen*
XIX	Analysis of Perception	*Smythies*
XX	Speech Disorders	*Stinchfield*
XXI	The Psycho-Biology of Language	*Zipf*

PRINCIPLES OF GESTALT PSYCHOLOGY

K KOFFKA

ROUTLEDGE

First published in 1935 by
Routledge

Reprinted in 1999 by
Routledge
2 Park Square, Milton Park, Abingdon, Oxon, OX14 4RN

Transferred to Digital Printing 2005

The publishers have made every effort to contact authors/copyright holders of the works reprinted in the *International Library of Psychology*. This has not been possible in every case, however, and we would welcome correspondence from those individuals/companies we have been unable to trace.

These reprints are taken from original copies of each book. In many cases the condition of these originals is not perfect. The publisher has gone to great lengths to ensure the quality of these reprints, but wishes to point out that certain characteristics of the original copies will, of necessity, be apparent in reprints thereof.

British Library Cataloguing in Publication Data
A CIP catalogue record for this book
is available from the British Library

Principles of Gestalt Psychology
ISBN 0415-20962-5
Cognitive Psychology: 21 Volumes
ISBN 0415-21126-3
The International Library of Psychology: 204 Volumes
ISBN 0415-19132-7

TO

WOLFGANG KÖHLER

AND

MAX WERTHEIMER

IN GRATITUDE

FOR THEIR FRIENDSHIP AND INSPIRATION

CONTENTS

I. WHY PSYCHOLOGY? 3
II. BEHAVIOUR AND ITS FIELD: THE TASK OF PSYCHOLOGY 24
III. THE ENVIRONMENTAL FIELD: THE PROBLEM. REFUTATION OF FALSE SOLUTIONS. GENERAL FORMULATION OF THE TRUE SOLUTION 69
IV. THE ENVIRONMENTAL FIELD: VISUAL ORGANIZATION AND ITS LAWS 106
V. THE ENVIRONMENTAL FIELD: FIGURE AND GROUND. THE FRAMEWORK 177
VI. THE ENVIRONMENTAL FIELD: THE CONSTANCIES 211
VII. THE ENVIRONMENTAL FIELD: TRI-DIMENSIONAL SPACE AND MOTION 265
VIII. ACTION: REFLEXES; THE EGO; THE EXECUTIVE 306
IX. ACTION: ADJUSTED BEHAVIOUR, ATTITUDES, EMOTIONS, AND THE WILL 368
X. MEMORY: FOUNDATION OF A TRACE THEORY. THEORETICAL SECTION 423
XI. MEMORY: FOUNDATION OF A TRACE THEORY. EXPERIMENTAL SECTION AND COMPLETION OF THE THEORY 465
XII. LEARNING AND OTHER MEMORY FUNCTIONS—I 529
XIII. LEARNING AND OTHER MEMORY FUNCTIONS—II 591
XIV. SOCIETY AND PERSONALITY 648
XV. CONCLUSION 680
BIBLIOGRAPHY 687
INDEX 703

PREFACE

The purpose of this book has been stated in the introductory and the final chapters. Therefore this preface can be brief. I conceived the plan of writing a book on gestalt psychology when after five years of pure research work I had to resume the work of teaching. It seemed to me to be the best way of systematizing my own knowledge if I presented it in book form. The final result has not been quite the book I had in my mind when I began to write the first pages. I hoped that I could produce a work which would appeal to a wider circle of readers than that of the trained psychologists, and which would at the same time contain enough concrete material to interest the more technical reader. To myself, and to some of my friends, I formulated this idea by saying that I planned a book which would have a position intermediate between Köhler's "Gestalt Psychology" and an ordinary text-book. I am afraid that all that has survived of this conception is that the book is neither the one nor the other.

In my original plan I intended to give as systematic a presentation of psychology as I was capable of doing. And to this part of my programme I have clung with a determination which to some readers may at times appear pedantic. By this I mean not completeness but consistency. I wanted to bring order into the great mass of facts discovered by modern psychology, by formulating clear-cut problems, showing their interrelationships, offering possible solutions, and exposing the gaps which these solutions leave unfilled. If I wanted to present a system of psychology, it was not a dead or finished system, but a system in the making, a system in the state of growth. From this point of view I divided the field and selected my material. My treatment, long as it has become, leaves out a great number of facts, many of them surely of great significance. But some selection there had to be, and although every selection is to some extent arbitrary and depending upon the person who selects, I have tried to choose my material with regard to the contribution it could make to my general plan. That I have drawn largely from gestalt literature is justified by the title which indicates my concept of systematization.[1] In rereading the book I found some parts much

[1] The greater part of this literature is in German and for this reason not easily accessible to English and American readers. In order to lift this barrier to their becoming familiar with the original literature Dr. W. D. Ellis is preparing a book in which he has assembled the condensed translations of some forty German books

more difficult than others. This is especially true of the treatment of the perceptual constancies contained in the sixth chapter. These constancies contain some of the major problems of today's experimental research and reveal in my opinion the power of the leading concepts of this book. But their discussion is not absolutely essential to the development of the system as a whole. The reader who is not sufficiently interested in them may therefore skip the sixth chapter without losing the thread of the general argument.

After saying what I intended the book to be I may add a few words in explanation of what it is not meant to be. In the first place it has no wish to be dogmatic. It lays before the reader a theory in a great number of applications, but it is for the reader to judge how effective this theory is. It would also be wrong to look at this book as the "authentic presentation of gestalt theory," for there is no such thing. I have done nothing that any psychologist could not have done equally well or better, had he wished to do so. The general theoretical equipment and all the facts were available to everybody. There exists no "secret of the guild" which would give me or other members of the so-called "gestalt school" a special standing. And therefore the book has to be judged not only as a "gestalt psychology," but also as a psychology.

Furthermore, the book does not want to be polemical except in an entirely impersonal way which should appear throughout its pages and is explicitly mentioned in the concluding chapter. Naturally, in order to establish a certain explanation of phenomena other explanations had to be ruled out. In many places such explanations have been presented in a form made up by myself in such a way as to give them the greatest plausibility. At times, however, it was expedient to quote from individual authors.[2] In these cases personal polemics were as far from my mind as in the others. I have chosen my opponents because of the value of their contributions; it would have seemed unfair to me to disregard their arguments, and often enough the criticism of their opinions has helped me in the development of my own hypotheses.

In conclusion it is meet to express my obligation to those without whose direct or indirect help this book could not have been written. Everybody knows, and my text reveals it in every chapter, what I owe to the two friends to whom I have dedicated it. Ever since the winter semester of 1910-11, when we three worked together at

and articles on gestalt psychology covering the period from 1915-1929. This collection, to be published in the near future, will be of great help to the student of gestalt psychology. (*A Source Book of Gestalt Psychology*, 1938, Kegan Paul).

[2] All references in the text refer to the bibliography appended at the end.

Frankfort on the Main, I have been guided by their creative ideas. I was sorely tempted to add to my dedication the quotation from *Faust* which Hermann Ebbinghaus inscribed on the page on which he dedicated his *Grundzüge* to Gustav Theodor Fechner, and only my reluctance to plagiarizing has prevented me from doing so. I owe a great debt of gratitude to President W. A. Neilson and to Smith College, first for appointing me Research Professor and thus granting me five full years in which supported by president and faculty I could devote all my efforts to pure research, and then making my load of teaching so easy that I could within little over two years write this book, thus utilizing the result of my five years' experimenting and thinking. I thank my students who patiently listened to these chapters as they were composed, and contributed by a number of well chosen criticisms, and my colleagues with whom some of the problems were discussed in seminar talks. Another colleague of mine, though not a psychologist, Professor W. A. Orton, has read a good third of the book, suggesting several valuable changes; he has also been of inestimable help in revising the final galleys. Dr. Julian Blackburn of the University of Cambridge, who spent six months with me as a Rockefeller Fellow, read the whole typescript and drew my attention to many places where the argument was not clear or lacked consistency. To my colleague at the Massachusetts State College, Dr. W. D. Ellis, I am indebted for his painstaking work in revising the proofs. But of all I have received the most active help from my former student, Dr. M. R. Harrower. To her not only the author, but also the reader, is greatly indebted. In scanning every line of the typescript and the proofs with the greatest care she thought constantly both of the content and of the reader. In many hours of discussion she made me reformulate a number of passages so that they carried meaning not only to myself but also to those who might take the trouble of studying the book. It is also due to her skill that the English of the text is as correct as it is.

I believe that psychology has entered a period of rapid and healthy progress so that this work will soon be antiquated in many parts. If it contributes even a small share to such progress, I shall feel rewarded for the labour it cost me to write it.

K. KOFFKA

Smith College
Northampton, Mass.
February, 1935

Principles of Gestalt Psychology

CHAPTER I

WHY PSYCHOLOGY?

An Introductory Question. Facts and Theories. Science and the Sciences. Science and Conduct. The Danger of Science. Science as Discipline. Function of Science. Special Function of Psychology. Nature, Life, Mind. Integration of Quantity, Order, and Meaning. The Common Principle in the Preceding Discussion. Generality of the Gestalt Category. Why Psychology?

AN INTRODUCTORY QUESTION

When I first conceived the plan of writing this book I guessed, though I did not know, how much effort it would cost to carry it out, and what demands it would put on a potential reader. And I doubted, not rhetorically but very honestly and sincerely, whether such labour on the part of the author and the reader was justified. I was not so much troubled by the idea of writing *another* book on psychology in addition to the many books which have appeared during the last ten years, as by the idea of writing a book on *psychology*. Writing a book for publication is a social act. Is one justified in demanding co-operation of society for such an enterprise? What good can society, or a small fraction of it, at best derive from it? I tried to give an answer to this question, and when now, after having completed the book, I return to this first chapter, I find that the answer which then gave me sufficient courage to start on my long journey, has stayed with me to the end. I believed I had found a reason why a book on psychology might do some good. Psychology has split up into so many branches and schools, either ignoring or fighting each other, that even an outsider may have the impression—surely strengthened by the publications "Psychologies of 1925" and "Psychologies of 1930"—that the plural "psychologies" should be substituted for the singular.

Psychology has been pampered in the United States, where for many years it has enjoyed great popularity, though it seems to me that its fortunes have somewhat ebbed and may be ebbing more; in England, the land of conservative change, it found for a long time as cold a welcome as any other loud and startling innovation, but has gradually gained ground and is, in my belief, still gaining; in Germany, where experimental psychology was born and had at first a period of rapid expansion, a strong reaction set in soon afterwards which very definitely kept psychology "in its place."

I confess that today I feel much less animosity towards the active enemies of psychology—or those of them who are serious and honest—than when I was younger.

The comparison of psychology as it is today with other branches of human knowledge has raised the question in my mind what contribution psychology has made through the very extensive and intensive effort of the men and women who devote their life's work to it.

No student of philosophy need fail to get some inkling of the great and deep problems which have beset the minds of our profoundest thinkers from ancient to modern times; no student of history need remain unaware of the terrific human forces that have been consumed in the making and unmaking of empires and have combined to create the world in which we are living at this moment; no student of physics need pass his final examination without some insight into the increasing rationalization of our knowledge of nature nor into the inexorable exactness of experimental methods; and no student of mathematics should leave his courses without having learned what generalized thinking is and what beautiful and powerful results it can achieve. But what can we say of the student of psychology? Must he have learned to understand human nature and human actions better at the end of his course? I am not ready to answer this question in the affirmative. But before I had an answer to the question, what it is that a student of psychology should be able to gain from his general course, what it is, more generally expressed, that psychology can contribute to the imperishable possessions of our race, I did not feel justified in writing a general book on the subject.

FACTS AND THEORIES

Nobody can reproach psychology with having discovered too few facts. A psychologist who knew all the facts that have been brought to light by experimental methods would indeed know much, very much. And such knowledge is today regarded as an aim in its own right. "Find facts, facts, and again facts; when you are sure of your facts try to build theories. But your facts are more important." This slogan expresses the creed of a philosophy which is widely accepted today. And indeed it seems very plausible. On the one side are the objective facts, independent of the scientist who investigates them; on the other are his hypotheses, his theories, pure products of his mind. Naturally we should attribute more value to the former than to the latter. In psychology such a view can claim a particular justification. For this science consisted of a number of simple and comprehensive theories and few scientifically established facts before the beginning of the new era. With the advent of experiment more and more facts were discovered which played havoc with the old theories. Only when psychology determined to become a fact-finding science did it begin to become a real science. From the state in which it knew little and fancied a great deal it has progressed to a state where it knows a lot and fancies little—at least consciously and with a purpose, though unawares it contains more fancy than many psychologists are aware of. To evaluate this progress we have to examine what it means to know much. The Latin adage *multum non multa* distinguishes between two meanings of the word "much." The one which it discards in favour of the other is purely quantitative. According to the latter a person who knows twenty items knows ten times as much as the person who knows only two items. But in another sense the latter person, if he knows those two items in their intrinsic relation, so that they are no longer two but one with two parts, knows a great deal more than the former, if he knows just twenty items in pure aggregation. Although from the point of *multa* this person would be superior, he would be inferior from the point of *multum*.

Now as I look upon the growth of science it seems to me that it began to find itself and thereby entered a new epoch when at the time of the Renaissance it changed from a chase for the *multa* to a search for the *multum*. Since that time science has continually striven to reduce the number of propositions from which all known facts can be derived. In this enterprise it has been more and more successful, and has by its new method also discovered more and more facts which otherwise would never have become known; it has simultaneously discarded as fancy many a piece of knowledge which was taken as fact, and has changed the systematic status of many other facts. It is a "fact" that heavy bodies fall more quickly than light ones, as anyone can test by dropping a pencil and a sheet of paper. But it is a complex, not a simple fact, whereas the simple fact is that all bodies fall with the same velocity in a vacuum. From this scientific fact the everyday fact can be derived but not vice versa. The very concept of fact, therefore, becomes problematical.

One can look at the progress of science as a steady increase in the number of facts known. Then one arrives at a position where much knowledge means knowledge of *multa.* But a very different aspect of scientific progress is also possible: the increasing simplicity—not of course in the sense that it is more and more easy to learn, but in the sense that to him who has mastered it the system of science becomes a more and more cohesive and unitary whole. Or otherwise expressed, science is not comparable to a catalogue in which all facts are listed according to an arbitrary principle, like the books in a library in the alphabetical order of their authors; science is *rational;* the facts and their order are one and the same; facts without order do not exist; therefore if we know one fact thoroughly we know ever so many more facts from the knowledge of this one fact. From this point of view, much knowledge is knowledge of *multum,* knowledge of the rational system, the interdependence of all facts.

SCIENCE AND THE SCIENCES

Of course science never succeeds in reaching its goal. At any one moment in its history there is a wide gap between its ideal and its accomplishment. The system is never complete, there are always facts, old and newly discovered, which defy the unity of the system. Apparent as this is within the compass of any individual science, it becomes even more manifest when we consider the variety of different sciences. They have all arisen from one common matrix. The first scientific impulse was not directed towards different special groups of topics but was universal. In our present terminology we can say that philosophy is the mother of all sciences.

Progressive specialization has marked scientific progress, and our science, psychology, was the last to gain her independence. This separation and specialization was necessary, but it has of necessity worked against the aim of unification of knowledge. If a number of separately established sciences have developed, then, coherent as each one may be in itself, what is their mutual relation? How can a *multum* arise from that *multa?* That this task must be accomplished follows from the very function of science. I am the last to see the value of science in its practical applications. The explanation of the shift of spectral lines coming from stars millions of light years distant, is in my eyes a much greater triumph of science than the construction of a new bridge with a record span or the transmission of photographs across the ocean. But for all that I do not believe that science can be legitimately regarded as the game of a relatively small number of people who enjoy it and get their livelihood from it. In some sense science cannot be wholly divorced from conduct.

SCIENCE AND CONDUCT

Conduct, of course, is possible without science. Humans carried on in their daily affairs long before the first spark of science had been struck. And today there are millions of people living whose actions are not determined by anything we call science. Science, however, could not but gain an increasing influence on human behaviour. To describe this influence roughly and briefly will throw a new light on science. Exaggerating and schematizing the differences, we can say: in the prescientific stage man behaves in a situation as the situation tells him to behave. To primitive man each thing says what it is and what he ought to do with it: a fruit says, "Eat me"; water says, "Drink me"; thunder says, "Fear me," and woman says, "Love me."

This world is limited, but, up to a point, manageable, knowledge is direct and quite unscientific, in many cases perfectly true, but in many others hopelessly wrong. And man slowly discovered the errors in his original world. He learned to distrust what things told him, and gradually he forgot the language of birds and stones. Instead he developed a new activity which he called thinking. And this new activity brought him great advantages. He could think out the consequences of events and actions and thereby make himself free of past and present. By thinking he created knowledge in the sense of scientific knowledge, knowledge which was no longer a knowledge of individual things, but of universals. Knowledge thereby becomes more and more indirect, and action, to the extent that it loses its direct guidance by the world of things, more and more intellectualized. Moreover, the process of thinking had destroyed the unity of the primitive world. Thought had developed categories or classes, and each class had its own characteristics, modes of behaviour, or laws. Concrete situations which demand decisions and prompt actions do not, however, fall into only one such class. And so action, if it were to be directed by scientific knowledge, had to be subjected to a complex thought process, and often enough such a process failed to give a clear decision. In other words, whereas the world of primitive man had directly determined his conduct, had told him what was good, what bad, the scientific world proved all too often a failure when it came to answering such questions. Reason seemed to reveal truth, but a truth that would give no guidance to conduct; but the demand for such guidance remained and had to be filled. Thus arose eventually the dualism of science and religion, with its various phases of double-truth theory, bitter enmity, and sentimentalization of science, one as unsatisfactory as the other.

THE DANGER OF SCIENCE

Is it the tragedy of the human race that for every gain it makes it has to pay a price which often seems greater than the gain? Must we pay for science by a disintegration of our life? Must we deny on week-days what we profess on Sundays? As a personal article of faith I believe that there is no such inexorable must. Science, in building rational systems of knowledge, had to select such facts as would most readily submit to such systematization. This process of selection, in itself of the greatest significance, involves the neglecting or rejecting of a number of facts or aspects. As long as scientists know what they are doing, such procedure is fraught with little danger. But in the triumph over its success science is apt to forget that it has not absorbed all aspects of reality, and to deny the existence of those which it has neglected. Thus, instead of keeping in mind the question which gave rise to all science, "what God is, what we are . . ." it holds up such questions to ridicule, and considers the men and women who persist in asking them as atavistic survivals.

This attitude, whose historical necessity and merit I plainly discern, must be rejected, not because it is inimical to religion, but because it would, if consistently maintained, block the progress of science itself by closing to its advance the gates that lead to the most essential of all questions. In my opinion no gate should be closed to science; by this I do not mean that today's or yesterday's science is capable of answering the fundamental questions, as so many radicals, men of the best motives, seem to think. Instead I believe that science, aware of its incompleteness, should gradually attempt to broaden its base, to include more and more of the facts which it found at first necessary to exclude, and thereby become better and better equipped to answer those questions which mankind will not be denied. As long as science misunderstands its task it will always be in danger of losing its position of independence and integrity. The illegal usurper of a throne will always find illegal pretenders. The denunciation of the intellect which has assumed such tremendous proportions in some parts of our world with such far-reaching consequences, seems to me the outcome of the wrong scientific attitude, although for that reason it is no less wrong itself. I shall revert to this theme in a later chapter (Chapter IX), and shall point out only that science if it follows the path which I have briefly indicated will assume a different face. But I hope that such a science will, slowly but surely, help to re-create that original unity which it had to destroy in order to develop.

A science, therefore, gains in value and significance not by the number of individual facts it collects but by the generality and power of its theories, a conclusion which is the very opposite of the statement from which our discussion started. Such a view, however, does not look down upon facts, for theories are theories of facts and can be tested only by facts, they are not idle speculations of what might be, but *θεωρίαι*, i.e., surveys, intuitions, of what is. Therefore in my presentation of psychology I shall emphasize the theoretical aspect; many facts will be reported, but not as a mere collection, or an exhibition of curious phenomena to be compared to Mme. Tussaud's waxworks, but as facts in a system—as far as it is humanly possible not a pet system of my own, but the system to which they intrinsically belong—i.e., as rationally understandable facts.

SCIENCE AS DISCIPLINE

Such a procedure would, however, be without value if it neglected another aspect of science, so far omitted from our discussion, viz., the greatest possible exactness in the establishment of facts. By its demand for exactness science frees itself from the personal wishes of the scientist. A theory must be demanded by facts; in its turn it demands facts, and if they fail to conform exactly to it, then the theory is either wrong or incomplete. In this sense science is discipline. We cannot do what we want, but must do what the facts demand. The success of science has tended to make us proud and conceited. But such conceit is out of place. He is the greatest master who is the greatest servant. Again and again we experience in the progress of knowledge how apt we are to halt and stumble, again and again we find how little we can *make* knowledge, how we must give our thoughts time to grow. Therefore the pursuit of knowledge, instead of making us proud and boastful, should make us modest and humble.

FUNCTION OF SCIENCE

To summarize: the acquisition of true knowledge should help us to reintegrate our world which has fallen to pieces; it should teach us the cogency of objective relations, independent of our wishes and prejudices, and it should indicate to us our true position in our world and give us respect and reverence for the things animate and inanimate around us.

SPECIAL FUNCTION OF PSYCHOLOGY

This is true of all sciences. What special claim can psychology make? To teach us humility, what science can do that better than astronomy and astrophysics which deal with times and distances far beyond the scope of our imagination? And what science can discipline us better than pure mathematics with its demands for absolute proofs? Could we then claim that psychology is particularly fitted for the task of integration, and give this as an answer to the question from which we started? I think we can, for in psychology we are at the point where the three great provinces of our world intersect, the provinces which we call inanimate nature, life, and mind.

NATURE, LIFE, MIND

Psychology deals with the behavior of living beings. Therefore, as every biological science, it is faced with the problem of the relation between animate and inanimate nature whether it is aware of and concerned with this problem or not. But to the psychologist, one special aspect of behaviour, in ordinary parlance called the mental, assumes paramount importance. This is not the place to discuss consciousness and mind as such. Later chapters will show the use we make of these concepts. But we will not reject at the outset a distinction which permeates our idiomatic speech as much as our scientific terminology. We all understand what is meant by the proposition that a prizefighter was knocked out and did not recover consciousness for six minutes. We know that during these fatal six minutes the pugilist did not cease to live, but that he lost one particular aspect of behaviour. Furthermore we know that consciousness in general and each specific conscious function in particular, is closely bound up with processes in our central nervous system. Thus the central nervous system becomes, as it were, the nodal point where mind, life, and inanimate nature converge. We can investigate the chemical constitution of the nervous tissue and will find no component that we have not found in inorganic nature; we can study the function of this tissue and will find that it has all the characteristics of living tissue; and finally there is this relation between the life function of the nervous system and consciousness.

Two Types of Solutions of the Problems Involved in This Relation Rejected. Anybody who would claim to have found a complete and true solution of our problems would expose himself to the just suspicion of being either an ass or a quack. These problems have occupied the best human minds for thousands of years, and therefore it is more than unlikely that a solution can be found by any other way than a slow and gradual approach. What I think about the mode of this approach I shall again defer to a later part of the book.

MATERIALISM. But here I shall reject two types of solutions that have been offered. The first is the solution of crude materialism, which gained great momentum about the middle of the last century and found its most popular expression in a book that around 1900 was a best seller and is now practically forgotten. I mean Haeckel's "Riddle of the Universe." I am not sure that the United States are not even now feeling the last ebbing wave of this flood which reached the shores of the New World long after its crest had passed from the Old. This materialistic solution is astonishingly simple. It says: The whole problem is illusory. There are no three kinds of substance or modes of existence, matter, life, and mind; there is only one, and that is matter, composed of blindly whirling atoms which, because of their great numbers and the long time at their disposal, form all sorts of combinations, and among them those we call animals and human beings. Thinking and feeling, why, they are just movements of atoms. Interfere with the matter of the brain and see what remains of consciousness. Although I have expressed this view very crudely, I believe that I have expressed it adequately, particularly when I add that this view is not only a scientific conviction, but as well, or even more so, a creed and a wish. It is the revolt of a generation that saw a strongly entrenched church hold on to dogmas which science, growing up like a young giant, had crushed—a generation that, by the successful applications of science to technical problems, had become vainglorious and had lost that feeling of awe which should accompany all true knowledge. Just as the victorious barbarians, be they vandals or Calvinists, destroyed thoroughly and passionately the creations most dear to their vanquished enemies, so our materialists developed a hatred of those parts of human philosophy that pointed beyond the pale of their narrow conceptions. To be called a philosopher was an insult, and to be a believer was to belong among the untouchables.

Now I bear no grudge against these men, much as I see their narrow-mindedness and their smallness of stature. For I believe that *malgré tout* they have served a good purpose. They have helped to build up an intelligentsia strong enough to stand out against the unwarranted interference of a reactionary church and pursue their own way, bringing up a new generation which was unhampered by theological restrictions and therefore had no axe to grind.

As to materialism itself, it is not necessary today to refute it. I will add only this: the materialist's claim that the problems of relationship or interaction between matter, life, and mind were falsely put may turn out to be perfectly valid. The hopeless error which the materialists committed was to make an arbitrary discrimination between these three concepts with regard to their scientific dignity. They accepted one and rejected the two others—their excuse being the intrinsic and extrinsic success of science and the absurdities of the contemporary speculative philosophy—whereas each of them may, as a conception, contain as much of the ultimate truth as the others, quite apart from the stage of development which each of them may have reached at a given time.

VITALISM, SPIRITUALISM. The other type of solution which I want to reject here does not deny the validity of our problems; rather it attempts to solve them by establishing two or three separate realms of existence, each sharply distinguished from the other by the presence or absence of a specific factor. One can discriminate three such attempts; the first draws the dividing line between life and mind, life and inanimate nature belonging together (Descartes), and mind, a new and divine substance, separating man from the rest of creation. The second, on the other hand, throws life and mind together as directed by a power not found in inorganic nature and therefore essentially different from it (vitalism). The third sticks to the threefold division and looks for special active principles in each of the three realms (Scheler). Of these three, vitalism has gained by far the greatest importance because many thorough and highly ingenious attempts have been made to establish it as a truly scientific theory. The problem of vitalism will therefore occupy us repeatedly in the following pages. Here I only explain why I must reject this whole type of explanation at the outset. The answer is simple enough, but will, without a wider context, appear somewhat unsatisfactory. The vitalistic type of solution is no solution, but a mere renaming of the problem. By renaming it, it emphasizes the problem, and is, in that respect, much superior to crude materialism. But by pretending that a new name is a solution, it might do a great deal of harm to science were it widely accepted. Characteristically, however, vitalism, not to mention the two other forms of our type, has never been popular among scientists, particularly not among those nearest concerned, the biologists. It required always a full share of personal courage to profess oneself a vitalist, and therefore let us honour the men who were willing to sacrifice their reputations and their careers in the service of a cause which they considered to be a true one.

Integration of Quantity, Order, and Meaning. By rejecting these types of solution I have implied the kind of solution our psychology will have to offer. It cannot ignore the mind-body and the life-nature problem, neither can it accept these three realms of being as separated from each other by impassable chasms. It is here that the integrative quality of our psychology will become manifest. Materialism tried to achieve a simple system by using for its interpretation of the whole the contribution of one part. To be truly integrative, we must try to use the contributions of every part for the building of our system. Looking at the sciences of Nature, Life, and Mind, we may extract from each one specific and particularly important concept, viz., from the first: quantity, from the second: order, and from the third: meaning or significance (in German: *Sinn*). Our psychology, then, must have a place for all of these. Let us discuss them one by one.

Quantity and Quality. Modern scientific psychology was started by quantification. Mental functions were shown to be expressible in purely quantitative terms (Weber's Law), and ever since then the quantitative interest has done as much harm as good to the further development of our science. On the one side, we find those who want to measure everything, sensations, emotions, intelligence; and on the other, those who deny that true psychological problems are amenable to quantitative treatment; to them, psychology is the domain of quality, excluding quantity. In my opinion this famous antithesis of quantity and quality is not a true antithesis at all. It owes its popularity largely to a regrettable ignorance of the essence of quantity as used in physical science.

Modern science, it is true, begins with quantitative measurement. The present-day physicist devotes the greatest efforts to making his measurements finer and finer; but he will not measure anything and everything, but only such effects as in some way or other contribute to his theory. It is impossible to discuss here all the functions of quantitative measurement in physics. But it is fair to say that a mere collection of numbers is never what the physicist wants. What he is frequently interested in is the distribution of measurable characteristics in a given volume and the changes which such distributions undergo. Both types of facts he describes by means of mathematical equations which may contain a few concrete numbers but in which abstract numbers are by far the most important constituents. And the mathematical formula establishes primarily a definite *relationship* between these abstract numbers. Measurement has then the rôle to test the validity of the equation for the process which it is meant to describe, i.e., of the relationship established. Such a relationship, however, is no longer quantitative in the simple sense in which any one concrete number is; its quantity is no longer opposed to quality. The misunderstanding arises when one considers only the individual facts with their measured quantities, overlooking the manner of their distribution. But the latter is no less factual than the former, and it indicates a property or quality of the condition or process under discussion. A simple example should clarify this point: In a soap bubble the forces of cohesion between the soap particles pull them as close together as possible. They are held in equilibrium by the air enclosed by the soap membrane, whose pressure would increase if the bubble contracted. The soap, therefore, must remain distributed over the outside boundary of an air volume, and the distribution will be such that it will occupy as little space as possible. Since of all solids the sphere is the one which has the greatest volume for a given surface or the smallest surface for a given volume, the soap will distribute itself on a spherical surface. A statement like this seems to me to be as much qualitative as quantitative; the latter, because it says of each particle that it is here and not somewhere else; the former, because it assigns a definite shape with all its peculiarities to our distribution. Once our attention has been drawn to this point we shall find it difficult in a great many cases to decide whether a statement is quantitative or qualitative. A body moves with constant velocity; truly quantitative, but equally truly qualitative, and the same is true whatever kind of velocity we attribute to the body. Thus when the velocity varies with the sine or cosine of time, the body executes a periodic movement which is qualitatively quite different from a mere translatory movement.

We conclude from these examples: the quantitative, mathematical description of physical science, far from being opposed to quality, is but a particularly accurate way of representing quality. I will, without proof, add that a description may be quantitative without being at the same time the most adequate one. Of the two analytic equations of the circle: $x^2 + y^2 = r^2$, and $r = constant$, the second expresses the specific quality of the circle more directly and hence more adequately than the first.

And we can now draw a lesson for our psychology: it may be perfectly quantitative without losing its character as a qualitative science, and on the other hand, and at the present moment even more important, it may be unblushingly qualitative, knowing that if its qualitative descriptions are correct, it will some time be possible to translate them into quantitative terms.[1]

ORDER. Let us now turn to "order," the concept derived from the sciences of life. Can we give a satisfactory definition of this concept? We speak of an orderly arrangement of objects when every object is in a place which is determined by its relation to all others. Thus the arrangement of objects thrown at random into a lumber room is not orderly, while that of our drawing room furniture is. Similarly we speak of an orderly march of events (Head) when each part event occurs at its particular time, in its particular place, and in its particular way, because all the other part events occur at their particular times, in their particular places, and in their particular ways. An orderly march of events is, e.g., the movement of the piano keys when a practised player plays a tune; a mere sequence of events without any order takes place when the keys are pressed down by a dog running over the keyboard.

"ORDER NOT AN OBJECTIVE CATEGORY." Both examples may give rise to a particular objection or may lead to a special theory of order. Let us take up the objection first: "Why," so an opponent, whom for the sake of convenience we shall call Mr. P, might ask, "do you call the motions of the piano keys in the second case less orderly than the first? I can," so he continues, "find only one reason, and that is that you like the first better than the second. But this subjective feeling of preference is surely not a sufficient reason for introducing a distinction allegedly fundamental, and for deriving from this distinction a new scientific category. And the same is true of your first example. You happen to like your drawing room, but I can well imagine a person, say a stranger from another planet, who would feel happier in your storeroom. Look at your two cases without any personal bias; then you will find that each object, whether in the drawing room or in the loft, is where it is because, according to mechanical laws, it could not be anywhere else; and just so is each key set into motion according to the stern laws of mechanics whether it be Paderewski's fingers or a frightened dog

[1] Wertheimer expressed a similar idea in an unpublished lecture from which Scheerer quotes (p. 272, fn. 1).

which run over the keyboard. But if the ordinary old mechanical laws explain these events, why introduce a new concept, order, which confuses the issue by creating an artificial difference between processes which from the point of view of mechanics are essentially similar?"

REFUTATION OF THIS VIEW BY VITALISM. To this argument another person (we will call him Mr. V) might reply as follows: "My dear fellow, it is very generous of you to disregard your own feelings in the matter, for I know how sensitive you are to badly furnished rooms and how fastidious your taste is with regard to piano music. I shall therefore exclude from my answer the person who is merely supposed to look at or live in one of our two rooms and to listen to the two sequences of tones, just as you said one should. But even so there remains a difference between the two alternatives in each of the two examples, and this difference is decisive, since it refers to the way in which the arrangement and the sequence have been brought about. In my ideal lumber room, each piece has been deposited as it happened to come without regard to any other. And since, as you pointed out yourself, every object in this loft is where it is according to strict mechanical laws, this lumber room is an excellent example of what mechanical forces will do if left to themselves. Compare this with our drawing room. Here, careful planning has preceded the actual moving of the furniture, and each piece receives a place that makes it subservient to the impression of the whole. What does it matter whether a table has at first been pushed too far to the left? Somebody who knows the plan, or who has a direct feeling for the intended effect, will push it back into its proper place: just so a picture hung awry will be straightened out; vases with proper flowers will be well distributed, all of course with the help of mechanical forces, but nothing by these mechanical forces alone. I need not repeat my argument for the two tone sequences, the application is too obvious. But my conclusion is this: in inorganic nature you find nothing but the interplay of blind mechanical forces, but when you come to life you find order, and that means a new agency that directs the workings of inorganic nature, giving aim and direction and thereby order to its blind impulses." And so Mr. V, in trying to answer Mr. P's argument, has developed the theory which I referred to at the beginning of this discussion. Remembering our previous discussion of nature and life, one will recognize this theory as a vitalistic one. As a matter of fact the strongest arguments for vitalism have been based on the distinction of orderly processes and blind sequences.

SOLUTION OF THE POSITIVIST-VITALIST DILEMMA. But let us return to the argument between Messrs. P and V. We have already pledged our psychology to a rejection of vitalism. But can we disregard V's answer to P's argument, his defence of the distinction between orderly and orderless arrangements and events? We can *not*. And that lands us in a quandary: we accept order but we reject a special factor that produces it. For the first we shall be despised by Mr. P and his followers; for the second we shall incur the wrath of Mr. V. Both reactions would be justified if our attitude were truly eclectic; we should then appear to accept two propositions that are incompatible with each other. Therefore the task of our system is clearly defined: we must attempt to reconcile our acceptance and our rejection, we must develop a category of order which is free from vitalism. The concept of order in its modern form is derived from the observation of living beings. But that does not mean that its application is restricted to life. Should it be possible to demonstrate order as a characteristic of *natural* events and therefore within the domain of physics, then we could accept it in the science of life without introducing a special vital force responsible for the creation of order. And that is exactly the solution which gestalt theory has offered and tried to elaborate. How that has been done we shall learn in the course of this book. But it is meet to point out the integrative function of the gestalt solution. Life and nature are brought together not by a denial of one of the most outstanding characteristics of the former but by the proof that this feature belongs to the latter also. And by this kind of integration gestalt theory contributes to that value of knowledge which we have called reverence for things animate and inanimate. Materialism accomplished the integration by robbing life of its order and thereby making us look down on life as just a curious combination of orderless events; if life is as blind as inorganic nature we must have as little respect for the one as for the other. But if inanimate nature shares with life the aspect of order, then the respect which we feel directly and unreflectively for life will spread over to inanimate nature also.

SIGNIFICANCE, VALUE. We turn to the last of our categories: significance. What we mean by that is harder to explain than the two previous concepts, and yet here lies one of the deepest roots of gestalt theory, one which has been least openly brought before the English-speaking public. The reason for this is easy to understand. There is such a thing as an intellectual climate, and the intellectual climate, just as the meteorological, varies from country to country.

And just as the growth of a plant depends upon the physical climate, so does the growth of an idea depend upon the intellectual climate. There can be no doubt that the intellectual climates of Germany and the United States are widely different. The idealistic tradition of Germany is more than an affair of philosophic schools; it pervades the German mind and appears most openly in the writings and teachings of the representatives of "Geisteswissenschaften," the moral sciences. The *meaning* of a personality prominent in history, art, or literature seems to the German mind more important than the pure historical facts which make up his life and works; the historian is often more interested in the relation of a great man to the plan of the universe than in his relations to the events on the planet. Contrariwise, in America the climate is chiefly practical; the here and now, the immediate present with its needs, holds the centre of the stage, thereby relegating the problems essential to German mentality to the realm of the useless and non-existing. In science this attitude makes for positivism, an overvaluation of mere facts and an undervaluation of very abstract speculations, a high regard for science, accurate and earthbound, and an aversion, sometimes bordering on contempt, for metaphysics that tries to escape from the welter of mere facts into a loftier realm of ideas and ideals.

Therefore when the first attempts were made to introduce gestalt theory to the American public, that side which would most readily appeal to the type of German mentality which I have tried to sketch was kept in the background, and those aspects which had a direct bearing on science were emphasized. Had the procedure been different, we might have incurred the danger of biassing our readers against our ideas. Living in a different intellectual climate they might have taken this aspect of gestalt theory for pure mysticism and decided not to have anything to do with the whole theory before they had had a chance of becoming acquainted with its scientific relevance.

At the present moment, however, when gestalt theory has been taken up as a main topic of discussion, it seems only fair to lift the old restriction and expose all its aspects.

THE DILEMMA OF GERMAN PSYCHOLOGY OUT OF WHICH GESTALT THEORY AROSE. To do this I shall revert for a moment to the origins of our theory and to the leading ideas of its first founder, Max Wertheimer. What I said about the German intellectual climate does not apply to German experimental psychology. Rather, experimental psychology had carried on a feud with speculative psychologists and philosophers who, not without reason, belittled its achievements and claimed that mind in its truest aspects could never be investigated by scientific methods, i.e., by methods derived from the natural sciences.[2] How could, so the argument would run, the laws of sensation and association, which then composed the bulk of scientific psychology, ever explain the creation or enjoyment of a work of art, the discovery of truth, or the development of a great cultural movement like that of the Reformation? The facts to which these opponents of scientific psychology pointed and the facts which the experimental psychologists investigated were indeed so far apart that they seemed to belong to different universes, and no attempt was made by experimental psychology to incorporate the larger facts in their system which was erected on the smaller ones, at least no attempt which did justice to the larger.

Weighing this situation in retrospect we are forced to take an attitude similar to that which we took with regard to the materialism-vitalism controversy. We must admit that the criticism of the philosophers was well founded. Not only did psychology exhaust its efforts in trivial investigations, not only had it become stagnant with regard to the problems it actually worked on, but it insisted on its claim that it held the only key to those problems which the philosophers emphasized. Thus the historian was right when he insisted that no laws of sensation, association or feeling—pleasure and displeasure—could explain a decision like that of Caesar's to cross the Rubicon with its momentous consequences; that, generally speaking, it would be impossible to incorporate the data of *culture* within current psychological systems without destroying the true meaning of culture. For, so they would say, culture has not only existence but also meaning or significance, and it has value. A psychology which has no place for the concepts of meaning and value cannot be a complete psychology. At best it can give a sort of understructure, treating of the animal side of man, on which the main building, harbouring his cultural side, must be erected.

On the other hand we cannot disregard the attitude of experimental psychology. Its position was this: for ages psychology had been treated in the way which philosophers and historians claimed to be the only true one, with the result that it had never become a true science. Clever, even profound, things might have been said about men's higher activities by speculative philosophers and "understanding" historians, but all these dicta bore the stamp of their authors' personalities; they could not be verified and could not produce a scientific system. Science wants an explanation in terms

[2] A good account of this side of German psychology is given by Klüver.

of cause and effect, but the kind of psychology they opposed gave explanations in terms of motives and values. This, the experimental psychologists averred, was no explanation at all, whereas their work was concerned with true causal theories. If it failed at the moment to include the cultural aspects, it did so only because it was so very young. But a building had to be erected from the bottom and not from the roof. "*Psychologie von unten*" was their slogan. And there is much to be said for this attitude. If we believe that the sciences, natural and moral, are not merely a collection of independent human activities, some players playing one kind of game, others another, but that they are branches of one all-embracing science, then we must demand that the fundamental explanatory principles be the same in all.

The dilemma of psychology, then, was this: on the one hand it was in possession of explanatory principles in the scientific sense, but these principles did not solve the most important problems of psychology, which therefore remained outside its scope; on the other hand, it dealt with these very problems, but without scientific explanatory principles; *to understand* took the place of *to explain.*

WERTHEIMER'S SOLUTION OF THE DILEMMA. This dilemma must have been prominent in Wertheimer's mind even when he was a student. Perceiving the merits and faults of both sides, he could not join either, but he had to try to find a solution of this acute crisis. In this solution two principles could not be sacrificed: the principles of science and of meaning. And yet these very two were the origin of the whole difficulty. Scientific progress occurs very often by a re-examination of the fundamental scientific concepts. And to such a re-examination Wertheimer devoted his efforts. And his conclusions can be stated in a few simple words, although they demand a radical change of our habits of thought, a change in our most ultimate philosophy. To explain and to understand are not different forms of dealing with knowledge but fundamentally identical. And that means: a causal connection is not a mere factual sequence to be memorized like the connection between a name and a telephone number, but is intelligible. I shall borrow a simile from Wertheimer (1925). Suppose we entered Heaven with all our scientific curiosity and found myriads of angels engaged in making music, each playing on his own instrument. Our scientific training would tempt us to discover some law in this celestial din. We might then set out to look for regularities of such a kind that, when angel A has played *do,* angel C would play *re,* then angel M *fa,* and so on. And if we were persistent enough and had sufficient time at our disposal, we might discover a formula which would make it possible for us to determine the note played by each angel at each moment of time. Many philosophers and scientists would say that then we had explained the music of the heavens, that we had discovered its law. This law, however, would be nothing more than a factual statement; it would be practical, making prediction possible, but it would be *without meaning*. On the other hand, we might try to hear the music as one great symphony; then if we had mastered *one* part, we should know a great deal about the whole, even if the part which we had mastered never recurred again in the symphony; and if eventually we knew the whole we should also be able to solve the problem which was resolved by our first attempt. But then it would be of minor significance and derivative. Provided, now, that the angels really played a symphony, our second mode of approach would be the more adequate one; it would not only tell us *what* each angel did at any particular moment but *why* he did it. The whole performance would be meaningful and so would be our knowledge of it.

Substitute the universe for Heaven and the occurrences in the universe for the playing of the angels and you have the application to our problem.

The positivistic interpretation of the world and our knowledge of it is but *one* possibility; there is another one. The question is: Which is really true? Meaning, significance, value, as data of our total experience give us a hint that the latter has at least as good a chance of being the true one as the former. And that means: far from being compelled to banish concepts like meaning and value from psychology and science in general, we must use these concepts for a full understanding of the mind and the world, which is at the same time a full explanation.

THE COMMON PRINCIPLE IN THE PRECEDING DISCUSSION

We have discussed quantity, order and meaning with regard to their contributions to science in general and to psychology in particular. We extracted each of our categories from a different science, but we claimed that despite their different origins, they are all universally applicable. And as a matter of fact, in our treatment of the issues involved in each of our three categories we have found the same general principle: to integrate quantity and quality, mechanism and vitalism, explanation and comprehension or understanding, we had to abandon the treatment of a number of separate facts for the consideration of a group of facts in their specific form of connection. Only thus could quantity be qualitative, and order and meaning be saved from being either introduced into the system of science as new entities, the privileges of life and mind, or discarded as mere figments.

GENERALITY OF THE GESTALT CATEGORY

Do we then claim that all facts are contained in such interconnected groups or units that each quantification is a description of true quality, each complex and sequence of events orderly and meaningful? In short, do we claim that the universe and all events in it form one big gestalt?

If we did we should be as dogmatic as the positivists who claim that no event is orderly or meaningful, and as those who assert that quality is essentially different from quantity. But just as the category of causality does not mean that any event is causally connected with any other, so the gestalt category does not mean that any two states or events belong together in one gestalt. "To apply the category of cause and effect means to find out which parts of nature stand in this relation. Similarly, to apply the gestalt category means to find out which parts of nature belong as parts to functional wholes, to discover their position in these wholes, their degree of relative independence, and the articulation of larger wholes into sub-wholes." (Koffka, 1931 b.)

Science will find gestalten of different rank in different realms, but we claim that every gestalt has order and meaning, of however low or high a degree, and that for a gestalt quantity and quality are the same. Now nobody would deny that of all gestalten which we know those of the human mind are the richest; therefore it is most difficult, and in most cases still impossible, to express its quality in quantitative terms, but at the same time the aspect of meaning becomes more manifest here than in any other part of the universe.

WHY PSYCHOLOGY?

Psychology is a very unsatisfactory science. Comparing the vast body of systematized and recognized facts in physics with those in psychology one will doubt the advisability of teaching the latter to anybody who does not intend to become a professional psychologist, one might even doubt the advisability of training professional psychologists. But when one considers the potential contribution which psychology can make to our understanding of the universe, one's attitude may be changed. Science becomes easily divorced from life. The mathematician needs an escape from the thin air of his abstractions, beautiful as they are; the physicist wants to revel in sounds that are soft, mellow, and melodious, that seem to reveal mysteries which are hidden under the curtain of waves and atoms and mathematical equations; and even the biologist likes to enjoy the antics of his dog on Sundays unhampered by his week-day conviction that in reality they are but chains of machine-like reflexes. Life becomes a flight from science, science a game. And thus science abandons its purpose of treating the whole of existence. If psychology can point the way where science and life will meet, if it can lay the foundations of a system of knowledge that will contain the behaviour of a single atom as well as that of an amoeba, a white rat, a chimpanzee, and a human being, with all the latter's curious activities which we call social conduct, music and art, literature and drama, then an acquaintance with such a psychology should be worth while and repay the time and effort spent in its acquisition.

CHAPTER II

BEHAVIOUR AND ITS FIELD

The Task of Psychology

The Starting Point. Definitions of Psychology. Molar and Molecular Behaviour. Molar Behaviour and Its Environment. The Geographical and the Behavioural Environment. In Which Environment Does Behaviour Take Place? Behaviour Defined. The Locus of Behavioural Environment. Behavioural Environment Only a Part of Direct Experience. Behaviour and Environment Summarized. The Field Concept. The Field in Psychology. Behavioural Environment as the Psychological Field. Inadequacy of Behavioural Environment as Psychological Field. The Balance Sheet. Relation Between Behavioural and Physiological Field Crucial. The Task of Our Psychology

THE STARTING POINT

We have developed a very ambitious programme and must now begin to carry it out. But where are we to begin, what is our starting point to be? Everybody knows the kind of facts in psychology which he wants to learn something about; there are all too many, and that makes it so difficult to choose one for a beginning. Why do we love our families, why can one person enjoy music while it is boring to another, why is it so difficult to understand mathematics, how does a great scientist hit upon his new ideas, why are some people extremely conservative, others extremely radical, how do children differ from adults, animals from humans? However, all of these questions presuppose a whole theoretical system which we have not yet developed. No such question can therefore stand at the beginning of a treatise on psychology. Should we then start by selecting fundamental facts? The difficulty remains the same, for which facts are fundamental, and how would the student to whom such an allegedly fundamental fact was presented know it to be fundamental? This is a very real difficulty which I remember all too well from my student days. When in the first lectures of my first course in psychology the professor talked about colour mixture, colour contrast, and the colour pyramid, I began to be very deeply disappointed with psychology, for I could not for the life of me see why these were fundamental psychological facts.

Before a fact can become a fundamental fact, a setting must have been prepared in which all facts take their more or less prominent places, be it on the ringside or in the gallery.

DEFINITIONS OF PSYCHOLOGY

Such a setting is usually given by a definition of psychology, what its subject matter is, what its methods are. Since the methods depend upon the subject matter we shall concentrate on a definition or, better, on a delineation of our science first. Three different definitions of our subject matter can be discriminated: Psychology as the science of consciousness, of mind, and of behaviour. Although psychology was reared as the science of consciousness or mind, we shall choose behaviour as our keystone. That does not mean that I regard the old definitions as completely wrong—it would be strange indeed if a science had developed on entirely wrong assumptions—but it means that if we start with behaviour it is easier to find a place for consciousness and mind than it is to find a place for behaviour if we start with mind or consciousness.

The swing from consciousness to behaviour is largely due to the work of American psychology, although, as far as I know, William McDougall was actually the first to define psychology in terms of behaviour. But what he meant by behaviour was something different from and much more inclusive than what is meant by the American school which takes its name from this term. Since their usage of the term is restricted and implies a *theory* of behaviour we must return to McDougall's usage, which is purely descriptive and therefore does not prejudge in favour of any theory.

MOLAR AND MOLECULAR BEHAVIOUR

The difference between McDougall's and the behaviourists' meaning of behaviour has been very appropriately described by Tolman as the difference between behaviour as a molar and a molecular phenomenon. Without going into a detailed exposition at this moment I will give a few examples to bring this difference home. A molar behaviour is: the student's attendance at class, the lecturer's delivery, the pilot's navigation, the excitement of the spectators at a football game, Mr. Babbitt's flirtation, Galileo's work which revolutionized science, the hunting of the hound and the running of the hare, the biting of the fish and the stalking of the tiger, in short, all those countless occurrences in our everyday world which the layman calls behaviour. Molecular behaviour, on the other hand, is something very different: the process which starts with an excitation on the sensory surface of an animal, is conducted by nerve fibres to nerve centres, switched over to new, efferent nerves, and ends in a muscle contraction or a gland secretion. Now the ordinary man, probably more than 99% of the population of the earth, knows nothing about the latter, whereas everyone knows the former; on the other hand, those who know anything about physiology will have to admit that molar behaviour always implies muscle contractions which in their turn set our limbs into motion and are activated by nervous impulses. It is very easy to pass from a statement like this to another: molar behaviour is a secondary phenomenon; it is but the last outwardly observable result of a great number of physiological processes; these are the primary events; these form continuous causal sequences; and, therefore, these alone can form the subject matter of a science. Therefore, for behaviourism molar behaviour supplies no more than the problems, the solutions must always be given in terms of molecular behaviour, so that the finished system of psychology will contain only molecular data, the molar ones having been completely eliminated. We are not yet concerned with the particular mode in which behaviourism tried to carry through its programme, but we may emphasize two aspects of its doctrine: (1) It attributes reality to parts, denying it to the wholes which these parts compose: the molar has to be resolved into the molecular; (2) as a result of this, psychology would forever remain exposed to the criticism of the Moral Sciences which we have discussed at the end of the first chapter. Meaning and significance could have no possible place in such a molecular system; Caesar's crossing the Rubicon: certain stimulus-response situations; Luther at Worms: so many others; Shakespeare writing "Hamlet"; Beethoven composing the Ninth Symphony; an Egyptian sculptor carving the bust of Nephretete, would all be reduced to the stimulus-response schema. What then holds our interest in these occurrences? If they are nothing but combinations of *one* type of events, stimulus-response sequences, why do we not take as much interest in the sequence of numbers that come out as winners on the roulette table, why do we not pore over a list of all the bridge hands that have ever been dealt? The behaviourist will explain this by saying that the sequence of stimulus-response situations in most of us has been such that now we react positively to Shakespeare and Beethoven, and negatively to statistics of rouge et noir. At this the historian would throw up his hands in despair, and would continue his work confirmed in the conviction that psychology, whatever else it might be, is perfectly useless for his purposes, and the behaviourist would let the historian continue writing his fiction, equally convinced that his was the only truth.

Clearly such a state of affairs is highly unsatisfactory to anyone who is not a sceptic by nature or profession. What can he do to satisfy the just claims of the two opposing factions, to prevent the disruption of knowledge into a number of incoherent sciences? If psychology is to be the science of behaviour, must it not have a real place for Caesar, Shakespeare, Beethoven, a place which gives to the behaviour of these men the same *outstanding* and *distinctive* position in his system which they enjoy in the estimation of the ordinary educated person and the historian? It is clear that such an aim cannot be achieved if psychology begins and ends with molecular behaviour. Let us try molar behaviour instead. Perhaps it will be possible to find a place for molecular behaviour in a system that begins and ends with molar.

MOLAR BEHAVIOUR AND ITS ENVIRONMENT

What is the most general statement we can make about molar behaviour? That it takes place in an environment, whereas molecular behaviour takes place within the organism and is only initiated by environmental factors, called the stimuli. Molar behaviour of the type we have chosen for our examples occurs in an external setting: the student's class performance occurs in the classroom in which the lecturer holds forth; conversely, the lecturer behaves in a room filled with students who at least understand his language, if nothing else; Mr. Babbitt flirts in a very definite *social* environment, to say nothing about the partner necessary for this accomplishment; the hound and the hare both run through the field, and for each of them the other is the outstanding object of the environment. All this sounds obvious and banal. But it is not quite as trivial as it appears at first sight. For in reality there are, in all of the cases just mentioned, two very different environments to be distinguished from each other, and the question has to be raised: In which of them has molar behaviour taken place? Let us illustrate our proposition by an example taken from a German legend.

The Geographical and the Behavioural Environment. On a winter evening amidst a driving snowstorm a man on horseback arrived at an inn, happy to have reached a shelter after hours of riding over the wind-swept plain on which the blanket of snow had covered all paths and landmarks. The landlord who came to the door viewed the stranger with surprise and asked him whence he came. The man pointed in the direction straight away from the inn, whereupon the landlord, in a tone of awe and wonder, said: "Do you know that you have ridden across the Lake of Constance?" At which the rider dropped stone dead at his feet.

In what environment, then, did the behaviour of the stranger take place? The Lake of Constance. Certainly, because it is a true proposition that he rode across it. And yet, this is not the whole truth, for the fact that there was a frozen lake and not ordinary solid ground did not affect his behaviour in the slightest. It is interesting for the geographer that this behaviour took place in this particular locality, but not for the psychologist as the student of behaviour; because the behaviour would have been just the same had the man ridden across a barren plain. But the psychologist knows something more: since the man died from sheer fright after having learned what he had "really" done, the psychologist must conclude that had the stranger known before, his riding behaviour would have been very different from what it actually was. Therefore the psychologist will have to say: There is a second sense to the word environment according to which our horseman did not ride across the lake at all, but across an ordinary snow-swept plain. His behaviour was a riding-over-a-plain, but not a riding-over-a-lake.

What is true of the man who rode across the Lake of Constance is true of every behaviour. Does the rat run in the maze *the experimenter* has set up? According to the meaning of the word "in," yes and no. Let us therefore distinguish between a *geographical* and a *behavioural* environment. Do we all live in the same town? Yes, when we mean the geographical, no, when we mean the behavioural "in."[1]

In Which Environment Does Behaviour Take Place? After having distinguished two kinds of environment we have to discuss the question more fully in which of them behaviour occurs. It will help to elaborate this latter concept if we raise the question: How does behaviour occur in an environment, what are the general characteristic relations between behaviour and environment? Take the example of the hound and the hare: the hare starts from a bush and runs across an open field in a straight line; the hound will follow him; when he comes to a ditch, the dog will change its running movement into a jumping movement and clear the creek. Now the hare changes his direction; at once the dog will do the same. I need not continue; what I have said will suffice to draw the inference that the behaviour is *regulated* by the environment. *Which* of the two environments does the regulating, the geograph-

[1] This point is lucidly developed in the beginning of Eddington's beautiful book.

ical or the behavioural? From our last example one might be inclined to answer: The geographical. But suppose now that the ditch were covered by a thin layer of snow, sufficient to bear the weight of the hare but not that of the hound. What would happen? The dog would fall into the ditch, i.e., he would not jump when he came to the ditch but would continue to run. He would, before his fall, behave in a ditchless environment. Since, however, the geographical environment contained the ditch, his behaviour must have taken place in another one, namely, the behavioural. But what is true of the few short moments in which the dog stepped on the treacherous layer of snow, must be true of his entire behaviour; he has been in that behavioural environment all along.

THE STIMULI AS A SUBSTITUTE FOR THE BEHAVIOURAL ENVIRONMENT. Against this argument one might raise the following objection. Nobody in his senses could expect that the dog would jump over a snow-covered ditch, or claim that any animal behaved with regard to the geographical environment per se. Obviously, two different geographical environments which are equal with regard to the manner in which they affect the animal's sense organs, are also equivalent for its behaviour. If, therefore, one substitutes the term stimuli for the term geographical environment, the whole difficulty disappears, and there is no need to distinguish a behavioural from a geographical environment.

Justified as this reasoning appears with regard to our example, it can easily be shown to be wrong. We choose a new type of behaviour. Two chimpanzees are separately brought into a cage from the ceiling of which an enticing banana is suspended. The cage is absolutely empty save for a box in a place ten feet removed from the spot over which the lure dangles. One of the animals will, after a longer or shorter delay, run to the box, carry it under the fruit, and using it as a stool, take possession of the banana. The other, less intelligent, after various unsuccessful jumps will resign himself and eventually ascend the box to sit there sunk in gloom. Both apes have behaved in a geographical environment that contained a box; for both, the stimulus situation was identical. And yet they have behaved differently, and the behaviour of each was regulated by the environment. The geographical environment, or the stimulus situation, cannot be the cause of the different behaviours. But this difference is explicable as soon as we consider the behavioural environments of our two animals. We could describe or explain the activities of either of them very well if we assumed that the behavioural environment of the one contained a "stool" and that of the other a "seat," or in more general terms, the behavioural cage of the one contained an object functionally alive with regard to the ape's present trend of action; that of the other an object functionally dead.

Individual Differences. My discussion of this example will meet with no less fierce opposition than that of the first. Far from admitting the validity of my inference about the behavioural environment of the two chimpanzees, the critics will say that I try to reintroduce the old anthropomorphic explanations which fortunately psychology had discarded for good, and that in addition I had overlooked a much simpler explanation. If two animals behave differently under similar stimulus conditions, then the explanation must be in the animals themselves; they are either by innate endowment or by their previous experience so different from each other that the one behaves in one way, the other in another. I shall not defend myself here against the first part of this attack and accept the proposition of the other. Certainly, if the geographical environment is the same for two animals and the animals behave differently in it, then the cause of this difference must be found in the ("geographical") animals. But I want to go beyond this conclusion, for it is incapable of explaining any actual example, just because it applies to any and every kind of behaviour. And clearly, when I view the *molar* behaviour of these two apes, I find that one *uses* the box as a stool; the other *uses* it as a seat. This description is as adequate as possible, for neither does the intelligent ape fumble about the box until after many vicissitudes he finds himself incidentally standing upon it, nor does the other behave similarly with the only difference that in the end the box is still in its old place and the ape drowsing upon it. No, their molar behaviour is truly described by saying that the one uses a stool, the other a seat. Certainly the two animals must be different animals, but we can now see that this difference must be such as to make of the geographical box two different *manipulanda,* to borrow another term from Tolman. What more do we say when we call these two manipulanda parts of the behavioural environments of our two apes? We started our whole discussion of molar behaviour with the proposition that it takes place in an environment. Since the geographical environment or the "stimulus-providing geographical environment" cannot be the immediate cause of the two behaviours, we must either deny our proposition and establish behaviour without environment—and then our manipulanda would have no place at all—or we must accept these manipulanda as realities, stick to our proposition, and then retain the behavioural environment as that kind of reality which contains the manipulanda and possibly other things as well. In other words, we maintain that the relation between behaviour and the geographical environment must remain obscure without the mediation of the behavioural environment.

Behaviour and Geographical Environment. Let us summarize what we have gained so far: behaviour takes place in a behavioural environment by which it is regulated. The behavioural environment depends upon two sets of conditions, one inherent in the geographical environment, one in the organism. But it is also meaningful to say that behaviour takes place in a geographical environment. What does this signify? (1) Since the behavioural environment depends upon the geographical, our proposition connects behaviour with a remote instead of an immediate cause. This may be useful in itself, and it will help to set our problem, for (2) the results of the animal's behaviour depend not only on his behavioural but also on his geographical environment, quite apart from the dependence of the former upon the latter. The geographical environment, not only the behavioural, is changed through all behaviour: the fruit is eaten and thereby ceases to exist as a fruit; the snow bridge is broken and gives place to a hole; the box is actually transported when the ape uses his "stool." As a matter of fact, in all our examples, and in a great many others, the behavioural result depends upon a geographical result. The type of behaviour which we have so far exclusively considered cannot occur in a behavioural world alone, although there are other types where this is more or less the case, as, for instance, when a man in delirium tremens catches nonexistent fish in his tub and shows them with great pride to the attendants. We gather from this that the relation between the two environments will present us with a fundamental problem in our future theories.

Behaviour Defined. (3) One particular aspect of the second point may be given a special mention: certain properties of the geographical environment will produce movements of the organism which we have not yet considered. Think of a mountaineer who breaks through a snow bridge, and not being roped to a companion, falls hundreds of feet into the icy chasm. Here we have a movement of an organism that is exclusively determined by the geographical environment. Before the victim loses consciousness he may make frantic efforts to stop his fall. These movements are still behaviour occurring in a behavioural environment, but at the same time the body drops whether there exists a behavioural environment or not and whether the man has retained or lost consciousness. This is again perfectly banal, and yet it gives us a means of defining behaviour: only such movements of organisms are to be called behaviour as occur in a behavioural environment. Movements which occur only in a geographical environment are not behaviour. It should be noticed that this definition does not claim that all behaviour is movement.

The Locus of Behavioural Environment. Let us now go one step further. So far the behavioural environment has been introduced as a mediating link between geographical environment and behaviour, between stimulus and response. These two terms denote objects which seem to have a very definite place in our system of knowledge; they both belong to the external world. But what is the locus of behavioural environment? To prepare for our answer we may discuss a new example, a series of experiments by Révész. Révész trained chicks to peck from the smaller of two simultaneously presented figures. Beginning with circles he then substituted rectangles, squares and triangles, taking good care that the relative positions of the two figures were continually changed; this is necessary, of course, in order to obviate the possibility that the animals, instead of learning to choose the smaller, might have learned to choose the "right" or the "left," the "upper" or the "lower." After this training was completed, he introduced as new figures two segments of a circle of different sizes presented in different positions; he then interspersed his critical experiments: two *equal* segments were presented so as to cause for us the well-known optical illusion called the Jastrow illusion. (See Fig. 1.) And in the vast majority of cases the hens pecked from the one which to *us* appears smaller. The whole course of this experiment is a demonstration of behavioural environment, for in terms of geographical environment it is meaningless to say that the birds learned to choose the *smaller* of two figures. "Of squares, parallelograms and triangles, the animal in the majority of cases chose the smaller figure *without any introductory training*" (p. 44). But for our present purposes the critical experiments are of particular interest. Why do the animals choose one of the two equal figures, when they have been trained to choose the smaller one? Described in these *geograph-*

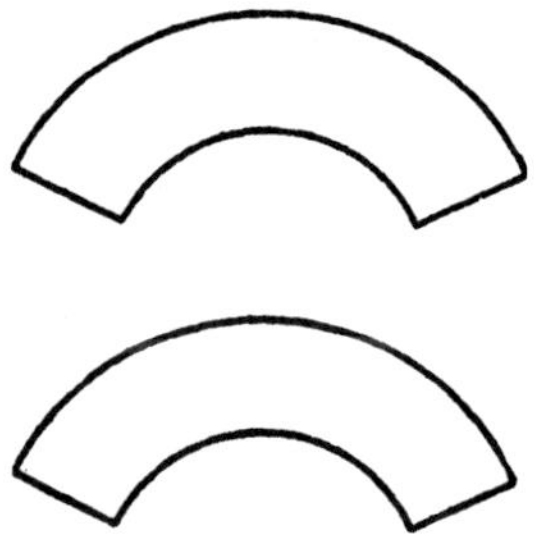

Fig. 1

ical terms their behaviour seems quite unintelligible, and neither stimulus properties nor experience can supply even the semblance of a satisfactory answer. But everything becomes perfectly plain and simple if we answer our question as every unbiassed layman would answer it, by saying: The animals chose one of the two equal figures because it *looked* to them smaller, just as it looks smaller to us. Or, in our terminology, the behavioural environment in the critical experiments was similar to the behavioural environment in the training experiments inasmuch as it too contained a larger and a smaller figure, although the critical geographical environment contained two figures of equal size. The behaviour of the hens cannot be explained in any way without the assumption that they were directed in their choice by a relation. Since this relation certainly does not obtain in the geographical environment, it must have been present somewhere else, and this somewhere else is what we call the behavioural environment. When now we remember what the layman had to say about this experiment, we see that our difference between the geographical and the behavioural environment coincides with the difference between things as they "really" are and things as they look to us, between reality and appearance. And we see also that appearances may deceive, that behaviour well adapted to the behavioural environment may be unsuited to the geographical. If, for instance, we were as naïve with regard to the Jastrow illusion as Révész's hens and happened to need two objects of equal shape and size we would not choose these two figures. I can illustrate the truth of this proposition by an experiment which I made in the summer of 1932 in a small village in Uzbekistan in Central Asia. I had shown the Jastrow illusion, using the pattern of the "Pseudoptics," to a young native who was the host of the tea house, the one meeting place of the male populace of the village. The man behaved as the hens did, apart from the fact that his reactions consisted not in pecking but in pointing to the larger of the two pieces of cardboard. I then put one on top of the other and gave them to him to handle. I wanted to see what explanation he would give to the curious discrepancy between their previous inequality and their now manifest equality. He said something like illusion, but without much conviction; and when I asked, "So you think they do not *really* change when you take them apart," he answered, "Oh, yes, I believe they *will* change a little."

FUNCTION OF BEHAVIOURAL ENVIRONMENT. Our argument, based on the Révész experiments, proved that the relation between the geographical environment, or the stimulus pattern, and behaviour is tremendously simplified by the introduction of the behavioural environment as a mediating link. This relationship is thus broken up into two different relationships, that between the geographical and the behavioural environment and that between the latter and behaviour. That this second relationship is, at least in many cases, intelligible, appeared from our example; if the upper of the two geographically equal ring sectors was behaviourally smaller, then the fact that the animals trained to choose the smaller of two figures selected the upper one offered no new problem.

We might have demonstrated the same fact in precisely the opposite way. It happens again and again that *different* stimuli produce the same reaction: this becomes perfectly intelligible if we know that under the given conditions of the case these different stimulations produce the same behavioural object. We shall discuss such cases later (Chapter VI) when we treat perceptual constancies, like those of size and colour, from the point of view of the relation between the geographical and the behavioural environments. At the moment we will only point out that, e.g., two surfaces may both look black, although one may reflect a thousand times as much light as the other; or expressed in terms of behaviour: two stimuli as different as those which we have just mentioned may lead to the same behaviour, for instance, if the task is to pick up a black object. To account in terms of stimulus response for this uniformity of behaviour in the face of the tremendous diversity of stimulation is impossible, particularly if one remembers that under other conditions a difference in stimulation of only 2% will lead to different behaviour.

In terms of the behavioural environment the difficulty disappears; behaviour with regard to two stimuli is identical when they produce two identical behavioural objects; it is different when the two corresponding behavioural objects are different. The problem which remains is no longer that of the relation between stimulus and behaviour, but that of the relation between the geographical and the behavioural environment. This problem can be solved systematically, but the problem of the pure stimulus-response relation can find no systematic solution as proved by the facts of constancy —identical behaviour with respect to different stimuli—and those of the Révész experiment—different behaviour with respect to identical stimuli.[2]

[2] This criticism applies with equal force to Tolman's definition of discriminanda and discriminanda capacities. (Pp. 86 f. and 91 f. See also Koffka, 1933, p. 448.)

CONSCIOUSNESS. In the beginning of this chapter I proposed to use behaviour as the primary subject matter of psychology. But in my distinction of geographical and behavioural environment, admittedly equivalent to that of reality and appearance, have I not smuggled in consciousness through a back door? I must deny this accusation. If we are forced to introduce the concept of consciousness, we have to accept it, whether we like it or not. But it is important to note that the *word* consciousness does not change the *meaning* of our own term behavioural environment. If anyone wants to speak of the animal's consciousness instead, he must apply this word to those objects which we call behavioural environment. Thus the dog's consciousness in chasing a hare would be "a hare running through a field," the ape's consciousness in trying to obtain the suspended fruit would be "a stool standing in that corner," and so forth. The field and the hare, the stool and the fruit, by being called conscious, or objects of consciousness, must not therefore be considered as something *within* the animal, if this has the meaning of a behavioural, or experienced, within. The behaviourists' aversion to consciousness seems to me to be largely founded on this misinterpretation. And their claim that they can write a psychology without consciousness can now be shown to be false. The animals they observe, the mazes and discrimination boxes they use in their experiments, the books in which they record their results, all these are first of all parts of their behavioural environments. Forgetting this fact, and believing that they are speaking of geographical environments only, they think that they can build a purely "geographical" theory without behavioural data. But every *datum* is a behavioural datum; physical reality is not a datum but a constructum. This confusion is obscured, and the general obscurity is increased by the use of the word stimulus, the vicissitudes of which we shall deal with later. Here I want merely to point out that it is easy to write a psychology without consciousness if one fails to recognize that one's own environment is a behavioural (conscious) and not a geographical (physical) one. I will add that there is some excuse for the behaviourists' error in the traditional treatment of consciousness about which we shall learn later. In consideration, however, of the possible misinterpretations, I shall use the term consciousness as little as possible. Our term behavioural environment, though it includes only a part of what is meant by consciousness, should escape misinterpretations; as fully equivalent with consciousness Köhler (1929) has used the term "direct experience" which we shall also adopt for occasional use. Our term has the advantage that it signifies the exact place which it has in the system, viz., the mediation between geographical environment and behaviour.

Behavioural Environment Only a Part of Direct Experience. But, as I said, it is incomplete; consciousness means more than behavioural environment. And it seems appropriate to indicate now at least the direction in which it is to be completed, although for a long time we shall be concerned only with the behavioural environment. This direction will be seen if we subject our term behaviour to the same analysis which we performed with regard to the term environment. We can, indeed, describe behaviour with reference to either of our two environments, and such descriptions may often be contradictory to each other. But whether they agree or not, behaviour itself must have a different meaning in these two descriptions: since behavioural and geographical environment belong to two different universes of discourse, the behaviours which occur within them must belong to the two different universes also. The man who rode across the Lake of Constance is a good example: his geographical environment was this big lake, his behavioural an ordinary snow-covered plain; accordingly, as we have pointed out before, although with regard to his geographical environment his behaviour was riding across the lake, his behaviour in regard to his behavioural environment was riding across a plain. Or in the terms of the layman: he *thought* he was riding over terra firma; he had no notion he was riding on thin ice.

Thus at first sight it seems as though the distinction between our two behaviours was completely analogous to that between our two types of environment: here the things as they look and as they really are, there the activity as the actor *thinks* it is and as it really is. But the similarity is not quite as great as it appears. Let us take another example: we observe three rats in the same maze, each starting at one end and finally emerging at the other. Then in a way we could say the three rats have run through the maze, a geographical statement. But our observation has convinced us that there were obvious differences in their behaviour: one ran for food, one to explore, the third for exercise or from general restlessness. These characteristics refer to the behaviour within the *behavioural* environment. A rat running for food does not do so only from the moment when it is near enough to see or smell it, but from the very beginning. Tolman's book gives ample experimental evidence for this statement. But the first part of the geographical maze does not contain the food, nor any stimulation emanating from the food.

If, nevertheless, the behaviour is directed towards the food, it must be so in its behavioural environment. The same is true of exploratory behaviour. We can explore directly only our behavioural environment, and indirectly merely, through the behavioural, the geographical one. And even in the last case, the behaviour for exercise or from restlessness is a behaviour in a behavioural environment since it is regulated by it. Now in all these cases it is no longer a true description of the two kinds of behaviour to say: behaviour in the geographical environment is the activity as it really is, in the behavioural as the animal thinks it is. For an excited behaviour is really an excited behaviour, an exploratory one really exploratory, and even a food-directed activity is really food-directed even if the experimenter has removed the food from the food box. In this last case, indeed, it is also true that the animal does not run towards the food, because geographically there is no food, and in some sense our distinction applies here as it did in the case of the Lake of Constance. But this is no longer a description of *behaviour*. I shall try to explain this by an example: a ball runs down an incline and finally falls into a hole. Now there may be water in the hole or not, and therefore I can say the ball falls into a hole with water or without water. But this difference does not affect the motions of the ball until it has reached that position in space where the water begins in the one case and not in the other. For the rest of the motion the presence or absence of water is wholly irrelevant; similarly, the statement that the rat does not run towards food when the experimenter has just removed it, is quite irrelevant to the run of the rat until it is near enough to notice the absence of food.

Behaviour and Accomplishment. If the description of behaviour with reference to the geographical environment is not truly a description of behaviour, what then is it? In order to simplify our terminology we shall from now on call behaviour with regard to geographical environment "accomplishment," and behaviour with regard to behavioural environment just behaviour. The name "accomplishment" indicates directly the reason for describing behaviour with reference to the geographical environment, because results of behaviour issue, as we have pointed out, in changes of the geographical environment. We are often interested in these results, which are the accomplishments of an animal. But we have learned just now that the knowledge of an animal's accomplishment is not knowledge of its behaviour. I will give a striking example where accomplishment and behaviour are in a sense opposed to each other. Suppose I see a person standing on a rock which I know is to be blasted away at this very minute. He is too far away for me to explain his danger to him, so I shout as loud and urgently as I can: "Come here, quick!" The person, if sufficiently Impressed by my command, will begin to run *towards me* behaviourally, but geographically, in running towards me, he runs away from the danger spot; geographically speaking, these two descriptions are absolutely equivalent. If I, however, afterwards relate this incident, I will say that he got away before the explosion occurred. I describe his accomplishment and not his behaviour; the latter was a motion towards something, the former a motion away from something. If the connection between behaviour and accomplishment were always of this kind, this world would be a strange place indeed, and it would certainly not be a world in which we would develop the concept of meaning. It might be a world of fairy tales; think of Aladdin who rubbed the lamp and accomplished thereby the appearance of the djinn. We shall see that experimenters have frequently put animals in situations where the behaviour and accomplishment were connected in a manner similar to the rubbing of the lamp and the appearance of the djinn. But even though as a rule behaviour and accomplishment do not hang together in this Wonderland way, the relation between accomplishment and behaviour is in one respect similar to that between the geographical and the behavioural environment: if we know one member of either pair we do not yet know the other. But whereas the first relation is one of the most important straightforward problems of psychology, the second has no such simple standing. As a general question, as may be deduced from our last examples, it does not, strictly speaking, enter psychology at all. Still it is a question of some interest which we shall take up again; furthermore, since the relation between accomplishment and behaviour is not, as a rule, of the fairy tale type, we may often be able to draw inferences from accomplishment to behaviour and *its* environment. The whole objective method makes use of this possibility; the time a rat takes to run a maze, the number of errors it commits, which blind alleys it will enter and which not, all such facts give us clues for an interpretation of behaviour and behavioural environment, but they are not in themselves statements about behaviour.

For we have seen that the only system of reference for describing behaviour proper is the behavioural environment. And thus we have so far failed to solve the problem that was set at the beginning of this long discussion, viz., to supplement our concept of behavioural environment so as to make it as comprehensive as the concepts of direct experience or consciousness. We shall now return to this question.

OUR SOURCES OF KNOWLEDGE OF BEHAVIOUR. How do we acquire knowledge of behaviour? Behaviour of an animal is part of our behavioural environment, and we know it as such, together with all the other objects and events in our behavioural environment. The question, how we can know *real* behaviour, is, therefore, no different in principle from the question of how we know any non-behavioural reality. It will not occupy us now; we could not answer it before we had learned something of the general relation between our geographical and our behavioural environment. At the moment, two remarks must suffice: (1) That we must assume the existence of real behaviour just as we must assume the existence of real tables and books and houses and animals. (2) Since we have shown that behaviour is always behaviour in a behavioural environment, not ours but the animal's which behaves, we can now settle one of the objections formerly raised against our procedure, viz., that it is anthropomorphic. We observe an animal's behaviour in our behavioural environment. If we assumed, without further evidence, that our behavioural environment and that of the animal were identical, then we should certainly be open to the criticism of anthropomorphism. The assumption, on the other hand, that the animal behaves in *a* behavioural environment, viz., its own, is not anthropomorphic at all. How far this environment is identical with ours, in what characteristic aspects it differs, are very important questions indeed, and in their solution we must be careful to avoid anthropomorphism. But let us return to our main argument: on the ground of an animal's behaviour in our behavioural environment, and by more indirect methods, we infer the nature of the animal's real behaviour. But we are behaving ourselves. And of this behaviour also we have knowledge. We find it happening in our behavioural environment, but the word "in" has now a different meaning from the one it had when we spoke of another animal's behaviour occurring in our own behavioural environment. The animal is a *part* of our behavioural environment, we ourselves are the centre of our environment, although not "of it." The environment is always an environment of something, so my behavioural environment is the environment of me and my behaviour. Just as I know my behavioural environment, so I know myself and my behaviour in this environment. Only if we include this knowledge with the behavioural environment have we gained a complete equivalent of what Köhler calls direct experience, or what is called consciousness.

This knowledge includes, to enumerate a few items, my desires and intentions, my successes and disappointments, my joys and sorrows, loves and hatreds, but also my doing *this* rather than *that.* An example of the last: my friend asks me, "Who is the lady you raised your hat to?" I answer, "I did not raise my hat to any lady; I just raised it because it was too tight on my head."

Real, Phenomenal, and Apparent Behaviour. We can now introduce a new terminology. We have seen that we must distinguish *two* classes of behaviour from real behaviour, my behaviour in somebody else's behavioural environment from my behaviour in my own behavioural environment; or, with an interchange of subjects, somebody else's behaviour in my behavioural environment from his behaviour in his own behavioural environment. We shall call the first of each pair *apparent* behaviour, the second *phenomenal* or *experienced* behaviour. The apparent behaviour may, as our hat-raising example shows, be misleading with regard to real behaviour, but it might also have been a true guide, e.g., if I had really bowed to a lady. The phenomenal behaviour, on the other hand, was a true index. No doubt phenomenal behaviour is a very valuable clue for our knowledge of real behaviour. Whereas the relation of apparent to real behaviour is of the same kind as that between behavioural and geographical environment, that between phenomenal and real behaviour is of a different nature. To some extent real behaviour reveals itself in phenomenal behaviour. But only to some extent. For phenomenal behaviour never reveals more than a fraction of real behaviour, and this fraction may not always be the most important one. We shall take up this point later. Now we draw the conclusion that it would be just as wrong to discard phenomenal behaviour for our knowledge of real behaviour as to use it exclusively and blindly.

Behaviour and Environment Summarized. We may, in concluding, schematize our discoveries about behaviour and environment. (See Fig. 2.) G is the geographical environment. It produces BE, the behavioural environment; in this and regulated by it, RB, real behaviour, takes place, and parts of it are revealed in PH B, phenomenal behaviour. In some sense BE, RB, and PH B occur within the real organism RO, but not in the phenomenal Ego, which belongs with PH B. RO is directly affected by G and acts back upon it through RB. Our schema does not indicate the dependence of BE and PH B upon the organism,

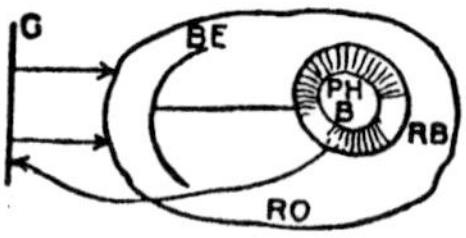

Fig. 2

neither does it contain the results of behaviour. But by RB affecting G two further changes occur: BE is changed and the phenomenal Ego is changed. When the ape has eaten the fruit, his behavioural environment has become "fruitless" and the animal itself "satisfied."

THE FIELD CONCEPT

So far we have clarified the concept of molar behaviour; we have seen that it takes place in a behavioural environment and that we have knowledge of it in two ways, the one revealing apparent molar behaviour, that of others, the other phenomenal molar behaviour, that of ourselves. Both types of knowledge are to be used for an understanding or explanation of real molar behaviour. Furthermore, we have gained some insight into the dynamical aspect of real molar behaviour. In this way we have laid the foundation for psychology as the science of molar behaviour. We must now elaborate this point. Which are to be the most fundamental concepts of our system? One of the postulates of our psychology was that it be *scientific*. Therefore let us try to discover one of the fundamental concepts of science which we can apply to our task. A short excursion into the history of science will lead us to our discovery. How did Newton explain the motion of bodies? According to him every change of motion is due to a force which arises either through impact—two billiard balls—or by an attraction exercised mutually by the bodies upon each other, according to his law of gravitation which gives a quantitative formula of this force. This force Newton assumed to act without time; it produced an action at a distance. There is the sun, here is the earth, nothing between them but empty space, nothing to mediate the attractive force of the sun upon the earth and vice versa. When, much later, the laws of magnetic and electric attraction and repulsion were discovered and proved to be quantitatively identical with Newton's law of gravitation, the same interpretation was given to them; they were interpreted as actions at a distance. This conception of a timeless action had been very uncongenial to Newton; he made it because he saw no other possibility, but by the time the first laws of electricity were discovered it had become a well-established concept and held a vested interest in the system of science. Therefore a young man whose brilliant experiments in the field of electricity and magnetism were duly recognized met with much contempt when he tried to explain his results in different terms, which excluded all action at a distance and explained electric attraction and repulsion of two bodies by processes occurring in the medium between them, the dielectric, propagated in time from place to place. But Michael Faraday's ideas were taken up, elaborated, and given mathematical form by Clerk Maxwell, who introduced the more general terms: electric and magnetic field, as the carriers of the forces, and who was able to deduce the velocity of the propagation of electric and magnetic forces, which in empty space proved to be identical with the velocity of light. The believers in the action at a distance put up a strong fight but were driven from their positions in the fields of electricity and magnetism, and the attack came to a temporary halt. One fortress remained in the hands of the enemy, Newton's gravitation. And not until the beginning of this century was this citadel forced to surrender. In Einstein's theory of gravitation the actions at a distance disappeared just as they had disappeared before from electromagnetism, and the gravitational field took their place. Empty space as mere geometrical nothingness vanished from physics, being replaced by a definitely distributed system of strains and stresses, gravitational and electromagnetic, which determines the very geometry of space. And the distribution of strains and stresses in a given environment will determine what a body of a given constitution will do in that environment. Conversely, when we know the body and observe what it does in a certain environment we can deduce the properties of the field in that environment. Thus we discover the magnetic field of the earth by observing the behaviour of magnetic needles in different places, their declination and their inclination; similarly we find out the gravitational field of the earth by measuring the period of a pendulum of given length in different places.

Thus the field and the behaviour of a body are correlative. Because the field determines the behaviour of bodies, this behaviour can be used as an indicator of the field properties. Behaviour of the body, to complete the argument, means not only its motion with regard to the field, it refers equally to the changes which the body will undergo; e.g., a piece of iron will become magnetized in a magnetic field.

THE FIELD IN PSYCHOLOGY

Let us return to our own problem. Can we introduce the field concept into psychology, meaning by it a system of stresses and strains which will determine real behaviour? If we can, we have at once a general and scientific category for all our explanations and we should have the same two kinds of problems which the physicist encounters: viz., (1) what is the field at a given time, (2) what behaviour must result from a given field?

Behavioural Environment as the Psychological Field. But where shall we find a field that plays the rôle in psychology which the physical fields play in physics? That it must be a different field is evident from our previous discussion. The physical field is the field of the geographical environment, and we have shown that behaviour must be explained by behavioural environment. Is this, then, to be our psychological field? Let us try how this assumption works. It means that our behavioural environment, qua determinant and regulator of behaviour, must be endowed with forces. For we shall stick to the axiom: no change of movement without a force. Does this determination rule out the behavioural environment as our required field? By no means. When we describe our behavioural environment adequately we have to indicate not merely the objects which are in it but their dynamic properties as well. We shall discuss a number of examples. Think of yourselves as basking in the sun on a mountain meadow or on a beach, completely relaxed and at peace with the world. You are doing nothing, and your environment is not much more than a soft cloak that envelops you and gives you rest and shelter. And now suddenly you hear a scream, "Help! Help!" How different you feel and how different your environment becomes. Let us describe the two situations in field terms. At first your field was, to all intents and purposes, homogeneous, and you were in equilibrium with it. No action, no tension. As a matter of fact, in such a condition even the differentiation of the Ego and its environment tends to become blurred; I am part of the landscape, the landscape is part of me. And then, when the shrill and pregnant sound pierces the lulling stillness, everything is changed. Whereas all directions were dynamically equal before, now there is one direction that stands out, one direction into which you are being pulled. This direction is charged with force, the environment seems to contract, it is as though a groove had formed in a plane surface and you were being forced down that groove. At the same time there takes place a sharp differentiation between your Ego and the voice, and a high degree of tension arises in the whole field.

If we take from this example chiefly the description of fields with regard to their homogeneity or inhomogeneity, we see that the former are much rarer than the latter, particularly for us over-active human beings of Western civilization. For action presupposes inhomogeneous fields, fields with lines of force, with change of potential. An exceedingly good and instructive description of a field with a very simple kind of inhomogeneity has been given by Lewin in his essay on the war landscape (1917). Here is a field which, apart from all details, has a polar structure in one direction: the enemy's land on the one side and home and safety on the other. This vectorial property is a primary characteristic and determines the entire field, no other characteristic being entirely free from it.

A number of other very instructive examples are contained in an article by H. G. Hartgenbusch on the psychology of sport. The author describes his own experience, or behavioural field, during several different sports. I select some instances from socker and one from weight lifting. "As they [the socker players] move towards the enemy goal, they will see the playing ground as a field of changing lines whose principal direction leads towards the goal." (1927, p. 50.) These lines are true lines of force in a behavioural field, changing continually with the changing configuration of the players and directing their actions. "All the motor performances of the players (as shiftings about on the field) are connected with the visual shifting. Certainly this is not a case of logical thinking, since thoughts, in the ordinary sense, are alien to a player. He knows nothing of them; in his tense state the visual situation produces the motor performance directly."

We must preface the next example with a more general observation. Our behavioural environments contain things and the holes between them. As a rule, the forces which regulate our behaviour originate in the former and not in the latter. Whether this is due to experience or not is a question we may leave open, although an affirmative answer seems to fit ill with the fact that the novice at cycling is attracted by all sorts of objects, although experience must have taught him the injurious effects of a collision. And yet, every prominent object in his behavioural environment will attract him, whether it be a woman pushing a perambulator or a heavy motor lorry. The mere fact that we speak of "prominent" objects in the environment indicates an inhomogeneity: where the object is, there is *more* than where the hole is. Of course the hole *may* become the most prominent part, and then there is *more* in the hole than in the objects around it, i.e., the hole is now the attracting mass. Another quotation from Hartgenbusch may elucidate this point: "The enemy's goal as seen by the attacking side was apparently walled-up except for a small hole at the left. From my position behind the threatened goal I saw how the attacking left halfback got hold of [8]

[8] Changed in conformity with the original. The English term would fit a rugger but not a socker game.

the ball, fixed his eyes on the hole, and with all his might kicked the ball through the one open spot. When I asked him afterwards what he had felt at that moment, the lucky player replied, 'I only saw a hole.'" However, football also gives us evidence for our first proposition that objects rather than holes are dominant points, centres of force. For the players have to *learn* to emphasize the hole and disregard the goal keeper: "When an expert . . . follows a football game attentively he will always notice that the goal keeper, standing before the comparatively large goal, is more often hit than can be accounted for by the mere adventitious kicking of the contestants" (p. 49), even when one takes account of the fact that the goal keeper whenever he can will try to intercept the ball. Our author then continues, "The goal keeper furnishes a prominent point in space which attracts the eyes of the opposing kickers. If the motor activity takes place while the kicker's eye is fixed on the goal keeper, then the ball will generally land near him. But when the kicker learns to reconstruct his field, to change the phenomenal 'centre of gravity' from the goal keeper to another point in space, the new 'centre of gravity' will have the same attraction as the goal keeper had before."

The next example from Hartgenbusch adds a new point, besides giving a very pretty illustration of the fact that behaviour takes place in a behavioural environment. It needs again a short introduction. If we exert muscular force, say, by lifting a weight, we must keep our body in balance; this presupposes a certain state of the general tonus of our musculature which will be determined by our task and the mechanical conditions under which it takes place. The neat point made by Hartgenbusch is that this poise, this fixation of our body on the ground, does not depend upon the geographical environment only, but also on the behavioural one and even on such aspects of it as have no direct mechanical or gravitational effect. He tells of a competition of "heavy athletes" where the performances, against all expectations, failed to reach even the earlier records. "One of the contestants found the solution of the puzzle. The place where the competition took place was a hall so brightly illuminated that there was no conspicuous fixation point on which the weight lifters could rivet their eyes. . . . The stability accompanying a fixed spatial orientation which is necessary for the lifting of heavy weights could not be attained under the conditions existing in the brightly lighted hall; the expected records did not appear" (p. 49). Thus we see that behavioural objects are dynamic, not only in the sense that they pull and push behaviour in various directions, but also that they can give purchase, stability, equilibrium.

My examples should have demonstrated the meaning of the term behavioural field with its dynamic properties and the usefulness of this concept. There are many branches of psychology where explanation need not go beyond it, others where it will need only little supplementation. Thus the description of a mentality different from our own, be it that of children, be it that of primitive peoples, will be complete if the behavioural fields of these beings, together with the behaviour which these fields demand, are adequately described. Such work as that done by Lévy-Bruhl on primitives and Piaget on children is truly such description. The question whether the descriptions of Lévy-Bruhl and Piaget are right or not does not enter here, for even if, or inasmuch as, they are wrong, a true description would be a description of the same kind; it would be a field description of the behavioural environment and the Egos within it. And Lewin's theory of behaviour, of action and emotion, contains this behavioural field as a nucleus, even though he has to go beyond its limits. Finally, when we or the novelists or the historians describe behaviour, we do it in terms of forces in the behavioural environment, although we, as well as they, use an entirely different terminology.

Inadequacy of Behavioural Environment as Psychological Field. However, there are imperative reasons why we cannot accept the behavioural environment as that psychological field which is to be our *fundamental* explanatory category. They derive from three sources: (1) the ontological status of the behavioural environment, (2) the relation of behavioural and geographical environment, (3) the insufficiency of the behavioural field. Let us discuss them one by one.

(1) Ontological Status of Behavioural Environment. I feel sure that in reading the description of the dynamic properties of the behavioural environment there will have been a certain reluctance felt with regard to accepting the behavioural environment as a truly explanatory concept. It may have been said that I was using a word with a well-defined meaning in a context where it cannot have this meaning. I am referring to the word force. "Force," it could be argued, "has a definite meaning in the physical world, but what can it mean in a behavioural environment? Force belongs definitely in the physical world, is a construct and not a datum; and yet has been treated as a property of the behavioural world also. It is introduced from its own universe of discourse into another where it has no place. Even if the descriptions are ade-

quate, even if it is admitted that one can speak of the attractive force exerted by a lure, the repulsive force exerted by a danger, this can be no more than a description; whereas force in physics is an explanatory term, the cause of change. But the explanatory meaning together with the descriptive meaning has been smuggled into the behavioural world. And a behavioural force has even been used in order to explain *real* behaviour, i.e., physical motion, whereas physical motion clearly can be produced by physical forces only. Furthermore, there has been no statement of *where* the behavioural world exists, what its ontological locus and status is. Are there two substances, a physical and a mental, the behavioural world consisting of the latter? If so, does this dualism imply an interactionism between mind and body; in this system, does a mental force interfere with the physical order of events? That the interactionism cannot be of the traditional kind where the soul as the Ego or the Self, a mental entity, controls the actions of the body, a physical entity, is clear; for in this system the body is also controlled by mental objects which are not the Self. But even though the interactionism would be of a new kind, it would still be a dualism, whereas in the introduction a system that contained separate realms of existence, like vitalism, was repudiated." I admit every word of this argument, although I must mention that there seems to be a possible way of escape from it which Lewin has indicated. One might argue that terms like force, field, and many others have a much wider significance than the one assigned to them in physics, that the latter is only one possible specification of the former. Simple examples will make this clear: if two containers are filled with water to different levels and then connected at the bottom, water will flow from the one vessel into the other because of a difference in pressure which gives rise to a force. This is a purely physical motion; but now consider the example: America had a great surplus of gold, Europe a great scarcity; what happened? Gold went across the ocean. Is not this example in its formal aspects quite similar to our hydrodynamic one? A motion takes place because of a difference in something which we call pressure in the physical case, a term which would fit the economic case equally well. Or another example: in Soviet Russia there has arisen an enormous new demand for all kinds of goods; the result is that factories are working day and night, and that more and more factories are being built; in the rest of the world supply exceeds demand, with the results that more and more factories decrease their output or shut down completely—this is not meant to be a description of our economic crisis but merely a simplified example. Thus we might raise the question: What produces the goods? The machines in the factory; yes, but also the demand for the goods; that is, a force in a meaning different from that in physics and yet identical in its application. To summarize: just as we have introduced a behavioural field, we might introduce an economic field, and that field too would have its lines of force. And therefore no objection should be raised against forces in the behavioural environment and not even against their producing actual bodily movements. For the demand makes the wheels turn and the ships carry gold and goods from coast to coast. Economic forces, then, which produce economic results, achieve this by producing mediating physical motions. At the same time the economist does not assume a special substance, say Trade with a capital T; therefore the psychologist treating of behavioural fields need not introduce a special substance, the Mind.

This is all excellent argument which may lead to consequences of great bearing on the philosophy of science. But personally I do not feel satisfied with it because, as it stands, it leaves the relation between the one kind of effect, the physical, and the other, the behavioural or economic, totally in the dark. I want one and the same universe of discourse in which *all* events can take place, since action is defined within a universe of discourse and not from one to the other. The argumentation which I have borrowed from Lewin may lead to a definition of such a general universe of discourse and may thereby radically affect our conception of reality. But before the development of his argument into a consistent, epistemological and metaphysical system, I prefer to meet the argument which I suggested might be raised against my use of behavioural forces in a different manner.

As I said before, I admit the cogency of the argument, i.e., I admit that in our *ultimate* explanations, we can have but *one* universe of discourse and that it must be the one about which physics has taught us so much. Not only is the energy which is consumed in our behaviour of chemical origin, the forces which are responsible for each individual motion must be considered as physico-chemical forces also. The organism is a physico-chemical system by itself, although depending for its existence upon a geographical environment, and its actions must be *ultimately* explained in terms of processes within this system. If an action is reducible to a causal sequence of organic processes, it becomes intelligible because it is then reduced to one universe of discourse which is the same as that in which its actual movements take place.

It would be misunderstanding the trend of this argument if it were thought that it had excluded the use of the field concept. The opposite is true; if the locus of behaviour is the physical world, then the field concept which is so powerful a tool in physics must be applied to behaviour. Our argument denies merely that this field concept can be identical with the concept of the behavioural environment.

(2) The Relation of Behavioural and Geographical Environment. Our second reason against this identification is based on the relation between the behavioural and the geographical environment. That the former depends upon the latter is a truism, although the manner of this dependency is by no means simple or unambiguous. But whereas this problem will occupy us in the next chapter, one aspect of it is relevant in this connection: we assume that this connection is a causal one, the geographical environment being a cause of the behavioural. But then the difficulty appears again that both belong to different universes of discourse. For how can a cause in one universe of discourse produce an effect in another? All our causal laws refer to events within the same universe of discourse, and therefore, since the geographical environment belongs to the universe of physics, we require its effects to belong to it also. So we are again forced away from the behavioural environment; we are compelled to substitute for it some occurrences in the real physical organism. Of course this question does not always interest us. We may take its answer for granted or leave it in abeyance and deal with other problems. Science always works at different levels, and the work at higher levels may proceed for a long time without reference to the work at the lower ones. Thus chemistry became a very advanced science before it became connected with physics, and even today it is by no means possible to reduce all chemical action concretely to the action of protons and electrons, although every scientist is convinced that in principle such a reduction is possible.

Our present argument, therefore, means only that as a fundamental concept at the lowest level, the psychological field cannot be identical with behavioural environment, because as a fundamental concept the field cannot be taken for granted but must be causally connected with the geographical environment. At the same time we have pointed out that psychology works at different levels, and that on some of them the behavioural environment may be, if not the whole field, yet a part of it.

(3) The Insufficiency of the Behavioural Environment. The totality of our behaviour is not explainable in terms of the be-

havioural environment. There are at least three different types of behaviour for which no proper behavioural environment can be found. We shall discuss them one by one.

(a) SO-CALLED REFLEXES. At every moment of our life the tonus of our musculature is regulated. Were it not, we could neither sit nor stand nor walk. But all these adjustments take place without our knowing about them; there is no behavioural environment for them. What is true of the tonic reflexes holds also for the so-called phasic ones: I send a strong beam of light into a person's eyes, and his pupils contract; I remove the light, and they expand again. Now it might be said that here a behavioural environment exists inasmuch as the person will see the light coming and going. But even so, his behaviour is quite unknown to him; he is entirely ignorant of the movements of his pupil before he has learned about them, and even then he remains unaware of them. Thus even though a behavioural environment may be present in these cases, phenomenal behaviour would be missing. Moreover whether one has a behavioural environment or not does not make any difference. The pupils of a boxer knocked unconscious will still react.

It is clear then that if the field concept is to be applied to such reflexes, it cannot be the same as that of behavioural environment. One might, of course, be tempted to exclude the field concept from the explanation of reflexes; that is what has been done. The reflexes were the prototypes of pure stimulus-response connections; they seemed clear cases of behaviour in a purely geographical environment. We shall see later (in Chapter VIII) why it is impossible to accept such an interpretation. It would mean that there were two sharply distinguishable types of behaviour, such as are field-conditioned and such as are not, just as there are behaviours that depend upon a behavioural environment and those that do not. However, there is no such absolute break. An action may be more or less determined by a behavioural environment, and there is no sharp dividing line. Correspondingly, we must feel reluctant to accept behaviour which is not in some way field-conditioned. But then, its field cannot be the behavioural environment.

(b) FORCES THAT DETERMINE BEHAVIOUR OUTSIDE OF BEHAVIOURAL ENVIRONMENT. The forces which determine our behaviour may not always be those we believe to be the determinants. We may do something in order to please X as we think, when in reality we do it to spite Y, when Y need neither be present nor in our thoughts. Psychoanalysis in its various forms has brought to light many such facts, and perhaps its general tendency may be said to be the proof that all our actions are of that type, reducible to a very few subterranean forces totally absent from our behavioural field. However far the psychoanalysts may overshoot the mark, it remains true that this type of action exists, that it cannot be explained in terms of behavioural environment, and that it is so similar to the rest of behaviour that it needs a common explanatory concept. Since the field concept is applicable to all behaviour, it appears again that the psychological field cannot be identical with the behavioural environment.

(c) MEMORY. There is memory. Now memory determines to a great extent our behavioural field, and in so far cannot serve as an argument against its universality. That I speak to A whom I met yesterday and not to B whom I never saw before is due to the fact that A is, in my behavioural environment, a familiar person, B a stranger. But there are other ways in which memory determines behaviour without the mediation of a behavioural field. The rapid and accurate activities of a trained typist are not explainable in terms of the actually present behavioural environment, as little as the playing of Kreisler or the tennis game of a Tilden or a Cochet. All their training goes into their present performances, but this training does not belong to the present behavioural environment. But skills are not the only memory effects that fall outside the scope of behavioural environment. I think of a person, a city, a mountain, but cannot recall its name. I want to very badly, but no effort seems to help. So I give up and do something else, when suddenly the name will appear. Again a type of behaviour which takes place without a behavioural environment but must, nevertheless, be the result of operative forces, a field process.

"UNCONSCIOUS." To call the facts adduced sub (b) and (c) unconscious or subconscious does not help us. Here we see the advantage of our terminology, for whereas the word conscious allows the formation of new words by the addition of prefixes like "un" and "sub," behavioural environment cannot become an "un"- or "sub"-behavioural environment without losing its meaning completely. And since we agreed that the word consciousness should be used only as an equivalent to direct experience, containing the behavioural environment and the phenomenal behaviour of the Ego, we must renounce the use of the terms un- and sub-conscious. However, there must be a reason why these words were coined and so widely accepted; why did not all psychologists simply distinguish between conscious and merely physiological processes? I believe the answer lies in the fact that the physiological processes were not treated as field processes, whereas the processes called un- or sub-conscious had very definite properties which in our terminology we call field properties. If, then, we retain the field properties in the physiological processes, we shall no longer be tempted to speak of unconscious processes. And if we survey in review the facts presented under the heading "the insufficiency of the behavioural field" we seem again to be forced to turn to physiological facts.

The Balance Sheet. What, then, is the balance of this discussion? We have gained and we have lost. Our gain consists in the establishment of a unitary universe of discourse. The physical field of the geographical environment acts on a physical object, the organism, and influences the physiological field within this organism; physiological field events take place which change the geographical field and thereby the physiological field. We have a pure problem of physics complicated by the relation of the two interacting fields, the physical and the physiological, and by the enormous complexity of the latter. But though complex, the problem is no longer obscure; we understand its terms, and as a matter of principle, we can follow each event from its beginning to its end over its whole course without jumping from one universe to another.

But our loss is equally obvious. We have, if we stop here, given up all the advantages which the behavioural environment brought to our system. We are no longer dealing with psychological facts at all but with pure physiology. As a matter of fact, this consequence will appear not as a loss but as a gain to many psychologists who will probably now be tempted to make the comment: "If you want to explain all behaviour in physiological terms, why did you ever introduce the behavioural environment?" We had set great hopes on our behavioural environment. With the help of this concept we thought we could build up a psychology which would be acceptable to the historian, the artist, and the philosopher as including motivation and beauty and rationality. And now we had to turn back and take refuge in mere physiology. Is that not equivalent to renouncing molar behaviour and putting molecular behaviour in its place? Are we not stultifying our own purpose? And lastly how can we hope to build a system of psychology in pure physiological terms when our knowledge of the central nervous system is almost a blank? Would not a new kind of speculative psychology supersede the experimental phase? Behavioural environment is something we know, but our physiological field is a totally unknown quantity.

So runs our balance sheet. And if we look at the assets and liabilities which have appeared on it through our commitment to the physiological field we see that they are the reason for the war waged between the different schools of psychology. Those who regarded the assets as the items that counted became behaviourists, thinking as lightly of their liabilities as debtors are ready to do. Those, on the other hand, who were conscientious debtors on whom the weight of the liabilities rested like an insupportable load, thought nothing of the assets and became "understanding" psychologists. Between these extremes we find all sorts of compromises. But all compromises were unsatisfactory because they failed to find a way of using the assets to meet the liabilities. That is what we must do if we want to be honest and pursue our business with a plan that carries us over a long period and saves us from the everlasting threat of an imminent bankruptcy. Or, to choose another metaphor, we must know where we are going and be convinced that the road on which we tread leads to our goal. I remember an episode in my student days. A colleague of mine with whom I was going home asked me the question: "Have you any idea where the psychology we are learning is leading us?" I had no answer to that question, and my colleague, after taking his doctor's degree, gave up psychology as a profession and is today a well-known author. But I was less honest and less capable, and so I stuck to my job. But because his question never ceased to trouble me, I was ready to grasp the first chance that offered to find an answer.

Relation Between Behavioural and Physiological Field Crucial. Therefore, if I have not forgotten that rather casual conversation, another conversation with another colleague remains in my memory as one of the crucial moments of my life. It happened at Frankfort on the Main early in 1911. Wertheimer had just completed his experiments on the perception of motion in which Köhler and I had served as the chief observers. Now he proposed to tell me the purpose of his experiments, of which, as a good subject, I had been entirely ignorant. Of course I had had many discussions with those two men before. One could not live in constant contact with Wertheimer without learning some aspects of gestalt theory, even in those old times. But on that afternoon he said something which impressed me more than anything else, and that was his idea about the function of a physiological theory in psychology, the relation between consciousness and the underlying physiological processes, or in our new terminology, between the behavioural and the physiological field. To state it in these new terms, however, is not quite fair, because this very statement was only made possible by Wertheimer's idea; before, nobody thought of a physiological or, for that matter, of a behavioural *field*.

TRADITIONAL PHYSIOLOGICAL THEORIES OF BEHAVIOUR AND CONSCIOUSNESS. For what were the current physiological assumptions at that time? Nervous processes were pictured as events of *one kind* only, excitations, starting somewhere, travelling along a nerve, being transmitted to another nerve, from that to a third, until finally they gave rise to a muscle contraction or a gland secretion. The enormous complexity of behaviour was not explained by an equal complexity of the processes as such, but only by the combination of a host of separate processes, all of the same general kind but occurring in different places. The *locus* of an excitation became the most important aspect of it; diversity of process was introduced merely to account for the different sense modalities and qualities, the first coupled with a local difference, the second not. Sound stimuli would produce excitations of fibres in the acoustic nerve which would be transmitted to the temporal part of the cortex and excite the ganglion cells there to their specific forms of response, corresponding to the attributes of tone sensations; and light stimuli would similarly produce excitations which would be propagated to the occipital cortex and would there produce cell excitations, which, because of the different nature of these cells, would be different from the processes in the temporal cortex. But one and the same occipital cell must be capable of different kinds of excitation. Since there is, in this system of physiological hypotheses, a fixed connection between a cortical cell and a cell in the sense surface, e.g., between a cell in the visual cortex and a cone in the retina, the same cortical cell will always be excited when the same cone is excited. Now the same cone can be excited by light of different wave length with the result that the organism sees different colours. Consequently the same nerve fibers and ganglion cells from cone to cortex must be able to react in different ways.

This, however, was the only qualitative variety granted to nervous processes; apart from that all complexity was explained by the combination of differently localized cell-excitations. No wonder that the question of brain localization loomed so large on the psychological horizon.

I have said that this form of physiological theory was prevalent in 1911; I must add that ten years before the great physiologist J. von Kries had given ample proof that it was utterly wrong. But he had not been able to put an adequate theory in its place, and so the old theory survived as though nothing had happened; indeed this theory has an iron constitution; it was still so vigorous in 1929 that Lashley, in his presidential address to the American Psychological Association, read before the 9th International Congress of Psychology at Yale, attempted to deal it a new death blow. The material against the theory had enormously accumulated since von Kries's famous speech; Lashley's onslaught looked deadly indeed, but the theory seems to have a charmed life; it seems to persist to this present day.

PHYSIOLOGICAL PROCESSES MOLECULAR, TOTALLY DIFFERENT FROM BEHAVIOURAL ONES. Therefore it is worth while to single out some of its salient aspects. In the first place it is what Tolman calls molecular. No molar characteristics can be found in the nerve excitations, the sum of which constitutes the nervous activity. In the second place, this theory of the physiological processes underlying behaviour with its behavioural environment, or, as it was formerly termed, underlying conscious phenomena, was constructed almost in complete independence of molar behaviour or conscious phenomena. The latter influenced it only by introducing the qualitative sensory differences we mentioned above. The facts of anatomy, interpreted in a particular way, seemed to reveal a number of separate structures, the neurones; and indeed anatomical facts are the main foundation of the theory. But not only is this theory independent of behavioural or psychological observation, it has exerted a decisive influence upon such observation. The description of behaviour as a combination of a multitude of reflexes, original or conditioned, and the description of the behavioural environment in terms of sensations as mental elements are both similar in form. When modern experimental psychology was created, the sensation theory was not created with it, but taken over from the older speculative systems. That it remained unquestioned for such a long time, that it became part and parcel of modern psychology, is without a doubt due to the physiological theory which originated in anatomical discoveries. Thus we see how facts are dependent on theories, how false, therefore, the claim is that a theory is nothing but a concise formulation of independent facts.

THEIR RELATION MERELY FACTUAL. In the third place, in this theory, as a consequence of the two characteristics just demonstrated, the relation between molar behaviour and behavioural environment on the one hand and the underlying physiological processes on the other, is merely factual. In essence they are totally different; did not Wundt emphasize the point that the sensation blue and the corresponding neural event had nothing, absolutely nothing, in common? Or could anything be more emphatic than the assertion: "Thought and feeling must be recognized, on any view, as fundamentally different from any material process, and the motion of the atoms and molecules of the brain as fundamentally different from thoughts and feelings" (Stout, 1913, p. 16). And does not Tolman write in his book published in 1932: "It will be contended by us . . . that 'behaviour-acts,' though no doubt in complete one-to-one correspondence with the underlying molecular facts of physics and physiology, have as 'molar' wholes, certain emergent properties of their own?" (p. 7). If we interpret this statement to mean that qua molar, behaviour is fundamentally different from the underlying molecular physiological processes, we link up this third point with our first.

On all three counts the theory has to be condemned. The assumption of merely molecular physiological processes is erected on much too slender an empirical basis; it results either in a molecular interpretation of behaviour and consciousness, which is contradicted by the facts, or it severs completely the two series of processes, physiological and behavioural or conscious, whereas at the same time it establishes the closest possible relation between them by considering the one as the correlate of the other, the nature of this correlation being left entirely in the dark.

WERTHEIMER'S SOLUTION. ISOMORPHISM. And now the reader can understand Wertheimer's contribution; now he will see why his physiological hypothesis impressed me more than anything else. In two words, what he said amounted to this: let us think of the physiological processes not as molecular, but as molar phenomena. If we do that, all the difficulties of the old theory disappear. For if they are molar, their molar properties will be the same as those of the conscious processes which they are supposed to underlie. And if that is so, our two realms, instead of being separated by an impassable gulf, are brought as closely together as possible with the consequence that we can use our observations of the behavioural environment and of behaviour as data for the concrete elaboration of physiological hypotheses. Then, instead of having one kind of such processes only, we must deal with as many as there are different psychological processes, the variety of the two classes must be the same.

MOLAR PHYSIOLOGICAL PROCESSES. However, this theory may appear merely verbal as long as one does not know what molar physiological processes are. Are we not introducing new entities into physiology, and thereby into science, which are incompatible with the principles of science? Is not physics a molecular science par excellence? Wertheimer saw that it is not; he knew the falsity of this objection. But it was left to Köhler (1920) to demonstrate the fallacy of this argument by showing that physics is a molar science. The name "atomic theory" seems to prove the opposite, but only to a superficial observer. Let us take the simplest example we can find: water is explained by the atomic theory as a compound of two elements, hydrogen and oxygen, in such a way that it consists of molecules, each of which is composed of three atoms, two of hydrogen and one of oxygen. Moreover, hydrogen occurs in nature in a form in which it is not composed of hydrogen atoms but of hydrogen molecules, each composed of two hydrogen atoms. Thus we have H, H_2, H_2O. This sounds like a straight molecular theory, but it is not anything of the kind. For H, H_2, and H_2O have all different properties which cannot be derived by *adding* properties of H's and O's. And in accordance with that, physics endeavours to construct models of atoms and molecules which are just as different from each other as the actually observed substances. The simple hydrogen atom consists of one proton and one electron in *very definite* dynamic relationship, expressed in terms of the Rutherford-Bohr theory by the orbits in which the electron moves around the proton.[4] In H_2 two hydrogen atoms have been combined. But what has happened? A completely new system has been formed with two protons and two electrons. And the motions of this new system, the forces which are active at every moment, are totally different from the motions in the H system. In the simple water molecule, what a complexity and what a difference of structure from the H and the O atoms! It is wrong to say that this system consists of two hydrogen atoms and one oxygen atom. For where are they to be found in it? Looked at in this way, chemical analysis which dissolves water into hydrogen and oxygen means only that one kind of system has been transformed into other kinds of systems and that in this transformation certain characters like total mass have remained constant. But it does not mean that water is just hydrogen plus oxygen combined in a certain proportion.

Molecular Theory and the Category of Substance. The fallacy contained in a statement like the last derives from a deep source. Man the builder assembles his bricks and erects his house. He knows that just as he made it he can destroy it, that he handled bricks

[4] Although the Rutherford-Bohr theory has been abandoned, the consequences which we draw from it are the same in the different forms of more modern theory. Therefore we use this simplest and most easily intelligible form of atomic theory in our text. See Eddington.

and that after all his house is just bricks. He forgets that he has piled these bricks in a gravitational field and that without this gravitational field he can build a house as little as without bricks. But the bricks are so much more palpable than gravitation that he thinks of them alone, and thus he models his concept of reality. Substance assumes for human thought the rôle of being the embodiment of the real. Molecular theory is nothing but an application of this idea. Fundamentally it derives from a selective principle applied to our appreciation of reality. In what does the reality of a house consist, or that of molar behaviour? The question becomes unanswerable when we attempt to solve it in terms of mere substance. Just so a molecule loses its reality if we describe it in terms of atoms only. We are left with the protons and electrons just as we were left with bricks in the case of the house and with our reflexes in the case of molar behaviour.

But this difficulty arises for the philosopher only, and not for the architect or the physicist. The physicist is far from such crude realism. As a matter of fact he finds it harder and harder to lay his hands on "substances." Organized fields of force assume for him the chief reality. The proposition: the world consists of protons and electrons, is as meaningless to him as the statement that Europe is inhabited by human beings is to the historian or politician. The second statement is incontestably true, but does it help to explain the history of Europe or the present political crisis? Europe is inhabited by British, French, Germans, and a vast number of other nations. Set a Frenchman on a deserted island, an Englishman on another, a German on a third, and so forth, then they will behave more or less alike; at least the fact that they are all human beings will be the main factor in the explanation of their behaviour. But the Frenchman in France, the Englishman in England, the German in Germany will be very different people. Why? Because not only human beings are realities, but also human societies with their institutions, forms of government, mores and customs, language and literature, art and music, social stratification and so forth. If we deny the reality of these we can neither be historians nor politicians, but as little can we be physicists if we deny the reality of the field forces in their distribution, or physiologists if we deny the reality of molar characters of physiological processes.

"Physiological Patterns." Perhaps one might object that nobody has done so, that the word "physiological pattern" is used in every book and treatise on the subject. True enough, but this word "pattern" obscures the issue. In what sense is this pattern considered

to be *real?* Only in what I shall call a geometrical or combinatorial sense, a sense in which it applies equally well to the throwing of dice. You shake six dice; each result can be called a pattern: 536224, 151434, 625251, etc., etc. Pattern means nothing here but combination of independent events. Such patterns may have very real results. I dial on my telephone the pattern 234 and the bell in the president's office rings; had I dialled 479 the psychology department would have been summoned, and so forth. This is the kind of reality which is attributed to the physiological patterns, quite different from the kind of reality I claimed for *molar aspects* of behaviour, physiological or physical events. An example which I have used in a previous discussion will contrast the two kinds of reality: "two insulated condensers of equal capacity are placed at a great distance from each other in a homogeneous dielectric. I convey to each of them the same amount of electricity E. Then they have an *equal* charge. But this equality is a purely logical equality. Nothing in the world compels me to compare just these two charges with each other. Physically, there is in this case no dynamic reality of equality. Indeed I can alter the amount of the charge in either of the condensers without thereby affecting the amount on the other. When, however, I join the two condensers by a piece of wire, the equality of their charges has become a physical, dynamical reality. Now this equality is no longer a relation which I can at will state or neglect, but has become a systematic property of the aggregate of conductors which can no longer be altered by changing the charge of one of the condensers" (1927 a, pp. 178 f.).

The equality in the second case is a true reality—but not in the first. "Physiological pattern," however, has been used in this first and not in the second sense, and therefore this term has nothing to do with the reality of molar properties.

Now we know what molar physiological processes are. They are not a sum or combination of independent local nerve processes, but nervous processes in extension such that each local process depends on all the other local processes within the molar distribution.

WERTHEIMER'S SOLUTION AND THE FACTS OF ANATOMY AND PHYSIOLOGY. The next criticism of Wertheimer's theory will challenge it with regard to its consistency with anatomical and physiological facts. These facts, at least, were duly preserved in the old physiological theory; do they not for that very reason invalidate the new one? Even the most cursory examination of these facts, however, will show this criticism to be nugatory. We might raise the question: What are the conditions under which a mere combination of local events takes place and what are those in which processes in extension are formed? The answer must run like this: when and only when the processes are totally insulated from each other so that they can run their course in absolute independence, only then is the first case realized. Thus the different connections that are made in a telephone exchange are a pattern of purely local events. A talks to B, C to D, etc., etc., but the fact that A and B talk together has no influence on the second fact that C and D exchange compliments or that E and F make a theatre appointment.

On the other hand, where the local processes are not *completely* insulated they will no longer be completely independent, and therefore what happens in one place will depend upon what happens in all the others. The degree of insulation will determine the degree of interdependence, so that we are now dealing not with one case as opposed to another, but with an infinite variety of cases. The question which any physiological theory of nervous processes ought to raise is, therefore: Are the individual nervous structures which anatomy has revealed, completely insulated from each other or not? Only if the answer were affirmative would the traditional theory of a mere additive pattern be possible. As soon as the insulation is found to be incomplete, a theory of molar distribution must take its place. Therefore the anatomical evidence so far adduced is insufficient to support the old theory. What, then, is the added evidence? If we look for an answer in the writings of the founders and supporters of the old theory we search in vain. For they never saw the dilemma; they never chose consciously between the two alternatives, but seduced by the gross anatomical facts, jumped at the one horn without being aware of the other. Although this is no true scientific procedure, it might have been the right guess. But as a matter of mere fact it was not. It is true that the nerve fibres are insulated from each other over long distances, but there are innumerable cross connections which probably connect every nerve cell with every other, a fact of which the old theory has made full use in order to explain the enormous variety of possible "combinations." But if it is so, then the events in this network of nervous tissue can no longer form a merely geometrical pattern; if they are interconnected, then the processes that take place within them can no longer be independent and we must consider them as molar distributions with a degree of interdependence varying inversely with the actually operative resistances. Physiological processes in extension, then, have not been invented in order to support a particular theory. They are demanded by the anatomical facts themselves. Two recent investigations from the psychological laboratory of the University of Kansas give direct experimental support to this view. They show that the action currents of the dog's cortex which result from localized stimulation are not restricted to small areas of the cortex but form a pattern pervading the whole cortex with areas of highest activity varying with the kind of stimulation. Perkins (1933) used sound stimuli; Bartley pain, motor and visual stimuli. Moreover "the records lead to the conclusion that the so-called passive animal exhibits a pattern of cortical activity of essentially the same order as exhibited by the active animal. In other words, there seems to be a basic pattern operating under all conditions of behaviour and that any experimental stimulation of the animal under controlled conditions does no more than modify this pattern" (Bartley, p. 47). The same author concludes that "in accordance with the facts and suggestions that have preceded, a field theory of the nervous system is demanded if its activities are to become intelligible" (p. 54).

BEHAVIOURAL DATA FOR PHYSIOLOGICAL HYPOTHESES. There remains one point in Wertheimer's theory which will meet with scepticism. I claimed as an advantage of this theory that it would use psychological observation, i.e., observation of the behavioural field and of phenomenal behaviour, as material for a physiological theory, thereby greatly augmenting its empirical data. This will seem an unwarranted and highly speculative assumption. The data for a physiological theory must, so it seems, be physiological. Only data from the physical world can be used for a theory about the nature of a part of the physical world, viz., the physiological processes. But this objection overlooks a fact which Köhler (1929) has emphasized, namely, that all observation is observation of behavioural facts of direct experience. Through a careful selection of such facts it has become possible to develop the science of physics, although the relation between the behavioural and the geographical environment is an indirect one. Between these two worlds and mediating between them are the physiological processes within the organism. If, then, we can use the behavioural world in order to obtain insight into the geographical, why should it not be possible also to derive insight into the physiological processes from such study? The way is shorter in the latter case than in the former; in the former, we jump across the mediating link, in the latter we take only one step. Moreover the connection between the behavioural world and the physiological processes is much closer than that between the latter and the physical world; do we not speak of "underlying" physiological processes or of the physiological "correlates" of conscious phenomena? Then, to quote from Köhler, "there is no reason at all why the construction of physiological processes directly underlying experience should be impossible, if experience allows us the construction of a physical world outside which is related to it much less intimately" (1929, pp. 60 f.). Furthermore, if B stands for the behavioural world, G for the geographical, and P for the physiological processes, BP ← G shows the relationship. Now P is in causal connection with G and in a more direct connection with B; the usual assumption, which we shall prove to be erroneous, was that P and G were in close geometrical correspondence, whereas B and P were totally different. Does not such an assumption make it totally unintelligible that B can give us information about G? For if B is totally unlike P, and P is very much like G, how can B lead to G? If, however, B and P are essentially alike, then it only depends upon the G-P relation when and how we can gain knowledge about G from P. And if it is so, then surely observation of B reveals to us properties of P. This theory, first pronounced by Wertheimer, was carefully elaborated by Köhler. In his book on the "Physische Gestalten" (1920) he has gone deeply into physics and physiology to prove the compatibility of the theory with physical and physiological facts; in his "Gestalt Psychology" he has formulated this theory of *isomorphism* in a number of special axioms. In his book (1920) he had formulated the general principle in these words: "Any actual consciousness is in every case not only blindly coupled to its corresponding psychophysical processes, but is akin to it in essential structural properties" (p. 193). Thus, isomorphism, a term implying equality of form, makes the bold assumption that the "motion of the atoms and molecules of the brain" are not "fundamentally different from thoughts and feelings" but in their molar aspects, considered as processes in extension, identical. Moreover the physiologist von Frey draws the following conclusion from his famous investigations on the sense of touch: "The progress achieved by the recent investigations lies, in my opinion, less in improved definition of concepts than in the conviction that the somatic processes which are co-ordinated to mental gestalten must have a structure similar to them" (p. 217).

OLDER FORMS OF ISOMORPHISM. That *some* isomorphism was necessary has been held by most psychologists since the times of Hering and Mach. Hering constructed his theory of colour vision in strict accordance with direct colour experience. The axioms underlying his system have been formulated as psychophysical axioms by G. E.

Müller (1896), but this isomorphism was almost casual though demanded by the scientific problem; it concerned the geometrical, or systematic, order of sensation and not the real dynamic order of living experience. For that reason it remained an isolated part, unrecognized as a fundamental psychological principle. Mach (1865) indicated a more far-reaching isomorphism, one that looks identical with that of Wertheimer and Köhler. Yet it played no rôle in the development of our science; it was so little known that Köhler, who refers to Hering and Müller, fails to mention Mach in this connection. I found the passage in Mach to my great surprise by mere accident. Again we need not look far to find the reason for this apparent injustice of history. Mach was an excellent psychologist, who saw many of the most fundamental problems of psychology which, a whole generation later, many psychologists failed even to understand; at the same time he had a philosophy which made it impossible to give fruitful solutions to these problems. And so his dynamic isomorphism had no effect on psychology because of his interpretation of dynamics in general.

ISOMORPHISM AND OUR BALANCE SHEET. And now, with the tool of a thoroughgoing isomorphism in our hands, we return to our balance sheet which we drew up after stating the reasons why, when we come to fundamentals, we must choose a physiological field rather than the behavioural environment as our fundamental category. We find, then, that we have lost none of our assets, but have succeeded in turning them to such use that they will meet our liabilities. We are no longer losing the advantages gained by the introduction of the behavioural environment, for we construct our physiological field in accordance with, and directed by, the observed properties of it. Thus we have a good reason for introducing and keeping the behavioural environment, even though we look ultimately for physiological explanations. Therefore, all the hopes raised by the introduction of our behavioural environment survive in our new system. If physiological processes are processes in extension, if they are molar instead of being molecular, then we have escaped the danger of abandoning molar behaviour in favour of molecular behaviour. And lastly, we are not advocating pure speculation. The opposite is true; we want to use *more* facts for our physiological theory than the traditional theory did, not less. The brain processes are terra incognita, no doubt about it. Shall we as workers in a young science resign ourselves to this state of affairs or shall we not rather try our utmost to improve it? Physiological theory, as we envisage it, will indeed be much more difficult than the old conception of telephone wires or railway tracks, but it will be just as much more interesting.

"Brain Mythology." In a very striking passage Köhler has defended his hypotheses against the criticism that they were purely speculative, mere brain mythology. I translate only a short but incisive passage: "In the third place it has to be said that the argument betrays a strange misconception of the actual procedure of empirical science. Natural sciences continually advance explanatory hypotheses, which cannot be verified by direct observation at the time when they are formed nor for a long time thereafter. Of such a kind were Ampère's theory of magnetism, the kinetic theory of gases, the electronic theory, the hypothesis of atomic disintegration in the theory of radioactivity. Some of these assumptions have since been verified by direct observation, or have at least come close to such direct verification; others are still far removed from it. But physics and chemistry would have been condemned to a permanent embryonic state had they abstained from such hypotheses; their development seems rather like a continuous effort steadily to shorten the rest of the way to the verification of hypotheses which survive this process" (1923, pp. 140 f.).

ADDED ADVANTAGE OF ISOMORPHISM. Thus we have met point by point the arguments which appeared on the liability side of our ledger. But we can add three more items to our assets. (1) We have gained an insight into the relation of molar and molecular facts. When we saw that a psychology built upon molecular facts could never hope to solve the most important psychological problems, those of the historian or the artist, we suggested that a science built on molar facts might find a place for the molecular ones. And our expectation has been fulfilled; for no real molecular fact disappears from our system; molecular facts merely cease to be independent events, the true elements of all facts. Instead they appear as local events within and determined by larger field events.

(2) Granted, then, that our theory will be a molar theory, nevertheless it is a purely physiological theory, even though mental facts, facts of direct experience, are used in its construction. Does that not reveal a materialistic bias, does it not imply a valuation with regard to reality in which the physical ranks higher than the mental? Is this theory not, after all, a posthumous child of materialism? Let me quote a very impressive paragraph from Wertheimer: "When one goes to the root of one's aversion to materialism and mechanism, does one then find the *material properties* of the elements which these systems combine? Frankly speaking, there are psychological

theories and many psychological textbooks which treat consistently of elements of *consciousness* and are nevertheless more materialistic, barren, lacking in meaning and significance than a living tree which possibly possesses nothing of consciousness. It cannot matter of what material the particles of the universe consist, what matters is the kind of whole, the significance of the whole" (1925, p. 20).

Thus the alleged materialistic bias of our theory disappears. A physiological theory which allows to physiological processes more than mere summative combination of excitations is less materialistic than a psychological theory which allows only sensations and blind associative bonds between them. But we can say even a little more. Is our theory really *purely* physiological? Would it not mean an abandonment of fact if it were? For the physiological processes which we construct as the correlates of consciousness are known to us in the first place through their conscious aspect. To treat them as though they were purely physiological, without this conscious aspect, would be to neglect one of their outstanding characteristics. True enough, this conscious side of the processes does not enter into our causal explanations, but it has to be recognized as a fact nevertheless. And that leads to the conclusion that it is of the warp and woof of certain events in nature that they "reveal themselves," that they are accompanied by consciousness. Why they are so, and what special characteristics a process must have in order to be so, these are questions that cannot now be answered, and perhaps may never be. But if we accept our conclusion, consciousness can no longer be regarded as a mere epiphenomenon, a mere luxury, which might just as well be absent. For in an aspect which we do not know, these processes would be different, were they not accompanied by consciousness.

(3) And this leads us to our last point. What about the consciousness of animals? That the behaviour of animals is molar and not molecular is a fact. Animal and human behaviour belong together; they are not totally different. On the other hand, we can never observe their behavioural environment, their consciousness. But the same is true with regard to any behavioural environment except our own. Directly, I can only know my own consciousness, you yours, yet nobody thinks of claiming a unique position for himself in the universe. Therefore the assumption of animal consciousness is nothing essentially new. However, if we do assume it, we are still faced with the problem, when shall we attribute consciousness to animals, when not? Is there, e.g., a definite point in the phylo-

genetic series where consciousness emerges? If so, where is it? Is an amoeba conscious? If not, a crab, a spider, a fish, a chick, a cat, a monkey, an anthropoid ape? Let us frankly admit that there is no answer to this question. Since we do not know what properties make a physiological process the correlate of a conscious one, we have absolutely no criterion by which we can decide with certainty whether any behaviour is conscious behaviour or not. All attempts to establish such criteria have begged the question by assuming a necessary relation between certain types of behaviour and consciousness.[5] But in our system this whole problem is of no importance. Have we not learned from Wertheimer that there are much more essential characteristics of behaviour than whether it is conscious or merely physiological? Molar behaviour will be a field process; by studying the behaviour we can draw conclusions with regard to the field in which it occurs; we can make molar physiological theories. Because of our isomorphism we can even go a step further; we can describe this field in behavioural rather than physiological terms. This is very useful, because we have a behavioural terminology for such field descriptions, but not a physiological one. When I said previously that a chimpanzee used a "stool," I employed behavioural terminology. How could I, at the present state of science, have used a physiological one? And yet I need not mean more by this terminology than a description of the physiological field, leaving it entirely outside the scope of science, whether a behavioural field corresponded to it or not. Thus we are even less anthropomorphic than we appeared in our last discussion of the problem. There we claimed that the assumption of a behavioural environment was not anthropomorphism; now we are willing to give up even the behavioural environment, substituting for it a physiological field, the properties of which can best be described in behavioural terms. Thus the issue between us and the behaviourists with regard to animal psychology is not conscious behaviour vs. purely physiological behaviour, but physiological behaviour of the *field* type vs. physiological behaviour of the mechanical connection type. This issue can and must be decided on the plane of pure science, and the decision cannot fail to affect the wider issues which distinguish gestalt theory and behaviourism.

One last remark in this connection: we said that physiological processes that are accompanied by consciousness must in some unknown aspect differ from physiological processes which have no such accompaniment. We must add that in other relevant aspects

[5] Compare my discussion of this problem (1928), pp. 13 f.

they must be alike. For they are all field processes. Our whole solution of the mind-body problem would help us nought if we restricted the field concept to conscious physiological processes. But we do not. We view these as part events in a much wider field event and thereby avoid the argument against the behavioural field as a fundamental category which we have termed the insufficiency of the behavioural field. Let us introduce for future use the term "psychophysical field," indicating by this term both its physiological nature and its relation to direct experience.

THE TASK OF OUR PSYCHOLOGY

And now we can formulate the task of our psychology: it is *the study of behaviour in its causal connection with the psychophysical field.* This general programme must be made more concrete. Anticipating, we can say that the psychophysical field is organized. First of all it shows the polarity of the Ego and the environment, and secondly each of these two polar parts has its own structure. Thus the environment is neither a mosaic of sensations nor a "blooming, buzzing confusion," nor a blurred and vague total unit; rather does it consist of a definite number of separate objects and events, which, as separate objects and events, are products of organization. Likewise, the Ego is neither a point nor a sum or mosaic of drives or instincts. To describe it adequately we shall have to introduce the concept of personality with all its enormous complexity. Therefore if we want to study behaviour as an event in the psychophysical field, we must take the following steps:

(1) We must study the organization of the environmental field, and that means (a) we must find out the forces which organize it into separate objects and events, (b) the forces which exist between these different objects and events; and (c) how these forces produce the environmental field as we know it in our behavioural environment.

(2) We must investigate how such forces can influence movements of the body.

(3) We must study the Ego as one of the main field parts.

(4) We must show that the forces which connect the Ego with the other field parts are of the same nature as those between different parts of the environmental field, and how they produce behaviour in all its forms.

(5) We must not forget that our psychophysical field exists within a real organism which in its turn exists in a geographical environ-

ment. In this way the questions of true cognition and adequate or adapted behaviour will also enter our programme.

Points (3) and (4) are the nucleus of a theory of behaviour; (1) and (2) are necessary for their solution. And therefore one cannot wonder that the two problems (3) and (4) have been much less studied than others; moreover, experimentation was started within the province of our first point, both in psychology in general and in gestalt psychology in particular. Therefore the reader must not be surprised when we devote more space to our first point than seems proportionate in consideration of its importance in the whole scheme. The value of theoretical concepts is tested by their application in actual research. The concepts which we have so far developed cannot be understood without a good knowledge of the concrete experimental research work in which they have played the leading rôle. But there is another point to remember. In our fifth item we have touched upon a fundamental philosophical problem. The studies in perception to which my last remarks referred will give us valuable clues for the solution of this philosophical problem. This must be kept in mind if perspective is not to be lost. There will be many experiments, which, though they appear neat and ingenious enough, will seem trivial when seen by themselves. Why such experiments? What can they contribute to a real knowledge of behaviour? The answer is that they serve as demonstrations of general principles; they are not meant to be of great significance in their own right.

CHAPTER III

THE ENVIRONMENTAL FIELD

The Problem. Refutation of False Solutions. General Formulation of the True Solution

The Environmental Field. Causal Relation Between Geographical and Behavioural Environment. Why Do Things Look as They Do? The First Answer. The Second Answer. The True Answer. What We Have Gained by Our Distinction of Process and Conditions. Summary

As the first step which our field psychology had to take we announced an investigation of the environmental field. The organization of this field depends evidently upon the geographical environment which can affect the sense organs of the animal. Therefore in discussing this problem we shall have to investigate the relationship between the geographical environment and the environmental field. But before we attack this problem we must become better acquainted with this field in order to understand the full scope of our investigation.

THE ENVIRONMENTAL FIELD

It is clear that at the outset, at least, we cannot describe this field in physiological terms, for the physiological field is a construct necessitated by our demands for an explanatory theory; but it is not an observed fact. If we want to start with facts we must fall back on our behavioural environment, fully aware that the behavioural environment is at best the counterpart of only a fraction of the total active environmental field.

What, then, do we find in our behavioural surrounding? It presents us with a motley of data, the systematization of which would prove a difficult problem indeed. We shall not attempt it, confining ourselves to an enumeration of a variety of different kinds of objects in our behavioural environment. There are things like stones and sticks and man-made things, like tables and dishes, houses and churches, books and pictures; there are people, animals, plants and ghosts; there are mountains, rivers, and oceans, but also clouds and fog, air, light and darkness, the sun, the moon and the stars, heat and cold, noises, tones and words, motions, forces and waves. This is hardly less heterogeneous than the cabbages and kings in Alice's world, and it cannot claim to be a complete list. But it seems enough for a beginning.

Things and Not-things. If one tried to bring some order into this medley, one would probably begin by distinguishing things and not-things, and among the former the living and the dead; among the dead, things made by man and things natural. Of course one must not forget that in making this order one should stay within the confines of the behavioural environment as one finds it, and that one must not use any indirect knowledge about it. Thus I have included ghosts as part of the behavioural world, although I know quite as well as anyone that ghosts do not exist, the spiritualists' contention to the contrary notwithstanding. And when we approach our material in this naïve way we shall find our classification much less satisfactory. For quite frequently we shall be in doubt whether one of our data is to be counted as a thing or not, or as a live or a dead thing. Are clouds things? If yes, is fog, air, light, cold? If clouds are things, they are surely things different in kind from stones and sticks, and the twinkling stars are again different. Air? The breath, the "pneuma," the "spirit" has thing-like qualities; did not God create Adam by imparting the breath of life to the dust of the ground! And does not the meaning of the word spirit indicate that it referred originally to a substance, a thing of finer texture? A fog which we see creeping up a mountain valley has a thing-like quality similar to that of clouds, but a fog which makes our ocean liner reduce speed and sound its piercing horn is not thing-like at all, as little as the mist from which we emerge when we climb a mountain. Light when it travels through the night as in the beam from a lighthouse is thing-like, or when it spreads across the sky at dawn. But the light here in this room is in no way a thing by itself; here is the same difference as between the air that surrounds us as opposed to the breath. Darkness may be a thing when storm-swept clouds cast a gloom over the land, or when we pause before entering a dark cavern. The same is true of heat and cold. We feel the cold drifting into our rooms—even though we know that it is cold air that is coming.

The river is a thing and yet old Heraclitus already said that we cannot bathe twice in the same river, only to be outdone by his pupil Cratylus, who denied that we can do it even once, for while we enter the water the water has already passed and is passing all the time. And yet we call a river a thing, or if we do not do it explicitly, we treat it as a thing.

Are words things? They seem completely un-thing-like, and yet, why do we write d—d, why do we speak of the dickens when we mean the devil? And the peal of thunder, has it not the character of a thing, threatening and awe-inspiring as it is? So noises and words may be things, but they need not. There remain the waves, the motions, and the forces. A wave certainly may have thing-character; the waves that send us sprawling on the beach or toss our ship about are mighty things indeed, and yet the argument of Heraclitus applies to the wave as much as to the river. Lastly, what about motions and forces? Even they may assume thing-like qualities: when two billiard balls cannon, do we not see the motion of the one pass into the other; does not motion in such examples have a character akin to the thing-quality of fluids? And even force may be experienced as something thing-like, to be sure not the force of the physicists, but something in our behavioural environment which we can name no better than force. The "potency" of a drug appears to the naïve person as something within the drug; we feel the force of the wind, a perfectly good *description,* not a metaphor, and what we feel is of the essence of things.

Now it cannot be the purpose of this argument to claim that every part of our behavioural environment is a thing. The very opposite is true: we must distinguish between things and not-things, but this distinction is not permanent in the sense that the same real objects will always appear either as things or as not-things. On the contrary, we have shown many objects which may be thing-like or not according to circumstances. But the fact that almost anything may at one time or another assume the thing-character reveals a significant feature of our behavioural environment: the parts of this environment must possess a strong tendency towards thing-ness, or, expressed without the precarious word tendency, qua part of our environmental field almost anything may acquire the character of thing-ness.

However, the term "thing" seems to have lost its meaning. To find it again, let us try to discover significant properties of non-thing parts of our environment. A dense fog which surrounds us is a good example. Comparing it with a fog drifting up a valley it has two distinct characteristics: it has no boundary or shape, and it is absolutely static, whereas the drifting fog has shape and motion. And when we compare our fog with a stone we discover still another characteristic: the stone is constant, i.e., tomorrow it will be the same as it is today; not so the fog.

Thus we may single out three characteristics of things which will severally and jointly be constitutive of things: shaped boundedness, dynamic properties, and constancy. Jointly these properties are manifest in living things before all others. And thus a thing in which these properties are blended will appear as a living thing, even when in reality it is dead, e.g., a corpse. One must be an anatomist or an undertaker to regard a human corpse as a thing of the same kind as a table or the fallen trunk of a tree.

One more word about the dynamic characters of things. It would be, descriptively and genetically, a grave mistake to assign to them a secondary rôle. The terrifying character of the thunder is its outstanding characteristic, its description as a noise of a certain intensity and quality, quite secondary; similarly, a snake is uncanny before it is brown or spotted, a human face happy before it is of a certain hue and chroma. All these descriptions imply something like a force, something that goes beyond the mere static thing and affects ourselves. Thus force, which may have the character of a thing, is also a property of things, or, otherwise expressed, thing and force, substance and causality, are, as parts of our behavioural environment, often not two separate objects but closely interrelated aspects of one and the same object. Discursive thought has separated what to naïve experience is in many cases a unity.

It is tempting to pursue this argument and to investigate different combinations of our three thing-characters, to see how far they would exhaust the richness of our behavioural field. But this would lead us too far away from our main problem. Therefore we summarize:

The thing category allows us to bring some order into the data of our behavioural environment. We have discovered three aspects of this category and have seen that things of different *kinds* exist according to the combination of these aspects, and we have also seen that the environment contains not only things, even if we use the term in the broadest sense, but also not-things. Particularly we find the things *within* something that is not itself a thing. The things do not fill our environment either spatially or temporally; there is something between them and around them. In order to have a convenient term for this we shall call it the framework, so that, disregarding the great variety of things, we can divide the behavioural environment into things and framework.

On the Phenomenological Method. Before we continue, a methodological remark may be in place. One can read many American books and articles on psychology without finding any such or similar description, whereas in German works one will meet with them quite frequently. This difference is not superficial, but reveals a thoroughgoing difference in the character of American and German work. Americans will call the German psychology speculative and hairsplitting; Germans will call the American branch superficial. The Americans are justified, when they find an author introducing such descriptions, refining them, playing with them, without really doing anything to them. The Germans are right, because American psychology all too often makes no attempt to look naïvely, without bias, at the facts of direct experience, with the result that American experiments quite often are futile. In reality experimenting *and* observing must go hand in hand. A good description of a phenomenon may by itself rule out a number of theories and indicate definite features which a true theory must possess. We call this kind of observation "phenomenology," a word which has several other meanings which must not be confused with ours. For us phenomenology means as naïve and full a description of direct experience as possible. In America the word "introspection" is the only one used for what we mean, but this word has also a very different meaning in that it refers to a special kind of such description, namely, the one which analyzes direct experience into sensations or attributes, or some other systematic, but not experiential, ultimates.

I can save myself and my readers the trouble of discussing this kind of introspection, since Köhler has done that admirably well in the third chapter of his "Gestalt Psychology." This kind of introspection became unpopular in America because American psychologists saw its barrenness. But in their justified criticism they threw out the baby with the bath, substituting pure achievement experiments and tending to leave out phenomenology altogether. That phenomenology is important, however, should appear from the preceding discussion. Without describing the environmental field we should not know what we had to explain.

There remains the question how this description is possible, what phenomenology as a part of behaviour is. The difficulties inherent in this problem have been frequently discussed; I may refer the reader to two articles of mine in which they are fully treated and in which a solution of these difficulties is attempted (1923, 1924).

CAUSAL RELATION BETWEEN GEOGRAPHICAL AND BEHAVIOURAL ENVIRONMENT

The Rôle of Light Waves in Vision. And now let us go one step further. We have described the environmental field as it is given; now we must ask for the causes that bring it into existence. Then it is quite clear that primarily the environmental field owes its existence to the affection of our sense organs. Since most of the descriptions we gave referred to aspects which were wholly or partially visual we shall begin with the organ of sight, our two eyes. Our eyes are stimulated by light waves which either come directly from the light sources or, more frequently, from physical bodies which reflect light emanating from one or several sources. This stimulation passes through a medium existing between our eyes on the one hand and the bodies and light sources on the other, and is modified in a certain way by a part of our eyes, the lenses, which assume such a curvature as to project what we call a sharp image of the objects on our retinae. Since we must take nothing for granted, we meet here with a first problem: Why do the lenses react in this strange way? What is it that makes them change their curvature in accordance with the real distance of the objects which are to be seen? Deferring the answer to this question to Chapter VIII (p. 311) we point out merely that if the lenses did not behave in this way, the objects would not be seen. As F. Heider has pointed out (p. 146): hold a photographic plate opposite an object, and expose it for the time necessary for the photochemical effect to take place, then the plate, when developed, will be virtually a uniform grey; there will be in no sense a picture of the object on the plate. If you want a picture you must have the plate in a camera that is well focussed. But even if you have taken a regular picture, what is on your developed plate? A picture? Yes and no; yes, when you include the person who looks at the plate in the situation, but *no,* if you consider the plate by itself. On this plate you have a great number of particles which, before the plate was developed and fixed, were sensitive to light and were affected according to the intensity of the light which struck them. The weaker the light, the more easily will they be removed by the developer, so that on the developed plate you have a layer of material of a thickness varying from point to point and depending on the amount of light which fell on each point at the time of exposure. Since this layer is composed of a finite number of separate particles, each of which is affected as a whole, the fineness of detail which your plate shows will depend on the fineness of its grain, i.e., the number of particles per unit area. But, however fine its grain, the developed plate can be adequately described if you divide it up into small areas and measure the thickness of the layer in each of these areas. A complete table of these thicknesses would be a complete description of the developed plate. There is *no* picture on it, if we mean by picture more than this complete table. Break off a corner of your plate, rub off a part of the photographic layer, the rest will remain as it was before, each point having its characteristics independently of all the others.

The "Picture" on the Retina. And now let us go back to our eyes. When they have focussed on an object, a snake, a cloud, a smiling infant, a book, what is on the retinae? Pictures of these objects? Yes, only when we mean by a picture just such a table as we have described in the case of the photographic plate; only instead of the individual particles we have to list the sensitive elements of the retinae, the cones and rods, and instead of the thickness of the layer the *kind* and amount of stimulation which each of these elementary receptors receives. But apart from this difference the immediate cause of our vision of any object is just such a mosaic of stimulation as that of the photographic plate. And that raises at once the problem: how the enormous richness and variety of our visual behavioural environment can be aroused by such a mere mosaic of light and shade and colour. I think, when formulated in these terms, the problem must appear thrilling by the very paradox which it seems to involve. How can such rich effects arise out of such poor causes, for clearly the "dimensions" of our environmental field are far more numerous than those of the mosaic of the stimulation?

Other Senses. The situation remains essentially the same if we include the other sense organs in our survey. Vibratory processes distributed in time affect our ears; we hear the rattling of an old Ford in the traffic noise, the song of a nightingale, the lecture of a professor, and the intertwined voices of a fugue played on the piano. In touch we have spatially and temporally distributed contacts between objects and our skin, and we "feel" hard and soft, dry and clammy, round and pointed objects.

WHY DO THINGS LOOK AS THEY DO?

And now we can take up the functional problem as to the relationship between the geographical and the behavioural environment. Concentrating on the world of sight we can formulate our problem thus: *Why do things look as they do?*

Two Aspects of This Question. This question has two aspects. Taken literally it refers to the things in our behavioural environment quite regardless of their being "veridical," i.e., leading us to reasonable actions, to adapted behaviour. In this first sense, then, the problem would apply to a world of pure illusion as well as to a realistic world. Illusory perceptions fall under it in the same way as non-illusory ones. If our world were such that all appearances were deceptive, the solution of this problem would have to be the same as it is now. If a pencil which we picked up for taking notes behaved like a snake, a bar of iron which we grasped turned out to be a ball of wax, a stone on which we stepped jumped at us like a wolf, and so on, still we would have to ask the question: Why does the pencil look like a pencil, the iron bar like a bar, the stone like a stone? But in reality our world is, fortunately, not such a burlesque nightmare; as a rule, things are what they look like, or otherwise expressed, their looks tell us what to do with them, although as a previous discussion of an optical illusion has shown, perception may be deceptive (see p. 33). And thus arises the second aspect of our question: Why is it that our behaviour, directed as it is by the objects in the behavioural environment, is, as a rule, also adapted to the objects in the geographical environment? This is a new question, falling under the fifth point of our programme (see p. 67-8). It is important not to confuse these two aspects of our general question, not to introduce facts which belong to the second aspect into our solution of the first. An example will make clear what I mean by this last warning. We shall later on raise the question: Why to the spectator does this actor on the stage *look* furious or embarrassed or grief-stricken? and in answering this question we must not introduce our knowledge of what he feels, whether he actually experiences the emotions of his part or whether he remains detached or full of glee. Only when we have answered our question can we turn to this second fact and try to explain why in this case our perception was possibly illusory. That means the second, the cognitive, aspect of perception can only be treated after we have exhausted the first, the qualitative aspect.

THE FIRST ANSWER

Why, then, do things look as they do? We shall systematically take up various answers that may be given to this question, although they have been implicitly refuted in our previous discussion.

A first answer would be: things look as they look because they are what they are.

Although this answer seems banal, it is not only utterly inadequate, but in many cases literally wrong. Let us single out a few aspects of behavioural things and compare them with the real ones. The pen with which I am writing is a unit in my behavioural environment and so is the real pen in the geographical. So far, so good. But if our proposition were true, to be a real unit would be a necessary and sufficient condition for a thing to be also a behavioural unit. But it is easy to show that it is neither necessary nor sufficient. If it were a necessary condition, it would mean: to every unit in my behavioural field there corresponds a unit in the geographical environment; for if behavioural units could exist without corresponding geographical ones, then the existence of the latter would no longer be necessary for the existence of the former. Nothing, however, is easier to point out than behavioural units to which no geographical units correspond. Look at Fig. 3. In your behavioural field it is a unit, a cross; in reality, in the geographical environment, there is no cross, there are just eleven dots in a certain geometrical arrangement, but there is no connection between them that could make them a unit. This is, of course, true of all pictures, equally true of the stellar constellations like Charles's Wain, a case which Köhler has chosen as an illustration of this point.

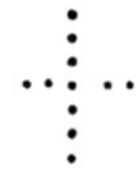

Fig. 3

If the visible existence of real units were the *sufficient* condition for the appearance of a behavioural unit it would mean that whenever our eyes were directed on a physical unit we should perceive a behavioural one. But this is not true either. Certainly, in most cases, this correspondence exists, but there are exceptions. As a matter of fact, it is possible to interfere with the real units in such a way that they will no longer look like units, an effect which we try to produce when we want to conceal certain well-known objects. If a gun is covered with paint in such a way that one part of it will "fuse" with the bole of a tree, another with the leaves, a third with the ground, then the beholder will no longer see a unit, the gun, but a multiplicity of much less important objects. Camouflage was an art well developed during the war, when even big ships were destroyed as real units in the behavioural world of the scouting enemy. Thus existence of a real unity is neither the necessary nor the sufficient cause of behavioural unity.

If we choose size as the aspect in which we should find correspondence we see at once that no direct relation between real and apparent size can exist, for the moon looks large on the horizon and small on the zenith.

And even for the aspect of motion it is easy to prove that the existence, within the field of vision, of real motion is neither a necessary nor a sufficient condition for the perception of motion. It is not a necessary condition, for we can see motion when no real motion occurs, as on the cinematographic screen, but neither is it sufficient, for apart from the fact that too slow and too fast real motions produce no perception of motion, there are many cases where the apparently moving object is really at rest, as the moon that seems to float through the clouds.

We forbear discussing other aspects because our material is sufficient to prove the first answer to our question wrong. That things are what they are does not explain why they look as they look.

Consequences Implied in the First Answer. Before we discuss another answer to our question we may for a moment consider what it would mean if the first answer were right. If things looked as they do because they are what they are, then the relation between the behavioural and the geographical environment would be simple indeed. Then for all practical purposes we could substitute the latter for the former. Conversely, since we know that the answer is wrong, we must guard against this confusion, which is not as easily avoided as one might think. To show how a disregard of our warning has influenced psychological theory, we will formulate our conclusion in still another manner. If things looked as they do because they are what they are, then perception would not contain in its very make-up a cognitive problem. Perception would, barring certain unusual conditions, be cognitive of the geographical environment. A cognitive problem might arise in the field of generalized thought, but as long as we remained in the field of direct perception we ought to be face to face with objective reality. The proposition, included in many philosophical systems, that the senses cannot lie, is a special form of this more general idea. To be sure, the existence of special cases where perception was deceptive was generally admitted. But these cases were treated as exceptions to the general rule, and for this reason the so-called geometric optical illusions received so much attention in the development of psychology. And when one reads the older literature on the subject, and some of the recent too, one will find explanations of this kind: if of two equal lines, one looks longer than the other, then we must look for special conditions which mislead our *judgment* about the relative length of these lines. Remove these distracting circumstances and the judgment will be correct, the normal state of affairs, in which the behavioural world corresponds to the geographical one, will be re-established. That is to say, illusory perceptions were not accorded the same rank as non-illusory ones; they presented a special problem, whereas the normal appearance presented no problem at all. This distinction between two kinds of perception, normal and illusory, disappears as a psychological distinction as soon as one becomes thoroughly aware of the fallacy which it implies, much as it may remain as an epistemological distinction. For each thing we have to ask the same question, "Why does it look as it does?" whether it looks "right" or "wrong."

Two Meanings of the Term Stimulus. These last considerations ought to have shown that our refutation of the first answer is not so banal as might have been thought. At the start it might well have been argued, How can the first answer be right, when the geographical things are not in direct contact with the organism? When I see a table, this table qua table does not affect my senses at all; they are affected by processes which have their origin in the sun or an artificial source of light, and which are only modified by the table before they excite the rods and cones in our retinae. Therefore, these processes, the light waves, and not the geographical objects, are the direct causes of our perceptions, and consequently we cannot expect a very close relationship between behavioural and geographical things. For the light waves do not depend only upon the things qua things, but also upon the nature of the source of light (which only in the case of self-luminous bodies belongs to them as their own property) and on the position of the things with regard to our own bodies. This last relation is regulated by the laws of perspective, the first by laws of light absorption and reflection. But perspective, light absorption, and reflection remain outside our organisms. The retinae receive a pattern of excitations, and it can make no difference to the retinae how these excitations have been produced. If, without a table and even without light (for instance, by electrical stimulation of the rods and cones), we could produce the same pattern of excitation with the same curvature of the lenses which is ordinarily produced on our retinae when we fixate a table, then the person on whose retinae these excitations were produced should and would see a table. This leads us to introduce a new terminological distinction. The causes of the excitations of our sense organs are called stimuli. We see now that this word has two different meanings which must be clearly distinguished from each other: on the one hand the table in the geographical environment can be called a stimulus for our perception of a table; on the other hand the excitations to which the light rays coming from the table give rise are called the stimuli for our perception. Let us call the first the *distant* stimulus, the second the *proximal* stimuli. Then we can say that our question why things look as they do must find its answer not in terms of the distant, but of the proximal, stimuli. By a neglect of this difference real problems have been overlooked, and explanations proffered which are no explanations at all. We shall see this presently in detail, but we can point out here how the confusion of distant and proximal stimuli can have such a fatal effect on psychological theory. The danger of this confusion lies in the fact that for each distant stimulus there exists a practically infinite number of proximal stimuli; thus, the "same stimulus" in the distant sense may not be the same stimulus in the proximal sense; as a matter of fact it very seldom is. Thus the sameness of the former conceals a difference of the latter, and all arguments based on identical stimulation are spurious if they refer to identity of the distant stimulus only.

THE SECOND ANSWER

The introduction of our term proximal stimulus has, however, given us a clue to the second answer to our question: things look as they do because the proximal stimuli are what they are. Now in its broadest interpretation this proposition is certainly true, but the interpretation usually given to it is distinctly limited and therefore false. In the widest interpretation our proposition means no more than this: any change in the proximal stimulation will, provided it be not too small, produce *some* change in the look of things, but *what kind* of change in the behavioural world will follow upon a change in the proximal stimulation cannot be derived from our proposition; whereas in the narrower interpretation the proposition also contains implicitly a statement about the kind of this change. Two objects project retinal images of different size on our retinae and appear to be at the same distance. Then the one which corresponds to the larger retinal image will look larger. We see two adjacent surfaces at an equal distance in front of us, the one looks a lighter, the other a darker, grey; then the retinal image corresponding to the former will contain more light than that of the latter. From these examples two conclusions might be drawn: the larger the retinal image, the larger the perceived object, and the greater the intensity of the image the more white will the object look; consequently when I change the stimulus corresponding to one object by making it smaller, the object should look smaller too, and if I reduce the intensity of stimulation the object should look blacker. These conclusions which have been actually accepted as axioms of sense psychology will seem very plausible. But neither do they follow from our examples, nor are they true. They do not follow from our examples because they only take in a part of the conditions of these examples and they are continually contradicted by the facts. Look at a white surface and then reduce the illumination of this surface; for a long time the surface wili remain white, and only when you have reduced your illumination to a very low point will it become greyish. As a matter of fact a surface which still looks white under a low illumination may send much less light into our eyes than a black surface in good illumination. Disregard for the moment such plausible explanations as that when the light is decreased the pupil dilates so as to allow more of the incoming light to fall on our retinae, and that simultaneously the sensitivity of our retinae increases so as to make the effect of light greater. As we shall see later, both these factors, which are admittedly real, have been ruled out as sufficient explanations of our effect, so for simplicity's sake we neglect them altogether in our present discussion. Have we then shown that a change in the stimulus, in our case a diminution of light, has no effect at all on the look of things? If we had, we should have contradicted our general interpretation of the proposition: things look as they do because the proximal stimuli are what they are, an interpretation which we have accepted. But we have shown no such thing; we have only shown that the particular effect which would follow from the narrower interpretation of our proposition has failed to materialize. But there is an effect notwithstanding. For when the illumination is reduced, we become aware of a *darkening* of the *room*. Comparing this case with our former example we see that a change in the intensity of the retinal image may have at least two different effects: it may make the particular object look whiter or blacker, or it may make the whole room appear brighter or darker.

And the same is true of our other example. Look at the moon, particularly when it is at the horizon, and compare its size with that of a shilling held at arm's length. You will find the moon looking very much larger, whereas the retinal image of the shilling is larger than that of the moon. At the same time you see the moon at a much greater distance. Therefore decrease in size of a retinal image may either produce a shrinking or a receding of the corresponding object in the behavioural environment.

Two old experiments confirm this conclusion. In both, the observer looks monocularly at a screen with a circular hole in it. At some distance behind the screen there is a well illuminated homogeneous white wall part of which is visible through the hole. In the first experiment (Wundt, II) a taut vertical black thread between the screen and the wall passes through the centre of the circle exposed by the hole. This thread is attached to stands which can be moved backwards and forwards in a sagittal line from the observer in such a way that the thread, whatever its distance from the hole, divides the circle into equal halves, the stands being invisible behind the screen. A movement of the thread has then no other effect than an increase or decrease of the width of its retinal image, apart from a possible blurring due to insufficient accommodation. Under these conditions the observer sees, as a rule, a sagittal motion of a thread with *constant* thickness, and not an increase or decrease of the thickness of an immovable thread. In the second experiment there is no thread at all, and the room is totally dark so that the light circular hole is the only visible object in it. The variable is this time the opening of the hole itself which is made by an iris diaphragm which can be opened or closed. The retinal conditions are still simpler than in the first case, the retinal area on which the light falls increasing or decreasing. Accompanying these retinal changes the observers see either a forward or backward movement of the light circle, or its expansion or contraction, or finally a joint effect in which expansion and approach, contraction and recession, are combined.

We can now present our argument in a more generalized form. If the answer: things look as they do because the proximal stimuli are what they are, were true in the narrower sense, two propositions should hold. (1) Changes in the proximal stimulation unaccompanied by changes of the distant stimulus-object should produce corresponding changes in the *looks* of the behavioural object, and (2) any change in the distant object which produces no effect in the proximal stimulation should leave the looks of the behavioural object unchanged.

That (1) is not true follows from the example we have discussed. A white surface continues to look white, a black one black even when the proximal stimulation to which they give rise varies over a very wide range; my pencil looks no bigger when I hold it in my hand than when it is at the other end of my desk, when its retinal image may be less than half the size of the image of the pencil in my hand; the seat of a chair looks rectangular, although its retinal image will be rectangular in a negligibly small number of occasions only. In other words the behavioural things are conservative; they do not change with every change of the proximal stimulation by which they are produced. The constancy of real things is to a great extent preserved in the constancy of the *phenomenal* things despite variations in their proximal stimuli.

Relation of the Two Answers. When we compare this argument with the one given in our discussion of the first answer which explained the look of behavioural things by the nature of the real things, we are struck with a somewhat curious relation between the two answers: According to the first the correspondence between real and behavioural things should have been much better than it really is, and according to the second it should be much worse.

Refutation of Second Answer Continued. Let us now turn to the second point. It is quite true that changes of the distant stimuli unaccompanied by any change in the proximal stimulation can have no effect on the look of things. Thus a third variant of the experiment just described has been introduced (Hillebrand). The hole in the screen is constant, and behind it is a movable black surface with a very sharp and smooth straight-edge which cuts through the centre of the visible circle just as the thread did in the first modification. Howsoever this surface is moved backwards and forwards, the observer will see a semicircle bounded by a sharp contour, and in this case, much more frequently, motion of the surface will remain entirely unnoticed, in accordance with the fact that, again apart from possible blurring of the edge due to inaccurate accommodation, the proximal stimulation remains unaltered by the process of moving the surface.

And yet the proposition of our point (2) does not tell us the whole truth, because its conversion is no longer true. The conversion of our proposition (2) would be: no change can occur in the looks of things without corresponding changes in the proximal stimuli. But this is not true. Fig. 4 will not preserve its appearance when you continue to look at it; if you see at first a black cross on white, you will later see a white cross on black, and these two phases will alternate. Puzzle pictures, reversible perspectives, demonstrate the same fact, and so does the experiment with the iris diaphragm described above in which the observer may at one time see a displacement, at another time a change of the size of the hole. From this we must draw the conclusion that the looks of things cannot alone depend upon the proximal stimulation, even if this dependence is considered in the broadest sense,

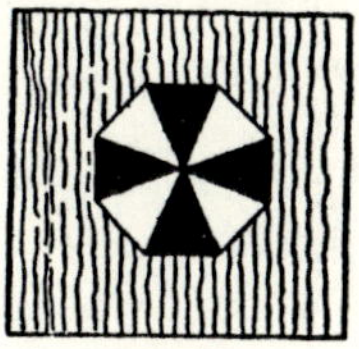

Fig. 4

but also upon sets of other conditions which must lie within the real organism.

Finally, many of the arguments used to disprove the first answer apply equally well to the second. Since the mosaic of proximal stimulation possesses no unity, the unity within our behavioural world cannot be explained by a corresponding unity in the proximal stimulation. And the argument derived from the cinema applies to proximal stimulation as well as to distant, so that, in this respect, the second answer is in the same boat with the first.

Reasons for the Survival of the Second Answer. It may seem strange that the view according to which there is a point-to-point correspondence between proximal stimulation and the look of things should have survived the evidence which we have presented and which is not at all new. But it is not difficult to explain the tenacity of this view which has by no means disappeared from present-day psychology. Two general features of traditional psychological thought mutually supported each other to keep it alive. The first is connected with the old physiological hypotheses about conscious phenomena which were discussed in the second chapter. It may be presented like this: the simplest experiments reveal that under standard conditions whiteness depends upon intensity of light, and apparent size on the size of the retinal image. If under other less simple conditions other correlations seem to obtain, these cannot be true correlations in the same sense in which our first are. For how should it be possible that one and the same nerve fibre should react once in one way, the next time in another way, when it receives the same stimulation in the two cases? The physiological hypotheses had no place for such a change (Stumpf, 1890, p. 10).

Current Theory a Combination of the Two First Answers; Sensation and Perception. Strongly entrenched as the physiological hypotheses were, this theory could hardly have survived the damning evidence of the facts without the second general feature mentioned above. The damning evidence consists in the fact that the things do not look as they ought to on the ground of pure proximal stimulation, and they differ from such an expectation by looking more like the distant stimuli, like the things with which we have real dealings. Therefore it was assumed that the *real* properties of things, that the distant stimuli, have something to do with the looks of things after all. The answer, that things look as they do because the proximal stimulation is what it is, had to be supplemented by the first answer, viz., that the fact that things are what they are must be included also in a final explanation. Current theory was, in this way, a sort of combination of our two answers, in which the second answer accounted for the immediate effect, the first for a secondary one. For according to this way of thinking, in dealing with things we acquire experience about them, and this experience enters our whole perception. Thus, according to this view, we must really distinguish between two kinds of behavioural fields, a primary and a secondary one, the field of sensations and the field of perceptions. The original primary field, the field of sensations, corresponded completely to the proximal stimuli—there was only one notable exception which we shall discuss later—for this primary field the answer that it looked as it did because the proximal stimuli were what they were, was true in a very narrow sense. But experience has changed this primary field and has substituted for it the secondary by virtue of the numberless experiences which we have had.

THE NETWORK OF TRADITIONAL HYPOTHESES. Let us see how this theory worked. Not so very long ago, in 1920, Jaensch explained Wundt's experiment of the approaching and receding thread whose motion we perceive, in the following manner: "In the case of the thread, judgment can rest only upon a change in the magnitude of the retinal dimensions which accompanies the alteration of the thread's distance, and although this change is too small to be directly noticed as a change of magnitude, still it must determine the judgment of distance." Several features of this explanation are worth noting. First it distinguishes between *effects* which can be *directly noticed*—even if they are not noticed at the time—viz., the change of the apparent thickness of the thread corresponding to a change of breadth in the retinal image—and *judgments* determined by such directly noticeable effects—viz., the greater or smaller distance of the thread. If we express this distinction by saying: the increasing thickness of the behavioural thread means, is interpreted as, approach, its decreasing thickness as recession, then we see that this is a clear-cut example of the "meaning theory" which Köhler has discussed with great brilliance in his book. What, so any unbiassed person ought to ask, is the reason for distinguishing in Wundt's experiment between a sensory, though unnoticed, breadth and a judgmental distance? Admittedly, experience presents us only with one fact, the change of distance; admittedly, because the change of breadth is called unnoticed, i.e., unexperienced; neither do we experience this movement as a judgment, but as a change of the same palpability as a change of width which we may experience at another time. That this particular change of distance is interpreted by Jaensch as a judgment is due to the fact that the proximal stimulation changed in breadth, and therefore implies the relation between proximal stimulation and the behavioural field assumed in the second answer. Thus we see the circular nature of this interpretation: in order to call the experienced change of distance a judgment, Jaensch must assume that a change of breadth in the retinal image produces primarily a change of breadth in the perceived object; but in order to reconcile this assumption with the observed facts he must interpret the actual experience of changed distance as a judgment.

CONSTANCY AND INTERPRETATION HYPOTHESIS. The general name for this assumption is "constancy hypothesis"—to be explained presently; we shall call the other the interpretation hypothesis—preferring this term to Köhler's "meaning theory" for no intrinsic reasons but merely for the practical one that we use the word "meaning," just as Köhler, in a very different sense and do not want to confuse the reader by an avoidable ambiguity. Then we can say: the interpretation hypothesis presupposes the constancy hypothesis, but also the latter the former. At the risk of appearing frivolous I will tell a joke which seems to me to give a perfect picture of the relation between the two hypotheses. A man and his small son are viewing with great interest an acrobat walking on the tight rope and balancing himself with a long pole. The boy suddenly turns to his father and asks: "Father, why doesn't that man fall?" The father replies: "Don't you see that he is holding on to the pole?" The boy accepts the authority of his parent, but after a while he bursts out with a new question: "Father, why doesn't the pole fall?" Whereupon the father replies: "But don't you see that the man holds it!"

NON-NOTICED SENSATIONS. Köhler, who has shown up this same vicious circle (1913), has emphasized what pernicious consequences it had for research, a conclusion which is also illustrated by our anecdote. But there is another point in Jaensch's explanation that deserves a special comment; the direct sensory experience is, according to him, too small to be noticed! And yet it is supposed to determine a judgment. This removes the last vestige of plausibility from this theory. We could at least understand what is meant by a judgment based on a perceived sensory experience. In the particular case under discussion the process would then be like this: the observer experiences a change in the thickness of the thread; he has learned, we do not know how, that often such a change is not a real change of the thread but merely due to a change of its position with regard to himself. Therefore he judges that in the present case too the thread has moved without changing its volume. I say that such a description would at least have a meaning, even though it must appear as a pure construction unsupported by facts which contain nothing of such an inferential judgment. But now the change of thickness is assumed to be unnoticed. Since I cannot judge about something I am not aware of, the term judgment must have a meaning different from the ordinary one; in fact it can have no definite meaning any more over and above the very general one: non-sensory process. But then it will not explain anything. For though we can understand how a judgment based upon a sensory experience may lead to a certain interpretation of this experience—we see smoke and we judge there must be a fire—we do not understand how a non-sensory process produces out of an unnoticed sensory process a noticed datum which has all the direct characteristics of a sensory process and is different from the non-noticed one.

Furthermore, the assumption of the non-noticed sensory experience is necessary only because of the constancy hypothesis which derives the looks of things from a universal point-to-point relation with the proximal stimulation. We have again the man on the tight rope and the pole. Without the constancy hypothesis we would not assume unnoticed experiences, and without unnoticed experiences we could not preserve the constancy hypothesis.

Why, you may ask, such a long discussion of so palpably bad a theory? My answer is that this theory has more importance than one would think. The fathers of our psychology incorporated it consciously into their systems, and the more systematic ones among them were at great pains to prove it (Stumpf, 1883). True enough it received its death blow in an article by Köhler (1913), but the passage which I have chosen for my discussion appeared seven years later, a sign of the tenacity of this way of thinking. I doubt whether at the present moment one would find a psychologist who would defend it explicitly, but that is not equivalent to saying that it has disappeared. The contrary is true. All applications of the interpretation theory contain it in some form or other. Therefore it will be advisable to eliminate it from our future discussion by disproving the interpretation theory with its distinction of original sensations and centrally modified perceptions. Our evidence will be experimental, for experiments have shown that the experience or interpretation theory explains in some cases too little, in others too much.

Special Refutation of the Interpretation Theory. It Explains Too Little. Let us return to the constancy of size. We saw that diminution of the retinal image instead of producing a shrinkage of the seen object may arouse the perception of its recession with conservation of its apparent size. If this effect is to be explained as a matter of perception and not of sensation, then the assumption must be that originally any diminution of the retinal image would produce a shrinkage of the seen object and that experience only can teach the organism that an object that seems to grow smaller need not really be shrinking. Or otherwise expressed: if of two objects the larger is so much further away from the animal that its retinal image is smaller, then, according to this view, originally the animal would see the larger as smaller and would only *learn* that it is bigger. We should then expect that it ought to be quite easy to find animals who would mistake large objects at a greater distance for small objects; we need only select animals which have not had much time to learn and have no great intelligence; for the acquisition of such knowledge as is implied in the theory is surely a high grade achievement. But this expectation has not been fulfilled. Thus human infants show a remarkable constancy of size. An infant of eleven months, e.g., who had been trained to select the larger of two boxes standing side by side, continued in her choice when the larger box had been removed to a distance at which its retinal image was less than $1/15$ of the area of the retinal image of the smaller, nearer box, which corresponds to a proportion of 4:1 in linear dimension in favour of the smaller box (Helene Frank, 1926). I doubt whether this result would have been foreseen by the defenders of the meaning theory. Once it has been obtained they are of course prepared to say that it proves the intelligence of the infant sufficiently great and the time he has lived sufficiently long to gain the necessary experience. Perhaps the faith of these psychologists will not be shaken either by Köhler's experiments published in 1915, which yielded the same results with chimpanzees. Although the species of animal used was sub-human the animals were older than the infants, and the greater time might compensate for the lower intelligence—an explanation tenable only as long as experiments with much younger chimpanzees have not disproved it. But such an experiment is hardly necessary, since Götz has proved that chicks only three months old show constancy of size in their behaviour. Since chicks choose spontaneously the larger grains first, it was not difficult to train them consistently to peck first at the larger of two simultaneously presented grains. For the purpose of the experiment it was necessary to go beyond this and train them to peck at the bigger grains *only,* a result that was safely though not quite so easily accomplished. Then in critical experiments the two grains were so deposited that the smaller was 15 cm. distant from the chick emerging from the door of an antechamber to the food box, whereas the bigger grain was at a greater distance. The chicks chose consistently the bigger one up to a distance of 73 cm. between the two grains; only at greater distances did they peck at the smaller one. Now objectively the proportion of the visible areas of the grains were 4:5, the proportion of their linear dimensions therefore 2:2.24; the fact that the chicks were so easily trained to select the bigger ones first, proves therefore a high degree of discrimination. But the results of the critical experiments are truly astounding, for in them the animals selected as the bigger a grain whose retinal image was but about ⅟₃₀ of the area of the smaller, corresponding to a linear proportion of 1:5.5! It may be mentioned that when, in control experiments, the larger grain was nearer, the smaller farther away, the chicks always selected the larger.

Such results are utterly incompatible with a meaning theory. Chicks must be geniuses if they can discover in the first three months of their lives that something that looks smaller is really bigger. Since we do not believe that they are endowed with such miraculous gifts we must conclude that they select the bigger because it looks bigger, even when, within wide but definite limits, its retinal image is smaller.

These experiments jointly, and the last one particularly, should prove beyond a reasonable doubt that the interpretation theory based on the constancy hypothesis is wrong. They have failed to prove the assumption of original sensations under conditions where everybody would have expected them who believed in this theory. And thereby they have positively proved that the relation between proximal stimulation and the look of things must be of a different nature, such that constancy of size follows as a natural and original result.

Our conviction is strengthened when we learn, without going into details, that so-called brightness-constancy has been proved to exist in infants, chimpanzees and chickens; i.e., trained to select the whiter or blacker of two objects, they will continue to do so when the blacker object reflects more light than the whiter. Suffice it to say that when Köhler published his results about the chimpanzees and chickens in 1915, they met with incredulity, and he had to make special new experiments (1917) in order to refute possible sources of error which had been thought out in order to preserve the old sensation-perception theory. We are apt to forget that certain experiments meant real theoretical decisions at the time they were made. Their results seem so evident today that we are apt to forget their theoretical implications.

The constancy phenomena, then, defy an explanation in terms of the sensation-perception or interpretation theory. But we might have used another experiment previously described to prove our point. I mean Révész's experiment which proved that chicks are subject to the Jastrow illusion just as we are. Here, experience which could account for meaning is excluded altogether. When the animals were presented with two equal segments one above the other for the first time, they had never seen this arrangement or a similar one before, and yet they selected the one which to us appears smaller, in accordance with their training to peck only from the smaller of two simultaneously presented figures. Here there is absolutely no reason why *sensory* equality should *mean* perceptual inequality.

Probably a diehard of the old school would give a different explanation for this case. He would say that the chicks failed to compare the areas and compared two proximate lines instead, viz., the lower line of the upper with the upper line of the lower figure. Since the former is shorter than the latter, they chose the upper figure. But this explanation, improbable as it is, does not explain other correct choices such as those between the figures represented in Fig. 5. For here, the upper contour of the lower and objectively smaller figure is still longer than the lower contour of the upper and larger one. In this case, then, the animals *cannot* have compared the length of lines but the size of areas. Why then should this training break down all of a sudden and give place to an entirely different behaviour when the animal is confronted with the critical figures? Surely, the animal did not know that these figures were critical!

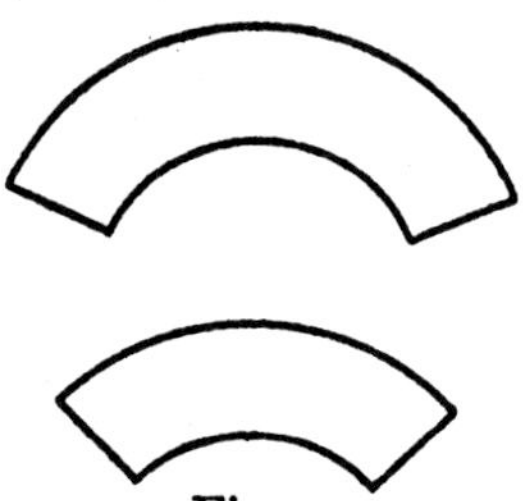

Fig. 5

In all the cases so far discussed, the interpretation theory explains too little. The observed facts cannot be derived from the theory even if it is burdened with a load of new hypotheses invented *ad hoc*.

It Explains Too Much. But we can choose the same kind of facts to prove that it explains too much. For constancy of size is not an all-or-none affair but a relative matter which can be measured quantitatively. A simple experimental procedure would be like this: an object of constant size is presented at a constant distance from the observer to serve as the standard. In a different direction and at different distances objects of varying sizes are presented, and the observer has to judge whether they seem larger or smaller than the standard or equal to it. The precaution to have standard and comparison objects in different directions, though it has not always been taken, is necessary because if the two objects are too close to each other in the visual field they will influence each other and so distort the picture of uninfluenced constancy. From these judgments one calculates for each distance the size of the object which is judged to be, on the ground of its looks, equal to the standard object. Although the first experiments of this kind were made in 1889 by Götz Martius, we have to the present day no complete knowledge of the quantitative relations, the range of distances over which the investigations have been carried out being rather limited. If we plot the distances at which the comparison objects are presented on the abscissa and the size of the objects which at these distances appear equal to the standard object on the ordinate, we obtain curves which under favourable circumstances, up to distances of as much as 16 m., are practically straight lines parallel to the abscissa. Somewhere after that distance the curves must rise at first slowly and then more quickly until finally they will approach the curve which illustrates the size of objects which at various distances project the same size of retinal image. To give a few figures: Martius found that a rod of 110 cm. at 6 m. distance appeared equal to a rod of 1 m. at 50 cm. distance, but there was no consistent change in the size of the stick between 4 and 10 m. The following table has been computed from Schur's experiments (1926), averaging the values of three observers. Both standard and comparison objects were circles projected by a lantern on screens, the rest of the room being dark, and only one circle being visible at a time, successive rather than simultaneous comparison being used.

TABLE 1

Distance in m.	*Straight ahead cm.*	*Above cm.*	*If constant angle*
4.80	18.3	19.7	21
6.00	20.2	23.4	26.25
7.20	22.4	27.7	31.5
16.00	32.4	41.6	70.

Standard circle diameter 17.5 cm. at 4 m. distance.

The figures in the second column show a slow though steady rise which would be much smaller if the room had not been totally dark, as test experiments at the distance of 16 m. have shown. The lower full line in the diagram of Fig. 6 shows how little the apparent size follows the retinal size, the upper full line representing the sizes which would produce a constant retinal image.

Our second diagram (Fig. 7) is taken from the extensive paper by Beyrl. These experiments were carried out in daylight and under

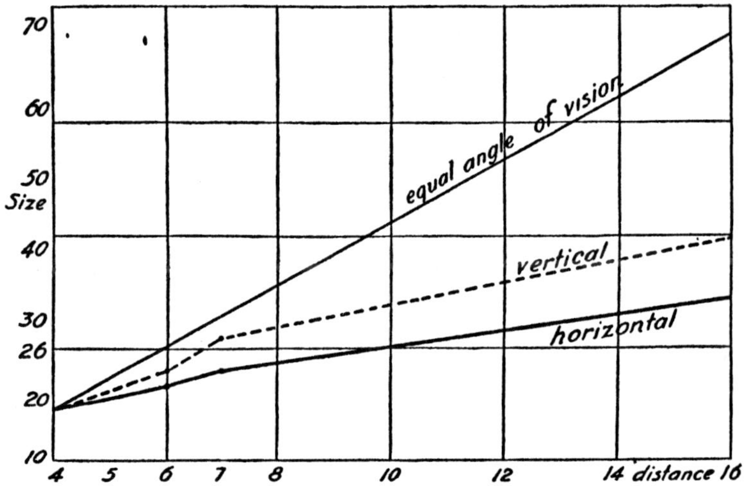

Fig. 6

conditions where the standard and comparison objects were close to each other in the field of vision. Two kinds of objects were used, cubic boxes 7 cm. high and circular disks of 10 cm. diameter; the subjects varied in age from two years to adulthood. Our curves refer to the results with boxes. The lowest is taken from the adults and shows absolute constancy from 1 to 11 m. The next shows the results of the two-year-olds, which still reveal an amazing degree of constancy if compared to the upper line which again represents the sizes of the boxes which would have produced a constant retinal image. But the curve for the two-year-old children does not do full justice to their achievements, as they were more strongly influenced by the close proximity of the two objects than the adults, as was proved by Mrs. Frank (1928). Beyrl's data contain another significant result, viz., the dependency of constancy upon the kind

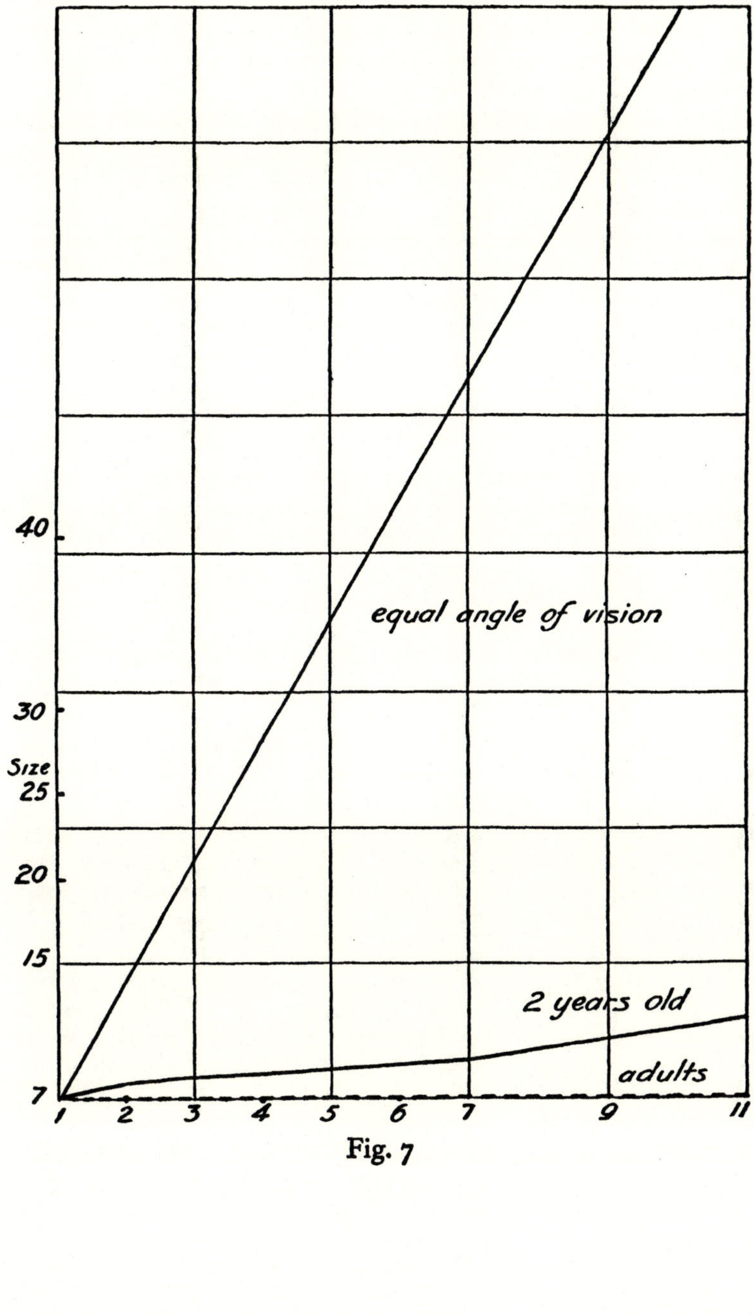

40
30
Size
25
20
15
7
1
2
3
4
5
6
7
9
11
equal angle of vision
2 years old
adults

Fig. 7

of object employed; it was more pronounced for the boxes than for the disks, the difference between disks and boxes being greater for the children than for the adults. I see no way of explaining this superiority of tri-dimensional objects over two-dimensional ones on the basis of the interpretation theory.

One more measurement before we continue our argument. Brown (1928) asked his subjects to equate an Aubert diaphragm at 1 m. distance with another one of 16 cm. diagonal at 6 m. The average diagonal chosen by four subjects was exactly 16 cm.

The new fact which must be introduced now is that the constancy curve is a function of the direction in which the objects are removed from us. In all the experiments so far related, this direction was the sagittal one, the two objects to be compared were in the same horizontal plane. Now, to a theory based on experience the direction should make no difference, whereas actually it does. The third column in Table 1 and the middle curve on Fig. 6 refer to cases where the two objects were at different distances *above* the observer. The constancy is distinctly worse, and that despite the fact that it was not possible to darken those high rooms in which these experiments were undertaken as thoroughly as the room in which the horizontal measurements were made. Since, as we have previously indicated, the constancy is greater in a lighter room than in a darker, the constancy in the upward direction was favoured relatively to that in the horizontal one; the true curve would rise at a steeper angle than the one in our diagram. Here, then, the meaning theory would predict too much.

If now the defender of this theory retorts that he cannot admit our imputation: naturally we should make less adequate judgments about vertical than about horizontal distances since we have so much less experience about them, I must mention some other facts: within the first four metres or so the difference between the vertical and the horizontal is very small and independent of the distance, while it increases very rapidly between 4½ and 14 m. and probably does not reach its maximum till somewhere beyond 70 m.

These data are taken from Schur's investigation of the moon illusion, for this illusion is but a special case of the general proposition that the constancy of size is a function of the direction. In our ordinary experiments we find that the smaller the retinal image of a distant object, which looks equally large as a near one, the better the constancy. Or, the constancy is the better, the greater the apparent size corresponding to a given retinal image. Now the retinal image of the moon is the same at the horizon and the zenith, therefore the fact that the moon looks larger on the first than on the second shows that, expressed in terms of constancy, the horizontal direction is favoured as against the vertical. In Schur's experiment artificial moons, usually circles projected by a lantern, were used, and it was found that between the distances of 3 and 33 m. the illusion increased from about 13% to about 50%, i.e., the circle straight ahead had to be decreased by 13% and 50% respectively in order to appear equal to the circle above. Of course in all these cases the angle of vision of the remote disk was kept constant at 1° 18′, corresponding to a diameter of 6.8 cm. at a distance of 3 m. And lastly, the illusion is a direct function of the elevation of the object, as appears from Table 2 summarizing experiments made at a distance of 4.80 m. with a circle 22 cm. in diameter, the figures indicating the average percentage of illusion of six subjects.

TABLE 2

(from Schur)

25°	35°	55°	70°	90°
0	1.1	5.4	8.2	15.2

That 25° of elevation yielded no illusion is due to the smallness of the distance. For at 25° of elevation the illusion was at different distances:

TABLE 3

(from Schur)

4.8 m.	5.6 m.	9 m.	16.5 m.
0	2.7	4.7	9.6

We find, then, very definite quantitative dependencies of the constancy upon the distance and angle of elevation. To account for these dependencies in terms of the interpretation theory would be equivalent to ascribing to any combination of *distance* and *elevation* which gives a lower degree of constancy than another a smaller number of experiences. This would impose upon the interpretation theory the task of proving that number of experiences at such combinations were exactly concomitant with the amount of constancy as illustrated in our tables—a task never undertaken and in my opinion more than unlikely to succeed.

We have adduced these various experiments which show the inadequacy of the interpretation theory, and thereby also of the constancy hypothesis, in order to give substance to our radical rejection of it. We might have taken a simpler course by showing directly how meaning does not account for constancy of size. I look at the bare hills that rise from the valley and on one of them I perceive a tiny object moving about. I know that it is a man: this tiny object in my field of vision *means* a man. Or I stand on the Chrysler Building in New York and look down into the street. I see hurrying ant-like creatures and tiny cars, but I do not doubt for a moment that these ants are men and women and the toys real automobiles and tramway cars. The meaning is as clear as it can be, but it does not affect in the slightest the size of the objects which carry this meaning. And that is what I had in mind when I said the interpretation theory explains too much: since the meaning is there, the interpretation theory implies that the sizes should be there also, but they are not!

We can summarize our discussion in this way: if "meaning" as employed by the interpretation theory has any assignable meaning, then it is neither the necessary nor the sufficient condition of discrepancies between the pattern of the proximal local stimuli and the perceived objects—not necessary because these discrepancies appear under conditions where we can exclude meaning, not sufficient because they fail to appear where meaning is clearly present. Thus the interpretation theory and the constancy hypothesis with which it is inextricably connected have to disappear from our system for good.

CONSTANCY HYPOTHESIS AND TRADITIONAL PHYSIOLOGICAL THEORY. LOCAL STIMULATION. In the beginning of this discussion we have claimed that the interpretation hypothesis is closely bound up with the traditional physiological hypotheses about brain processes. We can now make this claim more explicit. The interpretation hypothesis was demanded by the constancy hypothesis which we shall now formulate in a somewhat different manner. Recalling the arguments on which it was based we see that it correlated behavioural characteristics not with the total proximal stimulation but only with such parts of it as corresponded to the distant stimulus objects under discussion. In other words, it derived the characteristics of behavioural objects from the properties of *local* stimulations. In its consistent form the constancy hypothesis treats of sensations, each aroused by the local stimulation of one retinal point. Thus the constancy hypothesis maintains that the result of a local stimulation is constant, provided that the physiological condition of the stimulated receptor is constant (e.g., adaptation). This implies that all locally stimulated excitations run their course without regard to other excitations, in full accord with the traditional physiological hypotheses. When now we see that the constancy hypothesis has to be abandoned we know already what has to take its place, for we have demonstrated in our second chapter that physiological processes must be considered as processes in extension. But that means that no local stimulation can determine the corresponding excitation by itself, as the constancy hypothesis implied, but only in connection with the totality of stimulation. The form of the process in extension must depend upon the whole extended mosaic of stimulation, and all its parts become what they are as a result of the organization of the extended process. Only when we know the kind of organization in which a local process occurs can we predict what it will be like, and therefore the same change in local stimulation can produce different changes in the behavioural world according to the total organization which is produced by the total stimulation. Thus we can say: only when the total conditions are such that two visible objects will appear in *one* frontal vertical plane will the one whose retinal image is larger also look larger. The abandonment of the constancy hypothesis does not mean that we put in its place an arbitrary connection between proximal stimulation and the looks of things. All we intend to do is to replace laws of local correspondence, laws of machine effects, by laws of a much more comprehensive correspondence between the total perceptual field and the total stimulation, and we shall, in the search for these laws, find at least indications of some more specific constancies, though never one of the type expressed by the constancy hypothesis.

THE EXPERIENCE ERROR. There is one last aspect of the constancy hypothesis which must be specially emphasized, although we have discussed it already. Strictly speaking, the constancy hypothesis should refer to points only. In reality it has been used much less precisely; as a rule the local stimulus considered was the proximal stimulus coming from a definite distant stimulus object, the table, the thread in Wundt's experiments and so forth. But this looser use of the hypothesis implies a serious logical fallacy. Because the distant object is a thing by itself, the assumption is tacitly made that the retinal image corresponding to it is also. But as we have seen this assumption is by no means true. The stimuli at two adjacent points on the retina contain nothing qua stimuli that will make the two corresponding points in behavioural space belong to two different objects or to one and the same object. If an object in the behavioural field is a thing by itself, it must be an integrated whole separated or segregated from the rest of the field. The stimuli as a pure mosaic possess neither this integration nor this segregation. And therefore we saw that it is as misleading to speak of pictures of outside things being on our retinae as on a photographic plate. If we speak of pictures or images as stimuli we mistake the result of organization for the cause of organization, a mistake that is being committed again and again. Köhler has called it the experience error (1929). I have formulated the actual state of affairs by saying: we see, not stimuli—a phrase often used—but on account of, because of, stimuli (1926, p. 163).

THE TRUE ANSWER

The refutation of the two answers given explicitly or implicitly to our question has led us to the true answer. Things look as they do because of the field organization to which the proximal stimulus distribution gives rise. This answer is final and can be so only because it contains the whole problem of organization itself. Thus our answer, instead of closing a chapter in psychology, has opened one, a fact of which anyone who is acquainted with the psychological literature must be aware. It means that we have to study the laws of organization.

Process and Conditions. Now organization is a process and as such needs forces which set it going, but it also occurs in a medium and must therefore depend upon the properties of the medium. Let us clarify this distinction by a few simple examples from physics. Take, for instance, the sound field produced by a vibrating body, say a tuning fork. The motions of the prongs act as forces on the surrounding medium in which vibratory processes are set up. If the medium is entirely homogeneous, air of the same density and temperature all around, then the vibratory field will be quite symmetrical. If, on the other hand, the tuning fork is enclosed within a sound-proof box from which a single pipe starts, then the process will be confined to that pipe, and instead of spherical expansion we shall have virtually linear propagation. Again if the tuning fork is submerged in water, the process will travel much faster, and much faster still on an iron support on which the tuning fork may be fastened. The field may take on all sorts of shapes if the medium is inhomogeneous, varying in density either from point to point or at least in certain directions. No need to go into detail; the same force will produce different results according to the medium in which the process takes place.

The properties of the medium have three kinds of primary effects in this example by which they determine the final field organization: (1) an effect of constraining the process to a limited part of the field, (2) determining the velocity of propagation, (3) changing the process into another kind of process. The first effect is most clearly exemplified in a simple mechanical instance: a ball, if its support is removed, will fall straight to the ground following the vertical pull of the force of gravity. On the inclined plane, however, the same ball will roll down at an angle prescribed by the inclination of the support. Thus we see how the direction of a process produced by one and the same force may vary over a well-defined range. The second effect is of especial importance for organization of a field. If two processes are started in different parts, then their interdependence will depend upon the velocity with which each of them enters the sphere of the other. Since the medium between them may be such as to allow for all possible velocities, we see how the medium by this property alone can determine all degrees of interaction and thereby achieve an enormous variety of organizations. If the medium is totally impermeable, then these processes will never interfere with each other; the total organization will be the sum of the two part organizations. The last point is best illustrated by friction. The velocity of a ball running down an inclined plane depends on the roughness or smoothness of the plane and the ball. The rougher, the slower the motion of the ball will be, so that its kinetic energy at the end will be the smaller. Since, however, the potential energy at the beginning is quite independent of the nature of the plane, depending merely upon the absolute elevation of the starting point, some energy must have been lost; as we know, it has been turned into heat; directed motion has partly been transformed into undirected motion.

Applied to Psychophysical Processes. We have to apply these considerations to psychophysical organization, but in doing so we must remember that we are dealing with a special case, a case namely in which minimal energies give play to energies which are enormously larger. That this is true for all self-determined action is clear. The energies at work in my decision to climb the Matterhorn are minimal, but the energy expended in the achievement is well over 180,000 kgm. But the same is true of the receptor side of our behaviour. The energy of the light which falls on our retinae is not propagated to the brain as such, but liberates the energy stored in the nerves, and this energy liberates energy in other nerves and so forth.

How small energies can liberate and direct large ones is easy to understand: we need only think of ourselves driving a motor car. The slightest pressure on our accelerator increases the disposable energy and with it the actual forces that drive our car; an effortless small turn of the wheel changes its direction.

The organization which we are to study takes place between these nerve energies which are partly liberated by stimulation, partly by intra-organic processes, and which in their turn direct the much larger energies of our musculature. With these remarks in our minds let us apply the distinction of active forces and constraining conditions, and the more general one between the process and the conditions which determine it, to the psychophysical organization.

The Conditions of Psychophysical Processes. Let us first envisage the conditions. It is useful to distinguish between outer and inner, external and internal conditions, the first being those created on the sense surfaces by the proximal stimuli; the second being inherent in the nervous structure itself. Since there are receptor organs within the organism, in muscles and joints and the intestinal organs, outer and inner cannot mean outside and inside the organism, although in many cases, in the majority of those we shall discuss, that meaning will obtain as well. If we now scrutinize these conditions we see that all the outer conditions supply actual forces. What about the inner ones? Here we can distinguish between more or less permanent and momentary ones. The permanent ones are the structure of the nervous system as it has been inherited and as it has become through experience. As *structure* these conditions will be of the constraining and insulating sort; they will favour certain interdependencies rather than others, confine processes totally or preponderantly to certain parts of the system, co-determine the direction which the forces will take and so forth, although, as we shall see later (Chapter XI), this does not exhaust their function.

Among the momentary ones there are, first, freshness and fatigue. In order to form a conception of what these conditions are, I shall mention a few facts adduced by Sir Henry Head to support his concept of "vigilance." Referring to the work by Sir Charles Sherrington and his pupils, he writes:

"Suppose, for instance, that the spinal cord of a cat has been transected in the region of the medulla oblongata; twenty minutes later prick the hind paw with a pin and no general reflex results, but the toes make an opening movement. Gradually the response becomes more widespread, until the whole of the limb may be thrown into flexion, and the opposite one extended by a stimulus of the same nature and intensity. Not only has the motor response become brisker and more extensive, but the skin area from which it can be evoked has greatly increased. Pinching the superficial structures over any part of the limb may now cause flexion, accompanied by extension of the opposite extremity. The deep reflexes reappear rapidly and the character of the knee-jerk shows that the quadriceps has regained tone to a considerable extent. As the spinal preparation improves in excitability, even the scratch reflex may reappear. . . .

"When the spinal cord has reached this high condition of activity, the administration of chloroform causes rapid regression. Knee-jerk and ankle-jerk disappear, and finally the only reflex that can be evoked is a slight movement of the toes, elicited from the pad of the foot only. Pricking any other part of the limb no longer produces any effect." (1926, I, p. 482.) When the narcosis passes away, the reflexes regain their previous character. Quite similar are the symptoms in human beings whose spinal cord has been divided. At first all the muscles are flaccid and atonic and practically no reflex can be elicited. But with a young and healthy patient not only do numerous reflexes reappear, but the reaction assumes the nature of a "mass reflex." "The plantar reflex begins to assume a form characterized by an upward movement of the great toe. The field from which it can be evoked enlarges and finally, in successful cases, the spinal cord becomes so excitable that stimulation anywhere below the level of the lesion may be followed by a characteristic upward movement of the toes. But this now forms a small portion only of the reaction to superficial excitation; ankle, knee and hip are flexed and the foot is withdrawn from the stimulus applied to the sole. Not infrequently the abdominal wall is thrown into contraction, and every flexor muscle below the lesion may participate in an energetic, spasmodic movement. Stimulation of a small area on the foot has evoked a widespread response from the whole extent of the spinal cord below the lesion" (pp. 480, 481). "But if the patient develops fever . . . his condition may fall back to that found shortly after injury. . . . Even a gastro-intestinal disturbance, unaccompanied by fever, may produce the same signs of lowered activity" (pp. 481-482).

Two mutually inclusive interpretations are suggested by these and similar facts. The shock of an injury, narcosis, toxaemia, or other abnormal states, reduce the nervous activity far below the level which is attainable by the animal on the basis of its nervous structure. The fact that circumscribed reflexes take the place of mass reflexes suggests the possibility that the permeability of the nervous structure has been reduced so that the interdependence of its various parts has more or less diminished. Thus, what happens in one part may remain unconnected with what happens in another part. I find a good confirmation of this interpretation in the case of one of Head's patients "who had received a small wound in the left frontal region which injured the brain," and who "appeared to be in every way normal. In daily intercourse he behaved rationally and showed executive ability in the work of the ward, but he wrote a long letter asking detailed questions about his family, to his mother who had been dead for three years. He thought that there were two towns of Boulogne, one of which, on the homeward journey from the Front, lay near Newcastle; the other one in France was reached after you had crossed the sea" (pp. 493-494). This last observation particularly seems to show that the experience of passing through Boulogne, after the injury, occurred uninfluenced by the former experience of passing through that city on the way to the fighting lines.

And yet, this effect of reduced permeability can be only one side of the total effect. Head himself summarizes like this: "When vigilance is high, mind and body are poised in readiness to respond to any event, external or internal" (p. 496). That means that the energy at the disposal of the nervous system is variable, a conception which we shall find useful in later discussions.

We may now return to our concepts of freshness and fatigue as momentary inner conditions of psychophysical processes. Freshness might then be considered as a high, fatigue as a low, degree of vigilance, and therefore the interpretation which we have given to the different states of vigilance would apply to freshness and fatigue, which would represent smaller variations in the degree of vigilance than those on which Head has based his argument.

There is another momentary condition which, superficially at least, has some similarity with fatigue, but must be clearly distinguished from it. It may happen that a process results in the arousal of actual forces which impede and finally block its continuation. This condition, just as freshness and fatigue, may exert a decisive influence on perception as well as on action, but at this part of our exposition we cannot point out why we must assume it. We may remark, however, that it is not of the constraining kind, but contributes forces active in the production of processes. The same is true of other much more important inner conditions. All our needs, desires, attitudes, interests and attentions must also be considered as of this kind; the effect of these will be studied later.

What We Have Gained by Our Distinction of Process and Conditions. In our enumeration of the different conditions upon which psychophysical processes depend we have met with many familiar psychological concepts—like experience, attention, interest, fatigue, to name only some. What have we gained by calling them conditions? The critical and possibly sceptical reader will be inclined to think that this new term does not introduce a new meaning, and that therefore, inasmuch as we use the old terminology, we also use the traditional explanations. But a simple example will show that such an interpretation would be erroneous.

THE TRADITIONAL ASSIMILATION HYPOTHESIS. We choose the use made by traditional psychology of experience in the explanation of perception. Clearly the adherents of the constancy hypothesis could not and did not believe that the sum of sensations which according to their fundamental assumption constituted the result of any stimulation, was equivalent to the actually perceived things. We know that they did not, and that they attributed this difference to experience, the difference between sensation and perception often being defined as that between sensations uninfluenced, and sensations affected, by experience. Besides the interpretation hypothesis which we have already discussed, traditional psychology contained still another theory to explain the influence of experience on perception, the assimilation hypothesis of Wundt. This hypothesis, instead of explaining certain features of perception as illusions of judgment, acknowledges in many cases the truly perceptive, nonjudgmental character of the objects in our behavioural environment (however, it was never held to be incompatible with the interpretation hypothesis, so that both were included in the system, the different cases being distributed between them). The goal of the assimilation hypothesis determines its content. Since the senses, according to the constancy hypothesis, furnish only a sum of sensations, and since we find objects in our perceptual world, experience must have added something to that sum of sensations. But since we know only the actually perceived object the assimilation theory has to go further: not only must the group of sensations aroused by the present stimulation reproduce images of previous experiences, but these latter must fuse with the former into a unity in which many properties of the former are lost, and in which the two kinds of elements, sensory and imaginal, are indistinguishable. No part of this hypothesis has been verified; three of its constituents are by the very nature of the hypothesis unverifiable, viz., the primarily aroused sensations, the reproduced images and the process of fusion.

A fourth point seems to have escaped the notice of the assimilation theorists, although it seems to me to present an unconquerable difficulty. I will introduce it by starting with a very simple example. We perceive a snake in the grass; approaching cautiously we discover that it is no snake at all but a bent twig moved by the wind.

The assimilation hypothesis would explain the case like this: the stimuli coming from that stick were sufficiently similar to those which on former occasions had fallen on our retinae when they came from a snake. Therefore our present sensations were sufficiently similar to reproduce the image of a snake which we had formerly seen, and this image would inextricably fuse with those sensations so as to make us perceive a snake now. This seems very plausible, and yet it begs the question; for the stimuli coming from a snake should, according to the constancy hypothesis, produce nothing but a medley of sensations, of colour, position, and possibly movement. But the problem, we thought, was, How have these sensations become integrated into the perceptual snake? Of this problem we get no solution, not for the snake, not for the stick, and not for any other of the myriad objects in our behavioural environment. And I do not see how we can get such a solution. Perhaps the reader will grant that a solution in purely visual terms would be impossible, but he may object that we have overlooked our other senses; we may have touched the snake and heard its hiss. But even if we suppose that such is the case, what does it help? According to the constancy hypothesis, touching the snake would supply a number of touch sensations, but a snake as we know it is as little a number of visual plus a number of touch sensations as it is a number of visual sensations alone. In short, the theory presupposes what it is to explain, by assuming that the perceptions of previous stimulations are reproduced; for how did these previous perceptions arise?

A fifth and integral point, though verifiable, has not been verified; recent experiments have, to the contrary, shown it to be false. I mean the part, passed over rather hastily by the proponents of this theory, which deals with the reproduction of images. The assumption that stimuli which have produced a certain effect a number of times will under all conditions tend to reproduce the same effect is spurious, as we shall see later.

The assimilation hypothesis thus becomes untenable. Its main aspect was the addition of two kinds of mental elements, sensations and images. Experience was not only a condition but the source of special elements which were added to other elements supplied by the sense organs. How different the whole problem looks when we consider experience as an inner condition. Without experience, the nervous system has a certain constitution, with experience it has a different one. Consequently we can no longer expect that the same forces, the same proximal stimuli, will produce the same process in it. At one stroke we get rid of all the unverifiable parts of the assimilation hypothesis, the original sensations, the added imagery, and the process of fusion. At the same time we have freed ourselves from the last two difficulties since we do not assume that a mosaic of proximal stimulation produces a mosaic of sensations. And finally we have the advantage that we can now define the problem of experience in perception in clear terms. Thus it does make a difference to call experience an inner condition of a process, and what is true of experience is equally true of our other factors.

SUMMARY

Let us pause to see what we have achieved. We have stated our problem and have refuted two solutions of it which severally and jointly have had a firm hold on traditional psychology and have obstructed its progress. In the process of clearing the way we have eliminated a whole network of hypotheses, the constancy hypothesis, the hypothesis of non-noticed but effective sensations, the interpretation and the assimilation hypothesis, and we have shown up the experience error. We have formulated the true solution in general terms and have introduced our conceptual equipment for its concrete elaboration. It has become apparent that the true solution, without being in the least vitalistic, cannot be a machine theory based on a sum of independent sensory processes, but must be a thoroughly dynamic theory in which the processes organize themselves under the prevailing dynamic and constraining conditions.

CHAPTER IV

THE ENVIRONMENTAL FIELD

Visual Organization and its Laws

Organization and the Properties of the Behavioural World. General Characteristics of Stationary Processes. Law of Prägnanz. Simplest Condition: Stimulus Distribution Completely Homogeneous. Some Fundamental Principles of Space Organization. Primitive Perception Tri-dimensional. Inhomogeneous Stimulation. Simple Case of Only One Inhomogeneity in Otherwise Homogeneous Field. The Two Problems Involved in This Case. (1) Unit Formation. (2) The Problem of Shape. Points and Lines as Stimuli. Points. Factor of Closure. Factor of Good Shape. Good Continuation. Tri-dimensional Organization of Line Patterns. Consequences for the Theory of Space Perception. Nativism and Empiricism. Organization Theory of Tri-dimensional Space. Discontinuous Inhomogeneities of Stimulation, Lines, and Points. Proximity. Proximity and Equality. Closure. Organization and the Law of Prägnanz. Minimum and Maximum Simplicity. Organization from the Points of View of Quantity, Order, and Significance

ORGANIZATION AND THE PROPERTIES OF THE BEHAVIOURAL WORLD

The looks of things are determined by the field organization to which the proximal stimulus distribution gives rise. To this field organization we must, then, apply our research. What kind of organization is responsible for unit formation? Why is behavioural space three-dimensional? How does organization produce constancy of colour or size? These are a few of the questions we shall have to deal with. Historically these questions have been attacked in a random order, each experimenter choosing a field where he happened to see a real problem and a method of its solution. Needless to say, we have as yet no answer to many such questions and no complete one to any. But we possess now a sufficient stock of experimental evidence to warrant a more systematic procedure in our exposition. We shall select our material in such a way as to throw light on the chief problems in their interdependence.

GENERAL CHARACTERISTICS OF STATIONARY PROCESSES

Such a systematic attempt will succeed the better the more general our starting point. And therefore, before taking up any experimental evidence, we shall ask the question whether we do not know of any properties of organization which belong to all organizations. Since psychological organization is our problem, we cannot take our answer from psychological facts, psychological organization being the unknown quantity in our equation. And that means we must turn to physics. Do physical organizations, spontaneous distributions of process, show general characteristics of the kind we are looking for?

Maximum-Minimum Properties. When we turn to stationary distributions, i.e., such as no longer change in time, we do indeed find such characteristics. Stationary processes have certain maximum-minimum properties, i.e., a given parameter of these processes has not just any magnitude but the smallest or the greatest possible. A few examples may make this clear: if we have a number of different circuits between the poles of the same electric battery the currents will distribute themselves so as to produce a minimum amount of energy within the system. To take the simplest case of two part circuits only. Then Kirchhoff's law states that $\frac{i_1}{i_2} = \frac{r_2}{r_1}$, where i_1 and i_2 stand for the intensities of the two part currents, and r_1 and r_2 for the corresponding resistances in the part circuits. Now it is quite easy to show mathematically that these currents, i_1 in the circuit with resistance r_1, and i_2 in circuit with resistance r_2, produce less heat than if i_1 were greater or smaller, and consequently i_2 smaller or greater, than is demanded by Kirchhoff's law. (The sum of the two intensities must be constant, since the total intensity of the circuit depends only upon its electromotive force and its total resistance.)

Another example is the soap bubble. Why has it the shape of a sphere? Of all solids the sphere is that whose surface is smallest for a given volume, or whose volume is largest for a given surface. The soap bubble, therefore, solves a maximum-minimum problem, nor is it difficult to see why. The soap particles attract each other, they tend to take up as little space as possible, but the pressure of the air inside forces them to stay on the outside, forming the surface membrane of this air volume. So they must form as thick a surface lamella as they can, and the smaller the surface the greater can its thickness be, if the amount of mass is constant. At the same time potential energy of this membrane will be as small as possible.

Maxima and minima are of course always relative with regard to the prevailing conditions; the absolute maximum is infinite, the minimum zero. Thus in our last example the conditions were the amount of mass, i.e., the amount of soap solution, and the air volume. In the first example it is the total current intensity produced by the electromotive force with the total resistance.

Now we can understand a general proposition about all stationary distributions which I quote from Köhler: "In all processes which terminate in time-independent states the distribution shifts towards a minimum of energy" (1920, p. 250). Or the final time-independent distribution contains a minimum of energy capable of doing work. This proposition applies to the total system, and under certain conditions, to be discussed later, it demands that a part of the total system absorb a maximum of energy. (See Köhler, 1924, p. 533.)

Thus in physics we have found a characteristic of stationary distributions such as we have looked for. If nervous processes are physical processes, they must fulfil this condition whenever they are stationary or quasi-stationary; we cannot expect to find in our nervous system any processes which are entirely independent of time because the conditions never remain absolutely constant. However, within short periods of time this change of conditions will, in a great many cases, occur so slowly that the distributions are for all practical purposes stationary within such short periods; such processes are called quasi-stationary, and they can be treated as stationary ones. Thus we have found a general characteristic of all stationary nervous organizations: we know that they must possess certain properties merely because they are stationary organizations. This is in itself a great gain, but it does not give us any concrete insight into the actual nature of psychological organizations, since we have no means of measuring the energy of these processes. We might say, sacrificing indeed a great deal of the precision of the physical proposition, that in psychological organization either as much or as little will happen as the prevailing conditions permit.

Qualitative Aspects. But we can go one step further. Our statement is so far quantitative, but our behavioural environment reveals no such quantification; it is purely qualitative. How, then, can we bridge the gap between quantity and quality? We have answered this question in our first chapter: quantity and quality are not two different properties of events but only different aspects of one and the same event. Therefore we might ask: What is the qualitative aspect of stationary physical processes which satisfy the quantitative minimum-maximum condition? No perfectly satisfactory answer is possible; we have no general qualitative concept applicable in all cases. But there are enough special cases in which the qualitative aspect of stationary process becomes manifest (Köhler, 1920, pp. 257 f.). Physicists like Curie and Mach have been struck by the symmetry and regularity of many stable forms in nature, like crystals. Thus Curie formulated the proposition that "it is necessary for the occurrence of any physical process that certain elements of symmetry do not exist"; Köhler formulated the converse of this proposition that a system left to itself will, in its approach to a time-independent state, lose asymmetries and become more regular.

The terms of this proposition are clear enough as long as the conditions under which the process occurs are simple. What will happen when the conditions are less simple? A very instructive example is presented by drops of water. Suspended in a medium of equal density, they will be perfect spheres; lying on a solid support to which they have little adhesion the spherical shape is slightly flattened; falling through air they assume a new shape which, though less simple than the sphere, is still perfectly symmetrical and fulfils the condition that it offers the least resistance to the air through which it is passing, so that it can fall as fast as possible; in other words, the falling drop of water is perfectly streamlined; its symmetry corresponds again to a maximum-minimum principle. We see in this example how the shape of a stationary state becomes less and less simple the more complex the conditions under which the equilibrium is established. Therefore, when the medium is complex, varying in its properties from point to point in a complex manner, then the ensuing stationary distribution will no longer be regular or symmetrical in the ordinary sense, and we possess no concept to describe the qualitative aspect of such distributions. The concept would have to be such that ordinary symmetry would be a special case, realized under particularly simple conditions.

Although we have not gained very much, we have gained something. For we can at least select psychological organizations which occur under simple conditions and can then predict that they must possess regularity, symmetry, simplicity. This conclusion is based on the principle of isomorphism,[1] according to which characteristic aspects of the physiological processes are also characteristic aspects of the corresponding conscious processes.

Furthermore we must remember that there exist always two possibilities, corresponding to the minimum and the maximum; either as little or as much as possible will happen. Therefore our term simplicity or regularity will have a different meaning according to these two possibilities. A simplicity of a minimum event will be different from a simplicity of a maximum event. Which of these two will be realized in each concrete case must depend upon the general conditions of the process.

[1] Discussed at the end of the second chapter.

Law of Prägnanz. Thus we have gained a general, though admittedly somewhat vague, principle to guide us in our investigation of psychophysical organization. In the process of our research we shall make this principle more concrete; we shall learn more about simplicity and regularity itself. The principle was introduced by Wertheimer, who called it the *Law of Prägnanz.* It can briefly be formulated like this: psychological organization will always be as "good" as the prevailing conditions allow. In this definition the term "good" is undefined. It embraces such properties as regularity, symmetry, simplicity and others which we shall meet in the course of our discussion.

SIMPLEST CONDITION: STIMULUS DISTRIBUTION COMPLETELY HOMOGENEOUS

And now let us begin our study of concrete psychological organization. We begin with the simplest possible case, a case which has only of late received the attention of the psychologist. This simplest case is realized when the distribution of forces on the sense surface is absolutely homogeneous.

Why This Is the Simplest Condition. The Different Traditional View. To see this as the simplest case, natural though it may seem, required the radical change in our answer to the question, Why things look as they do, which we have discussed in the preceding chapter. As long as one expected the answer to our question from an investigation of the effects of local stimulation another case seemed the simplest, viz., that in which only one point of the retina was stimulated. Experimental evidence, which we shall discuss later, has shown the falsity of this assumption. The same conclusion follows directly from our third answer. If perception is organization, i.e., a psychophysical process in extension depending upon the total stimulus distribution, then homogeneity of this distribution must be the simplest case and not the traditional one which contains a discontinuity. We can express the two kinds of stimulation mathematically, by plotting the intensity of stimulation as a function of the place on the retina. Since the retina is a surface, each of its points can be represented within a plane with reference to a Cartesian system of co-ordinates. The intensity at each point would then have to be represented as a point above this plane, and all intensities would lie on a surface whose shape would depend on the distribution of the intensities. Now if the intensity is homogeneous, this surface would be a plane parallel to the x y plane, the higher above it, the greater the intensity, and at the distance nought, coinciding with it, if the intensity is nought. If, on the contrary, we have only one point of the retina stimulated, then our surface would no longer be a plane as a whole. The greatest part of it would still coincide with the x y plane, but at one point it would rise abruptly to the intensity with which this point is stimulated only to drop back into the x y plane at the next point. If we do not want to use perspective we can only reproduce a two-dimensional cross-section of these distributions. Then we can plot on the abscissa all the points along one line of the retina, say, the retinal horizon (roughly speaking a horizontal line passing through the centre of vision when the eye is in a normal position looking straight ahead), and the intensity on the ordinate. Then Fig. 8*a* represents a homogeneous distribution of the intensity *i*, and *b* the distribution if one point only is stimulated. In *a* the upper line represents the distribution, in *b* the whole graph, since the *x* and *i* lines coincide except at the one point. The first corresponds to a perfectly flat plane, the second to a plane with a pole projecting from it. What, then, shall we see when our retinae are stimulated by neutral light according to the first figure?

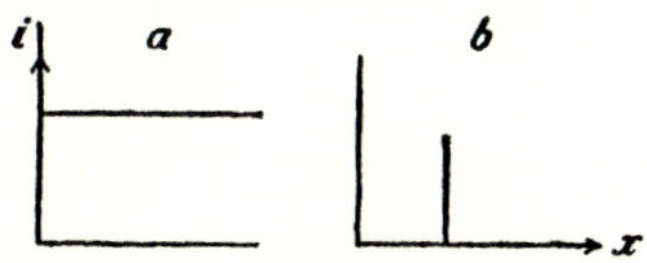

Fig. 8

Homogeneous Distribution of Neutral Light. I had to modify the general question by the new condition that the light be neutral, because the only experiments which have been made with such stimulus distributions have used neutral light. We shall give later on a hypothetical treatment of the case in which the light is not neutral.

THE DIFFERENT DISTANT STIMULI WHICH PRODUCE SUCH HOMOGENEOUS STIMULATION. The answer to our question is quite simple: under these conditions the observer will "feel himself swimming in a mist of light which becomes more condensed at an indefinite distance" (Metzger, 1930, p. 13). Let us consider how we can produce such uniform distribution of intensity over the entire area of our retinae; in other words, what distant stimuli we must use in order to obtain homogeneous proximal stimulation. Of course we might put our subject in the midst of an actual fog which would be perfectly evenly illuminated, and in that case his behavioural field would be a fairly good representation of the geographical one; the mist seen would correspond to the real fog. Even so, the increasing condensation would be a feature belonging to the behavioural, and not to the real, fog. But we can produce the same proximal stimulation by quite different means. Any surface in front of the observer, provided each of its points sends the same amount of light into his eyes, will fulfil our condition. And therefore it cannot make any difference to the observer whether he is in front of a plane vertical wall or in the center of a hemisphere or in an actual fog; he will always see space-filling fog and not a plane. Furthermore it cannot make any difference what the albedo of the surface is, provided that the light reflected from it remains constant. The albedo is the coefficient of reflection, the amount of light reflected from a unit area divided by the amount of light it receives; and the amount of reflected light is the product of the light falling onto the unit area and the albedo. If L stands for the albedo, i for the intensity of the reflected light, and I for the intensity of the light falling into the unit area, $L = \frac{i}{I}$, and $i = IL$. Since no surface reflects all the light that falls on it, L is always < 1. i remains constant if L changes in inverse ratio with I. $i = LI = (Lp)\frac{I}{p}$, where p means any positive number.

Whiteness Constancy Under These Conditions. Therefore under conditions of absolutely homogeneous stimulation the appearance of the fog can only depend on i and must be the same if i is constant, quite independent of L. Otherwise expressed, two surfaces, one ten times as bright as the other but receiving only 1/10 of its light, must produce exactly the same perception. And that means that there can be no constancy of whiteness under these conditions, for constancy means that, apparently, the actual appearance is a function of the albedo; under normal conditions a black surface in full light reflecting as much light as a white surface in shadow does not look equally bright, a point which we have discussed in the last chapter.

Whiteness and Insistency. The negative statement that with totally homogeneous stimulation no constancy can occur involves the positive proposition that all constancy presupposes inhomogeneity of stimulation and gives us the first clue for the explanation of constancy. On the other hand, this negative statement leaves us with a problem; if two homogeneous surfaces arouse the same perception when with albedos L_1 and L_2 they receive the amounts of light I_1 and I_2 in such a way that $L_1I_1 = L_2I_2$, what will this perception be like? Will they look white or grey or black? We could answer this question only if we knew the dependence of the appearance on *i*, the intensity of the reflected light. But this function is still more or less unknown. What we can say with certainty is that the dependent variable of this function, the appearance of the mist, has several aspects which are to be treated as separate variables. We must distinguish at least its "whiteness" and its "impressiveness" or "insistency."[2] By the former we mean its similarity to a member of the black-white series, by the latter a characteristic which does not concern the behavioural object alone but also the Ego, a relation between the Ego and the behavioural object (Metzger, p. 20). As early as 1896, G. E. Müller defined "impressiveness" by "the power with which sensory impressions attract our attention" (p. 20 f.). If this is meant as a direct description, it seems equivalent to the statement in our text which we have taken from Metzger, who also quotes Müller, and Titchener's three terms bring out the object-Ego relation still more clearly. We shall discuss characteristics similar to insistency when we introduce the Ego, but it is significant that we cannot even begin our discussion of the environmental field without being forced to refer to the Ego. It is a characteristic of the environmental field that it is the field of an Ego, an Ego which is directly influenced by this field.

EFFECT OF INTENSITY OF HOMOGENEOUS STIMULATION. However, we must return to our problem, the relation between the appearance of the fog and the intensity of the stimulation. Since our knowledge is still very incomplete, we disregard the effect which adaptation, in the ordinary sense of dark- and light-adaptation, has on this relation. Then we can conclude from Metzger's results under conditions of absolutely homogeneous stimulation that *insistency* varies much more with intensity than whiteness. Metzger gives the following description of the events in the field when, starting from absolute darkness, it is gradually lightened. "At first it grows lighter to the observer in the sense of less heavy, not in the sense of less dark; he feels the disappearance of a pressure, as though he could again breathe freely; some see at the same time a clear expansion of space. Only then it grows rather quickly lighter in the sense of less dark, at the same time the space-filling colour recedes" (p. 16). As he was not able to produce a perfectly homogeneous stimulus distribution at higher intensities, we cannot determine the dependency of the depth of seen foggy space on the intensity of stimulation, but we see that the onset of stimulation and its first intensification produces a marked expansion. Again

[2] The latter is Titchener's translation of the German "Eindringlichkeit"; two other terms which he proposes are "self-assertiveness" and "aggressiveness."

this expansion is Ego-related; note the relief from pressure which is the very first result of stimulation.

METZGER'S APPARATUS. It is now time to describe briefly Metzger's apparatus. The observer sat in front of a carefully whitewashed wall of 4 x 4 m. sq. area, at a distance of 1.25 m. Had he been seated directly opposite its centre, this wall would not have filled the entire field of vision which corresponds to a visual angle of about 200° in the horizontal and 125° in the vertical, whereas the side of the wall would have filled only an angle of 116°. Since the observer sat on a chair which stood on the floor of the room, but fixated a point about 1.50 m. above the floor, the dimensions of the wall were not sufficient in either direction; therefore wings bent towards the observer had to be added on all four sides, care being taken that the inhomogeneities thereby introduced were as small as possible. Actually the edges where wall and wings joined were either invisible from the start or became so after a very short while. The illumination was supplied by a projection lantern with a specially constructed set of lenses.

Stimulation with Microstructure. The results so far reported were gained with this apparatus, as long as the intensity of illumination remained below a certain level. If, however, the illumination was increased, something new happened. The fog became condensed into a regularly curved surface which surrounded the observer on all sides; its appearance was filmy like the sky, not surfacy, and similar to the sky it was slightly flat in the centre. The apparent distance of the furthest part of this boundary is approximately the same as that of the wall when seen under normal conditions. If the illumination is further increased the surface straightens out into a plane whose apparent distance may increase very definitely beyond the real one.

Why this change from space-filling fog to a plane surface? Very ingenious experiments of Metzger's, too complicated to be described here, give the answer. The cause lies in the "grain" of the whitewashed surface, or in terms of proximal stimulation, in the fact that at higher intensities the stimulus distribution was no longer perfectly homogeneous, but possessed what we will call a microstructure. Now the microstructure of the distant stimulus object is, of course, independent of the illumination; why, then, does the proximal microstructure depend upon it? The answer is to be found in accommodation. The inhomogeneity due to microstructure is so small that it disappears if the eyes are not perfectly focussed, and as long as the illumination is low, accommodation is no longer perfect—a point to which we shall return a little later. For the moment we accept the fact that a *surface* is seen only when the proximal stimulation is no longer quite homogeneous, and that microstructure is a sufficient inhomogeneity to produce this effect.

Some Fundamental Principles of Space Organization. (1) Primitive Perception Tri-dimensional. These facts reveal a number of fundamental principles of psychophysical organization. (1) Under the simplest possible conditions of stimulation our perception is three-dimensional; we see space filled with neutral colour stretching into a more or less indeterminate distance, which may vary with the intensity of the stimulation, although this point is not yet clearly settled.

This very simple fact does away with a number of answers to the question why we see a three-dimensional space, although our retinae are two-dimensional only. Berkeley, as a matter of fact, gave what he considered conclusive proof that we could not possibly *see* depth and that therefore our perception of depth could not be sensory. "It is, I think, agreed by all that Distance, of itself and immediately, cannot be seen. For distance being a line directed endwise to the eye, it projects only one point in the fund of the eye, which point remains invariably the same, whether the distance be longer or shorter" (p. 162).

Two interdependent false assumptions are necessary to make this argument conclusive. In the first place, it contains the constancy hypothesis in assuming that we can investigate the whole of perceptual space by examining its individual points separately one by one. Space is not treated as process in extension, but as a sum of independent local processes. In the second place the argument correlates the dimensions of the stimulus distribution with those of the effects of stimulation. The retina being two-dimensional, seen space must be two-dimensional also. But the retina is the boundary surface of the tri-dimensional optical sector of the brain, and the forces set up in this boundary surface determine a process extended over the whole tri-dimensional sector. Berkeley's argument proves only that under certain conditions two points which are objectively at different distances may appear at the same distance, but it does not prove that this distance must be zero, since it contains no indication whatever about the distance at which the two objects must appear (cf. Koffka, 1930).

A fallacy similar to the one of Berkeley's argument has been committed in other fields of sense psychology also. The argument has frequently been put forward that if a given stimulus modality had a certain number of dimensions in which it could vary independently, then the corresponding behavioural data should have the same number of dimensions and no more. Thus, to our statement about the double effect of intensity of light, whiteness and insistency, one might have objected that to one stimulus variable there could correspond only one perceptual variable, although, as far as I know, the argument has not been applied to this particular case. But this argument has been used in acoustics where one concluded from the double variability of pure sinusoidal waves, frequency and amplitude, that the corresponding auditory effects, the pure tones, could also have only the two attributes. The fallacy of this argument is obvious. If an electric current is sent through an electrolyte, the electrolyte is decomposed and heat is generated, both effects depending directly upon the intensity of the current. There is in other words no logical connection between the dimensions of the cause and the dimensions of the effect (Köhler, 1923 b, p. 422). And yet, both in space perception and in acoustics, this false assumption has decisively influenced experimentation and theorizing. No more need be said about it after we have eliminated it once and for all from our principles of explanation.

Primitive Tri-dimensional Space not Articulated. Let us return to three-dimensional space. In its most primitive form it appears almost homogeneous; not quite, since the density of the fog increases with distance. But apart from that, the whole visible space volume is filled with the same material, grey fogginess. How different is our space under normal conditions, and even in Metzger's experiments with stronger illumination! There one sees a white wall at a certain distance, the whiteness being restricted to that plane surface, the space between observer and wall not appearing white but simply transparent as "pure space." Thus we see that primitive space lacks that articulation which normal space possesses. We see at the same time that articulation of the proximal stimuli, mere microstructure, may produce a much richer articulation of the perceptual field, empty space terminated by a coloured surface.[8] Since articulation requires inhomogeneity of stimulation, i.e., special forces which are responsible for the articulation, we must further conclude that homogeneous tri-dimensionality, the fog, is a simple effect, the simplest of which our sense of sight is capable. And we are tempted to say that absolutely homogeneous stimulation causes a minimum

[8] It is very convenient to use the word "colour" so as to refer to neutral colours as well as to the proper or chromatic ones. Where no misunderstanding is possible, and where this usage helps to make the text simpler, it will from now on be adhered to.

event in the nervous system; as little will happen under these conditions as is possible.

(2) A Surface the Product of Strong Forces of Organization. To see a surface is, according to the preceding discussion, the effect of a higher degree of organization, presupposing special forces. That forces presuppose inhomogeneities is a truism. Nothing will happen within a system in which all parameters have constant values. How, more specifically, inhomogeneous stimulation produces forces in the physiological field has been shown by Köhler (1920), a demonstration which requires some physico-chemical detail and must, therefore, be omitted here.

These forces, due to the microstructure of the proximal stimulation, produce the organization of empty space and bounding plane surface; i.e., the colour, which before was dispersed over the whole space, becomes concentrated on a surface where it is held by real forces, disappearing from the rest of the space. It seems the simplest thing in the world to see a plane surface; we know nothing of the forces which bring it into existence, and yet this simple perception is a highly dynamic affair which changes at once if the forces which maintain it are interfered with. It is important to emphasize this point, since the traditional treatment of space perception, even by the men who have made the most valuable contributions to our knowledge, is fundamentally undynamic, i.e., purely geometrical, each point having its own "local sign," while the appearance of a surface is held equivalent to the sum of specially distributed local signs.

WEAKENING OF THE FORCES THROUGH BRAIN LESIONS. Interference with the forces which produce the plane surface changes its appearance. We have seen what happens when the forces are lost through a loss of the inhomogeneity of the stimulation. But we can interfere with the forces in yet another manner. The actual psychophysical process depends, as we have seen, on the external and the internal conditions. Let us keep the external ones constant and change the internal ones; let us interfere with the brain of our observers. Of course we shall not do it intentionally just to satisfy our scientific curiosity. But accidental injuries, of which the war produced a horrifying number, will serve our purpose. It can be said without exaggeration that all brain injuries affect the organization of the psychophysical processes, but the symptomatic manifestations of such effects will depend upon the place and the amount of the lesion (Head, 1926, Goldstein, 1927). Since with human beings we cannot make systematic extirpation experiments, we must study the cases which chance delivers into our hands. Now it has happened that Gelb (1920) found two patients whose organization was disturbed in the very aspect which interests us now. They could not see any real surfaces at all, i.e., the colour processes which occurred in their psychophysical field were never concentrated in one plane but always possessed a certain thickness which varied inversely with the brightness of the distant stimulus. Thus if a black surface appeared as a layer of black 15 cm. thick, a white surface would be seen as a layer of 2-3 cm. thickness only. A black circle on a white background would therefore not appear in the plane of the white; it would project from it towards the observer and away from him. Moreover it would appear larger than for us; the patients, if asked to point to the lateral boundaries of the circle, would point a few millimetres outside its rim. Therefore the forces which make and shape the figure are weaker in all directions, not in the third dimension only. That the spread is so much greater in the third than in the first two dimensions is, of course, due to the fact that the white colour prevents the black from spreading far in radial directions, whereas it does not exert a similar influence in the third dimension.

(3) Different Stages of Organization. To return to Metzger's experiments: Between the two stages of a fog-filled space and the appearance of a vertical plane lies a stage in which all the colour is condensed on one surface, which, however, is not a plane but a hollow *bowl* which surrounds the observer on all sides. In agreement with the preceding argument we must conclude that such a curved surface is easier to produce than a plane, that it corresponds to weaker forces than the latter. In accordance with this interpretation is the further fact that this bowl, if the observer remains sufficiently long in it, begins to dissolve into fog (which, however, does not spread to the observer but leaves a clear transparent layer in front of him), for continued exposure to one and the same stimulation reduces the forces exerted by the stimulation. Thus we have the following series of organization produced by stimulations which imply an increasing strength of the effective forces: (1) Colour equally distributed over a certain visible volume. This effect has not been reported; whether it is realizable or not must be determined by further experimentation. (2) Colour distributed over the whole of a certain visible volume, but becoming denser with increasing distance from the observer. (3) Colour confined to the further end of the visible volume where it forms a bowl-shaped fog. (4) Colour condensed on a filmy surface which surrounds the observer like a bowl. (5) Colour condensed in a vertical frontal parallel plane with true surface character (as opposed to filminess). Nos. (3) to (5) presuppose inhomogeneities of stimulation, microstructure; (2) and possibly (1) occurs when the stimulation is really homogeneous.

(4) The Forces that Produce and Maintain Behavioural Space. From the three preceding points we conclude: all phenomenal space is the product of actually effective forces; phenomenal space may be likened to a balloon whose size depends upon the gas pressure within, and not to a metal sphere. According to this view, which is held by Metzger, space becomes as small as possible, particularly in the third dimension. This view is based on the fact that in Metzger's experiments, space expanded with increased illumination, and that space produced by completely homogeneous stimulation possesses a very small depth as compared with ordinary space.

Two aspects of this hypothesis have to be distinguished, a general and a special one. The general is the interpretation of visual space as a dynamic event instead of a geometrical pattern, and this aspect will be whole-heartedly accepted into our system. The special aspect assumes that *expansion* of space requires force, and that space will therefore be the smaller the weaker the forces are which support it at a given moment. This part of the hypothesis seems at least very probable for the particular kinds of spaces which Metzger has investigated. But at the present moment I should feel loth to generalize it beyond these limits. There exists also the other possibility that under other conditions space will be as large as possible and that therefore it will require special forces to *constrain* it, an effect achieved by bringing either the boundary or any part-object nearer to the observer.

(5) The Rôle of Accommodation. We draw attention to the rôle of accommodation. In Metzger's experiment the stimulation would be inhomogeneous, possessing microstructure, only if accommodation was perfect. With imperfect accommodation the stimulus distribution would be perfectly homogeneous. The action of the lenses, therefore, is such as to create conditions for a process of higher rather than of lower articulation. If it were a general law that the visual sector will always produce the least possible reaction, then accommodation should work in the opposite way to that in which it really does; it should not focus the eyes on objects but should throw them out of focus so as to create the most homogeneous stimulus distribution possible. But even under the extreme conditions of Metzger's experiments it does not; it makes the stimulus distribution as inhomogeneous as possible, and thereby the actual process distribution as articulate as possible. We shall take up this point when we discuss the relation between field organization and behaviour (in Chapter VIII).

(6) Instability of Homogeneous Space. Homogeneous space and even sufficiently large homogeneous parts of space are not so stable as well articulated space. Everybody knows the spots and streaks of light that begin to swirl before his eyes when he stays in a completely dark room. Similar phenomena occur in homogeneous light space, although not often spontaneously; when, however, the observer begins to scrutinize the field to test whether it is really homogeneous, he may see points of light or cloudlike structures shifting through his field. The forces which produce these phenomena originate inside the nervous system, but under normal conditions of good articulation the total organization is so stable that these forces either cannot arise or, if they do, are incapable of affecting the firmly established structure.

Temporal Inhomogeneity of Stimulation. Before we leave the discussion of organization under the conditions of homogeneous stimulation we must lift a restriction which so far has limited our argument. Homogeneity of stimulation has been understood to mean spatial homogeneity. We were concerned only with the period of time during which the spatially homogeneous stimulation lasted. But each such period has periods which precede and which follow it, and the period of time which we have singled out must be considered also in the context of its past and future. Otherwise expressed, we shall apply our concept of homogeneity to time as well as to space, and then we see that the onset of a spatially homogeneous stimulation introduces an inhomogeneity in the temporal stimulus distribution; the organism must do something new, and this new organization will, in some of its aspects, depend upon the preceding organizations. Perfect homogeneity would be both temporal and spatial. Would it be too bold to say that if all, not only visual, stimulation were completely homogeneous, there would be no perceptual organization at all? What happens when we are in the dark and close our eyes? We see a dark grey, little extended, space at first, but after a while we do not *see* any more. The world of sight has ceased to exist for the time being. I am not sure whether the same effect cannot occur if we are in a totally homogeneous space that is not entirely dark.

Coloured Homogeneous Space. However, it is not because of this speculation that I have introduced the topic, but in order to remove a limitation of our previous discussion. We restricted our problem to the case of neutral light. Let us now lift that restriction. What shall we see when, in a set-up like Metzger's, the light that is projected on the wall is passed through coloured filters? The experiment has not been made, so we do not know. But it is possible to hazard a guess. For simplicity's sake we assume that the observer finds himself in a normally illuminated room before the experiment begins. Then the homogeneous coloured illumination breaks in upon a space which was "normal" and therefore will be seen with reference to normal neutrality, coloured in correspondence with the colour of the respective filter. But if the observer stays sufficiently long within the homogeneously coloured field, will it continue to look coloured? Most probably not; it will, according to my expectation, gradually become neutral. Why I expect it to become so and what the effect, if it occurs, means will be discussed later (see Chapter VI, p. 256). It is mentioned here only to indicate at least the possibility that continued homogeneous coloured stimulation will eventually produce the same result as neutral stimulation, in accordance with our proposition that under homogeneous stimulation as little as possible will happen. For colour is *more* than neutral grey; it is an added event, an extra effect. In support of this view I will only mention that both of Gelb's patients described above were colour blind, one totally, the other partially, and that as a general rule disturbances of spatial organization are accompanied by disturbances of colour vision.

My hypothesis does not go so far as to claim that the result of homogeneous coloured stimulation is quite identical with that of homogeneous neutral stimulation. I expect it to be different in the object-Ego relation which was touched upon previously. Thus I expect the subject to feel in a different mood in homogeneous red and violet fields, even if both appear as grey fog. For the moment it must suffice to note that colour in all its aspects may appear to be one side of the total organization.

Behavioural Space Not Purely Visual. One last word to exclude a misunderstanding. It would be wrong to suppose that in Metzger's experiment the seen space depended only upon the visual stimulation. Behavioural space is a much more comprehensive organization which is supported by other than visual forces, notably those which arise in the vestibular organ of our inner ear and those which derive from so-called deep sensibility. And of course what we have said about this more comprehensive organization of behavioural space holds not only for Metzger's experiments, for space produced by homogeneous retinal stimulation, but for every kind of visual space. Functionally space is never purely visual.

The choice of our first experiment was easy enough, because the "simplest" case of stimulation could be deduced from the definition of our problem. Our next step has to be more arbitrary. Of course we could follow up the lead which the first experiment has given us. We saw that organization of space into surfaces at different distances requires special forces, and we saw further that if these forces are produced by mere microstructure of an otherwise homogeneous stimulation we shall see a homogeneous vertical plane bounding our visual space.

Localization of the Plane Produced by Homogeneous Stimulation with Microstructure. A first question which we might ask now is: At what distance will this plane be seen? Unfortunately we have no sufficient experimental data to answer that question. Metzger's experiments proved only that the perceived distance depends to some degree on the intensity of stimulation, and that it need not be the same as the "real" distance. This expression is of course a mere abbreviation. Strictly speaking we cannot compare real and phenomenal or behavioural data. When, for brevity's sake, we use this incorrect terminology we mean that the behavioural quality which appears in a particular situation is different from the behavioural quality under more normal conditions. In the case of the distance of our homogeneous plane it would mean that the homogeneous plane appears at a different distance from a plane which was objectively at the same distance, but which formed part of a more richly articulated field. Since our behaviour is determined by our behavioural field, it will mean also that in such cases our behaviour would be badly adapted to the geographical field, or that there would be discrepancies between behaviour and behavioural field. More concretely, if we were to touch this plane with a stick, we should begin by pushing the stick not sufficiently far; but since "touching" means a very definite experience which would not occur before we brought the stick into contact with the real wall, we would then go on moving the stick against the data of our visual space. Thus the two patients described by Gelb were liable to fall when they alighted from a tram because, owing to the spread of colour, the ground seemed too near to them and they innervated their muscles accordingly. Thus discrepancies between the real and the behavioural world can always be described in terms of behaviour, which, as we have seen in our second chapter, depends on both the behavioural and the geographical environment.

But to return to our question at what distance the homogeneous plane surface will appear. Even though the seen distance was not entirely constant and would at higher intensities of stimulation be greater than the real one, it had definite limits. In Metzger's experiment the distance between the eye and the nearest point of the wall was about 1.25 m. The maximum distance estimated was not quite twice that amount. Therefore the range of distances at which the plane appeared, if not the distance itself, is well determined. Does it depend upon the real distance? Unfortunately we do not know, since in Metzger's experiments this was kept constant. There exists, then, the possibility that the behavioural will depend on the real distance. Of course the real distance cannot affect behavioural distance directly. Something must mediate between them. There are only three factors which can assume this mediating rôle. The first influences the stimulation directly: if the distance is too great, the grain will become too fine to be effective; the microstructure will disappear, stimulation will be homogeneous, and we shall see fog-filled space.

This first factor, therefore, cannot account for a positive correlation between real and perceived distance in the case of a homogeneous wall. Thus there remain only the two factors of accommodation and convergence. Accommodation, as we have seen, is possible only where there is inhomogeneity. And convergence has no direct determinant under the conditions of our experiment. We cannot substantiate this last statement since we are not yet prepared to state the direct determinants of convergence (see Chapter VIII), but convergence and accommodation are to some extent coupled together so that, when there are no opposing forces, a given accommodation will insure a certain convergence.

Inasmuch, then, as the apparent distance of the homogeneous wall will depend upon its real distance, it must do so through the mediation of accommodation and convergence. Although many experiments have been carried out to determine the influence of these two factors on the localization of objects in an articulated space, it would be dangerous to draw inferences from these cases for our case of a homogeneous plane even if the results of these experiments were univocal. As a matter of fact, such an inference becomes impossible since the results of these experiments are highly contradictory. We have no adequate knowledge as to the rôle of our two factors. But we can say this much: Assuming the apparent distance of our plane depended upon its real distance and therefore upon accommodation and convergence, this dependence would be a direct and not an indirect one. The early investigators held the opposite opinion; they thought that accommodation and convergence could influence perceptual data only if they gave rise to separate sensations of their own which interfered or fused in some way or other with the visual sensations. We cannot accept such a view. On the one hand, we do not normally experience such sensations, on the other this theory involves a kind of mental chemistry which has no place in our system built on actual scientific concepts. The direct influence which we have in mind is the state of the nervous system itself which corresponds to a given degree of accommodation and convergence. It requires energy to accommodate and to converge to a near object, and within limits the nearer the object the greater the energy. This fact, or other facts of a similar nature, may directly influence the organization of space, which, as we have seen (cf. p. 119), is itself a dynamic process consuming energy. Later on we shall see that such an influence, where it exists, is not very considerable, and therefore it is not very probable that the dependence of the phenomenal distance of the homogeneous plane upon its real distance can be very extensive.

INHOMOGENEOUS STIMULATION. SIMPLE CASE OF ONLY ONE INHOMOGENEITY IN OTHERWISE HOMOGENEOUS FIELD

We must now turn to non-homogeneous stimulation; a possible procedure would be to take the next simple case in which the stimulation varied uniformly from point to point in one or several directions. Leaving this till later, we discuss now the case where, within a homogeneous stimulus distribution on the retina, there is a circumscribed area of a different stimulation. Unfortunately, we cannot treat this case without limitations. No experiment has been made in which the conditions were fulfilled that both the enclosing and the enclosed area were absolutely homogeneous. Next to it comes an experiment by Metzger. The wall was illuminated with such an intensity that it appeared like a bowl. In the centre of the wall a small square was left unilluminated which, since the observer had to raise his eyes, was projected on the retina as a trapezium. The observer saw a black trapezium on the surface of this bowl, which in the region where the trapezium appeared was frontal parallel to the tilted head, that is, inclined towards the vertical.

In this case the enclosing stimulation possessed a microstructure, while the enclosed was homogeneous. Yet this latter did not give rise to the perception of a space-filling fog; the part of the field corresponding to it appeared in the same surface as that corresponding to the enclosing one. In other words, the surface was constituted as a whole by the microstructure of the enclosing stimulation and this determined the effect of the small homogeneous enclosed area.

However, interesting though this result is, it does not satisfy our curiosity about the effect of a discontinuity in an otherwise homogeneous stimulation. For in this case the production of the surface was due not to the discontinuity but to the microstructure of the enclosing stimulation. We still need to know the minimum discontinuity that would destroy the primary effect of fog-filled space.

Conditions Specified: The Field Appears as a Plane. Since this question has not yet been answered, we must limit our original problem. We shall consider those cases in which the surrounding field appears as a plane surface, whether because of microstructure or because of general field articulation, and we shall centre our interest on the effects produced within this plane surface by the enclosed discontinuity. Therefore we modify our postulate of a homogeneous *total* field so as to mean a homogeneous field that is *relatively* large and which contains somewhere within its boundaries a homogeneous discontinuity. In practice we shall use plane surfaces with spots upon them as distant stimuli. Let us look at any such spot, produced, for instance, by splashing ink on a white piece of paper. We see the ink blot: no problem seems to be contained in this simple case. There is the ink blot and we see it. But we have learned that the answer to our first question, why things look as they do, is wrong. There is a very real problem here which is only concealed by the fact of the universality of such experiences. And the appearance of the ink blot in our new example is as much of a problem as the appearance of the fog-filled space under conditions of perfectly homogeneous stimulation. To see an ink blot is the result of an organization just as the fog-filled space was. Of course it is a different kind of organization, and we must first describe some of its aspects.

The Two Problems Involved in This Case. (1) Unit Formation. In the first place, then, our blot is seen as a *unit, segregated* from the rest of the field, and in the second place it has a *shape*. Both descriptions have their theoretical implications. Why is the blot a unit; how does it become segregated from its surroundings? The answer seems obvious: because it is differently coloured. Certainly this is the right answer if one gives the right meaning to the word "because." For in and of itself, difference of coloration is not the same as unit formation.

First Law of Unit Formation and Segregation. If we ascribe segregation and unification of parts of the field to the fact that each part is in itself homogeneously coloured and differently coloured from its environment, we imply a general law of unit formation and segregation, viz., if the proximal stimulation is such that it consists of several areas of different homogeneous stimulation, then the areas which receive the same stimulation will organize unitary field parts segregated from the others by the difference between the stimulations. In other words the equality of stimulation produces forces of cohesion, inequality of stimulation forces of segregation, provided that the inequality entails an abrupt change. These are truly dynamic propositions, and our explanation of the unification and segregation of the blot is no longer banal if interpreted in this way.

The Forces of Unification and Segregation. The critical reader will be inclined to ask for some substantiation of our dynamical proposition. He will argue that it follows directly from the fundamental premises of our theory, but that he wants to know facts on which it is based. Let us satisfy our critic. We claimed no peculiarity for psychophysical organization which would not belong to physical organizations, and therefore we shall point out that exactly the same proposition holds in physics. Thus, to use one of Köhler's examples (1929, p. 138), if oil is poured into a liquid with which it does not mix, the surface of the oil will remain sharply determined in the violent interaction of molecules, and if the liquid has the same density, then the oil will form a sphere swimming in the other liquid. But, the critic will say, there are liquids with which oil does mix, therefore not *any* kind of difference will produce such forces of segregation in physics. Have you got anything similar in psychophysical organization? We have, and this fact proves more than anything else that unification and segregation are really dynamic events produced by forces and not mere geometrical patterns.

liebmann effect. I refer to an effect discovered and investigated by S. Liebmann. A coloured figure (coloured now in the ordinary sense), say a blue one, on a neutral ground, begins to lose sharpness and definition, and simplifies its shape, if it be intricate, when its luminosity approaches that of the ground on which it lies. When the two luminosities are equal the shape is completely lost; a vague and vacillating blotch is seen, and even that may disappear completely for short periods of time. Therefore difference of stimulation between an enclosing and an enclosed area, if it is a mere colour difference, has, to say the least, much less power to produce a segregation of these two areas in the psychophysical field than a very small difference in luminosity. Thus two greys which look very similar will give a perfectly stable organization if one is used for the figure and the other for the ground, whereas a deeply saturated blue and a grey of the same luminosity which look very different indeed will produce practically no such organization. This proves that difference of stimulation is not in itself equivalent to segregation of area; the latter, far from being a mere geometrical projection of a retinal distribution, is a dynamic effect which occurs with some stimulus differences more than with others and may fail to appear at all with very large stimulus differences when these are not of the kind to produce the forces necessary for organization.

HARD AND SOFT COLOURS. The physiological processes produced by two surfaces of different luminosity can then be compared to two liquids that do not mix, and two surfaces of equal luminosity but different colour to two liquids that do mix. This discovery by Liebmann has been amplified in an investigation carried out by M. R. Harrower and myself. We found that not all colours are alike in this respect, but that a colour will mix the better with an equiluminous grey, the shorter the wave-length of the light which produces it. Thus red is the colour which segregates best and blue the one that segregates least. We have therefore introduced the distinction between hard and soft colours, red and yellow belonging to the former, blue and green to the latter. We also made a quantitative comparison between the capacity of organization possessed by colour and brightness differences (I, pp. 159 f.). The observer sat in front of two revolving grey disks of the same luminosity. In each of these disks a ring could be produced by mixing either colour or a grey of a different brightness with the grey of the ground. On the one the ring contained a given amount of colour, say 20° of blue, of a highly saturated blue paper. This gave the appearance of a faint ring. On the other disk the ring was made either lighter or darker by the introduction of a lighter or darker grey paper, and the observer had to decide how much of this lighter or darker grey was necessary to produce a ring equally clear and marked as the coloured one on the other disk. In the example indicated the amount of the lighter grey needed in the neutral ring was such as to add only one degree of white to the rest of the disk.

Talbot's Law. A few words to explain the procedure. According to Talbot's law a spinning colour wheel composed of different sectors, if it rotates fast enough so as to fuse completely, looks like a non-rotating colour wheel on which the qualities of the different sectors are spread uniformly in amounts proportional to their respective sectors. Otherwise expressed, a rotating disk of several sectors is equivalent to a stationary one whose quality is the average of the qualities contained in the sectors of the different luminosities l_1 and l_2. Then if α is the angle of the sector with the grey l_1, and β the angle of the sector of the quality l_2, $\beta = 360 - \alpha$, the rotating disk is equivalent to a stationary disk with the luminosity $l = \frac{\alpha l_1 + \beta l_2}{360} = \frac{\alpha l_1 + (360 - \alpha) l_2}{360}$. From this formula we can calculate the luminosity of the ring if we know the luminosities of the disk and the grey paper introduced into the ring. We express the luminosities with regard to the luminosity of white. Calling the luminosity of 1° of white unity, a whole white disk has the luminosity 360.

In the example I have just mentioned, the grey, equiluminous with blue, had the value 47 white. The grey ring, equal in clearness to a ring of 20° blue and 340° of this grey, had the luminosity 48, i.e., it was only about 2.1% lighter than the rest, whereas the coloured sector in the other ring was 5.2% of the whole ring.

In another experiment, where green, less saturated and lighter than our blue, was used, the figures are: the neutral ring, equally clear as a ring of 8.3% of green (30°), was about 3% lighter than the rest of the disk. The Liebmann effect, i.e., the blurring of the ring, is not as marked under these conditions as I have described it above. There are at the boundaries other slight inhomogeneities which produce a better organization than the mere colour difference would be capable of bringing about.

DEPENDENCY OF LIEBMANN EFFECT UPON INTENSITY OF STIMULATION. Another general result of our experiments is relevant in this connection. The set-up was quite different from the one described last. An irregular coloured figure was seen in a uniform neutral surrounding, the intensities of the figure and surrounding being varied independently. Under these conditions we found the Liebmann effect stronger under low than under high illumination or, otherwise expressed, the greater the intensity of the illumination, the greater the unifying and segregating forces. Furthermore it was found that white is a harder colour than black even when it reflects the same amount of light into the observer's eyes, a result previously obtained in experiments carried out by Dr. Mintz and myself (see Chapter VI). Consequently a saturated red figure on a highly illuminated white ground would show practically no Liebmann effect at all; the figure would lose none, or only the faintest trace, of its articulation at the "coincidence point"; that is the point at which figure and surrounding are of the same luminosity (Koffka-Harrower II).

Now the result that intensity of stimulation increases the forces of organization may possibly modify our conclusions based on Metzger's experiments. Although without a doubt in his experiments the effect of greater intensity was largely due to the effectiveness of the microstructure, we have to consider the possibility that it has a direct result as well, so that possibly a very bright and totally homogeneous field would look less foggy than a less bright one. Furthermore, these results explain why, for Gelb's two patients, the thickness of colour in front of a surface varied inversely with the whiteness of the surface.

(2) The Problem of Shape. After having proved that unit formation and segregation is a dynamical process which presupposes forces produced by discontinuities in the proximal stimulation, we must turn to the second aspect of our problem. Our blot has a shape. Although it is perfectly true that the shape is produced by the same process which is responsible for segregating the unit, it would be wrong to suppose that for this reason no more need be said about shape. A simple demonstration will show that shape introduces a new problem.

Fig. 9

Look at the accompanying Fig. 9, taken from Bühler (1913). It can appear in three different shapes, two bi-, one tri-dimensional. It may look (a) like a sort of square with curved sides, or (b) tri-dimensional like a sail blown up by the wind, or (c) when the main axis of symmetry is diagonal from the right bottom to the left top corner, like a kind of kite. In all three cases unification and segregation occur along the same boundary lines; consequently unification and segregation *per se* does not explain shape.

Reality of Shape Proved. And yet, shape is no less real than the unit itself. In the preceding section we have proved the reality of the unit; accordingly we shall now prove the reality of shape. We shall do this by showing that shape has functional effects, indirect and direct ones. We owe the first proofs to an experiment by L. Hartmann, who investigated the influence of shape on the critical fusion frequency. We have already briefly referred to the fact that a periodic stimulation, if the period is short enough, has the same result as a continuous stimulation, the relation between the two being regulated by Talbot's law. This law was originally proved for colour wheels, but it holds, of course, also in the case when a light figure is projected on a wall and an episcotister rotates in front of the lantern's objective. An episcotister may be either a disk with holes in it, or an ordinary colour wheel from which one or more sectors are completely missing, so that the light can pass unobstructed to the screen when the opening of the colour wheel passes in front of the lantern. Objectively this produces an alternation between light and dark on the screen, the proportion of the light and dark periods being determined by the size of the open sector or sectors. But if the episcotister rotates fast enough, no such alternation, not even the trace of a flicker, is visible; fusion has been attained, and the lowest velocity which produces fusion is the critical fusion velocity, or, if we count the number of different exposures per unit of time, we establish the critical fusion frequency. The experiment to be described presently can indeed be made with such an apparatus. Hartmann's procedure, however, was different, yielding greater quantitative differences. Instead of a periodic succession of exposures interrupted by periodic intervals of darkness he used *two* exposures only; before the first and after the second exposure the whole field was totally dark, and between the two exposures there was a dark interval. He used a Schumann tachistoscope—a wheel with a wide rim rotating in front of a telescope. The rim has two slits, variable in size and at variable distance from each other. When these slits pass in front of the telescope, the observer sees an object exposed behind the wheel, and the time of the exposure is determined by the length of the slit and the velocity of rotation. If, then, two slits with a black interval pass between the telescope and a light figure, the experience of the observer will depend upon the velocity of the rotation. Without going into detail I mention only the two extreme cases: with very low velocities the observer sees the figure twice and in between an interval of darkness; with sufficiently high speed, however, the observer sees one figure only without the slightest flicker. It is easy to determine the lowest velocity at which this effect occurs, viz., the critical fusion velocity. Among many other figures Hartmann exposed also our Fig. 9 and instructed his observers to see it either in shape (a) square, or shape (c) kite. The result is summarized in Table 4, the figures giving the duration of one whole rotation of the wheel and of one whole period, the two exposures plus the interval between them, at which one complete fusion occurred, in $\sigma = 1/1000$ sec.

TABLE 4

(from Hartmann)

	period of rotation	*period of total exposure*
"square"	1190	116
"kite"	1080	105

I shall add the figures for another pattern used by Hartmann. Fig. 10 can be seen either as a square with a heavy diagonal line or as

Fig. 10

(In the original experiment the parts printed here in black were white and vice versa.)

two triangles. The critical fusion periods of this pattern are given in the next table, which is in all respects similar to the preceding one.

TABLE 5

(from Hartmann)

	period of rotation	*period of total exposure*
"square"	1260	123
"2 triangles"	1170	114

In the first pattern the difference between the critical fusion periods is a little more than 10% of the total period, in the second, a little less. And in each case the higher figure corresponds to the phenomenally *simpler* pattern, a point to be remembered. That these values reveal significant differences was also proved qualitatively. If the critical velocity had been reached for the simpler of the two possible figures so that it was seen without flicker, and the observers were then asked to change over to the other less simple one, this shape flickered invariably, until the period was further reduced by increasing the velocity of the rotating wheel. The second figure yielded still another qualitative observation, in that before fusion was reached the black strip looked different if it was a part of the square or the "dead space" between the two triangles. Objectively this particular part of the field was black all the time; the passing of the slits made not the slightest difference. Therefore, in and by itself, it should show no flicker at all. But this was true only when it appeared as the space between the two triangles, whereas it participated in the flicker of the whole figure when this was seen as a square, proving again the reality of the actually perceived units.

In the first example, the Bühler figure, the two patterns differ from each other in shape only, in the second, in shape and unification. Thus the first table proves the reality of shape, and the second the reality of shape and unification compounded.

But Hartmann discovered also a more direct effect of shape than the one previously described. Under his conditions of double exposure and with a somewhat more elaborate technique he found that the brightness at which figures fuse perfectly depends upon their shape, less articulated figures appearing darker than more articulated ones.

The Shape-giving Forces. What does it mean to have proved the reality of shape or form? We have shown that the critical fusion frequency is not an affair that concerns each nerve fibre separately but pertains to a whole segregated unit, and that with a given unit it still depends upon the shape of this unit. Both results prove that fusion depends upon the dynamic aspects of the fusing part of the field, upon the forces which keep it together and separate it from the rest of the field and upon the forces which give it its shape. The figures which we produced by intermittent stimulation correspond to physiological areas under stress, and the distribution of these stresses is a factor that determines the ease with which fusion occurs. What, then, is the relation between unit formation and shape? Let us return to the example from physics which we selected in our discussion of segregation. We saw that oil, immersed in a liquid with which it will not mix, will separate itself from it by the forces within and between the surfaces of the two media, and that the same surface forces will also give shape to the oil, under specially simple conditions, the shape of a sphere. The forces which segregate the oil from the other liquid are at the same time forces which hold the oil particles together, and these forces are not in equilibrium until the final shape is reached; before, there are pulls along the surface and in the interior which change the shape of the oil until it is in equilibrium with the surrounding fluid. If we apply this to our problem of perceived form we must conclude that the shape of our ink blot or of any other figure is the result of forces which do not only segregate the figure from the rest of the field but hold it in equilibrium with the field. There are then forces within the figures and along their contours, a conclusion which we had drawn directly from our experiments. However, this point is fundamental; in the last section of our second chapter we formulated the task of psychology and indicated the steps which we would take in order to develop a system of psychology. The point which concerns us now is the first part of the first step, the discovery of the forces which organize our environmental field into separate objects.

EXPERIMENTAL DEMONSTRATION OF THESE FORCES. We have already discovered some of these forces, and we shall now add some experimental evidence to prove that the organized objects or units are really dynamically different from the rest of the field, that each such unit has its specific distribution of forces. Our first examples are taken from the field of so-called contrast. It is well known that a small grey field looks whiter when it is surrounded by a black than by a white field. This in itself would be a proof of our proposition, if it were proved that the black and white fields, as *units* and not as mere sums of "black-white events," were responsible for the effect. For in that case the different appearances of the grey field in the two different environments would prove that the larger, black and white, fields exerted forces on the inlying grey fields so as to change their whiteness. However, according to the traditionally accepted contrast theories, which all have their origin in Hering's theory, the contrast effect has nothing to do with unity or shape of the fields but merely with the amount and proximity of the brightnesses outside the inlying field.

TRADITIONAL CONTRAST THEORY. According to this theory a white process induces black process in its whole surrounding, the strength of the influence decreasing according to an unknown function with distance. In the more modern form of this theory there is, except under special conditions, no similar influence exerted by black, since there is no local stimulation which produces black. If, therefore, a grey inlying field appears whiter when it is surrounded by a black field than when it lies within a field of its own brightness, this is not explained as the result of a whitening effect of the black environment, but by a darkening effect of the "equivalent" grey one, the term "equivalent" meaning "of equal whiteness." According to this view two equal excitations will weaken each other, each inducing black process in its neighbour and thereby decreasing the intensity of the white process produced by the incoming light. The fact that small grey patches on any background look lighter than large ones is explained by this principle which is called "Binnen-Kontrast" in German, which can be translated as "internal contrast." Even if our grey field were surrounded by a darker grey field it would still be *darkened* by it, since the white process, which is still aroused in the surrounding field by the incidence of light, produces contrast, i.e., black process in the inlying field.

It is characteristic of this theory that contrast is a *summative* and an *absolute* affair; it depends upon the mere amount and geometrical distribution of the excitations and upon their absolute intensity, unit formation and shape being excluded as effective factors as well as the *relation* of the stimulations of the two fields.

We shall later show the falsity of the second aspect of this theory, its character of absoluteness. At the moment we must prove that its summative aspect is wrong; for that disproof contains the proof of the forces operative within a unified and shaped field part.

Before doing so I must remind the reader that besides mere brightness contrast there exists also a colour contrast in the strict sense. A small grey field within a large red one looks green or greenish, within a green, red or reddish, etc. I also want to add that I am using the term contrast merely as a description of the facts reported and in no way as an explanation. Therefore the reader should not, in following my argument, connect any theory with the term contrast, but judge the argument for what it is worth as a conclusion from facts.

EXPERIMENTAL EVIDENCE AGAINST THIS THEORY. The first experiment is quite old. Wertheimer told me of it at the beginning of the war and I published it in 1915 (p. 40). Benussi had discovered the effect at about the same time (1916, p. 61 n.), and in his publication he pointed out that similar experiments had been made long ago in Wundt's laboratory by Meyer, who, however, drew very different conclusions from them. The form in which it is represented in Fig. 11 is a combination of Wertheimer's and Benussi's patterns. On a ground half red, half green, lies a grey ring. Looked at naïvely, it will appear more or less homogeneously grey. Now divide the circular ring into two semicircular ones by laying a narrow strip of paper or a needle on top of the boundary between the red and the green fields. At once the semicircular ring on the red field

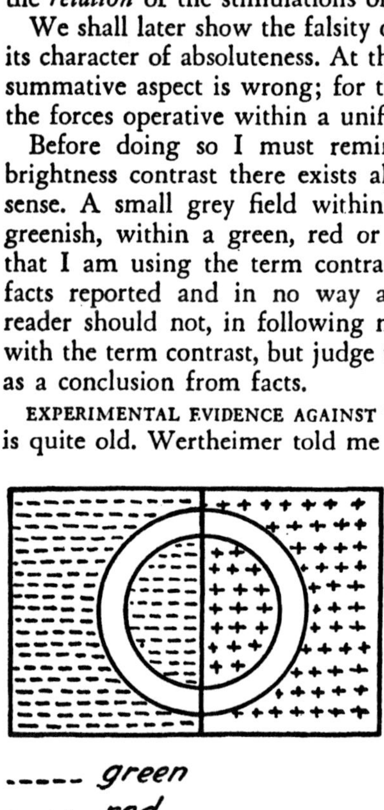

Fig. 11

will look distinctly greenish, that on the green field, distinctly reddish. We may express the result of this experiment thus: a unified figure will look uniform under conditions where two segregated figures produced by the same stimuli will look different from each other. What is the theoretical relevance of this experiment? On the stimulus side we have three uniform areas in definite geometrical relationships: a red, a green and a grey, so arranged that the one half of the grey interrupts the red, the other the green. From what we know, we should expect to see three units, a red, a green, and a grey one, an expectation that is fulfilled in the first part of the experiment. We then introduce a new inhomogeneity which divides our ring into two half-rings. And now something new happens; the hitherto ineffective circumstance that the two halves lie within different surroundings, interrupt different homogeneities, changes their own quality; in other words the leap of stimulation between the ring parts and their environment now becomes effective. These leaps of stimulation have existed in the first part of the experiment as well, therefore the forces which in the second part give to the two half-rings a different colour must have existed all the time. If, then, the whole ring looked grey, this can only be due to the fact that the forces of cohesion which hold the ring together are so strong as totally or partially to resist the influences of the other forces which would make the ring inhomogeneous. This leads us to a new principle of organization which is the conversion of one of our old ones: a strongly *unified* part of the field will look as *uniform* as is possible, i.e., as much as the prevailing conditions allow. For this proposition there is abundant proof. (Fuchs, 1923, Koffka, 1923, Tudor-Hart, G. M. Heider.)

To return to our experiment: still differently expressed, we produce two kinds of forces, such as will make the ring uniform and such as will make it look different in its two parts. When the ring is seen as one, the first forces are stronger, and only when they have been weakened, the other forces will gain supremacy, effect a change of colour and with it a change of shape; two figures are seen instead of one. A slight modification will bring out the rôle of shape in this process of organization. A ring is a perfectly balanced figure with no articulation within it. It is plausible to assume that it is this property which makes the forces of cohesion so strong that the forces of articulation remain without effect. If this is the true explanation, then our experiment should yield a different result if we substituted for the ring a figure which has two clear subdivisions like an eight. If this new figure is so placed on our red and green field that the boundary line of the two colours divides the figure symmetrically then before the dividing line is introduced these two parts should look more different from each other than the two parts of the ring. And this is the case. Indeed, one might derive a method of measuring the forces of cohesion belonging to a given shape from such experiments.

That the shape of the inlying field determines the amount of contrast colour it takes on from a surrounding field was also shown in certain experiments of G. M. Heider's (p. 52). On three large blue fields of equal size she introduced one small grey figure, a circle on one, a ring on the second, and 12 very small circles arranged on the circumference of a larger circle on the third. The dimensions of the figures were such that the total amount of grey was the same on all three blue fields. Now according to the summative theory these three figures should have looked yellowish to a different degree, the last one most and the first least, because in the last, the grey parts were in closest contact with the blue, each little circle being entirely surrounded by it, while in the first figure, a relatively large mass of grey is relatively far removed from the blue. The facts belie this expectation, the first figure, the full circle, looking most, the last figure least, yellow. It is the figure with the greatest cohesion that becomes most coloured, a new indication of the close relation between the degree of organization and coloration.

Of course there is no contradiction contained in the fact that in the Wertheimer-Benussi experiment the most cohesive figure was the least coloured, while here it is the most coloured, for in that experiment the uniformity which was enforced by the great cohesiveness had to be a neutral uniformity, while in Mrs. Heider's experiment, no such connection between uniformity and neutrality exists.

Another experiment, extremely ingenious, devised by Wertheimer and carried out by Benary, later repeated with modifications by W. H. Mikesell and M. Bentley and by J. G. Jenkins, reveals the forces of organization in a new way.[4] They show that the forces within a (behavioural) figure are different from those outside its boundary. In the two Figs. 12 *a* and *b,* a small grey triangle, identical in both patterns, lies either on a large black triangle (*a*) or outside

[4] The two later investigations fully confirm the results of Benary and his theory, although the authors of the first of them hold a different opinion. The relation in which these two papers stand to Benary's has been very ably summarized and discussed by W. Metzger (1931).

in a niche between the arms of a black cross (*b*). Both small triangles border on black and white. Actually the little triangle has more white in its neighbourhood in *a* than in *b*, *a* being produced out of *b* by parts of the black being cut away, as indicated in *c*. Therefore, according to the Hering theory of contrast, the little triangle should look darker in *a* than in *b*, whereas in reality it looks darker in *b* than in *a*. The reason is obvious. Phenomenally the triangle lies *on* the black in *a* and on the white in *b*, but this matter of belonging either to the black or the white is entirely a matter of organization, and not of the geometrical distribution of the proximal stimuli. For again, in each of our two patterns, the

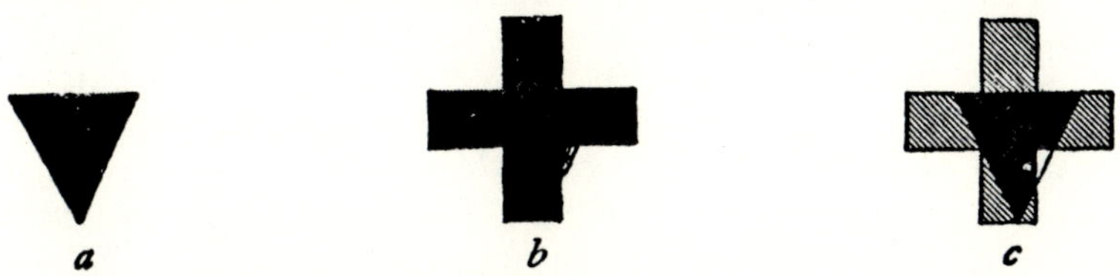

Fig. 12

proximal stimulation corresponding to it consists of three homogeneous areas all different from each other; that each of these homogeneous areas produces a special unit in the behavioural space we know already to be a result of organization. *A fortiori* the mutual relations of these units are products of the organizing processes. Therefore to lie on a particular field-part means to be subject to the forces which hold this field-part together as a unity and to be more or less shielded against forces from the outlying field. It would be wrong to assume that this isolation is complete. Benary's original experiments and the contributions of the later experimenters prove that these forces are also operative, but the result, as formulated in the preceding sentences, has been confirmed with a great variety of different patterns by Benary and the American investigators.

This experiment proves not only the reality of the forces of unification and segregation, but also the reality of shape. For what is it that makes the little triangle lie inside the larger figure in one case and outside in the other? The answer is: because in (*a*) the total large triangle, of which the small triangle is a part, is a well-balanced good form; the form of the black part alone is much less satisfactory. And conversely, in (*b*) the cross without the little triangle has by far the better shape than the figure which includes the small figure. Otherwise expressed: organization depends upon the resulting form. Of several geometrically possible organizations that one will actually occur which possesses the best, the most stable shape. This is, of course, nothing but our law of prägnanz.

OTHER DIRECT EFFECTS OF SHAPE. Thus we have established a first direct effect of shape. We shall now adduce more experimental evidence for this direct effect manifest in the process of organization itself. In the Wertheimer-Benary experiment the effect occurred under somewhat more complex conditions than those from which we started; instead of having two homogeneous fields with a leap of quality between them, there are three such fields in this experiment. To return to the simpler case we shall revert to our example of the oil which assumes the shape of a sphere within a liquid of equal specific density with which it does not mix. Let us ask the following question: If a spherical distribution of a certain kind of material within a different material is the most stable, why do we not see a sphere or at least a circle whenever there appears a spot of any shape in a homogeneous field? (We can exclude the sphere because we are assuming that in our experiments the conditions are such as to concentrate all colour processes in one plane.) But why do we not see a circle? The answer is very simple, and yet it will lead us to a new proof of the reality of form. The drop of oil becomes a sphere when, owing to the constitution of the surrounding liquid, there are no forces which prevent it from yielding to the forces on its own surface and in its own interior. As far as the surrounding liquid is concerned, any shape would be as good as any other. When, however, we stimulate our eyes by an irregular black spot on a white surface, the conditions set up on the retina which start the whole process and keep it going do exert just such an influence on the shape of the resulting distribution of process as was absent in the case of our oil sphere. For the stimulation determines not only the amount of black which is produced within the white—if it did only that, we should indeed expect to see a circle whatever the shape of the spot—but also very definite spatial relations of the ensuing distribution. The dynamic form of the process distribution depends upon a geometrical form of stimulus distribution.

TWO KINDS OF ORGANIZING FORCES, EXTERNAL AND INTERNAL ONES. In our psychophysical case, then, we have two kinds of forces, those which exist within the process in distribution itself and which will tend to impress on this distribution the simplest possible shape, and those between this distribution and the stimulus pattern, which constrain this stress towards simplification. We shall call the latter external, the former, internal forces of organization, external and internal referring to that part of the whole process which corresponds to our perceived form.

If this hypothesis is true we should expect very stable organizations whenever the two kinds of forces act in the same direction, if, e.g., our spot has circular shape. Conversely, if the forces are in strong conflict, the resulting organization should be less stable. Can we verify these conclusions?

EXPERIMENTS BASED ON THIS DISTINCTION. The general principle of such verification is easy to discern. We must expose irregular figures which would produce the conflicting forces just described and watch the result. In our choice of figures and general experimental condition we can pursue two aims, either to make the forces which prevent a stable organization very small or to make them very great. In the first case we would expect the internal forces of organization to be strong enough to overcome these external forces, in the second case we should expect unstable end-products, that is, perceived figures which change while we look at them, or which are not clearly structured over their entire extent. Experimental procedure has chosen the first modes of procedure, and chance observations have been made when the same special conditions were fulfilled. We shall discuss these results presently.

External Forces Strong. But at first we shall stick as closely as possible to the case of stimulation with which we started, viz., one spot in a larger homogeneous field which can be looked at without time limits. In this case the forces issuing from the retina are particularly strong. If, then, we bring them into strong conflict with the internal forces of organization, what will happen? We expose for our purpose a blotch with as irregular an outline as we can produce. The result is somewhat disappointing. Unless our spot is very large it will look clear and stable enough with all its irregularities. What conclusions can we draw from this result? In the first place it proves the strength of the determining forces, which prevent a large dislocation in the interest of a better organization. Without any other evidence we should even apparently be justified to suppose that these retinal forces were the only operative ones, that our percept were nothing but a geometrical projection of the retinal stimulus pattern. But even without further knowledge, such an assumption would not be quite in harmony with observation. For when we see such an irregular patch, we do not see its whole geometrical shape in the same way. We see first of all a general form, more or less symmetrical in outline, and then dents and protuberances which interfere with or modify this general outline; a distinction which is nowise contained in the geometrical pattern as such, but is the effect of those very organizing forces which we set out to find. However, I admit that this evidence alone would scarcely be sufficient to prove our point. Let us analyze our result a bit further to see whether we cannot discover why any more noticeable effect of the internal forces of organization failed to appear. We accepted it as proven that the external organizing forces excluded any great dislocation of parts. Let us assume, then, that smaller ones are possible. Now in many totally irregular patterns, small dislocations of parts would not make them any more regular, and therefore there is no reason why under these conditions they should occur. But this argument guides us to a new experiment: make our objective patterns such that small dislocations would make the figure more regular. When you look uncritically at Fig. 13 so as to see it as a whole, you will see a figure which is not quite a circle but very nearly so. In reality it is a polygon with 12 corners, and not an entirely regular one, since only four of the central angles are exactly 30°, the others all slightly less or more. Here slight dislocations of parts in the right direction will produce a much more regular organization, and here indeed these dislocations occur; you see a regular figure.

Fig. 13

Another way of demonstrating the same effect would be to make our spot very nearly, but not quite, a square so that, let us say, the two lower angles are of 89° only, the two upper of 91°. Such a figure will look like a square as long as one does not scrutinize it very carefully.

Demonstrations of the effectiveness of the internal organizing forces like the last one occur at practically every moment of our lives. We are surrounded by rectangular things which look to us rectangular. Even when we disregard the fact of perspective distortion, each one of these cases is a point in hand: for what real rectangle is a mathematically exact rectangle? The deviations will, as a rule, be considerably smaller than in our last figure, but they are there, and yet we see perfect rectangles. Now it will be objected to this argument that in the cases of everyday life the differences between the angles are so small as to be subliminal. But what does this objection prove? That two angles, say one of 90° and one of 90.5°, are subliminally different means that they will look alike, but it does in no way imply that they must both look like right angles, as they actually do; as far as the facts of threshold go, they might both look just the tiniest bit obtuse. Therefore the objection is no objection at all, and the fact that we see rectangles everywhere is due to the fact that the true rectangle is a better organized figure than the slightly inaccurate one would be, and that only a very slight dislocation is necessary to change the latter into the former.

But we can demonstrate the internal forces of organization under conditions of strong external forces in still another manner. Instead of producing actual distortions these forces may be made to produce completions and in that way interfere with the external forces. Fig. 14 may be seen as a very irregular form but also as two identical and symmetrical forms, one partly upon the other. In the second case, lines appear indicated in the seen form to which no changes of stimulation correspond. Therefore the unifying forces which are produced by the homogeneous stimulation of the whole dark area are overcome by segregating forces which arise from the unification of well-shaped figures, each one of the two figures being of a better shape than the one irregular figure with homogeneous colouring. It is easy to shift the relative position of the two figures so as to make it practically impossible to see them as two, and that happens when the one figure is simpler than in our pattern or when the protruding part of one of them is not a characteristic part of a part-figure.

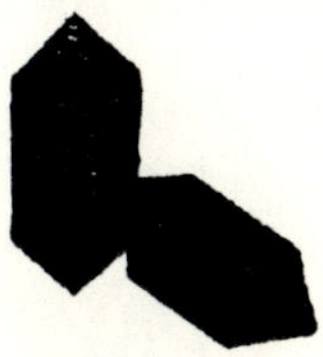

Fig. 14

External Forces Weak. And now let us turn to the evidence which has been accumulated in experiments in which the external organizing forces were reduced in strength. A number of different methods were used for this purpose, (1) short time of exposure, (2) low intensity, (3) small size, (4) after-images. The result has been the same throughout: simple, well-balanced figures are perceived when irregular figures are actually exposed. A few words about each of these methods. Lindemann exposed figures for 20 σ several times in succession and asked his subjects after each exposure to make a drawing of what they had seen. Fig. 15 shows a series of such drawings, the last being the one actually exposed, the others successive reproductions. The two next, Figs. 16 and 17, are taken from an article by Granit (1921), who used a method similar to Lindemann's except that he did not ask for consecutive drawings. The first of them shows the original and a drawing made by an 11-year-old child.

The second requires a word of comment. Here the original is not a single figure produced by a single inhomogeneity, a spot, but by a pattern of dashes. Although we shall discuss the process of organization occurring under these conditions a little later, we include this

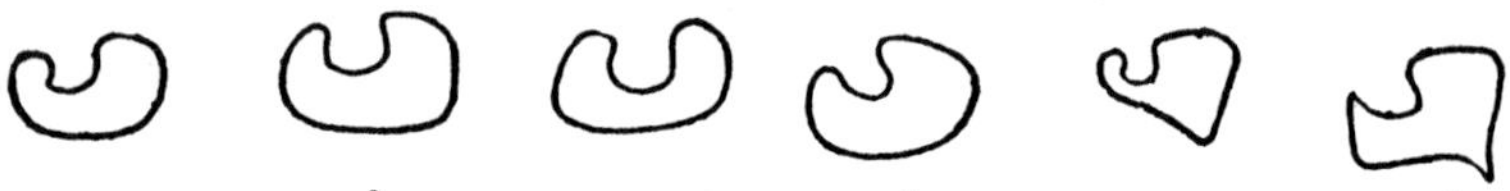

a b c d e f

Fig. 15

and similar examples from other investigators in the present discussion because, from the point of simplification of form, these examples are identical with the others. Our figure represents the original and two reproductions by two different adults.

The simplification is as clear in Granit's as in Lindemann's cases. Lindemann employed still another method in order to prove the greater stability of simple forms under conditions of short exposure, by exposing a circle and an ellipse in such a way that parts of these figures were exposed for different time intervals. Under these conditions the ellipse was deformed, assuming, for instance, the shape of an acorn, while the circle was either not affected at all, or, when the difference in exposure times was too great, disintegrated into two parts.

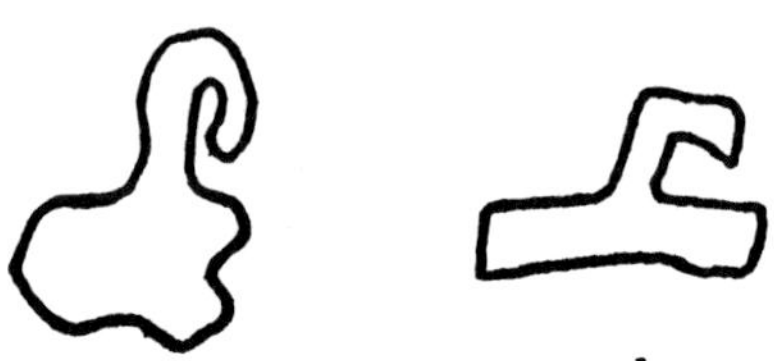

a b

Fig. 16

Lastly we recall Hartmann's experiment described above in which a figure was given two exposures separated by a short interval and the total exposure time measured which just made the figure appear unitary and without flicker. It was found that a stimulus pattern which could be perceived in two different shapes fused more readily when the perceived shape was the simpler of the two possible ones. In the light of our present knowledge and in conformity with our previous conclusions we can interpret this by saying that the internal stresses in the simpler figure were smaller than in the less simple one, and that this reduced internal stress facilitates the fusion of two processes into one process.

An experiment in reduced intensity was made as early as 1900 by Hempstead in Titchener's laboratory: the figures were projected on a moderately illuminated screen, and an episcotister with a variable opening rotated between the lantern and the screen. By gradually increasing the opening of the episcotister the figures were made more and more clear. With the smallest opening no figure at all was seen; when it began first to appear, it was strongly deformed compared with the stimulus pattern, being simpler, more symmetrical, with rounded instead of pointed corners, gaps closed, and even lines which were demanded by the general shape but absent in the stimulus filled in. Wohlfahrt, who worked with figures which were at first reduced in size almost to invisibility and then gradually made larger, found quite similar results; he stresses the phenomenal instability which appeared as a direct observable property of the figures; they appeared charged with internal forces which ever and anon would lead to actual jerks and jumps within them.

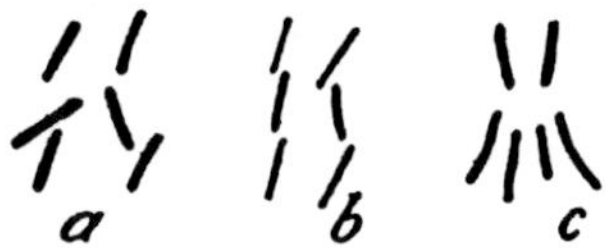

Fig. 17

All these experiments amply confirm our expectations. With weak external organizing forces the internal ones are strong enough to produce considerable dislocations which lead to more stable shapes. These same forces can even produce new material processes if thereby the figures become more stable; new lines may be added, a phenomenon which we shall study with some detail a little later.

We turn now to the after-image experiments. The after-image occurs when the stimulus is removed, and, in the simplest case, a homogeneous surface is substituted for it. It must be explained by forces which arise from the effects of the originally occurring processes in the nervous system. One might think of reversible chemical processes, material having been decomposed, and the products of this decomposition now recombining themselves to form the original substance by a reverse process. At any rate, the forces are entirely within the organism, their place is no longer impressed by outside agencies, and therefore they are more free to rearrange themselves. An old observation described by Goethe, which everyone can repeat, confirms this conclusion: the after-image of a square will gradually lose its sharp corners and become more and more circular.

Still more significant are experiments performed by H. Rothschild because, in these experiments, the occurrence of an after-image itself depended upon the fact whether it made a good shape or not. Instead of using surface figures he used contour figures for his patterns. If such contour figures were simple they produced very good after-images; as a matter of fact, the after-images were improvements on the original, inasmuch as all slight irregularities would disappear. If, on the other hand, the lines formed no simple shape, the after-image would either be a better shape or several of the lines would not appear in the after-image at all. The first is proved by an experiment with two parallel lines arranged as in Fig. 18. If both lines appeared in the after-image, their displacement in regard to each other was greatly reduced, so that they formed two

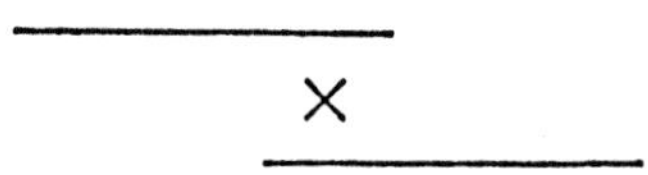

Fig. 18

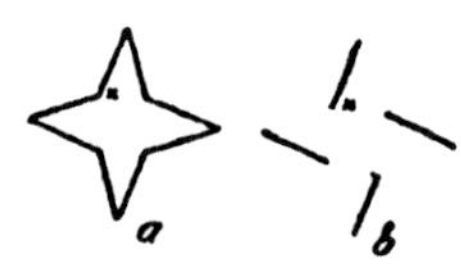

Fig. 19

sides of an incomplete rhomb. Frequently enough, however, the two lines did not appear simultaneously, but alternated with each other; and this brings us to the second possibility of which the next figures are a still better example. While Fig. 19*a* gave a clear and complete after-image, Fig. 19*b* did not. Here either only the line that lay closest to the fixation point, marked in our figures by x, appeared, or two lines came in alternation, and yet the four lines of Fig. *b* are identical with four lines of Fig. *a*.

These experiments, then, prove the influence of shape, and thereby the operation of the internal forces of organization on the total organization process.

External Forces Reduced to Zero. (1) *Experiments on the Blind Spot.* The anatomical structure of our eye permits us to go even a step further and to reduce the external forces to absolute zero. At a distance of about 13° from the fovea on the nasal side lies the blind spot, an area practically, if not entirely,[5] insensitive to light. This spot has a somewhat irregular shape, its horizontal extent is about 6°, its greatest vertical extent slightly more. The fact that even in monocular vision no hole in our phenomenal space appears has intrigued physiologists and psychologists for a long time, and many experiments have been made to find out what exactly is seen in the

[5] For experiments which seem to prove that the blind spot is not absolutely insensitive, see A. Stern, N. Feinberg, and H. Helson (1929).

region of the blind spot. The theoretical interpretation of the experiments suffers frequently from the implicit assumption, a special case of the constancy hypothesis, that what happens under a particular set of conditions must happen under all conditions. Without this assumption it is not difficult to bring order into the great variety of experimental data. For our purposes it is sufficient to recall one experiment which goes back to Volkmann (1853) and Wittich (1863). A cross is viewed in such a way that its centre falls into the blind spot while the arms stretch well into the sensitive region of the retina. Under these conditions the complete cross is seen, and when the two arms are of different colour the centre appears in the colour of either of the two arms, preferably in that of the horizontal. A figure in which the blue vertical arm passes over the red horizontal one is a good example, for the centre here appears red, although it is objectively blue. If one turns the figure so that the blue arm is horizontal, the centre will appear blue. The superiority of the horizontal arm can be overcompensated if one makes the vertical arm relatively longer.

What is the meaning of these results? The very first experiment reveals that the area of the psychophysical process is larger than that of the stimulated area. Therefore, what happens in this part of the psychophysical field which is not affected by direct stimulation, cannot depend upon external forces of organization at all but must be entirely determined by the internal forces of organization obtaining between those field events which are aroused by direct stimulation. Such field events, then, as are symbolized in Fig. 20, where the blank centre corresponds to the unexcited area of the blind spot, are not in equilibrium, but, owing to the fact that no external forces determine what is to happen in their centre, they can and will produce a complete "cross-organization" in which equilibrium is attained. If the two arms are of different colour, then the horizontal arm will determine the colour of the centre because this arm, falling in part on retinal areas which are more central and therefore more functionally efficient, will be better organized, look clearer, than the vertical one. Possibly there are other reasons for the dominance of the horizontal; however that may be, this dominance may be overcome by making the vertical more impressive in other respects. The organization of the centre is, then, dependent upon the forces of the parts outside; we have, in this case, isolated the internal forces of organization.

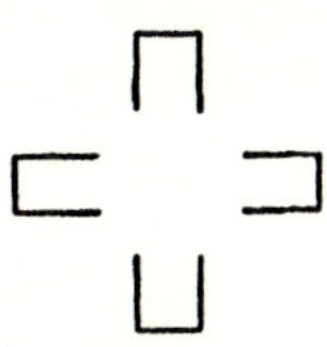

Fig. 20

(2) *Experiments with Hemianopics.* Experiments on the blind spot have one drawback; its location is so peripheral that objects seen in its neighbourhood are never very clearly structured. The familiar inferiority of the periphery of the retina in comparison with the centre is an inferiority of organization, combined, as any other inferiority of organization, with inferior colour vision. Therefore it would offer many advantages if we could perform similar experiments at the centre of vision where no such lack of clarity makes exact observation difficult. This possibility is supplied by certain pathological cases, mostly due to brain injuries, in which one half of the field of vision becomes totally blind. Many such cases of hemianopsia have been carefully investigated, but apparently it was Poppelreuter (1917) who discovered first that such completions of figures as had been observed in the blind spot could be demonstrated more easily in the blind half of an hemianoptic field of vision. I shall report here some experiments of Fuchs's which corroborated Poppelreuter's findings, but gave them an interpretation which was then (1921) entirely new, the interpretation which we have given above for the effects in the blind spot. Experiments with hemianoptics, if they are to reveal the effect, must be made with short exposures, because otherwise the patients move their eyes and thereby destroy the effect. With many, though not with all,[6] hemianoptic patients, phenomena such as are brought to light by our blind spot experiments appear. We choose a patient for whom on both eyes the left side of the field of vision is invisible, that is, for whom a test object is visible in no part of the space to the left of his line of regard, and we expose to him, tachistoscopically, a full circle whose centre he fixates. Then the patient reports that he has seen a full circle. Since, however, only the right half of the real circle can have anything to do with his perception of the circle, we may as well remove the left half and the effect will remain the same. The same experiment can be repeated with a few other figures, like square, ellipse, star. Only with an eight-armed star, however, was it possible to expose as little as one half; with other figures, more than one half had to be exposed if the patient was to see the whole; thus of a square three fourths and even more had to be shown.

Now these figures are both simple and familiar. Therefore, the completion might be due either to their simplicity or to their familiarity. Only if the first were true would these experiments

[6] The reason why not all hemianoptics show completions of the type described in the text cannot be given here.

prove the influence of shape on organization; if familiarity were the decisive factor, our explanation would, at least for these cases, have to be abandoned. Fuchs's results, however, decide quite unambiguously in favour of the first alternative. Figures less simple than the ones mentioned first, however familiar by previous acquaintance and however much practised in special experiments, were never completed in the slightest. Letters, words, pictures of a dog, a face, a butterfly, an inkwell, and similar ones were tried with the same negative success. The patients recognized every one of these objects but reported that they had not been complete.

Thus these experiments of Fuchs's gave a perfect proof for spontaneous organization in simple shapes, a proof which at that time was of enormous value to gestalt theory.

The Generality of Our Conclusions. A Word About Induction. After having established unit formation and shape as dynamic aspects of organization we can now trace them in new conditions of stimulation. Our present condition of two different homogeneous areas, one enclosed by the other, is an experimental artifact, as much almost as our first condition of entirely homogeneous stimulation. And yet both artifacts have supplied us with very important insights into the factors effective in organization. The question might here be raised, how far the results obtained under these artificial conditions can be generalized. We cannot here adequately discuss the universal problem of induction, the problem how we can ever be justified in asserting from the knowledge of a limited number of cases propositions about all possible cases. But a few words with regard to our own procedure will be in place. From the analysis of a small number of cases we have concluded that at a boundary line between two different stimulations forces of segregation and unit formation arise. In our cases the boundary line divided two homogeneous areas. Are we then justified in expressing our conclusion as we have just done without any reference to this special condition? To decide this question we must first clarify what the difference between the general and the specified proposition is. It may seem as though they were one and the same proposition, different only in their claim of validity, the first general, the second particularized. But in reality they are two different assertions. The first says: abrupt discontinuity of stimulation produces segregating and unifying forces. If this is true, it does not matter what the areas at either side of the discontinuity are otherwise. The second, and modified, on the contrary, says: *homogeneous* areas of different quality will at their boundary line produce such forces. And that means: the mere abrupt discontinuity of stimulation is *not* the sufficient cause of these forces, as the first proposition claims; it is discontinuity with something else that is responsible for their arousal. The question, which originally seemed to be merely a question of generality, has turned into a question of truth. Either the first proposition is true and then it is general, or it is not. Induction, i.e., the procedure of producing more empirical evidence, does not, therefore, consist in increasing the number of cases in which a certain proposition is true, but in deciding whether an explanation of case *a* is true by examining case *b*. Again, in terms of our experiments: if discontinuities between inhomogeneous areas do not produce the effects which we have found in our experiments with homogeneous ones, then our original conclusion was wrong; if they do, it is right, and as such universal. It is hardly necessary to say that the latter is true. An ink blot is by no means a perfectly homogeneous area, and yet it has its unity and shape because of the discontinuity at its boundary.

POINTS AND LINES AS STIMULI. (1) POINTS

We shall then apply our principles to some other cases, finally to such as abound in our normal experience. We begin by modifying our last condition, one area of uniform stimulation enclosed in another, without alteration of its character, by reducing the size of the enclosed area, first in one, then in both, dimensions. The first procedure leads us to lines, straight or curved, the second to mere points. The last is that condition which older theories have taken as the simplest case, as we have previously explained (see above, p. 110). It appears now as a special case, a case which would have been a bad case to start from; for a seen point, though geometrically it may be a very small circle or square, has phenomenally no shape at all. It is just a point. Therefore, in using the point as our standard case we should have overlooked the rôle of shape in perception, as traditional psychology has done. In considering the point as a special case of a more general condition, we do not only, however, avoid this mistake, we also gain a new positive insight into the processes of organization. Single points are unstable structures which tend to disappear.

Attitudes. Moreover, frequently enough their appearance requires definite attitudes on the part of the observer. One may look at a white sheet of paper for a long time unaware of a point on it, and only when one becomes suspicious and examines the paper carefully will one discover it. What does this mean? Without a critical attitude the inhomogeneity of stimulation corresponding to the point was not sufficient to break the homogeneity of the well-defined unit in the visual environment. It required a new factor, an attitude, to bring the point into existence. Had the inhomogeneity been greater in size it would have enforced the appearance of a visible object without a special attitude. Thus we learn two new facts. In the first place, we find the field organization under certain circumstances dependent upon attitudes, i.e., forces which have their origin not in the surrounding field at all, but in the Ego of the observer, a new indication that our task of investigating the surrounding field alone is somewhat artificial, and that we shall understand its organization completely only when we study the total field which includes the Ego within its environment.

Why Points Are Unstable. In the second place we must raise the question why single points are so unstable, why they may remain invisible. Formulated in this way, the question can meet only spurious answers, like those given by an older generation of psychologists who would have explained this fact by the hypothesis of the non-noticed sensations (see Chapter III). But the inadequacy of this explanation is quite evident in our case. When we fail to see the point, we see a homogeneous surface instead; i.e., if it is a black point on a white surface we see white when we fail to notice the point. This, the hypothesis of the non-noticed sensations fails to explain, for *not* to notice something black is not equivalent to noticing something white. We said just now that our question was badly formulated. Our last proposition gives us a clue as to how to formulate it better. Instead of asking why we do *not* see something, viz., the point, we should ask why we see something else, viz., the homogeneous surface, instead. We can fall back for our answer on the Wertheimer-Benussi contrast experiment described above. There we saw how a strongly unified whole resists forces which would make it inhomogeneous as to colour (see pp. 134 f.). In our present case there exists a force to break the uniformity of the surface, and if it does not accomplish this result, this failure must be due to other and stronger forces, those which make the uni*fied* area also uni*form*. These latter forces have their origin in the homogeneous coloration of the entire unitary surface in which the point is the only inhomogeneity. Around the point homogeneous processes occur in close proximity, all over the rest of the surface in contiguity. As we shall see very soon, proximity of equal processes produces the same kind of forces as contiguity. Therefore the unifying forces must be very strong in our case, and the single inhomogeneity will often not be strong enough to overcome them without an added force.

One conclusion of our discussion is that to see a point is not a primitive but a high grade achievement. Only in specially developed systems will such a slight inhomogeneity be capable of producing articulation; in others it will give rise to a simple homogeneous field.

(2) LINES

We turn now to the consideration of lines. Ordinary lines, whether straight or curved, appear as lines and not as areas. They have shape, but they lack the difference between an inside and an outside and are in that respect another special case of our general one. Geometrically, each straight line that we draw is a rectangle; psychologically, it is not. Shape, on the other hand, is a very important characteristic of lines, an assertion which we shall prove by experimental evidence a little later.

Closed Contour Figures. The consideration of lines, however, introduces a new point of view. If a line forms a closed, or almost closed, figure, we see no longer merely a line on a homogeneous background, but a surface figure bounded by the line. This fact is so familiar that unfortunately it has, to my knowledge, never been made the subject of a special investigation. And yet it is a very startling fact, once we strip it of its familiarity. Therefore, we want a functional proof for our claim that a figure surrounded by contours is an entity different from the field outside the contours, which in all other respects produces the same stimulation. We possess methods by which a difference between a contour figure and its surroundings could be established, but these methods have not been applied to our problem. We might measure the threshold of a small figure produced either inside or outside the contour of our original figure, e.g., by projecting such a figure on the contoured surface and having an episcotister between the lantern and the surface, an apparatus like that employed by Hempstead (see above, p. 143). If then the little figure required a greater episcotister opening in order to become visible inside than outside the contour, we should have proved a greater cohesiveness of the enclosed area as compared with its surroundings, which would make it more difficult to produce a new figure on it. Unfortunately this experiment has never been made, although from two similar experiments, one by Gelb and Granit and the other by Granit, our assumed result seems predictable.

The Dynamic Causes of Contour Figures. But our main problem appears when we accept this difference as a real one. For we want to know the causes which separate not only the contour from the rest of the field, but at the same time the enclosed figure from its surroundings. Our principle of discontinuity certainly does not explain it. For the discontinuity between the contour and the surface on which it is drawn is the same in either direction, towards the inside and the outside. From our old principle we can only explain why we see lines as lines, i.e., as units segregated from the rest, but not the case which concerns us now, viz., when we see the area enclosed by a line, or a pattern of lines, segregated from the rest of the field and not in the same way segregated from the contour. Although discontinuity of stimulation still has a segregating effect and in so far is in harmony with our law, this segregation is asymmetrical. What is the reason of this asymmetry?

Factor of Closure. Unfortunately this question has not been treated. But since a mere profession of ignorance might raise some doubt in the minds of the readers as to the validity of our general principle, we shall try to point out some factors which might possibly explain the phenomenon. The first point we would raise is the fact that closed, or almost closed, lines or patterns of lines have this peculiarity, whereas it is lacking in unclosed ones. This seems to indicate that the process of organization depends upon the properties of its result, in strict accordance with the general law of prägnanz. Closed areas seem to be self-sustaining, stable organizations, a conclusion which will be reached independently later on the basis of special experiments.

Factor of Good Shape. Secondly, we might try to find out whether there are closed lines or patterns of lines which will more readily be seen as mere lines than others. Although no experiments have been made to decide this point, I am inclined to believe that such differences exist, and that, e.g., a circle will be more easily seen as a mere line than a triangle, the latter appearing as a triangular surface rather than as three lines meeting each other at their terminal points. If this is true, we might attempt to connect this fact with our law of good shape. The circle is a perfectly good figure as a line. Each piece of it contains the principle of the whole. Not so the triangle, where no small piece demands to be continued in such a way that a triangle results. On the contrary, each part of each side will by itself demand a continuation in its own direction, the three corners being breaks in this mode of continuation. As lines, then, the contours of a triangle are not "simple," and therefore, we may tentatively conclude, not stable. Contrariwise the surface of a triangle, particularly if it is an isosceles or an equilateral one, is simple, possesses symmetry, and the reason for the segregation of the whole area may well be this symmetry, which should be accompanied by stability.

Briefly, then, we propose as a tentative hypothesis that the contour bounds a figure rather than segregating itself as a line from the rest of the surface, because this is the better, the more stable organization.

With this explanation we do not introduce a new principle. For we have seen before how factors of shape, as factors of stability, will organize a field against the mere effects of discontinuity of stimulation. Nevertheless I should be the last to be satisfied with my hypothesis. Not only does it, as yet, lack experimental evidence, but it is not explicit enough, it contains no statement about the actual forces along the contour line and their asymmetrical function.

Organizations Produced by Line Patterns. But we must let the matter rest at that. The fact remains that areas can be unified and segregated from the rest of a homogeneous field by mere closed lines. And this fact helps us to study the factor of shape in new ways. We shall now consider the specific principles according to which line patterns produce organization, line patterns which are still special cases of our general one: the field divided up into two different parts, each in itself homogeneous or practically homogeneous. Any one of the patterns to be discussed now fulfils this condition; the field consists of a continuous white part, the ground of the page, and a continuous black part, the lines. All these patterns might be produced by first making a large black spot and then removing some of the black.

Our question is: Given a certain line pattern, what figures shall we see? What are the general principles that govern this relation? Two papers from the Berlin laboratory contain a wealth of material, one as an integral part of a study devoted to a different problem by Gottschaldt (1926), the other, directly concerned with our problem, by Kopfermann. We shall choose our examples from the latter.

When our line pattern is such that it simply separates one part of the surface from the rest, no new problem arises. We shall now consider patterns such in which the separated area itself contains lines which divide it geometrically into two or more smaller areas. What shall we see? We have come across this same problem already under simpler conditions, when we dealt not with line-, but with surface-figures. If the enclosed homogeneous area had a special shape it would appear not as one figure but as two overlapping ones (see Fig. 14, p. 141).

Problem of Unum and Duo. Taking this case as a starting point we can ask the question: When will an outline figure be seen as one, with lines in its interior, and when as two or more? Figs. 21 and 22 give examples for either case; in the first, one sees a rectangle with a line passing through it, in the second two adjoining hexagons. The reason is clear: in the first the total figure is a better figure than either of the two part figures, whereas the opposite is true in the second. Moreover, in the first figure, the upper and lower side of the rectangle are continuous straight lines, while these same straight lines have to be broken up if the two irregular quadrangles are to be seen.

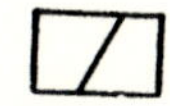

Fig. 21

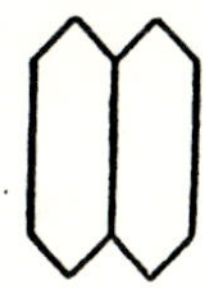

Fig. 22

Good Continuation. The first factor we have already encountered; the second would mean that, as we have also pointed out previously, a straight line is a more stable structure than a broken one, and that therefore organization will, *ceteris paribus,* occur in such a way that a straight line will continue as a straight line. We may generalize thus: any curve will proceed in its own natural way, a circle as a circle, an ellipse as an ellipse, and so forth. This aspect of organization has been called the law of good continuation by Wertheimer (1923). We shall meet with many examples of it in actual organizations. Here we add another one, in Fig. 23, taken from Bühler (1913), in which the external forces prevent the good continuation. The result is an esthetically unpleasant impression, because the proper continuation of the four semicircles is interrupted.

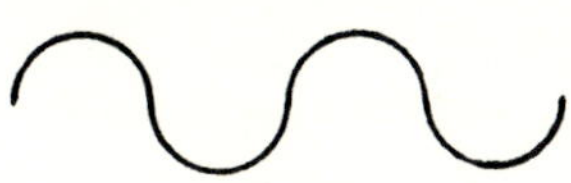

Fig. 23

If in a line pattern the "unum" and the "duo" organization are equally good with regard to shape of the areas and continuation of the lines, is there a preference for either of these? Kopfermann thinks there is, in favour of the unum, a preference for a single all-enclosed figure, for an all-enclosing contour. However, her figures are all such that the other factors, notably that of good continuation, enter in favouring the unum, so that she has not proved her claim. As a matter of fact it is at least extremely difficult, if not impossible, to produce

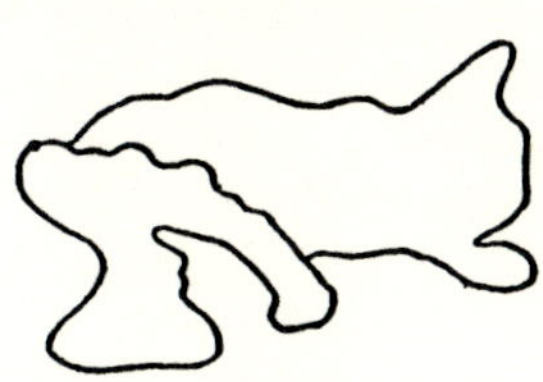

Fig. 24

such patterns as will fulfil our conditions (see Fig. 24), and the result with the best of them is very ambiguous. I am, therefore, not sure whether such a factor exists or not.

Duo-Organization. Our distinction of unum- and duo-organization, even if we include within the latter the cases where more than two figures are seen, does not do full justice to the variety of actual

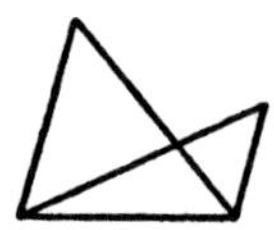

Fig. 25

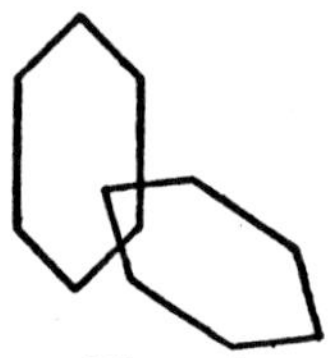

Fig. 26

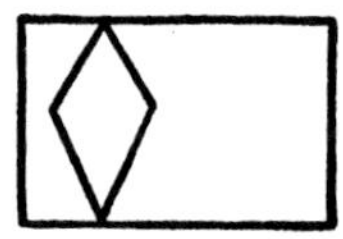

Fig. 27

organizations. On the one hand, most duo-formations have at the same time a unum-quality, and on the other the duo-formation may be of various kinds. The duo-figure of the two adjoining hexagons (Fig. 22), e.g., has at the same time a definite whole-character; so has Fig. 25, although it appears as two partially overlapping triangles. The unum and the duo of an organization may be in perfect harmony with each other, indeed such a harmony can be achieved in an indefinite variety of ways. At the one extreme we

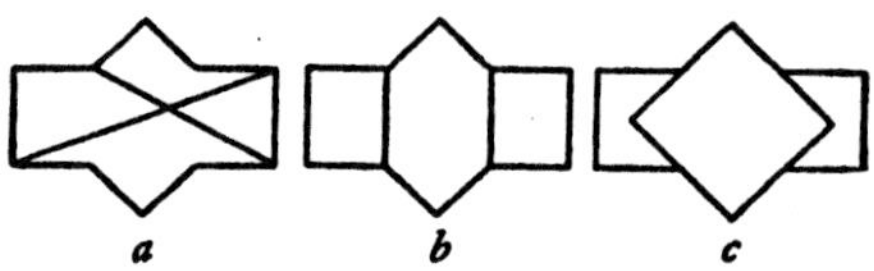

Fig. 28

have dominance of the unum, the duo being perfect parts of the whole, as in a figure 8. At the other extreme we have strong dominance of the duo, the unum being the more or less fortuitous combination of the parts as in Fig. 26, our two preceding examples (Figs. 22 and 25) lying somewhere between them. The duo itself can be of various kinds. We distinguish two notable cases, (a) exemplified by Fig. 22, in which the two parts are co-ordinated, (b) exemplified by Fig. 27, where one figure lies "on top" of another. This case will be taken up at greater length in the next chapter. Fig. 28 shows how one and the same outline pattern can be made by internal lines to appear either as unum (Fig. 28*a*), or as duo (a) (Fig. 28*b*), or finally as duo (b) (Fig. 28*c*). Good shape and continuation explain all these cases.

THE EMPIRICIST'S OBJECTION. We could consider our experimental proof of the effectiveness of our organizing factors as amply sufficient, had we not to contend with the vested interests of an old theory which claims to explain all our facts as well as we do, but without the assumption of all these different organizing forces. I mean the empiristic theory which would say: we see in an individual case such figures as we have frequently seen before; the stimulus conditions of our present cases are sufficiently similar to the stimulus conditions of previous and frequently repeated cases to produce the same results. Perfectly true, if two alternative theories are proposed for one and the same effect, a decision between them must be reached by weighing their relative merits against each other and, if possible, by crucial experiments.

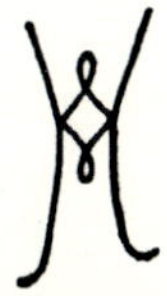

Fig. 29

Let us then weigh the claims of the empiristic theory with regard to our problems of perceptual organization. Look at the series of three figures, Fig. 28. An empiricist would have to say: "We see in *a* the decagon with two lines in its interior because we have seen such a figure more frequently than the four other irregular small figures; in *b* we see two oblongs with a hexagon between them because they have been seen more frequently than the decagon, which was seen in the first figure, and finally in *c* both square and oblong have been seen more frequently than the decagon and are therefore seen now." The explanation seems plausible. But in 1923 Wertheimer met such an objection by constructing figures like Fig. 29, in which the initials of his name, M W, are concealed, and Köhler has published a number of other figures (1925 and 1929).

EXPERIMENTAL DISPROOF OF THE EMPIRISTIC THEORY. More systematic proof was furnished by Gottschaldt (1926). In his experiments the subjects were presented with 5 simple line patterns (*a* patterns) which were projected on a screen for 1 second each, with an interval of 3 seconds between two exposures. They were told to learn these figures as best they could, so that when tested later they would remember them and be able to draw them on paper. After a certain number of presentations, different for two groups of subjects, new patterns (*b* patterns) were shown for 2 seconds each; the subjects were told that the learning experiments were to be continued later, meanwhile they were being shown a new set of pictures which they were merely to describe, mentioning if anything particular struck them about these pictures. Now each *b* picture was so constructed that geometrically it contained an *a* picture, but that under normal circumstances the *b* picture would not be seen as containing the shape of the *a* pattern. Fig. 30 gives one example, the most difficult

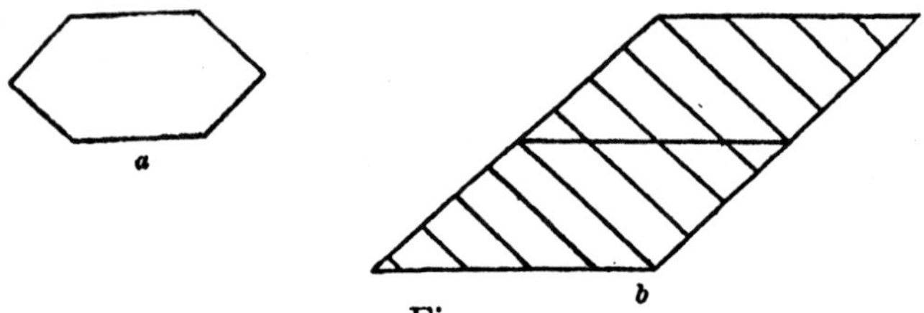

Fig. 30

one in the series. To each *a* figure there corresponded six or seven *b* figures; e.g., to the *a* figure of our last diagram also the much easier *b*, Fig. 31. Now if the empiristic theory were right, practice in seeing the *a* figure should make the *b* figure look like *a* plus something else. In order to test this assumption three subjects were shown the *a* figure three times only and eight subjects 520 times. Of the 3 subjects in the first group 2 saw the *b* figures as new figures on all 30 occasions, and of the 8 subjects of the second group 5 gave the same result. The outcome of this experiment is not changed if one lumps all the subjects of one group together.

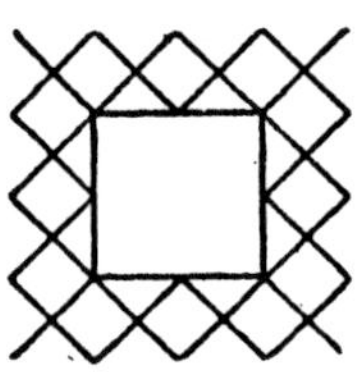

Fig. 31

To do this one has to distinguish a number of different possibilities. (1) The *a* figure would be seen at once when the *b* figure was presented. This happened only once in the 92 experiments of the first group and 4 times in the 242 experiments of the second. (2) It was discovered later either at the end of the exposure or afterwards in the image. 5 such cases occurred in the first and 3 in the second group. (3) The subjects did not really see the *a* but they guessed correctly that it was there, no case in the first group, 5 in the second. There is a (4) in which the subjects guessed at an *a* figure but made a wrong guess, and finally a (5), in which they only saw the *b* figure.

In Table 6 we give in percentages of the total number of cases the combined number of cases 1-3 in which some influence of the *a* figure can be traced and those of cases (4) and (5) where no such influence was apparent.

TABLE 6

(from Gottschaldt)

	3 repet. *92 cases*	*520 repet.* *242 cases*
a has some influence	6.6	5.0
a has no influence	93.4	95.0

The assumption has been disproved. There is absolutely no significant difference between the two groups. The very few cases, moreover, in which an influence of the *a* figure was apparent, cannot be due to mere experience either; first of all they do not increase with an increase of experience, and secondly the subjects who showed that influence were not in an entirely neutral attitude, but expected to find the old figures again, as is evidenced by the wrong guesses made by two of the four subjects concerned.

The conclusion is that experience does not explain why we see a line pattern in the shape in which we see it, but that direct forces of organization, such as we have analyzed, must be the real cause.

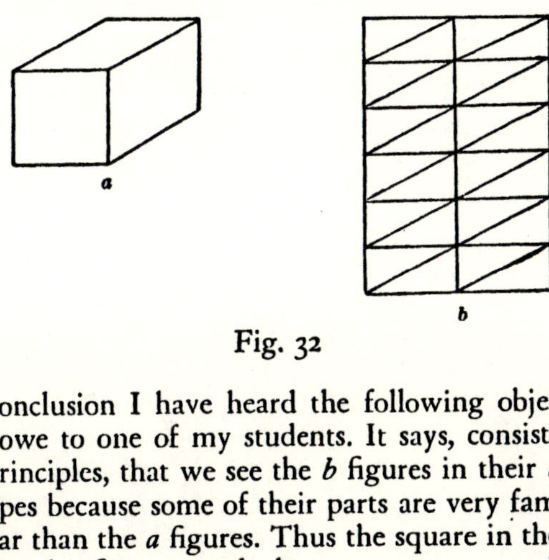

Fig. 32

To this conclusion I have heard the following objections made. The first I owe to one of my students. It says, consistent with the empiristic principles, that we see the *b* figures in their *b* shapes and not as *a* shapes because some of their parts are very familiar figures, more familiar than the *a* figures. Thus the square in the second and the "grill" in the first example have a greater experience behind them than the hexagon of the *a* figure. The first answer to this objection is that it does not explain why the difference between 3 and 520 repetitions of the *a* figure should have made no difference whatsoever for the result. A second point is that not in all cases were shapes of *b* figures more familiar than the shapes of *a* figures as demonstrated by Fig. 32. True enough the simple shapes are as a rule the familiar shapes, a coincidence which makes the empiristic theory so plausible, a coincidence which is, moreover, by no means fortuitous. Naturally if the laws of organization are true laws, we must expect the products of human activity to be simple, since they owe their existence to organized processes; and therefore the simple will be the frequent. Because of this connection between simplicity and familiarity it was of such fundamental importance when Fuchs proved that not the familiarity but the simplicity of certain figures was the cause of their completion (see above, pp. 146 f.). We can add a third point to our answer: Gottschaldt devised an ingenious method for measuring the degree of difficulty which each *b* figure offered to the finding of its *a* figure. Now if the objection were right, those *b* figures which contained the most familiar parts should be the most difficult ones. Nothing of the kind is true. Fig. 31 is much easier than Fig. 30, and yet the square is much more familiar than the grill. And one of the three easiest of Gottschaldt's *b* figures has the shape of a well-known pattern. This objection, clever as it is, cannot, therefore, stand the test of the facts.

The other objection runs like this: there was no experience of *b* figures, the *a* figures when experienced were always in a different setting and one must of course include the "total situation."

The "Total Situation." This argument has the semblance of plausibility because of the term "total situation," which in reality means nothing. For in each "total" situation there are always parts that are relevant to the particular effect we are studying, and some that are not. And thus the term "total situation" obscures the problem. Turn back to our series of figures, Fig. 28 on p. 154, to which we applied the empiristic theory. In this application there was no mention made of total situation, and indeed we could not have seen the decagon, the oblongs, the hexagon and square very often, if at all, in those particular "total situations." The argument rested entirely on the fact that we had seen these figures *per se* more frequently than the other figures whose shape did not appear in those patterns. And the empiristic argument would have to be this, for otherwise it would beg the question. If, for instance, it claimed that we saw the decagon with its internal lines in the first pattern of our series because we had seen this, or similar, patterns before, then we should ask, *Why*

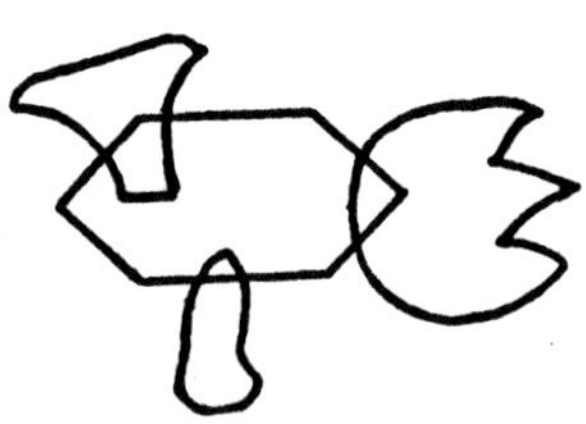

Fig. 33

have we under these stimulus conditions seen just this shape and not the others? In other words, if the empiricist were to argue like this, he would commit what we have called the experience error.

Finally, it is quite easy to produce total situations which are entirely new and which will not in the least interfere with the recognition of the *a* figure. Köhler has given a very good demonstration of this fact in his book (1929, p. 210). Fig. 33 demonstrates the same with a pattern we have frequently used before. If, then, some "total situations" do not (or very little) interfere with the shape of a special part, while others obliterate it completely, there must be some specific factors in those "total situations" responsible for this difference. These factors we have singled out in our laws of spontaneous organization.

Tri-dimensional Organization of Line Patterns. These laws explain even more than the two-dimensional shape we have so far considered. Of the three patterns of Fig. 34, *a*, when presented without *b* and *c*, is a plane figure, a hexagon with diagonals, or a sort

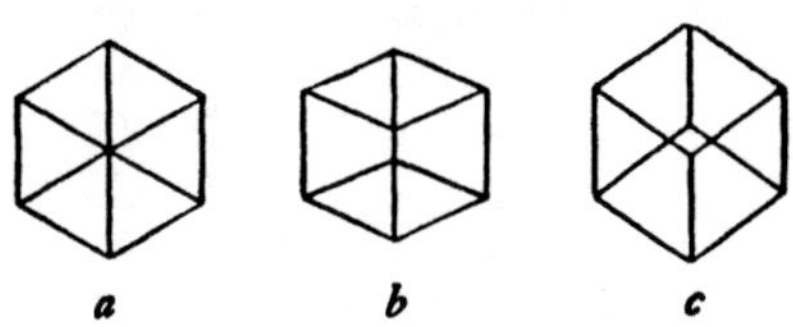

Fig. 34

of cross or star-like figure; Fig. *c*, on the other hand, appears tri-dimensionally as a cube, and *b* can appear either bi- or tri-dimensional: in the former case one sees the pattern of Fig. 35 lying on top of a hexagon, in the latter, it is a cube. All three figures are projections of one and the same wire-edged cube, either of them could therefore be the retinal image of such a cube. A simple application of our laws will show why these different projections have such different effects. On account of both good shape and continuation, *a* as a plane figure is perfectly simple and symmetrical, whereas as a cube the long straight lines are broken up. The opposite is true of *c* where the plane figure is very irregular, without any simple plan, and therefore very hard to see. In *b* the forces are more balanced, both the bi- and the tri-dimensional aspect being regular. The greater symmetry of the cube is in favour of tri-dimensionality, while the continuation of the central vertical line favours bi-dimensionality. For

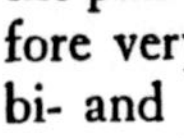

Fig. 35

this reason *b* is more ambiguous than either *a* or *c*. Kopfermann has developed these ideas with a number of other figures; I have tried to show why an empiristic explanation is false, using arguments similar to the last employed in the refutation of the empiristic theory of tri-dimensional shape (1930).

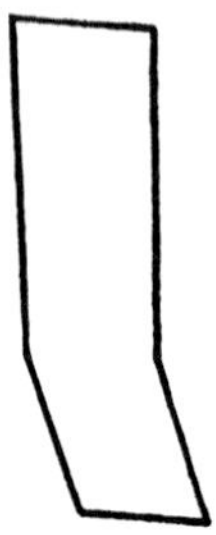

Fig. 36

Perhaps the simplest demonstration of all is the following. Fig. 36 will look like a somewhat distorted oblong. Hold the page against the light [7] and you will see it as *two* surfaces, one in the plane of the paper and the other stretching toward or away from you. Here the introduction of one line into a simple enough figure produces this difference. Without the line the area was unified, with it, it is divided, and the relationship of the parts is better in the tri- than in the bi-dimensional appearance.

Consequences for the Theory of Space Perception. Nativism and Empiricism. These experiments throw a new light on the theory of depth perception. The tri-dimensional aspect of figures like the cube and other perspective drawings has always been explained by experience. Even the nativists who admitted that there was *sensory* depth caused by the disparity of retinal stimulation, the binocular parallax, considered this only as a slender basis on which the structure of our tri-dimensional space, as we actually perceive it, is created by experience. There was no disagreement between nativists and empiricists about the great contribution which experience made to our space perception, the only difference being that the latter denied *any* original depth perception, while the former accepted it as a basis for the rest. The functional point of view in American psychology has accepted this state of affairs, but has added to the obscurity of its theoretical significance. Thus Woodworth speaks of "signs of distance" which are "utilized together in the visual perception of three-dimensional space" (p. 400). While most of these signs are learned, i.e., the results of experience, our author holds it to be "quite possible that some sign of distance, probably the binocular sign, does not have to be learned." This "functionalist" theory of depth is clearly a case of the interpretation theory which we have rejected in our third chapter. The obscurity which it adds arises from the "sign" concept. For we must ask what is the sign and what is the significate. Are both of them given in direct experience? If so, what is, e.g., the binocular sign? If not, what right have we to hypostatize one of them, presumably the sign, as a part of experience and as a sign?

[7] I borrow this method from Bühler.

Organization Theory of Tri-dimensional Space. Against all these theories our hypothesis claims that three-dimensional shapes are matters of organization in the same way as two-dimensional ones, depending on the same kind of laws. We are far from denying the importance of binocular parallax as a cause of tri-dimensionality, but as we shall show later, we shall prove it to be the cause of forces of organization which may either co-operate or conflict with other forces of organization. I should also be very wary in denying that experience has any influence on depth. Only, before we know what experience means, the introduction of experience has no explanatory value, and only when we understand experience as a process of organization itself will it help us in our present problem.

Organizing Forces and Binocular Parallax. For the moment, our main claim is that there are other forces of tri-dimensional organization than binocular parallax, forces that may be stronger than this last factor. Two proofs for this last claim: the first is contained in all our last experiments in which bi-dimensional figures look tri-dimensional. For in all these cases the lack of binocular parallax is a force to organize the visual processes in one plane. For if any parallax has a positive or negative depth value, then the parallax nought has the depth value nought; that is, all parts of the field seen without parallax should appear in one plane. All our drawings have the value zero of binocular parallax, and therefore the fact that they are seen as tri-dimensional shows the strength of the other organizing forces. These forces have to overcome not only the lack of parallax but also that of the other conditions which tend toward organization in one plane. The page on which these figures are drawn is strongly organized as a plane surface, and the lines belong in a way to this surface. And yet they produce tri-dimensional effects. Thus we have in all our examples cases where bi- and tri-dimensional forces [8] conflict. Remove some of the bi-dimensional ones, and the tri-dimensional effect should be stronger. That this simple deduction is true is proved by the well-known fact that perspective drawings look more tri-dimensional when one closes one eye. Nevertheless, a fact also frequently referred to, a perspective drawing, even when viewed monocularly, does not give the same vivid impression of depth as the same drawing if viewed through a stereoscope with binocular parallax. Again this must be so, if our hypothesis is right, for in the stereoscope the tri-dimensional force of the parallax co-operates with the other tri-dimensional forces of

[8] This is an abbreviation for "forces which, alone, would produce bi- or tri-dimensional organization respectively."

organization; instead of conflict between forces, stereoscopic vision introduces mutual reinforcement.

The second proof that binocular parallax can be overcome by other forces of organization was given in special experiments of Kopfermann's. In these experiments different parts of a line pattern

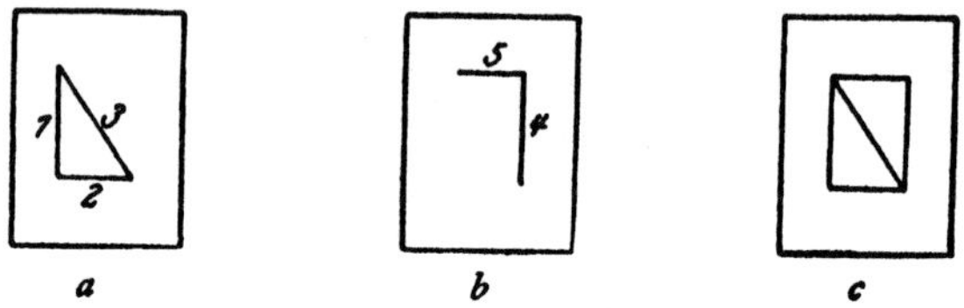

Fig. 37

were objectively presented at different distances by having them drawn on glass plates which were inserted in a box one behind the other at a distance of 2 cm. The observer looked into the box and had to describe what he saw. If each of the plates had a pattern unconnected with those of the others, figures were always seen in their correct relative distances. But if the patterns of the different planes would make one common pattern, this pattern would be dependent upon the forces of organization which we know. If the forces work

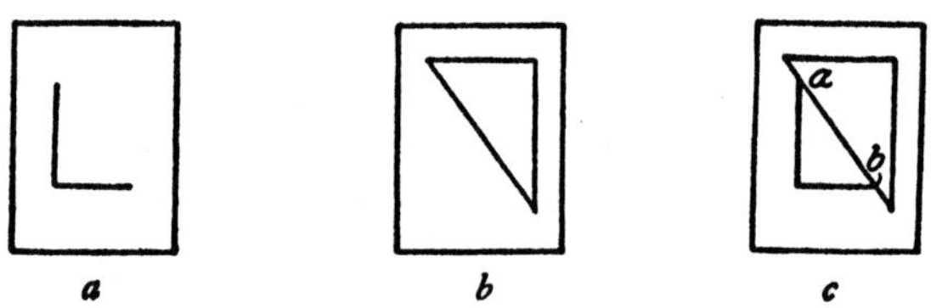

Fig. 38

in the same direction as those due to the parallax, correct depth will be seen, if not, the effect will depend upon the relative strength of the respective forces. In Kopfermann's experiments the patterns were such that the internal organizing forces were stronger than the parallax. We give three examples: In Fig. 37, *a* and *b* are pictures of the two slides presented one behind the other, *c* the figure actually seen. The simplicity of the figure has destroyed the depth effect. In Fig. 38, which is geometrically but little different from the preceding one, the resulting figure is less unified; even as a plane drawing it would lead to a duo, not to a unum, organization. Correspondingly, as a rule, the two parts were seen as one behind the other. Finally the three patterns, *a, b* and *c* of Fig. 39, were always seen as a cube, *d,* i.e., as a tri-dimensional object, the base of the cube being com-

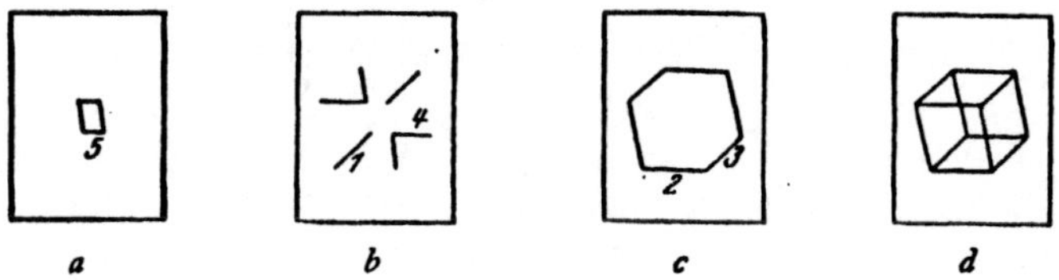

Fig. 39

posed of the lines 1 2 3 4 5, which are distributed over all three glass plates.[9]

"PRIMARY" AND "SECONDARY" CRITERIA OF DEPTH. The theory of tri-dimensionality as a particular form of organization is consistent in itself and with experimental facts. It demands that the difference between primary, "innate," and secondary, empirical, criteria be abandoned in favour of a theory of external and internal forces of organization. All the traditional secondary criteria, like overlapping of shapes, shadows, lack of clearness, and so forth, must be interpreted as factors of organization, not as items of experience in their own right which carry a special meaning. Here we will only point out that even in a pattern like that of Fig. 40, which is an example *par excellence* of the influence of empirical criteria and which corresponds schematically to the impressions which we get from a distant range of mountains, we must find its explanation in terms of direct organization. We actually see in reality, and to some extent in our figure, the partly covered mountains *behind* the nearer ones, although binocular parallax plays no part, the distance being far too great in the case of the real mountains for parallax to become effective.

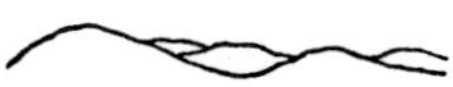

Fig. 40

Our discussion makes us turn back to the beginning of the chapter where we discussed Berkeley's argument against the possibility of seeing depth. We have now become acquainted with a new set of facts to support our criticism. Formerly we saw that without constraining forces produced by inhomogeneities of stimulation the colour in the field of vision will distribute itself in all three dimensions; now we have seen that internal forces of organization may also produce tri- rather than bi-dimensional forms. The second step

[9] This discussion will be continued in Chapter VII.

really follows from the first. For it is by no means evident that all distributions of forces which destroy the homogeneously filled space should transform it into a plane surface. Some distributions will do that, while others will transform it into tri-dimensional bodies.

DISCONTINUOUS INHOMOGENEITIES OF STIMULATION, LINES, AND POINTS

We shall now include in our discussion also such patterns as are no longer continuous, lines and points. These will give us the promised proof of two principles of organization which we have already mentioned, viz., proximity and closure. For a full discussion the reader should turn to Wertheimer's original article (1923) and to Köhler's essays (1925, 1930).

Proximity. The factor of proximity is quite easy to demonstrate. In the patterns of Figs. 41 and 42 the dots and the lines form pairs

Fig. 41

in which spontaneously the nearer ones unite. Indeed one can, particularly if the difference of the distances is not too great, see at will also the other pairs, but never more than one or two at the same time, and the more of such units there are, the more difficult it is to see the more distant ones together, whereas the other pairs gain

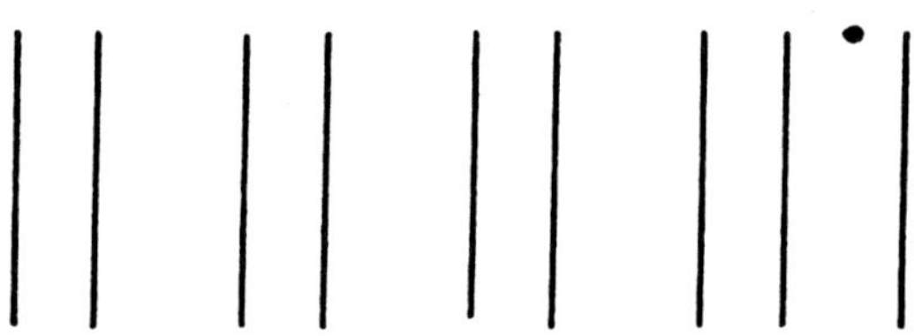

Fig. 42

in stability by multiplication. Furthermore, it is clear that proximity is a relative term; one and the same distance which in one pattern may be an intramembral distance may in another be an intermembral one. Of course there are limits to this law; when the distances become too great, no unification will occur, and the shorter the intramembral distance the more stable will the unit be.

Proximity and Equality. It is not quite so easy, however, to formulate the law of proximity. So far, we have only demonstrated that when the field contains a number of equal parts, those among them which are in greater proximity will be organized into a higher unit. This organization must be considered as real as the organization of a homogeneous spot. Just as we explained the latter by actual forces which hold the uniform area together and segregate it from the rest of the field, we must think of our group formation as due to actual forces of attraction between the members of the group. This is not a mere hypothesis, much less a mere name, for

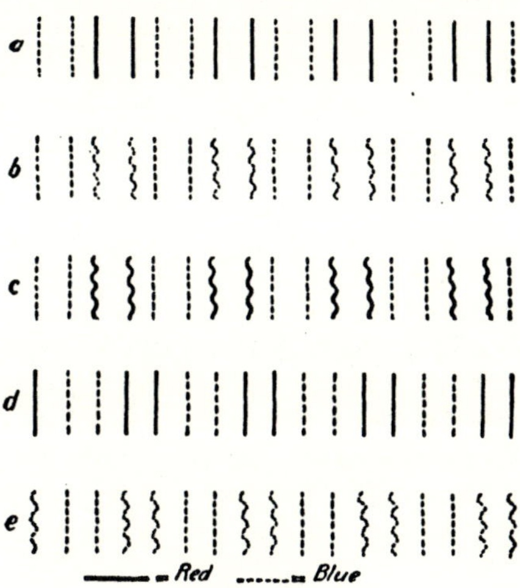

Fig. 43

these forces have demonstrable effects, as we shall see later when we study the reaction of the organism to these forces in the field.

However, our law of proximity is so far dependent upon the equality of the parts in proximity. Even with this limitation it is important enough. But we shall try to see how far we can generalize it beyond this limit. In Fig. 43*a* the principle still determines grouping. We see the groups as composed of one blue and one red line but not of two blue and two red lines respectively.[10] In Fig. 43*b*, however, the result is doubtful. The pattern is more ambiguous; we can see the groups with near and those with equal parts. The former seem slightly to predominate, at least I can see all lines in this grouping rather easily, whereas in the latter I tend to lose either the straight or the sinuous ones. Although, then, the proximity

[10] Since I had to dispense with coloured reproductions, the reader, if he wants to verify the text, must draw these figures for himself according to the patterns of Fig. 43.

still seems to dominate over equality, this preponderance has diminished, owing to the new kind of difference we have introduced, form vs. colour. We find equality of form a stronger factor of organization than equality of colour. In Fig. 43*c* both factors have been combined, and now equality clearly overcomes proximity, the groups are now formed by equal and not by proximal lines. In these three patterns the relative distances have been like 1 to 3. A measurement of the relative strength of these factors would be possible, as Wertheimer has already suggested, by varying these relative distances. If we make them all equal, we isolate the factor of equality. This is done in Fig. 43*d* and *e*, where again *e*, with differences in form, is more stable and less ambiguous than *d* with mere difference in colour.

This discussion seems to demand the following formulation of the laws of proximity and equality: two parts in the field will attract each other according to their degree of proximity and equality. If this statement were true, no attraction, and therefore no grouping, should take place if either of the two factors, proximity or equality, had the value zero. For proximity this is easy to prove, for the degree of proximity, or rather its opposite, distance, can easily be varied quantitatively. We need only remove two field parts sufficiently from each other and the force of attraction will, at least for all practical purposes, vanish. The degree of equality cannot as yet be measured, and therefore it is not possible to decide experimentally whether no grouping will take place when the two field parts are totally different. However, we can limit this last statement. Never was the particular segregated part grouped together with the surrounding ground; all grouping occurred between figures upon the ground. In that respect, then, namely qua figures, there must be equality, if grouping is to appear. This gives a very important determination of the term equality. In so far, at least, equality is on the same footing as proximity; no equality in this respect, no grouping, just as there was none with no proximity.

The purpose of this argument is the claim that proximity qua mere proximity, proximity between events of *any* kind, does not produce forces of organization, but that their arousal and the strength of these forces depend upon the processes that are in proximity. The latter part of this sentence has been proved by our last demonstrations: the organization at constant proximity conditions depended upon the degree of equality and difference between the processes in organization. That the first part is true also, that proximity alone is not a sufficient condition, can be derived from the figure-ground articulation which will be discussed at greater length in the next chapter. If proximity alone were a cause of organization, we should be at odds with all we know about organization in physics. "Wherever an A and B have anything to do with each other in physics, the effect is found to depend upon the properties of A and B in their relation to each other" (Köhler, 1929, p. 280).[11] Thus two bodies attract each other according to their masses, and of course the more, the nearer they are together, but two bodies may be as near to each other as they like without exerting any *electric* forces on each other, if they are electrically neutral. Therefore in our psycho-

Fig. 44

(Solid = red, hatched = blue, see footnote 10, p. 165.)

physical organization, when two heterogeneous parts form a group because of proximity, there must be some aspect in which they are equal and therefore able to influence each other.

As a matter of actual fact we can by mere proximity combine practically any kinds of parts in a group, provided that these parts are sufficiently removed from others. Our Fig. 44 gives one more example. But this does not mean that by mere proximity anything whatever will hang together, but that these parts have qua parts a common property which accounts for their interaction.

A last word about proximity and equality. In Fig. 43 (*a-e*) the alternative groupings were both approximately equal with regard to the ensuing shapes, and the total patterns resulting from either kind of grouping were regular and consistent. How proximity and equality will work when no regular or simple pattern can be the result has not yet been investigated. In this, as in many other respects, our knowledge is still incomplete.

Closure. Let us now turn to closure. We averred in a previous discussion (p. 151) that closed areas were more stable and therefore more readily produced than unclosed ones. We shall prove this by producing closed organization against the factors of proximity and

[11] Köhler's argument is directed against the traditional concept of association, but it applies equally well to our problem of spatial organization. It is well to remember it for our future discussion of association.

of good continuation. Fig. 45, taken from Köhler[12] (1929), exemplifies the first. Predominantly not those vertical lines which are in closer proximity form the groups but those which enclose space, although in Fig. 45 their distance is three times as great as that of the nearer ones, the distance between the ends of the short oblique lines being equal to that of the nearer vertical ones. And in Fig. 46*b* the parts A B C D of Fig. 46*a* are contained, but whereas in *a*, according to good continuation, B is the continuation of A, D of C, in *b* the two closed areas appear as subwholes, so that A is no longer continued by B, nor C by D. That closure does not always win out over good continuation is shown by several patterns in Wertheimer's paper which I shall omit here, where I want to demonstrate the effectiveness of the closure principle.

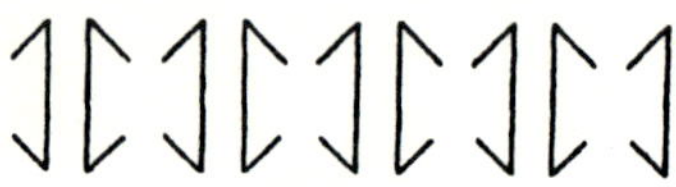

Fig. 45

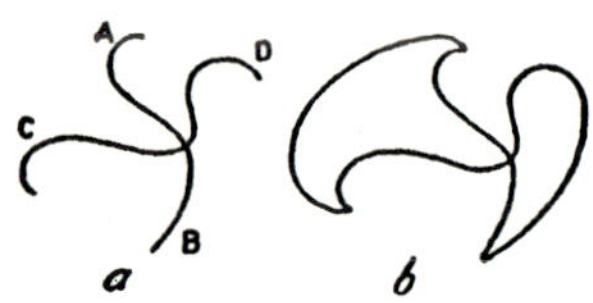

Fig. 46

I take one last example from point-patterns to show that not all closures are equally good, demonstrating at the same time that unit formation and shape are two different aspects of organization. Of the two patterns of Fig. 47, *b* will be familiar, recalling the constellation of the plough, whereas the former will look entirely new. And yet both figures have been constructed by Hertz by connecting the seven points of the plough in different ways. The one, *b*, is that connection which we all make when we see it in the sky, the other is in one respect even simpler, inasmuch as it produces a single closed figure, and yet nobody has ever seen it, because the closed figure is so irregular, while the closed part of the other is very simple.

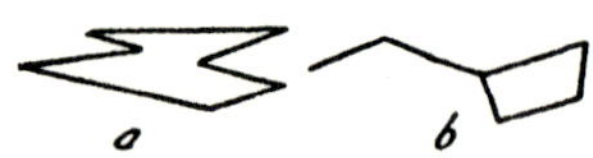

Fig. 47

[12] It has been slightly modified to exclude the factor of good continuation which in Köhler's pattern works in the same direction as closure.

OTHER INHOMOGENEOUS STIMULATIONS

We shall close this discussion by considering some less artificial stimulus conditions. Normally neither entirely homogeneous distributions occur, nor such that different homogeneous areas constitute the whole stimulus pattern. As a rule, the areas between which leaps of stimulation occur are not homogeneous in themselves. We consider two special cases of such inhomogeneities. The simplest is that kind of inhomogeneity where the stimulation is constant in one direction, but varies as a linear function of the distance from a given point in the other dimension, e.g., a graded disk which grows uniformly lighter or darker from the centre to the periphery. As Mach discovered in 1865 such distributions will look uniform provided, we must add, that the area over which they occur give rise to a well-defined unit in our field of vision. In reality two cases must be distinguished; in the first the uniformity is complete, and in this case the seen quality of the area is the same as if the average of the stimulation had been uniformly distributed over it. In the second case the uniformity is not complete but refers to one aspect of the colour only, its quality, and not to another, its "brightness" or "illumination." A white wall in a large room looks white all over, but "darker," "less illuminated," where it is further away from the source of light. Deferring the discussion of this second case to a later chapter, we return to the first. If we divide the area with the uniformly changing stimulation into two or more areas by introducing fine contours, then the uniformity of colour disappears in the whole area and is only retained in the newly formed part areas which now look different from each other, each according to its own average stimulation (Koffka, 1923 a). The same may also be true when the change of stimulation is not uniform; in this case the *rate* of change varies from point to point. Whereas in the first case $i = f(x)$, where i stands for the intensity (or any other well-defined characteristic) of the stimulation, and x for the distance from an arbitrary origin, and $\frac{di}{dx} = const.$, in the second case, not only is $i = g(x)$, but also $\frac{di}{dx} = \varphi(x)$. If then the absolute value of the second derivative $\frac{d^2 i}{dx^2}$ is not too great, the area will still look uniform. Under these conditions the average of the stimulation will again become effective, as I have proved.

But if the change of the rate of change is too great, something new happens, and that is the second case I intend to discuss. To understand it better we shall use the graphic representation of the stimulus distribution which we have introduced in the beginning of this chapter (p. 111). Uniform change is then represented by a straight line inclined towards the *x*-axis, as in Fig. 48*a*, whereas distributions of the second type are exemplified by Figs. 48 *b* and *c*. If we single out a point *p* its stimulation will be the same as the average stimulation in its neighbourhood, when the change of stimulation is constant (Fig. 48*a*). But when the rate of change varies with *x*, this will no longer be true. Thus in Fig. 48*b* point *p* will receive

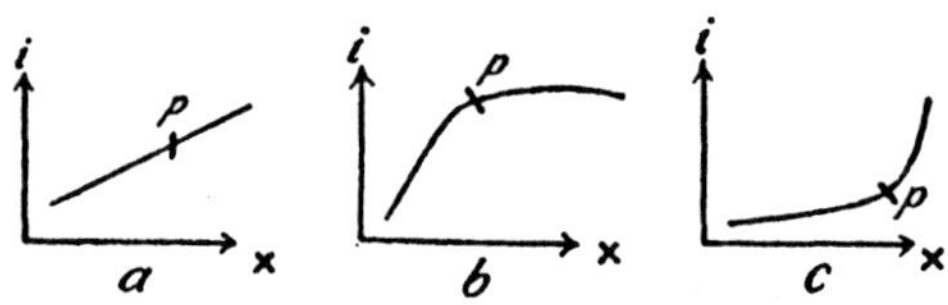

Fig. 48

more stimulation than the average of its surrounding, in Fig. 48*c* less. Under these conditions, provided that the difference between the stimulation of *p* and the average of its neighbourhood is sufficiently great, a curious and significant effect will appear, which Mach discovered almost 70 years ago. When the stimulation of *p* is stronger than the average stimulation of the neighbourhood, a *light* line will appear at *p*, when it is weaker a *dark* line, although in both cases the stimulation is weaker than the stimulation of *p* on the one side, and stronger on the other. When these stimulations are provided by rotating disks, then these lines are naturally rings. Thus the Mach rings prove, as Mach himself pointed out very clearly (1865, 1885), that the local effect is not the result of local stimulation only, but depends upon the stimulus distribution over a large area. We have to amplify Mach's theory in one respect only. Mach considered this effect as an affair of the pure colour sense, and his experiments as a final proof of the physiological theory of contrast as opposed to Helmholtz' psychological theory; as such it appeared in a good many of the older textbooks, while the more modern ones are apt to omit it. But the appearance of a ring, i.e., a new shape within an area, is a matter of organization. From this point of view the problem was taken up by M. R. Harrower and myself (I), and we definitely established the fact that conditions which are favourable for organization of a special shape will produce Mach rings, while these rings will fail to appear or be less marked, when the general circumstances are less favourable to such organization. We have learned from the Liebmann effect that luminosity differences are more powerful in producing segregation than mere colour differences. Therefore Dr. Harrower and I concluded that, if the Mach rings are effects of organization, mere colour changes should not produce them. Thouless had already made a few such experiments which confirmed this conclusion; in a set of rather elaborate experiments we corroborated Thouless' findings and established at the same time the efficacy of the difference between hard and soft colours for the production of Mach rings.

ORGANIZATION AND THE LAW OF PRÄGNANZ. MINIMUM AND MAXIMUM SIMPLICITY

We have now reached a certain stage in our discussion. Organization has been studied under a number of different conditions, and a number of active principles of such organization have been established. It is meet to compare our accomplishments with the introduction of this chapter in which we formulated a guiding principle for our investigation, the law of prägnanz, which related the resulting stationary organizations to certain maximum-minimum principles. As a matter of fact this law has pervaded our whole discussion; we have encountered it in various forms, as unity, uniformity, good continuation, simple shape, and closure. But there remains one point which was mentioned in the beginning and not followed up in the later discussion, viz., the difference between what we called the simplicity of a maximum and a minimum event. We must now envisage our discussion from this point of view and add some more evidence in order to give more substance to our distinction.

Roughly speaking, a minimum simplicity will be the simplicity of uniformity, a maximum simplicity that of perfect articulation. In our examples both kinds have figured; the first kind in after-image experiments and in the other effects of reduced external forces of organization; the second in examples of good shape and continuation. Can we derive a hint as to the causes or conditions which make for either of these two effects? Unfortunately we lack a special systematic investigation of our problem, but we may tentatively derive some conclusions from the facts familiar to us, if we supplement them by a few others. When we look at a portrait photograph, we see a face with its form and expression; but if we try to develop an after-image of it, all we see is a blurred patch. The after-image is much less articulated, much more uniform than the perception, the former shows simplification of the minimum, the latter of the maximum kind. It is, however, not impossible to produce an after-image of a face, but then the original must possess

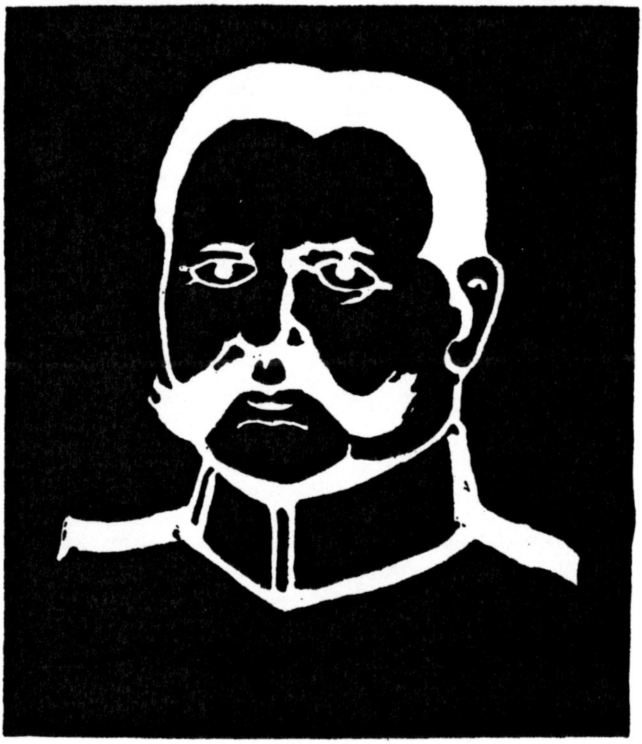

Fig. 49

much stronger contrasts than any ordinary photograph; thus Fig. 49 will yield a very good after-image of President von Hindenburg.

Secondly, look at the pattern of Fig. 50.[18] At a casual glance you will see it as a chaotic jumble of lines. But when you are told that this pattern is a real picture and make an effort to discover it, you will find the face of a good-humoured portly gentleman.

For my last example I return to our discussion of accommodation (p. 119 f.), where we learned to understand this function as a motor

[18] The picture has been taken over, in a slightly simplified form, from Hazlitt.

response in the service of articulation. Now remember an occasion when you were very tired but had to attend an evening lecture which bored you more than ordinarily. What happened? The lecturer on whom you would rivet your eyes to keep awake would lose his shape like the black poodle in Dr. Faust's study, would grow in extent, and finally fuse more or less with the wall of the room. Evidently your accommodation had given way and had now acted in such a manner as to give you the minimum amount of articulation, the greatest amount of uniformity.

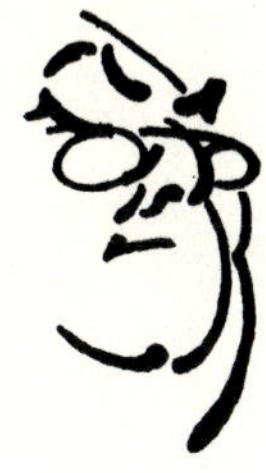

Fig. 50

These examples suggest the following kind of conclusion: when the organism is active, at a high degree of vigilance, to use Sir Henry Head's term, it will produce good articulation; when it is passive, in a state of low vigilance, it will produce uniformity. In our interpretation of vigilance, given at the end of Chapter III (p. 102), we suggested that high vigilance means that the organism has much energy at its disposal. And if we apply this interpretation to our last cases it means that simplicity of the maximum kind, high articulation, will occur when the disposable energy of the organism is great, and simplicity of the minimum kind, uniformity, when it is small. All our three examples fit into this explanation. That fatigue, low vigilance, is a condition of lowered energy has been our starting point. The second case, where the attitude of searching for a meaningful picture produced articulation, is also clearly a case of greater disposable energy, since here the Ego-system with its store of energy is brought to bear on the organization. The first case is the most difficult to understand. But the comparison between the negative effect of an ordinary portrait and the positive effect of the Hindenburg pattern clears up the difficulty. The external organizing forces are much stronger in the second case than in the first, owing to the greater jumps of stimulation between the different field parts, and the greater articulation is due to these greater forces. Therefore, if greater articulation implies that more energy is consumed in the process, then these greater forces must have liberated more energy, just as an electromotor doing work against forces uses up more energy than an idling motor.

I have stressed this connection between energy and articulation on what may seem rather insufficient evidence, because it is theoretically sound. Let us repeat a quotation from Köhler: "The final time-independent distribution contains a minimum of energy capable of doing work" (see above, p. 108). This is true in all cases but needs a very important corollary in a special one. Suppose the system whose changes we are considering consists of a relatively small sub-system and a large reservoir from which it can draw as much energy as it needs. In applying our proposition to this case we must take as the system whose final energy becomes a minimum the total system, composed of the sub-system and the reservoir. We find that in this process the small sub-system draws as much energy as possible from the reservoir, so that after the process its own energy content is greater than it was before. Köhler (1924) applies this principle to organic growth and its increasing articulation. It seems equally applicable to our present problem: if the special reacting system can draw on much energy, it will do so, and thereby achieve articulation, i.e., simplicity of the maximum kind; if it is cut off from, or limited in, its supply of energy, the minimum kind of simplicity will result.

ORGANIZATION FROM THE POINTS OF VIEW OF QUANTITY, ORDER, AND SIGNIFICANCE

The reader who has not by now forgotten the programme of this book as it was announced in the first chapter, may well wonder whether the author has not lost sight of his general point of view in the amount of detail discussed in this chapter. Let us therefore halt and see what contributions, if any, we have so far made to the problems stated in the beginning. We saw the special value of psychology in its integrative function, our science being at the nodal point where nature, life, and mind converge. Has our discussion contributed to this integration? We had abstracted three leading concepts from the sciences of the three converging realms, the concepts of quantity, order, and meaning. What does our discussion mean in these terms?

Quantity. I think that as far as quantity goes our discussion has borne out the inferences which we reached when we first investigated the relation of quantity and quality. Our law of prägnanz has a quantitative character which is at the same time qualitative. As a maximum-minimum principle it is the first, and as a simplicity principle it is the second. Clearly, the quantitative and the qualitative character are not two separate characteristics, but only two aspects of one and the same principle. In actual experimentation the qualitative aspect had the lead; not for any real organization are we as yet able to give the exact quantitative formula. But as real organizations, units and shapes must have a formula which will express them quantitatively, just as physical gestalten have their formulas. Our qualitative knowledge is different from such desirable quantitative knowledge in the degree of preciseness, but not in kind.

Order. The laws of organization which we have found operative explain why our behavioural environment is orderly in spite of the bewildering spatial and temporal complexity of stimulation. Units are being formed and maintained in segregation and relative insulation from other units. Think for a moment what happens to a retinal element while your eyes roam around as they continually do: in quick succession, and without any order whatsoever, this element will be stimulated now by white light, now by greenish light; one moment the stimulation will be strong, the next very weak; green will be followed by red or blue, a kaleidoscopic change. And what corresponds to this whirl of stimulation of the retinal points? A perfectly steady and orderly world; the cigarette box on my desk remains a cigarette box, the calendar a calendar, while my eyes move along; I experience no change in my behavioural environment, though I experience a change within "myself," feeling my eyes moving over the stationary objects. True enough, we have not yet explained this particular effect, but we see that without our principles of organization the objects could not be objects, and that therefore the phenomenal changes produced by these changes of stimulation would be as disorderly as the changes of stimulation themselves. Thus we accept order as a *real* characteristic, but we need no special agent to produce it, since order is a consequence of organization, and organization the result of natural forces. In this way our discussion has made manifest how nature produces order.

Significance. Lastly, our discussion has given us a basis for the understanding of significance. Good continuation and good shape were powerful organizing factors, and both were in the true sense "understandable": a line carries its own law within itself, and so does a shaped area or volume. Violations of this law due to external forces are felt as violations; they conflict with our feeling of the fit, hurt our sense of beauty. The shapes which we see at any moment are not adequately described by allotting a local value to each of their space elements, but only as consistent wholes; they are like the celestial music heard by Wertheimer's visitor to heaven, and not like the table or purely empirical formula of tones which his other explorer of paradise might be able to elaborate.

Our discussion has dealt with very elementary objects, objects which as such are far removed from those manifestations of the mind in which the "understanding" psychologists are justly interested. But even these humble objects reveal that our reality is not a mere collocation of elemental facts, but consists of units in which no part exists by itself, where each part points beyond itself and implies a larger whole. Facts and significance cease to be two concepts belonging to different realms, since a fact is always a fact in an intrinsically coherent whole. We could solve no problem of organization by solving it for each point separately, one after the other; the solution had to come for the whole. Thus we see how the problem of significance is closely bound up with the problem of the relation between the whole and its parts. It has been said: The whole is more than the sum of its parts. It is more correct to say that the whole is something else than the sum of its parts, because summing is a meaningless procedure, whereas the whole-part relationship is meaningful.

CHAPTER V

THE ENVIRONMENTAL FIELD

Figure and Ground. The Framework

Things and Framework. Figure-Ground. Double Representation. One-sided Function of Contour. Functional Dependence of Figure and Ground. Ground as Framework. Functional Proofs of the Figure-Ground Differences. Dynamics of Figure-Ground Articulation. Why Is the Ground Simpler Than the Figure? General Aspect of Figure-Ground Articulation. Peripheral and Central Vision; the Former a "Ground-," the Latter a "Figure-Sense." Figure-Ground in Normal Behavioural Environments. Why We See Things and Not the Holes Between Them

THINGS AND FRAMEWORK

So far our discussion has dealt with relatively simple aspects of our behavioural environment. We have mostly dwelt in the world of artifacts well adapted to reveal the laws of organization, to show the effectiveness of forces. But it is a long way from these simple shapes to our environments as we know them. It is time to remember the beginning of the third chapter, our discussion of things, not-things, and framework. We have, in the meantime, contributed something to that discussion. We have discussed the nature and origin of one not-thing, the space-filling fog which arises from completely homogeneous stimulation, and we have discussed one attribute which we found characteristic of things, viz., "shaped boundedness." Thus in presenting the laws of unit-formation and segregation and of shape we have made a first contribution to the thing-problem. But we have to do more, we must take up the other thing-characteristics and include the framework which we have so far completely neglected.

Figure-Ground. If things are shaped may we conclude that the framework is not? And if it be not, whence comes this difference? For systematic and historic reasons it is expedient to study our problem in two dimensions before we include the third. For the same distinction holds with regard to surfaces, where, since the pioneer work of Rubin (1915), it is called the distinction between figure and ground.

Duo Formation: One upon Another. For us the best way of introducing it will be to take up a thread which we dropped in the last chapter. We discovered there that several kinds of duo-formation are possible and deferred the discussion of one of them, the formation of "one figure 'upon' or 'within' another." Turn back to Fig. 27, page 154, and the point will be clear. It is this form of duo which we will investigate now. We see a leaf-like quadrangular figure within an oblong. This simple description implies a number of important consequences.

Double Representation. In saying that the small figure lies on an oblong, we maintain that the larger figure is a unit, and that means that the larger figure does not cease to be where the smaller is, that it stretches behind or underneath the smaller. This again means that a part of the total field, coinciding with the area of the small figure, is *twice* represented in our environmental field, once as the small figure itself, and once as a part of the larger oblong.

A word about this double representation. It always involves, in however low a degree, a third dimension of space. Two things in the same direction must be at different distances if they are to be two. Thus our oblong is *behind* the small figure. In our example, however, the depth difference is the smallest possible, and it is clear that it must be so, since we are dealing with bi-dimensional patterns, i.e., with organizations in which the general dynamic conditions demand plane shapes without depth. As soon as we change our conditions, we obtain clearer tri-dimensionality. Thus the book on the table does not destroy the unity of the top of the table, which is clearly behind it. This leads to another question about the double representation. My book is red, the top of the table is black. I see the red book on the table, and yet where I see the book I see no black colour, although at the same time I do not see the table as broken.

representation without colour. How can we solve this seeming paradox? Traditional psychology would have given a solution in contradiction to the *observable* facts. For traditional psychology had established the dogma: what we see has colour. Therefore, where there is no colour, we do not see. And hence the table behind the book had to be explained as a contribution from some non-sensory part of the organism. Such an explanation would have seemed so self-evident to traditional psychology that it never troubled to discuss this case, not, at least, as far as I know. Traditional psychology was all too ready to explain what obviously appeared as A as B or C. Never was a psychologist prouder than when he could say: A is not really A but something else. The best-known example is perhaps the James-Lange theory of emotions, according to which an emotion is not really an emotion but a set of kinesthetic and organic sensations aroused by responses to the emotional situations. All such explanations fail to explain why we think that A is A. For, even when the psychologists told us that A really was B, we stubbornly persisted in calling it A and in treating it as A and not as B. Was it entirely due to our perverseness and lack of willingness to learn from the expert when we continued to speak of the sad mood of an adagio or the virile hilarity of a Beethoven scherzo, instead of speaking of our different organic sensations? Why are we so hopelessly stupid as to call the colour of our tablecloth on the candle-lit dinner-table white, when Helmholtz told us that it was yellow? Helmholtz (Vol. III) tried to explain the reason for this second stupidity, but it remained in his explanation an error which we constantly committed and persist in committing when we know that it is an error. We shall discuss this second example in another place and see that we can describe and explain the facts ever so much better when we rule out the concept of error altogether. For in the long run it has proved to be more profitable to accept an A as an A and explain it as such. And that is what we shall try to do with our example, the red book on the black table.

Accepting A as A, we admit that we see the red book and the table behind it, although where we see the book, we see no black. To accept this proposition is equivalent to rejecting the traditional dogma that everything we see has colour.[1] Positively expressed, this means: visual objects that are devoid of colour may appear in our behavioural environment. And that again implies that visual organization may take place without participation of those chemical reactions which we correlate with the appearance of colour. There is nothing impossible in this conclusion. Rather is it probable that in the brain field the beginning of organization precedes the actual arousal of the colour processes. It would require too detailed a discussion of the neural hypotheses and would therefore interrupt our present argument too much were I to explain this side of organization.[2] But in the very first paper in which gestalt theory was expounded, this possibility was clearly envisaged. The "phi-phenomenon" which Wertheimer described in his famous paper of 1912 is a striking example; we may see motion without seeing anything that

[1] Colour of course in the general sense in which it includes the neutral with the chromatic.

[2] The reader may find the necessary explanations in Köhler, 1920 and 1932 a.

moves, not even a colour. To end with a literary reference: from the point of view of this theory Alice's grin without the cat is not sheer amusing nonsense, but may be a good phenomenal reality, as Lewis Carroll probably knew perfectly well.

Again we must pause to guard ourselves against a misunderstanding. We claimed that the table was seen behind the book. But what would a cross-examining counsel make of such a statement? We can easily imagine the following scene being enacted in court: Counsel: "Where was the book?" Witness: "On the table, sir." Counsel: "And what was underneath the book?" W.: "The table, sir." C.: "How do you know?" W.: "But I saw it, sir." C.: "Are you willing to testify under oath that under the book there was no opening in the table through which a revolver might be dropped?" W.: "Certainly not, sir." C.: "Why not?" W.: "Because I could not see it, the book being where it was." C.: "And yet you say that you saw that the table was under the book? Thank you."

The counsel for the prosecution is perfectly right but the truth of his proposition—"you could *not* see what was under the book"—is in no contradiction with our or the witness's statement, that we and he see it there. For, obviously, what the counsel means by seeing is not the same as what we mean by it. Our witness switched during his examination quite naturally from our to the counsel's meaning and thereby gave the appearance of contradicting himself, which in reality he did not. *We* mean by seeing a thing that it appears in some form or other in our visual behavioural environment; counsel means by seeing the appearance of an object in a visual environment under *such conditions* that it could not appear in the behavioural without having its counterpart in the geographical environment. The counsel is interested in the latter exclusively, the behavioural world of the witness is for him only a means of getting at the geographical. We on the other hand are interested in the behavioural environment itself. For us it is an end and not a means, or if it is a means then a means for finding out something about the brain field, but not about the geographical environment. And yet the psychologist who claims today that he sees the table behind the book is apt to be treated by his critics just as our witness is handled by the examining counsel. For although the critics are psychologists, and therefore should know better, they also use the cognitive meaning of "to see," based in their case on an implicit use of the constancy hypothesis, instead of the purely descriptive or phenomenological meaning.

DOUBLE REPRESENTATION CONTINUED. After this excursion into the law courts, let us return to double representation. The case in which one of the representations is devoid of all colour is only one of the possible cases. The other extreme is the case of a transparent surface in front of an object, a wire screen or a glass, coloured or uncoloured, through which we see. The problem of transparency will occupy us later. Here we introduce it only to connect our kind of double representation with other kinds which descriptively are much more palpable. One might doubt that cases of transparency are in the same sense cases of double representation because here are really *two* objects, each of which is represented, whereas in our initial case, the smaller figure within the larger, there is only one. But then one commits the experience error. On the retina the conditions are essentially alike in this case and in the case of an opaque object behind a transparent one. For on the retina, we have no more than differently stimulated areas, to some of which not one but *two* objects correspond in the behavioural environment. Double representation will occur more easily under certain conditions than others, as Kopfermann has found, and thereby double representation becomes also a shape-determining factor, and should be added to the factors which we discussed in the last sections of the fourth chapter.

ONE-SIDED FUNCTION OF CONTOUR. But double representation of the kind we are interested in now has still another highly important aspect, well illustrated in our figure. One of the representations is, as we said before, a whole figure, the other, on the contrary, only a *part* of a larger figure. The "same" part of the field which is segregated from the rest in one of the representations is connected with it in the other. The contour shapes its inside, but not its outside, or, as Rubin has described it, the contour has a one-sided function.

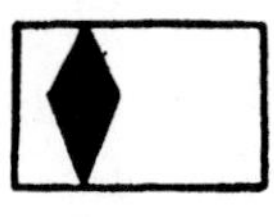

Fig. 51

We came across another asymmetry of the contour in our last chapter (pp. 150 f.), which though related to the one we are discussing now, is not identical with it. Then we spoke of contour figures and considered the fact that a closed contour line, although separated from the rest of the field on either of its sides by the same leap of stimulation, *belonged* to the enclosed figure and segregated it from the surrounding field. The asymmetry we are concerned with now does not refer to contour figures only, it applies equally well to surface figures, whose contours are their boundaries. If we modify Fig. 27 so as to obtain Fig. 51, the same kind of duo organization still occurs, a small leaf-like figure on an uninterrupted rectangle. The contour or the boundary is a boundary only to the smaller, but not the larger, figure, the pentagons at either side of the central figure are normally not seen.

One-sided function of the boundary or contour and double representation are thus only two aspects of one and the same process of organization; they indicate the establishment of more than one organized area in the same region of the field. Wherever the contour has a two-sided function, this double organization does not occur; instead we have the duo of co-ordination, as in our old Fig. 22. Therefore, special forces must be responsible for making the contour one-sided, for doubling part of the field. In our example these forces are easily discovered. The larger figure, bounded by the rectangular contour, is a simple shape in itself, and this simple shape

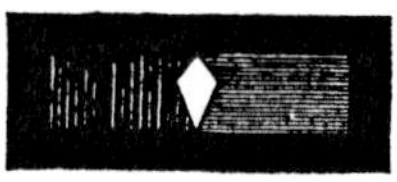

Fig. 52

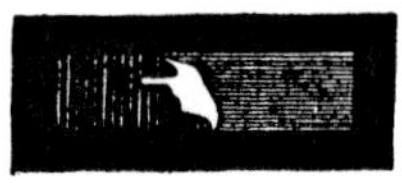

Fig. 53

resists disruption by the introduction of the smaller shape. Moreover, apart from the inset it is uniform in colour, so that the factor of equality also contributes to its unity. If this equality is destroyed by colouring the right and the left part of the large oblong differently, as in Fig. 52,[3] its unity is destroyed. The main feature of the new pattern is the central shape, while the rest is much more difficult to describe. One thing, however, seems clear, viz., that the disappearance of the double representation has not brought about a clear double-sided contour function. At least I find it very difficult to see all three figures, the red, the white, and the blue, at the same time. This is truer still if the inset figure is less regular, as in Fig. 53. Systematic experiments in the field are lacking, and therefore one must practise great caution in drawing inferences from the scant material here presented. Still it seems safe to say that just as the one-sided function of the contour needs special forces to become effective, so does the two-sided. It is not a case of a simple logical distinction: the function of the contour must be either one- or two-sided; if it is not the one it must be the other. Reality defies such handling by primitive logical precepts. We know of cases where the general conditions of organization produce a one-sided contour function with double representation, and others

[3] Compare the footnote on page 165.

where the conditions make the contour double-sided and create a co-ordinated duo. When neither of these conditions is realized, a much less clear and stable organization results, a fact from which at the moment we can conclude no more than this: organization in several parts which have no intrinsic relation to each other, but are merely one plus one plus one, is extremely difficult and not frequently realized.

ONE-SIDED FUNCTION OF CONTOUR AND SHAPE. Let us return to the one-sided contour function. It has, necessarily, the property of giving shape only to one part of the field which it bounds and not to the other. Therefore, if there are other shape-producing factors in these two fields, their effect will be different according to the effect of the contour. To prove this, we make use of a method invented and largely used by Rubin, viz., of producing patterns which are ambiguous with regard to their duo-character. For simplicity's sake, we will now introduce Rubin's terminology, calling the larger figure, upon or within which the smaller is seen, the ground, and the latter one the "figure." How useful this terminology is will appear later; now it helps us to define the ambiguity of our patterns: they are so constructed that the same field parts may appear either as figures or as ground. We have made use of such a figure before (Fig. 4, p. 83). We now introduce a modification, varying slightly one of Rubin's patterns. One can see either the sectors cross-hatched with arcs as the figure, or those that are cross-hatched with straight lines. In either case, one will see a cross. The difference appears in the lines of the hatchings. In the first case, the arcs will be arcs, in the second, they will be parts of whole circles, and correspondingly the straight lines will be bounded by the arms of the cross in the second case, and filling without interruption the whole circle in the first. The double representation is amazingly manifest, just as the one-sided function of the contour which bounds and shapes the figure but not the ground. This pattern illustrates a last point. It is easier to see the full circles than the uninterrupted straight lines, a proof that the arcs demand their continuation more strongly than the straight lines, a fact corroborated by several other experiments. In the beginning of this chapter we raised the question, whether, things being shaped, the framework was shapeless. We have now taken the first step towards answering this question. True enough, we are dealing with special cases in which the

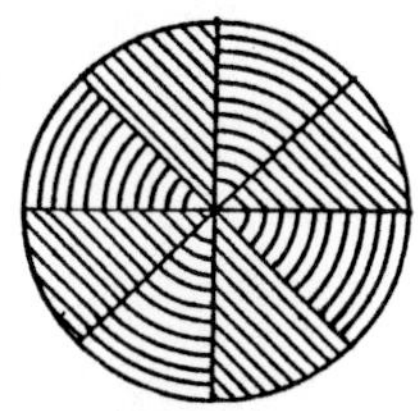

Fig. 54

concept of framework has not yet appeared; but it is clear and will be discussed shortly, that there is a connection between things and figures on the one hand, and ground and framework on the other. With this in mind, we can now express our last results in this way: the contours which shape the figure do not shape its ground; if the latter has a shape, it owes this to other forces than those which produce the figure upon it.

The one-sided or asymmetrical function of the contour can also be described by saying that contours have an "inside" and an "outside." This description is not arbitrary, but compelled by the organization itself. In ambiguous figures the same side may be either the inside or the outside, but when it is the one it is not the other; the inside or outside character belongs in each case to the contour and not to "us."

FUNCTIONAL DEPENDENCE OF FIGURE AND GROUND. GROUND AS FRAMEWORK. We have so far described the figure-ground relation by saying that the figure lies upon the ground. But this description, though it is complete enough as regards the actual experience, the product of organization, leaves out a decisive aspect of the process of organization itself. The figure depends for its characteristics upon the ground on which it appears. The ground serves as a *framework* in which the figure is suspended and thereby determines the figure. The more we generalize our ground concept, the more application shall we find of this rule. Here, restricting ourselves to smaller figures on larger ones, we can demonstrate the framework character of the ground by its influence on the shape of the figure.

We make use of the fact that a square may have two different shapes depending upon its spatial position, either the shape of a square or that of a diamond. That these two shapes are really, functionally, different has been proved by Hartmann with the help of his flicker-fusion method (see Chapter IV, pp. 129 f.); the diamond has a greater critical fusion rate than the square. Which of the two shapes will actually be realized depends to a large extent upon the orientation of the figure; resting on one side it will appear as a square, standing on one corner as a diamond; or, the same condition differently expressed, when one pair of sides is horizontal, the square will be seen, when one diagonal is horizontal, the diamond. But this last formulation is not equivalent with the first; indeed, it is not an adequate formulation at all. In the two accompanying figures, taken from Kopfermann, we see in the *b*-members indeed the diamond, where one diagonal is horizontal, and the square where two sides are, but in the *a*-members, these relations tend to be reversed, although these patterns are more ambiguous than the others. 55*a* appears most decidedly as a square, although its diagonal is horizontal, 56*a*, at least quite easily, as a diamond, although two of its sides are horizontal. The reason is easy to understand. In Fig. 55*a* the sides of the small figure are parallel to the side of the frame, in Fig. 56*a* the diagonal is. Orientation, as a factor which determines the shape of our figure, is, then, not an absolute matter, but relative with regard to the frame. Still, the *a* figures are more ambiguous than the *b* ones. This again is easy to understand, for the larger figure itself is in a frame, the page of the book, so that there are at least two frames operative. In the *b* figures

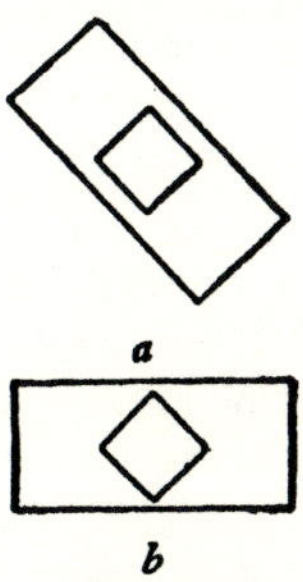

Fig. 55

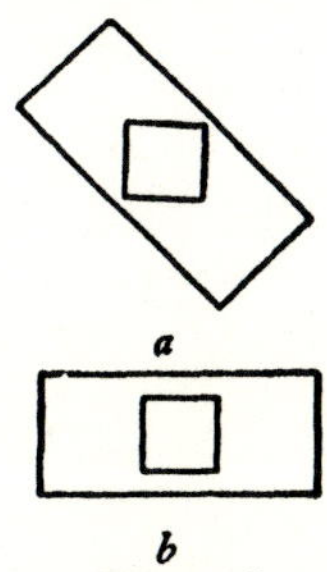

Fig. 56

these frames coincide in their main directions, and therefore in their effects; in the *a* figures they conflict, the smaller frame being the nearer to the critical figure, the larger frame farther removed. Because of this conflict between the frames, the figures are more ambiguous in these patterns than in the others. Finally, the square effect seems to be more easily realized against the "absolute" orientation than the diamond effect, 56*a* is fairly easily seen as a square. This, in a way, completes our picture, since we know from Hartmann's experiments that the square is simpler than the diamond. In reality, then, we have to distinguish three operative factors in our patterns: the two frames[4] and the simplicity of the ensuing figure. The reader may make a chart for himself in which these three factors are combined for our four patterns.

Figures and Things. The framework appeared in our previous discussion as the non-thing like part of the behavioural environment. Has the figure correspondingly thing-character? Just this has been

[4] In reality there are more frames than the two mentioned. We live continually in a definite "space-level" (see below), which acts as a very large frame.

claimed by Rubin, when he first introduced our distinction, and has been confirmed by later authors (see Köhler, 1929, p. 219). In changing from ground to figure a field part becomes more solid, and in the reverse change more loose, as observation of any of the patterns here presented will prove. Furthermore, it is the figure we are "concerned with," the figure we are remembering, and not the ground. Thus we find a beginning of the thing–non-thing difference in the figure-ground articulation of the field. How much more it can tell us about the thing quality we shall see when we have described more properties which distinguish figure and ground from each other.

Shape of Figure and Ground Compared. When, in the ambiguous figures so far presented and in Fig. 57, we compare the figure and the ground parts with each other, we always find the latter ones to be simpler, in the sense of greater uniformity, less articulation, than the former. In the cross patterns, where in both aspects the figures are crosses, the grounds are circles (in Fig. 54) or "squares with cut-off edges" (in Fig. 4). In our last pattern the black and white figures differ in shape also, T's vs. leaves, but the respective grounds are much more similar to each other, both being stripes, the black one on its lower side bounded by a sinuous line.

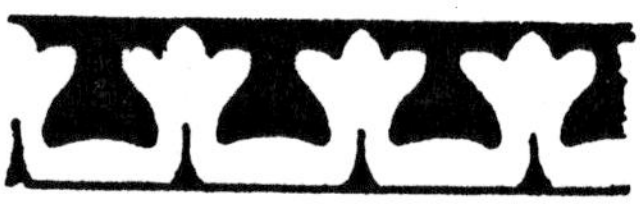

Fig. 57

Colour of Figure and Ground. This difference in articulation between figure and ground is universal, and appears not only in their shapes but also in their colours. We have previously encountered the connection between high degree of articulation and colouring. Therefore we should expect the same field to look more coloured when it is figure than when it is ground. And that is confirmed by fact. If one makes figures like Fig. 54 with alternate green and equivalent grey sectors, so that the sectors, instead of differing by their hatchings, differ in colour, then the change from the one cross to the other is accompanied by clearly noticeable colour changes. A green cross on a grey ground changes into a distinctly red cross on a dull green ground. Thus, the green parts *lose* colour in their transition from figure to ground, and the reddish parts gain colour by the opposite transition. The red is a contrast red, and therefore this experiment proves anew the insufficiency of a purely summative contrast theory, which we have discussed in our last chapter (p. 134). Our results have

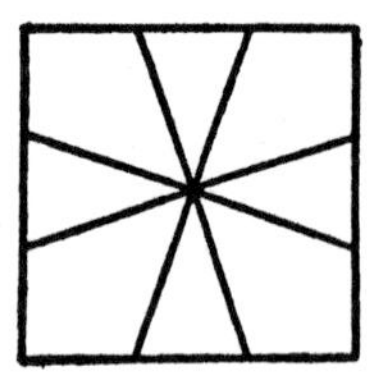

Fig. 58

been confirmed by a neat experiment by Mrs. Frank (1923). She cut out of coloured paper a figure corresponding exactly to the central cross of Fig. 58 and asked her subjects to develop an after-image of it, which then was projected on the design of our figure. If in this design, the central part appeared as the figure, the after-image upon it looked much more coloured than when it appeared as the ground of the oblique propeller-like shape.

Functional Proofs of the Figure-Ground Differences. Clear and impressive as these differences are in simple observation, it would greatly improve their status as *real* could we prove that there existed functional differences corresponding to them. Such proof has been given in so many different ways that we select a few outstanding examples.

Our first idea will be to apply the Hartmann test to our distinction. Expose a white-black cross twice in quick succession and measure the critical exposure time at which flicker ceases when either the white or the black parts appear as figure. Hartmann did this in such a way that as before (see p. 131) only the white parts provided the objective conditions for flicker, the black being black all the time. The result was that in the average of four series the critical exposure time had to be 12.3 σ shorter for the white cross than for the white ground, a difference of about 12% of the shorter of the two exposures. The difference in readiness to fuse between a field when it is ground and when it is figure is, therefore, the same as that between a more or less simple figure.

One of our descriptive differences was that the figure was more solid (thinglike), the ground more loose (stuff-like). If this is true, the figure should be held together by stronger forces than the ground, i.e., it should offer greater resistance to the intrusion of another figure. This deduction was verified in ingenious experiments by Gelb and Granit. The observers looked through a tube at Fig. 59 which filled the entire tube opening. The pattern is that of a grey cross on a grey background, the cross being either darker or lighter than the ground. By a simple device, using light reflection, a small coloured spot could be produced either on the lower arm of the cross or on the ground to the right of it, and the amount of light necessary to make this spot visible could be measured. Of course, the darker the field the less the intensity of the coloured light required, therefore a comparison of two such measurements would say nothing about the difference between figure and ground, since the two field parts which would be compared would be of different luminosity. The procedure was therefore more complex.

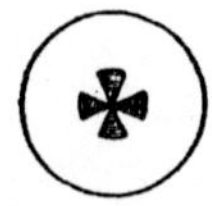

Fig. 59

To any figure-ground combination there was always added a second in which the luminosities of figure and ground had changed their places. Thus, for each combination of luminosities four thresholds had to be determined. If *d* stands for the darker and *l* for the lighter grey, *f* for figure and *g* for ground, the four thresholds are respectively (1) *lf*, (2) *lg*, (3) *df*, (4) *dg*, in which the two extremes and the two middle ones belong to the same pattern respectively. By comparing (1) with (2) and (3) with (4) we can directly determine the influence which the organization of the field exerts upon the arousal of a new figure within it, for in these comparisons the luminosities are kept constant. The result was unambiguous: the even combinations consistently gave lower thresholds than the corresponding odd ones, which is a verification of our deduction that a figure field is more strongly organized than a ground field.

As a matter of fact, this conclusion is not quite compulsory, since the figure field is in this pattern always the smaller of the two fields, and since previous investigators have found that a threshold determined within a larger field is lower than that within a smaller, a result which has been interpreted in a rather complicated manner as a mere summative contrast effect. However, a second experiment carried out by Granit (1924), the description of which I will omit, makes this interpretation virtually impossible, so that these two experiments in conjunction establish sufficient proof for our deduction.

A number of facts brought out by M. R. Harrower and myself add proof to the specific functional difference of figure and ground. Our investigation, concerned with the Liebmann effect, led to the discovery of the difference between functionally hard and soft colours, the latter showing the Liebmann effect more markedly than the former. This much was reported in the last chapter (p. 127). But since we investigated the Liebmann effect by making a figure equiluminous to its ground, the question arose whether it makes any difference whether the figure or the ground is hard or soft. In order to answer this question, we first reversed the figure-ground combination, by using now coloured grounds and neutral figures, and then proceeding to put colour into both figure and ground. The results were quite unambiguous: softness and hardness are much more important in the figure than in the ground. Consequently, if *h* stands for hard-coloured and *s* for soft-coloured, and *f* and *g* again for figure and ground, the following combinations represent a rank order of organization, the top giving the clearest articulation, the bottom the best Liebmann effect:

	f	g
(1)	h	h
(2)	h	s
(3)	s	h
(4)	s	s

This rank order which was discovered in qualitative experiments, was confirmed in discrimination and legibility experiments. I shall briefly describe the latter. On grey papers, 30 centimetres square, a number of letters 10 millimetres high and one millimetre wide were produced, letters and ground being equivalent, one of them coloured, the other neutral. For each colour, red, yellow, green, and blue, two such papers were used, one grey with coloured letters, the other coloured with grey letters. A pair of these was attached to the wall of a long room. The subjects were initially put at a distance of thirty feet from the wall and asked to describe what they saw. They then went three feet nearer, gave a new description, and continued in such stages of three feet until all the letters had been read. The following table gives the average difference in feet for each of the pairs, the colours referring to the letters, not to the ground:

red-grey	3.3
yellow-grey	1.2
grey-blue	7.9
grey-green	3.8

This means that the red letters on a grey ground could be seen on the average at a distance greater by 3.3 feet than the grey letters on a red ground, etc. One sees: the coloured letters are superior when they are hard, otherwise they are inferior to the grey letters, which in their turn become hard on soft and soft on hard ground. Thus we see that hard figures on soft ground give a better articulation than soft figures on hard grounds. That the hardness and softness of the ground is also effective appears from our rank order: the differences between (1) and (2) and between (3) and (4) respectively are mere differences in the ground, and in both cases the harder ground gives the better articulation, as was also proved in the discrimination experiment just mentioned.

The figure is harder, more strongly structured, and more impressive, the last determination apparently being closely related to the two former ones, impressiveness depending upon the density of the energy within the area. This greater impressiveness of the figure can also be demonstrated functionally, e.g., in binocular rivalry. The ground part produced in the tract belonging to one eye will be more easily disturbed or expelled from the actual field of vision than a figured part, as I have indicated in a very simple experiment which I omit here, a fact which appears also from older experiments of Hering's (1920).

Dynamics of Figure-Ground Articulation. We must now raise the question as to the laws which determine the figure-ground organization, a question which has two sides, (1) why is the field structured in this particular way, and (2) which parts of the fields will become figures, which ground? Very little experimental work has been done from which we can collect data for the solution of this problem. And the little that has been done refers to the second aspect. It is important to have a complete survey of all the conditions obtaining in any one case. Therefore we shall proceed step by step, starting with special cases and gradually limiting our restrictions.

Let us begin with such ambiguous figures as we have used in the preceding discussion. The simplest are the various forms of crosses, and for these it is characteristic that, apart from the cross-hatchings, all the contours of the figure are also contours of the ground, while the figure has contours which the ground has not. Are there conditions which, in patterns defined by this last condition, determine which parts shall belong to the figure, which to the ground? In the completely symmetrical patterns which we have so far made use of, there can, evidently, be no such conditions. Under these circumstances if we neglect the difference in colour [5] no objective factor exists which will favour either of the two organizations. But we can change these patterns slightly and thereby favour one organization at the expense of the other.

(1) Orientation as a Determining Factor. We orient them differently so that one cross lies in a favoured position, with one pair of arms vertical, the other horizontal, while the arms of the other are in oblique positions. Then the former is favoured over the latter. This fact, discovered by Rubin, has never been proved by statistical experimentation; but from mere inspection, I have no doubt that it is a true fact. Its importance is considerable, for it shows that the organization of a small field depends upon factors far outside, such as general orientation. More correctly it indicates

[5] Unpublished experiments by M. R. Harrower indicate an influence of relative brightness. But the completion of these experiments must be awaited before definite conclusions can be drawn.

that there are *main* directions in space, the horizontal and the vertical, and that these directions exert an actual influence upon the processes of organization by making figural organization easier in the main than in the other directions. We can formulate our result this way, because, whatever cross we see, the ground is always symmetrically distributed in all directions, forming a complete circle or square underneath the cross.

(2) RELATIVE SIZE. We vary the relative width of the arms of our cross. Then, again, the result is clear: the cross with the narrower arms will preponderate over that with the wider, and that the more, the greater the difference in width, as has been quantitatively proved by Graham. Fig. 60 may serve as an illustration;[6] relatively the white cross is more easily seen in 60*b* than in *a*. Here we have a law intrinsic to the organization itself: if the conditions are such as to produce segregation of a larger and a smaller unit, the smaller will, *ceteris paribus,* become the figure; the larger, the ground.

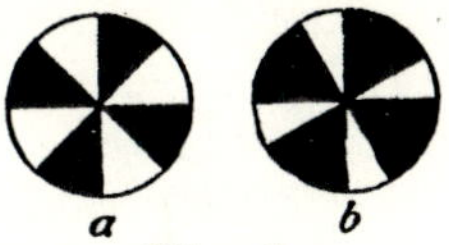

Fig. 60

This formulation, plausible as it sounds, is not really adequate. On the one hand it omits a necessary condition, on the other it begs, strictly speaking, the question. We will begin with the last point, because it will lead us directly to the first. We have seen that the ground is not interrupted by the figure, that it stretches behind it, and is therefore always larger than the figure. Thus in our last pattern, when the cross with the wide arms is seen as the figure, the ground is still larger, because, owing to double representation, it comprises not only the narrow arms, but the wide ones as well. Our law of size could therefore be formulated only thus: if the conditions are such that a smaller or larger figure can be seen, then, *ceteris paribus,* the former will be realized. But such a statement gives us no insight into the actual dynamics of the process. We can, however, state our law still differently: if the conditions are such that two field parts are segregated from each other and *double representation ensues,* then, *ceteris paribus,* the figure will arise in such a way that the difference between its area and that of the ground is a maximum, or still simpler: the figure will be as small as possible. This formulation is more than

[6] Owing to the fact that these figures are printed on the white page, the black and white parts have not an equal chance of becoming figure, the black ones being favoured in this respect.

a mere statement of fact, it contains a dynamical reason, as we shall see when we further investigate double representation. Without double representation our law of relative size no longer holds, as in Fig. 61 where the small black strip no longer lies upon the white ground of the rectangle. Here both the white oblong and the black stripe are figures, we have duo-formation in co-ordination. Before we continue this discussion, we shall introduce a new factor.

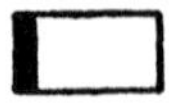

Fig. 61

(3) Enclosing and Enclosed Area. In Fig. 62 the part inside the angular contour is seen as the figure and not that outside, although the latter is smaller than the former. Rubin had already stated the law that if two areas are so segregated that one encloses the other, the enclosing one will become the ground, the enclosed one the figure. This law can be understood from the dynamics of organization. We know that the ground fills the whole area by virtue of double representation. Ground is seen, in other words, in places where there is no local stimulation corresponding to it. Thus the organization of the ground is a process similar to that which we studied in the blind-spot experiments and those with hemianopic patients (see pp. 144 ff.). And thus we understand now the factors of relative size and of enclosing. The greater, within a given area, the part that is to become ground, the less "completion" does it require. And the ground closes more readily from the outside toward the inside than vice versa. In the former case an area determined on all sides has to be filled by convergence, in the latter by divergence. Convergence has its limit defined by the part missing within the ground itself. The limit of divergence is not so determined; if, as in our Fig. 62, it should be determined by the circle contour, the segments between it and the polygon being then the figure, this determination would arise from the boundary of the figure and not that of the ground. The ground would have to *reach* this boundary, but it would not be drawn towards it, it would be pushed from the core.[7]

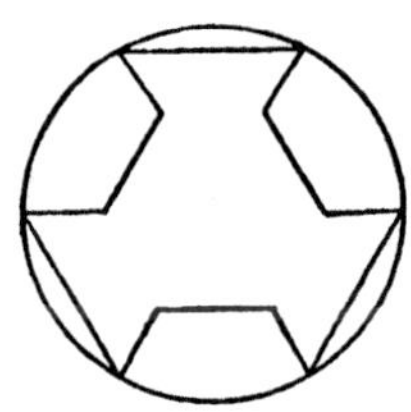

Fig. 62

These purely theoretical deductions find a counterpart in description. Von Hornbostel has emphasized as universal the difference between the concave and the convex, the embracing and the aggres-

[7] Enclosedness is not the only factor which accounts for the figure-ground distribution in Fig. 62. If this distribution were reversed, six unconnected figures would appear in place of the one coherent figure actually perceived.

sive, which correspond to the ground-figure difference. It is as though the dynamics of each field part, the forces to which they owe their existence, were at least vaguely revealed in consciousness, i.e., in properties of the behavioural environment.

(4) DENSITY OF ENERGY. Whereas our first factor determined the figure-ground articulation primarily by determining the former, our third evidently works directly through the latter. What about the second, the relative size? So far we have treated it also as a "ground determining factor," but relative size will also work directly through the figure. Under certain conditions it is, as Köhler (1920) has shown, plausible to assume that within a certain area the process energies of figure and ground are equal. Then if we have a small figure on a large ground it follows that the *density* of energy must be greater in the figure than in the ground, proportional to the ratio between the ground and the figure area. Therefore the figure would be defined by the greater density of energy, a definition which tallies well with experimentally proved figure characteristics (threshold and binocular rivalry experiments; see above, pp. 187-90). It is clear that the smaller the area of the figured part in a constant field, the greater its relative energy density with regard to the ground part. If the condition that the energy density in the former is greater than that in the latter is a necessary condition, then the smaller part must be the figure. This condition can, however, be taken as necessary only if it applies to the ground both outside and behind the figure, otherwise it would have been violated by our last pattern. But then our principle of small figure loses its value because the figure is always smaller, as we have agreed above. But if we could state as a law that organization takes place, at least under certain conditions, in such a way that the figure is as much of a figure as possible, then of course relative size would have a direct figure effect by its effect on energy-density. This implies that there are degrees of *figuredness,* which we could define by the ratio of the energy densities, which indeed depends upon the ratio of the areas. The threshold experiments by Granit are most compatible with such an interpretation, as also the general dependence of a figure threshold upon the size of its ground.

It is no use going any further since our theoretical deductions would lack experimental confirmation. Perhaps some reader will take up the thread where we are dropping it, and increase our knowledge of fact.

INTERNAL ARTICULATION OF FIELD PARTS. We proceed by taking up the clue derived from relative size: the figure has the greater density of energy. This was derived under simple conditions under which the total energy contained in the figure and the ground processes could be considered to be equal. But we can introduce new articulations within certain parts of the field, e.g., every second sector in our cross patterns, which though they increase the energy of the figure do not at the same time increase the energy of the ground. For if they did, its relative energy density and thereby its degree of figuredness should remain the same, whereas, as we shall see, we can easily produce patterns where the articulated sectors preponderate as figure over the homogeneous ones. However, not any kind of articulation will produce this effect. I can only go by my

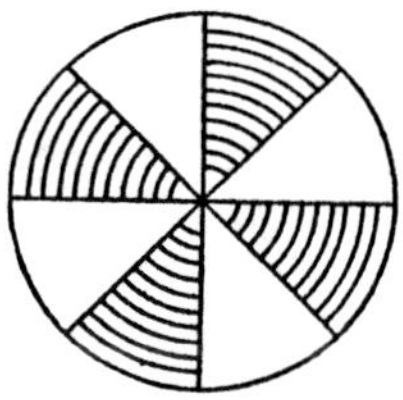

Fig. 63

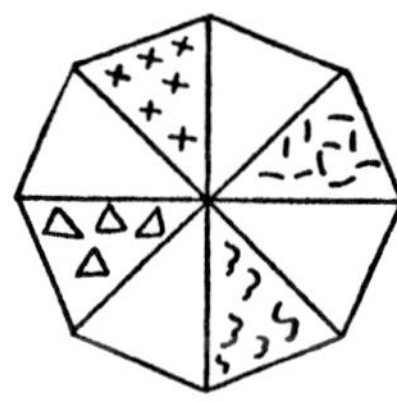

Fig. 64

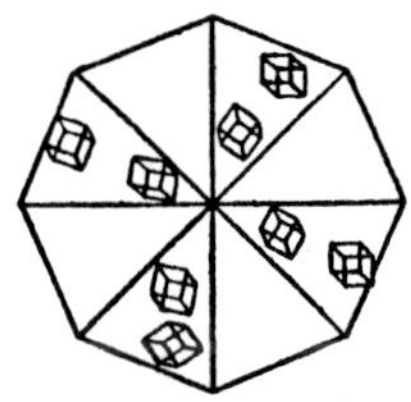

Fig. 65

own impressions, confirmed by results of class-room experiments; statistical data, if *properly collected,* might reveal finer differences which must escape pure qualitative observation; but I doubt that they can controvert it. I had thought in constructing Fig. 63 that the sectors with the hatchings would appear more readily as figures than the uniformly white ones and remain as figures for a longer time. As a matter of fact, the reverse seems nearer the truth. If the arcs form the closed circles of the ground, they are amazingly stable, at least as much so as the arc-hatched cross on the white ground. One has, therefore, not only to consider what articulation will do to the figure, but also its effects upon the ground. Even Fig. 64 shows no strong preponderance either way, but 65 does distinctly. Here one may well see the white cross, but this cross is never on a clear and well-shaped ground, and it will disappear as soon as one tries to discern the shape of its ground. But then we have reached a new and very general factor of figure-ground articulation: those parts which have the greater internal articulation will, *ceteris paribus,* become figures. A good example of this law are the sea charts on which, contrary to ordinary maps, practically all the detail is on the sea and not on the lands, with the result that now the seas become the figures, the lands grounds, and thereby look perfectly strange to us.

(5) SIMPLICITY OF RESULTING ORGANIZATION; SYMMETRY. A fifth factor concerns the organization in its totality, being a direct consequence of the law of prägnanz. The figure-ground distribution will,

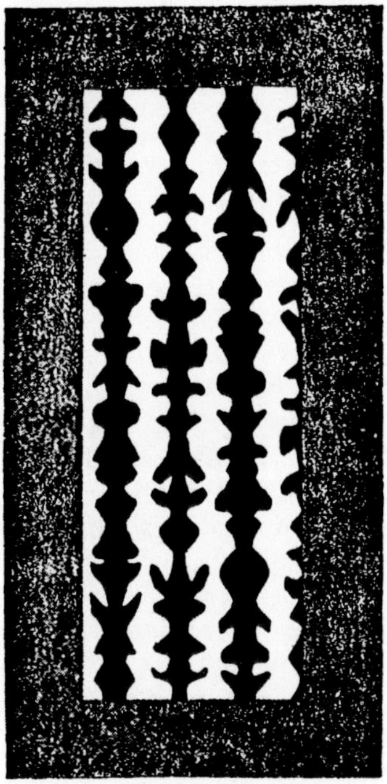

Fig. 66

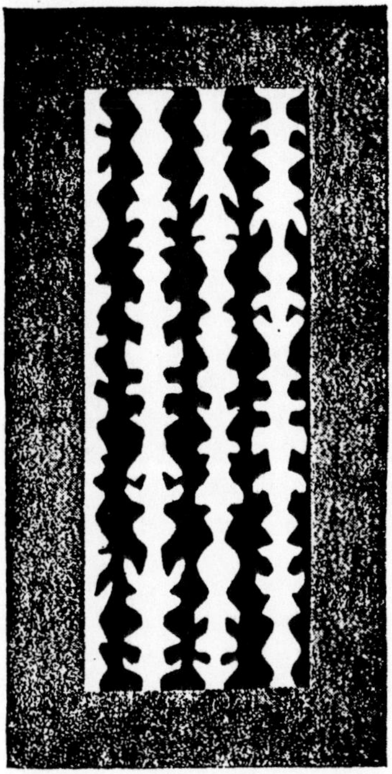

Fig. 67

ceteris paribus, be such that the resulting shapes are as simple as possible. This has been proved for the aspect of symmetry in pretty experiments by Bahnsen, a student of Rubin's. He presented patterns like Figs. 66 and 67 to his observers who were instructed to describe what they saw. Now in Fig. 66 one can see either black ornamental symmetrical or white asymmetrical stripes, while in Fig. 67 the white stripes are the symmetrical, the black the asymmetrical. The grounds, whether black or white, are always perfectly plain. 64 subjects observed 4 such patterns, one half having white, the other black symmetrical stripes. In 57 cases, i.e., 89%, the symmetrical stripes were reported, in one case only the asymmetrical, the remaining 6 (9.4%) being unstable and ambiguous.

What this result means may be best understood when we compare the possible organization of these patterns as determined merely by the colour difference between their various parts with each other. Then we find a survey like this:

I. Duo in co-ordination, black and white stripes, the whole field inside the grey frame composed of highly articulate figures, half of which are symmetrical, half not.

II. Figure-ground articulation, asymmetrical stripes visible; i.e., uniform simple ground, one kind of articulated figures, asymmetrical.

III. Figure-ground articulation, symmetrical stripes.

III is the simplest—in III the forces are in the best balance, and the fact that III is strongly favoured over all the others, proves that it is this best balance which determines the result. Moreover, the results indicate the reason, not only why *one* figure was seen more frequently than the other, but also why the figure-ground articulation occurred, No. I not having been reported a single time, and being at the same time the least simple of the three possibilities. To determine the meaning of simplicity further, it would be useful to investigate patterns such that in the figure-ground reversal not only the shape of the figure but also that of the ground was affected. This is true in our leaf-T pattern (Fig. 57), but the particular combination of changes which I have in mind is not realized in this pattern, viz., a combination of high uniform simplicity of the ground with asymmetry of the figure, and of less simplicity of the ground with symmetry of the figure. Which factor would be stronger, simplicity of the ground or symmetry of figure?

EFFECT OF ONE ORGANIZATION UPON ANOTHER. Leaving this question open till it can be answered on the basis of experimental data, I return for a moment to Bahnsen's experiment. Of course in this experiment only *one* figure was shown at a time, and the different presentations were separated by a sufficiently long interval. Looking at the two figures on the preceding page will be very unconvincing. Supposing you have looked at Fig. 66 first and have seen the symmetrical black stripes and turn then to Fig. 67. As likely as not you will see again the black stripes although now they are asymmetrical. Your first organization influences your second. I am convinced that functionally this influence is very complex, and as such in need of special investigation. One factor, however, can be analyzed with certainty: when you saw the black stripes, the black parts of the field formed the figure, it was they you were concerned with, and when you now turn to the second figure you are, or you may be, still in the attitude of being concerned with the black parts. We have seen before that the figures become the objects of our interests, and conversely: where the centre of our interest lies, there, *ceteris paribus,* a figure is likely to arise—this interchangeability of cause and effect is quite general. I recall merely the relation of unity and uniformity (see Chapter IV, p. 135). An old class-room experiment of mine illustrates this point well. I divided my class into two groups, and told the one to watch the screen for something black to appear on it, and the other to watch for something white. Then I projected on the screen for a short time the leaf-T pattern. The result was always the same: the first group saw the T's, the second the leaves, and the members of the different groups were much surprised when they saw each other's drawings of the pattern that had appeared on the screen.

Again we had to transcend the behavioural environment and to include the Ego. Forces starting in the Ego can take effect in the field and codetermine its articulation.

Why Is the Ground Simpler Than the Figure? We can now try to answer in a general way the question why the ground is simpler than the figure for those cases in which the ground contours are also figure contours. Since not all figure contours are also ground contours, the conditions for the ground are simpler and therefore the result must be simpler too, and the question only remains why these contours have their one-sided function. We have discussed this point in one example, and there it followed from the law of prägnanz. But a simpler example will lead us a step further. Why is it so difficult to see the pattern of Fig. 68 without the figure-ground articulation as eight triangles with a common apex? Why does the contour have the one-sided function even here, although geometrically it is surrounded by equal areas on either side? We shall apply the same method which we used a short while ago, i.e., we shall compare any triangle with regard to its properties which it has either as an arm of a cross, or as a part of the background, or finally as one of eight equivalent triangles. Since the latter is the effect in closest correspondence with the geometry of the pattern, we shall use it as our standard. Then we see that it gains articulation, solidity, definition, by becoming the arm of a cross, while it

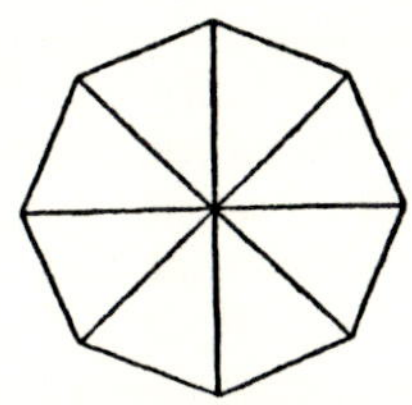

Fig. 68

loses in any of these aspects by becoming a part of the background. The cross organization, then, differs from the eight-triangle organization by being more articulated in one half of its parts, and less so in the other half.

ORGANIZATION IN THE AFTER-IMAGE. This is still mere description. A simple experiment will help us to turn this description into an explanation. Once I constructed a pattern like the last one, except that the area of the large octagon was blue, and the edges and diagonals yellow and somewhat wider than the lines of our pattern. I then developed an after-image of it and found, to my great surprise, that in the after-image the cross pattern failed, as a rule, to appear, being replaced by the monotonous eight-triangle pattern —or by a plain yellow circle with four dark blue lines on top of it.

What does this mean? The fixation of the original pattern which produces the perceptual organization, if continued for a sufficiently long period, gives rise to new forces. On the one hand, even during the period necessary for the development of an after-image, one or two reversals will take place, a proof, as Köhler has pointed out (1929, p. 185 f.), that the processes of organization produce conditions which interfere with their continued progress and thereby lead to other organizations. But the effects of fixation responsible for the arousal of an after-image must, at least in part, be different in kind. The organization of the after-image in this last experiment does not seem in the least to depend on the form of the perceptual organization. This latter depended on processes originally started in the retina by the incoming light rays. The result of the last experiment, as those of Rothschild's and Frank's, seem to me best explained by the assumption that the after-effect is one primarily in the *conditions* of the process rather than in the process itself, i.e., in those processes which *give rise* to organization, and not in the organization itself. Through continued fixation the peripheral conditions have become so changed that when the pattern is removed and replaced by a homogeneous surface, peripheral processes will take place, opposite in direction to the original ones, but in that respect similar to them that they provide the conditions for the organization in the psychophysical field.[8] We may, then, conveniently speak of the retinal image of an after-image, and correlate the actually seen after-image with its retinal image just as we correlate the actual perceived objects with their retinal images. And then the difference in this relation becomes apparent. Apart from the fact

[8] It is irrelevant for our argument whether these reversed processes occur actually in the retina or in some higher centre.

that the colours are exchanged, the original retinal image and that remaining after its removal are identical. And yet as a rule they lead to different organizations, the one arising from the latter having a simplicity of the minimum kind, that from the former of a maximum kind. We have found before that after-images will be distinguished by simplicity of the minimum kind and have ascribed this result to the smaller amount of energy consumed in the production of an after-image.[9] The figure-ground articulation, then, in our example, is one of higher energy as compared to the mere juxtaposition of equal parts. It is at the same time more stable. It can be achieved only by the contours assuming a one-sided function. This latter, which, as previously noted, entails the greater simplicity of the ground, finds therefore its explanation in its function of producing a stable organization whenever the disposable energy suffices.

New Condition: Figure Entirely Within the Ground Area. As a rule, however, the conditions which we have just discussed are not realized, figure and ground do not have common contours, but the contour of the figure lies completely within that of the ground, as in our standard pattern for the organization of the "one-on-top-of-the-other." Here our explanation no longer holds. For here figure and ground have each their own shape-determining factors, and it may well be that those of the ground are more complex than those of the figure. This case has not been investigated. Fig. 69 is an example, which I constructed more or less at random in order to see what would happen. Now the amazing thing in this pattern seems to me that the little circle does not necessarily, I should even say not spontaneously, appear as a figure on the ground formed by the larger figure, which in its turn lies on the plain circular ground. Rather do I see the circle as *part* of the larger figure, its concave and not its convex contour performing the function of segregation, so that the inside of the circle belongs together with the rest of the general background. As far as this one example goes, it shows that the articulation—simple figure on a less simple ground—is not very easy to achieve. In reality, many such cases may occur. But in most of them, I should sus-

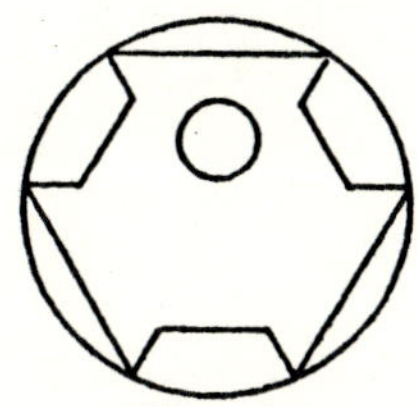
Fig. 69

[9] That this assumption was not quite arbitrary is proved by the fact, seldom sufficiently appreciated, that in ordinary life we see after-images so rarely, and that it is not always quite easy to demonstrate after-images to the layman, the explanation being that these processes of low energy have to give way to processes of higher energy.

pect, the less simple figure which serves as ground for the simpler would be much larger or separated from it by special forces. If it is much larger, it is by its very size of a relatively low degree of figuredness, so that the simpler but smaller figure may surpass it in that character. Of other forms of segregation, I have in mind chiefly tri-dimensional ones. Put a penny on a star and that penny will not appear as a hole in the star unless you look at it from a great distance. Here the penny protrudes from the star, which will, like a good ground, stretch behind it. How much the fact that a figure is the ground for another figure affects the degree of its figuredness we cannot tell. Possibly no such effect exists, possibly, and I should say probably, such an effect will sometime be proved and measured.

Other Cases. With all this detail, we have not by any means exhausted all the possibilities. There may be lines on the ground which are not in the figure, such as in our patterns 63 and 64. Their rôle in the first of these two has been discussed, their rôle in the second and in many similar ones (familiar from wall-papers) must be omitted. Our theory would have to be too far ahead of empirical facts to make it worth while to discuss it. Besides this is not a monograph on the figure-ground articulation. All we wanted to show is the interplay of forces in this fundamental organization. But here, as everywhere, where we try to get an adequate conception of the actual dynamics, we are hampered by the enormous complexity of the conditions and by the insufficiency of our knowledge. One must not blame psychology for this scarcity, for only within the last twenty years has dynamics become a psychological problem.

General Aspect of Figure-Ground Articulation. Finally we shall now take up a new functional side of the figure-ground problem. Does it pertain to our behavioural environment in all its sensory aspects or is it the domain of vision alone? Our answer must needs be brief, again because of the lack of experimental data. But we shall have to admit that the distinction holds for all the senses. For audition, it is clear; we can hear speech on the background of the patter of the rain, or the roaring of a mountain stream.

Other Senses. Clear enough as this distinction is here, it becomes more difficult when we approach the other senses. It is always easy enough to demonstrate the figures, the hard or soft objects we touch, the taste of this morsel of well-cooked steak, or the aroma of the wine of a choice vintage which we have sipped; the smell of this violet, the hot or cold feel of this piece of metal. All these experiences are figure-like, but what is their ground? Here is a problem which I do not pretend to solve. Let one indication be sufficient: we spoke of the ground of the roaring stream against which the words of our friend appeared. But often, though for city dwellers not often enough, this auditory ground is "stillness." In favour of the claim that stillness is not, or need not be, simply nothing, but will frequently serve as ground I shall only adduce the fact that stillness may become figure, as when we leave the city and spend our first nights in the lonely mountains. It seems to me quite likely that ground qualities of similar kinds exist for the other senses as well, though it is probable that they are more functional than descriptive. That means the grounds of these senses will functionally influence what actually appears in our behavioural environment without having any direct counterpart in it comparable to visual ground. This will ultimately mean that our most general ground is supersensory in the sense that it owes its existence to the contributions of potentially all senses. In saying this we are far from ascribing the same importance to all senses for our general framework.

Only a few additions, before we return to vision. We had no difficulty in pointing out figures in different sense modalities. But some senses will also provide us with grounds that are more than "emptiness." I am thinking particularly of smell, which may envelop us like a soft cloak or the blue walls of a rotunda in the castle of a fairy-king. And the ground of these other senses is often not only, not even chiefly, the ground of the figures of these same senses, but determines *our* relation to these figures and to all figures or things in our given behavioural environment. The "atmosphere" of a room is as good an example as I can give. Thus these backgrounds are more comprehensive than the purely visual ones so far discussed, since they are grounds for the Ego as well as for the things with which it finds itself confronted. Our conclusion then is that the figure-ground distinction, though it is applicable to all senses, offers new problems when we go beyond vision, problems which are of great significance for the theory of behaviour, but which as yet are in too embryonic a state to deserve further discussion.

Peripheral and Central Vision; the Former a "Ground-," the Latter a "Figure-Sense." Let us then return to sight. All modern theories of vision acknowledge two kinds of receptors, the rods and the cones, of which the latter alone are found in the fovea centralis, while the former increase in proportion towards the periphery. At the same time it is a well-known fact that the centre is functionally distinguished from the periphery by its higher articulation both in form and colour. Moreover, usually three zones can be distinguished on the retina, one totally, one partially colour-blind, besides a central area with its normal colour sense. The articulatory power measured, e.g., by the two-point limen, decreases rapidly towards the periphery, so that segregated field parts, being produced exclusively by peripheral stimulation, lack detail of both colour and shape; in other words, the periphery of the retinae provides us with such field parts as have distinctly the characteristics of ground, while the central part of the retina causes our perception of figures. Thus it seems plausible to say that the periphery is a ground-sense, the centre a figure-sense.

THIS DIFFERENCE FUNCTIONAL AND NOT MERELY ANATOMICAL. This description of our organ of sight unifies the different parts by assigning a common cause to them. No doubt there is an anatomical reason for the distinction, but the anatomical difference has to be considered as a secondary, not as a primary fact. Let us elaborate this point. (1) We saw that *ceteris paribus* the enclosing part of the field will become the ground, the enclosed the figure. Should we then consider it as a mere coincidence that the centre of the retina mediates figure-perception while the surrounding periphery supplies the ground? Is it not a much more plausible hypothesis to assume that the centre is the figure-sense *because* it is the centre and that its anatomical properties derive from this function? If it were so, then the anatomical centre should no longer be the region of highest articulation when it is no more the centre. This deduction is amply confirmed by experiments performed with hemianopic patients.

CONFIRMATION BY FUCHS'S EXPERIMENTS WITH HEMIANOPICS. The clearest demonstrations to this effect we owe to W. Fuchs (1920, 1922). In the hemianopic field of vision the anatomical fovea lies at the right or left margin. This anatomical centre is, for many hemianopics, no longer the functional centre with regard either to localization or articulation. Instead they develop a pseudo-fovea, i.e., a new point on the retina, well within the intact region, becomes the place of greatest articulation and clearness. "This new place of clearest vision has no constant position on the retina, but constitutes a functional centre, i.e., a centre determined by the actual visual data, changing its location with the actual shape or size of the objects, or the form of the total field which confronts the patient" (1922, p. 158). Therefore, hemianopic patients, before being examined, have no idea of the nature of their affliction. They complain about not seeing so well as they used to, but their phenomenal field of vision is quite different from their functional field of vision. Whereas the latter has a quasi-semicircular shape, the bounding diameter passing through the fovea, the former is more or less like our own, i.e., quasi-circular. Furthermore, the extent of their field of vision varies with the particular task to which they are put. We shall keep this in mind now when we discuss a few of Fuchs's results. Several letters about one inch high were projected on a screen and at their side a black mark which the patient had to fixate, i.e., to regard in such a way that it fell on his fovea. He was then to indicate which of the letters appeared to him most clear. Now, when the patient sat at a distance of one metre from the screen, he chose a letter about six centimetres from the fixation point, and when his distance was doubled, he chose a letter only slightly further out, viz., 6.5-6.7 centimetres from the fixation point. At the same time the limit of his field of vision toward the periphery was approximately as far away from the clearest letter as that from the fovea. Two conclusions are obvious: the place of clearest vision lies in the centre of the actual field of vision, and it does not correspond to a definite part of the retina, for if it did, from a distance of two metres the patient should have seen the clearest letter twice as far from the fixation point as from the distance of one metre.

In the next experiment the distance of the patient was kept constant, and the size of the letters varied. The result was that if one increased the size of the letter, one had to remove it further from the fixation point in order to keep it at its highest degree of clearness. The changes are quite considerable, the smallest letter, having one-twelfth of the size of the largest used in the first experiment, was clearest at a distance of 1.1 cm. from the fixation point as compared to the 6 cm. of the largest. The small letters determine a small field of vision and thereby a centre close to the fovea on the margin. In a third experiment, both distance of the observer and size of the letter were varied, but in such a way that the angle of vision remained constant, letters twice as large being observed from a double distance, and so forth. Again, the objectively larger letters had to be further away from the fixation point than the smaller, the constancy of the visual angle having no effect at all. Thus we see how clear articulation appears as a function of the total field and its properties, not as the result of pre-existing anatomical conditions. Of the many other highly instructive experiments, I will mention only one to corroborate the last statement that the actual units, produced by organization, determine the structure of the whole field and thereby the clearness of its parts, and not the arrangement of stimuli or the factor of attention. If a large broken vertical line (Fig. 70) was moved so far out from the fixation point that it appeared in full clearness, and the observer was then asked to concentrate his attention on one of the centre parts of this line, the result was that this part, instead of gaining in emphasis, shrank and became blurred, and if the dimensions of the whole and its pieces were properly chosen, would disappear completely, so that the observer saw a gap in the rest of the still visible line. By isolating a part from its structural unity, the patient destroys this part, an absolute proof that it was the large unit as an objective fact which produced its visibility, and not an attitude of the observer's.

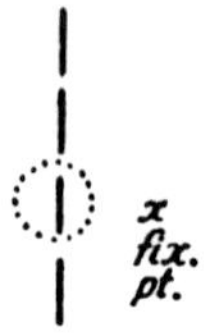

Fig. 70

THE PERIPHERY'S CONTRIBUTION: FUNCTIONAL GROUND, AND FIGURES OF STRONG INTERNAL FORCES OF ORGANIZATION OR CO-OPERATION BY THE CENTRE. (2) When we say that the periphery is a ground sense, we do not mean that it can under no condition produce or co-operate in the production of figures, as little as our claim that the centre is a figure sense denies that it can co-operate in the production of ground. But this remains true: the periphery alone can produce a ground while the centre alone cannot, even when the periphery has lost all capacity of producing figures by itself. The latter statements are confirmed by two kinds of disturbances of sight. If, through retinitis, the field of vision has shrunk so much that only the centre remains functional, the patient is for all practical purposes as good as blind. On the other hand, perimetric tests of certain hysterical patients, or patients with special functional psychoses, reveal a field of vision restricted to a minute central area, which may be smaller than the area which makes a patient with retinitis practically blind. And yet these patients can orient themselves visually without too great difficulties.

One short word about the perimetric examination. The patient fixates a point while the examiner introduces from the periphery small disks of various shapes and colours. The patient has to indicate as soon as he sees something, and what shape and what colour the object he sees in the periphery has. By this method, which tests the arousal of figures, the three different colour zones of the retina are discovered.

This examination tests, then, the production of figures in the periphery by the periphery alone. It is very important to know this.

For if we keep in mind the kind of performance we are testing we shall not be surprised to find the results depending upon the kind of test material we use, rather we should expect better performances with such objects as give rise to good organizations when looked at directly than with objects which under these more favourable conditions produce poorer articulation. Furthermore, we should not be surprised that field parts which are produced jointly by centre and periphery, should have, provided they are strongly unified, the characteristics which they derive from the centre. Both these expectations are amply confirmed.[10] Even in the ordinary examination of visual acuity, in central vision, the result depends to a large degree on the test object employed. Thus M. R. Harrower's and my discrimination experiments referred to above proved, e.g., the dependence of acuity on hardness and softness of figure and ground. For the periphery Gelb (1921) has made a neat experiment. A black double ring, outer diameter 36 cm., width of the black lines 8 mm., width of the intervening white space 5 mm., is drawn on a large cardboard. The subject fixates, monocularly, the centre of the ring. Then another white cardboard with an open ring sector of about 12 degrees is placed on top of the first[11] and the cardboard moved so near to the observer that the two small arcs fuse into one, completely obliterating the intervening white space. When then the masking cardboard is withdrawn the entire double ring with the white circle between the two black ones becomes clearly visible. Similarly, if instead of a black double ring one uses a coloured single ring, and pushes the test object so near to the subject that he sees under the mask a neutral short line, the subject will see a full *coloured* circle when the mask is removed. The opposite effect takes place when instead of rings and circles one uses double straight lines. If from a distance ascertained in the preceding experiments, one end of such a line is fixated, then without the mask the line will fuse at a distance of about 10 cm. from the fixation point, while a small bit of it will still appear double at a distance of about 20 cm. This proves that the *degree* of organization of a field part depends upon its *kind* of organization, its shape. Good shapes will be better

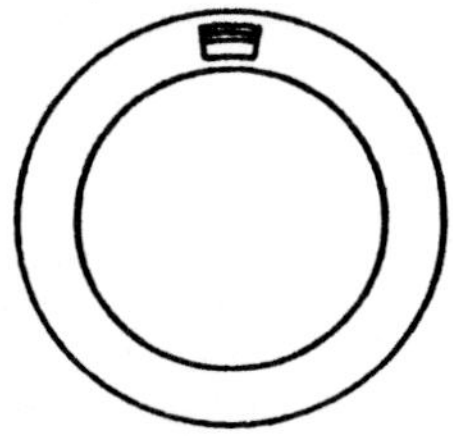

Fig. 71

[10] See C. Berger for a psychological treatment of modern literature on visual acuity.
[11] Fig. 71 represents schematically the double line visible through the opening in the "mask."

figures, i.e., more articulated and coloured than poor shapes. The fact that the small part of the straight double line is superior to the whole line is due to the concentration of attention on this small part. Attention, like attitude, is a force which starts in the Ego, and must therefore be discussed later. But we should extract from this experiment the fact that attention, adding energy to the particular field part, will increase its articulation, if it is not articulated as well as it might be. Since with the circles the small parts are inferior to the whole figure, although they must be as much favoured by increased attention as the small parts of the straight lines, the internal forces of organization must be stronger than the effect due to the added attentional energy.

We shall draw from this discussion one more conclusion. Oculists test visual acuity as a part of their standard examination. This test is a test of *organization* under particular conditions, it is *not* directly a test of anatomical structures of the retina, a view which still seems prevalent among oculists (see Berger). The results of the test may indicate also certain anatomical facts, but only indirectly; we conclude backwards from the process of organization to its conditions, of which the anatomical ones are only a fraction. It seemed wise to add this remark in order to prove that our experimental and theoretical discussions also may have their immediate practical value.

Centre Co-operating with Periphery. We noted above that the field parts produced jointly by central and peripheral stimulation would have properties of purely centrally aroused parts. When we lie on our backs on the soft grass of a hill and look into the sky, we see the sky blue over its whole extent although the periphery of the retina is colour-blind; or when we stand opposite a red or a green wall, the wall does not become grey at a certain distance from the fixation point, although a zone between the totally colour blind area and the centre is red-green blind. That is, we must always distinguish between the periphery as acting alone and as co-operating with the centre. The blind-spot experiment previously discussed with the cross with blue and red arms should be considered from this angle.

CAUSAL RELATION BETWEEN STRUCTURE AND FUNCTION OF CENTRE AND PERIPHERY. (3) The gist of our two first points can be summarized like this: the organization of the visual field was proved to depend on two sets of factors, the internal forces of organization within the field and the anatomical differences within the optic sector. For, even though clearness and articulation can be produced by peripheral parts, the centre is superior in these respects. Now, when we claimed the centre to be a figure- and the periphery to be a ground-sense we established a connection between these two factors, based on the fact that a central area, surrounded by another area, would tend to become the figure on the surrounding ground. We must now examine what kind of connection this can be. Why is the centre the figure- and the periphery the ground-sense, why has the anatomical structure of the retina, and probably the brain, developed in such a way? This is distinctly a genetic and biological question and can find its final answer only when we know very much more about the actual occurrences of phylogenesis than we do now. But a general outline may be attempted at the present moment. We can explain the morphological status of any organism or of any of its members if we can derive it from a less (or more) structured state as a consequence of the behaviour in that less (or more) structured state; briefly, if we can derive the organ from the function. As a matter of principle this is by no means impossible, as Köhler (1924) has shown.[12] A process will leave traces in the form of chemical products, and must do it in such a way that it will facilitate its own recurrence. If, then, the same kind of process occurs again and again, in the same region, this region will gradually be changed so as to make the occurrence of similar processes more and more easy. Apply this general idea to our problem of vision. Since the enclosed part will tend to become more easily figured than the enclosing part, the centre of the retina has a greater chance to produce figure processes than the periphery, even when they are anatomically equal. However, there are so many other factors operative in the figure-ground articulation that possibly the superiority of the centre due to its central position might not be sufficient to give it a significant advantage over the periphery.

The Factor of Frequency. But another factor enters. If the field conditions are such that the resulting organization is one figure on a ground, and this figure lies at the periphery, the field of vision is not so well balanced as in the case in which the single figure is in the centre; being enclosed makes a field-part a figure, this factor added to others will increase its degree of figuredness, and the field with its pressure towards highest possible articulation will therefore be more stably organized when the figure is as much a figure as possible. We might also say: just as enclosedness makes for figure organization, thus will figure organization press towards enclosed-

[12] A somewhat different hypothesis to explain this connection between structure and function was advanced by Maccurdy (p. 217 f.).

ness. This pressure can be relieved. For the relation of the eye to the stimulating object, and thereby to the distribution of the proximal stimuli on the retina, is not fixed; eye, head, and body can move and by such movement shift the stimulus distribution. Therefore we shall expect such a solitary figure to give rise to eye-, head-, or body-movements until its proximal stimuli fall into the centre. We shall take up this fundamental point when we discuss the theory of behaviour. At the moment we derive from this argument that the frequency with which a figure-organization is started from the centre of the retina must be much greater than we originally had reason to expect. And, therefore, according to the general principle just enunciated, we must expect this region to turn into a region particularly favourable for the arousal of figure-organization.[13] Of course, this gives us no insight into the actual details of the process, it does not say how it has come to pass that the density of receptors is so much greater in the fovea than in the periphery, nor does it attempt to derive the difference between the rods and the cones. But, incomplete as our theory is, it is at least a beginning. And even in this beginning a great number of facts, hitherto merely coexistent, become unified and intelligible.

Figure-Ground in Normal Behavioural Environments. We now apply the figure-ground category to the normal behavioural environment. It is created by retinal stimulation which is *in kind* the same as that operative in the cases discussed so far, but ever so much more complex in its distribution. Furthermore, new factors of organization are usually introduced by binocular parallax. However, since the main features of the behavioural environment are not essentially different in one-eyed persons from those with binocular vision, we shall disregard this factor for the moment. All normal fields of vision have a great amount of depth detail apart from the detail of form. At the same time in all normal fields the contours have the one-sided function. We see, to use von Hornbostel's phrase, the things and not the holes between them.

WHY WE SEE THINGS AND NOT THE HOLES BETWEEN THEM. We can now attempt an answer to the question why we do so. Two of the factors of organization which we have so far discussed seem to me to be the most important causes of this effect. In the first place, the segregation and unification which occurs will separate areas of different degrees of internal articulation, and according to our law,

[13] The idea that phylogenetically the histological structure of the fovea had to be connected with its psychophysical function was already developed by Fuchs, 1920, p. 163 fn.

the more highly articulated ones will become figures, the rest fusing together to form the ground. Look at any landscape photograph. You see the shape of the things, the mountains, and trees and buildings, but not of the sky. The second factor, equally important, is that of good continuation and good shape. The things which we see have a better shape, are bounded by better contours, than the holes which we might see but do not. Therefore, when in exceptional circumstances these conditions are reversed, we see the hole and not the things, as the shape of a gap between two projecting rocks with sharp profiles, which may look like a face, an animal, or some other object, while the shape of the rock disappears.

Refutation of the Empiristic Answer. This explanation is radically opposed to traditional ways of thinking. Whereas to traditional psychology the articulation of our field into things, or into figures and ground, appears as a clear example of experience or learning, our theory considers this articulation as the direct result of the stimulus distribution, i.e., as the spontaneous organization aroused by the stimulus mosaic. Let us, therefore, examine in detail what the empiristic explanation of this articulation implies, a task which has been neglected by the empiricists who never thought of doubting the truth of their theory. The empiristic theory could either accept or reject our description of the figure-ground difference as a matter of organization. If it accepted it, but reduced it to experience, it would have to say that originally the chances were even *which* side of the contours would have the segregating function, whether holes or things would be seen. Experience would continually favour the one at the cost of the other. The first claim, equal chance for hole and things, is in strict contradiction to the laws of figure-ground articulation which we have derived from empirical evidence. Were it true, then patterns for which we had no experience should be absolutely ambiguous with regard to the figure-ground articulation. And this deduction contradicts experimental evidence. And the second claim of the empiricist, that experience turns the scales in favour of one of several possible figure-ground organizations, lacks any kind of substantiation. Neither do we know what kind of experiences are to have this effect, nor how they are to bring it about. Perhaps the empiricist might here raise the point that the shape of the things is constant, while that of the holes is changeable, because of the same things being in different places and next to different other objects. The answer is again very simple, viz., that this argument commits the experience error. The retinal images of the things change with every change of position between thing and observer; the conditions for the arousal of one and the same thing are as little constant as those for the arousal of the holes. The fact that despite this change of proximal stimulation the perceived things are constant is a problem, not a fact to support an empiristic theory. Experience with things or figures can be had only after things or figures have been established as parts of the behavioural environment.

If the empiricist rejects our claim that the figure-ground articulation is a matter of organization, then he must first explain what it is. Since the only explicit attempt of this kind I know of is the attention-hypothesis, the inadequacy of which has been shown a great number of times, I forbear to discuss this any further (see, e.g., Koffka, 1922).

The empiristic reader, even if he feels the strength of these arguments, will not readily abandon his theory. For these arguments have failed to show why empiricism is such a popular doctrine; therefore the reader will not yet see explicitly how the new theory explains those particular facts or aspects of facts which make his empiricism so dear to him. This gap will be filled in later when we discuss "constancy" problems (pp. 223 f.), where the advantage of empiricism seems particularly obvious, and where empiricism is as false as it is here. To avoid misunderstanding: by rejecting an empiristic explanation of the figure-ground articulation as such, I do not imply that experience may not be one of the several factors which determine any such given articulation. If under certain conditions, equivalent with regard to two figure-ground articulations, one of them has occurred once or several times, it may be that the same kind of articulation will occur under the same conditions. Rubin thought he had proved such a "figural after-effect"; however, certain experiments of Gottschaldt's (1929) throw some doubt on the validity of this proof. For, as we have seen before, it is not so easy to prove the influence of experience as the empiristic theories would lead us to believe. It is, however, my personal opinion that experience may influence the figure-ground articulation in the sense that one such actualized articulation may facilitate similar ones. Future experiments must show whether my belief is justified, and under what conditions such an influence, if it exists, takes place.

CHAPTER VI

THE ENVIRONMENTAL FIELD

The Constancies

The Framework. Shape and Size of After-Images. Localization. General Dependence of Localization on Framework. General Principle: the Main Directions of the Field Constitute the Framework. Localization of the Ego Through Constitution of Framework. Application of the General Principle to Our Various Examples; the Invariants. The Special Case of Ego Localization. Constancy of the Framework (Constancy of Direction, Size, and Shape). Theory of Perceptual Constancies. Constancy of Shape. Constancy of Size. Whiteness and Colour Constancy

THE FRAMEWORK

In the last chapter, we proposed to discuss things and frameworks, and we introduced the figure-ground articulation as a part of that more general problem. We can now generalize, beginning with the framework and adding our theory of thingness at the end.

All Perceptual Organization Is Organization Within a Framework. Therefore, we shall now prove that all perceptual organization is organization within a framework and depending upon it, and shall then demonstrate some salient aspects of the frameworks.

For our proof we can resume a thread which we dropped in the last chapter, when we gave some demonstration of the functional dependence of figures on their grounds. There we saw how the shape of a small figure would depend upon the ground on which it appeared. The same fact can be demonstrated with the help of after-images. If the after-image of a circle is projected on a plane which is not frontal-parallel, it will appear as an ellipse.

Shape and Size of After-Images. What is true of shape is equally true of size, the size of an after-image being a direct function of the distance at which it is projected. That this relation depends also on the direction of the projection, we have learned in Chapter III, the size being the smaller the greater the elevation of the line of regard against the horizontal. But apart from this major factor, there are also minor factors, depending upon the shape and the articulation of the after-image itself, which interfere with a strict proportionality of size and distance of the after-image, a proportionality which had been discovered by Emmert, and has since played a considerable rôle in the investigation of eidetic images.[1]

It is much more important for our present purpose that the distance of the ground upon which the size of the after-image depends is not the objective or geographical, but the phenomenal or behavioural distance. Mrs. Frank (1923), influenced by an old experiment of Volkmann's, had her subjects project after-images on a plane surface on which a perspective drawing of a deep tunnel had been made. Then the size of the after-image varied with the place on the sheet of paper on which it was projected; if it fell on a part corresponding to a near part of the tunnel it was considerably smaller than when it was thrown on a part corresponding to a remote part of the tunnel; the enlargements obtained were of the order of magnitude of 3:1. This is not surprising, for a well-known so-called optical illusion shows the same effect. Of two objectively equal objects drawn inside such a tunnel the one appearing nearer will also appear smaller.

Localization. But the framework will also influence localization. Indeed, without a stable framework, there is no stable localization, a fact which is fundamental for the theory of space perception. Let us briefly describe Hering's theory of localization in order to develop our point. In this theory, each point of the retina has by itself a definite pair of space values, a height and a breadth value, corresponding to the direction at which any point will appear if with head erect the eyes are focussed on an infinitely far point in the centre of a horizontal plane passing through the two eyes. Thus the centre of the retina will have the space value "straight ahead," i.e., both breadth and height values are nought. Points vertically above and below will still have the breadth value zero, but negative and positive height values, if positive means that they appear below and negative that they appear above the point straight ahead. Similarly, points horizontally to the left and the right of the centre have a height value zero, and increasing breadth values towards the right and left. Finally in this theory, amount of retinal disparity gives to each point a depth value. We shall discuss the theory of depth perception later, therefore we restrict ourselves to the two first dimensions.

How could such a theory of the fixed space values of retinal points be tested? Witasek (1910), a firm believer in the theory, suggested

[1] See for this my review of work done on eidetic imagery (1923c) and the two papers by myself (1923b) and Noll in which exceptions from the Emmert law are demonstrated.

the following experiment. Put your subject in a totally dark room with one point of light in front of his eyes as his fixation point. Then expose one after the other a number of different points and have the subject indicate the direction at which these points appear. The experiment was deemed necessary by Witasek because it does not at all follow from Hering's theory that the height and breadth values of a retinal spot increase proportionally with their distance from the centre. It may very well be that the relation is less simple, that in other words the system of the phenomenal space values of the retinal points is not an adequate map of the geometrical position of these points. Thus the well-known over-estimation of a vertical as compared to a horizontal line was, in this theory, explained by the assumption that the height values increase more rapidly than the breadth values.

But let us return to Witasek's experiment. It has never been performed, and that for a simple reason: it *cannot* be performed. If you stay for any length of time in a totally dark room with only one point of light visible, this point will soon begin to move around in the most erratic manner, making excursions up to 90 degrees. During the whole time fixation is as perfect as can be, no more than the minute normal tremor movements of the eyes taking place with an excursion under 1 degree as was proved by Guilford and Dallenbach. These "auto-kinetic" movements, then, prove that no fixed retinal values belong to retinal points; they produce localization within a framework, but do so no longer when this framework is lost. That this is the true explanation of the auto-kinetic movements is borne out by the fact that after continual observation of these movements, the rest of the framework which is still preserved in our experiment begins to lose its stability also; the floor under one's feet, the chair one sits on, begin to sway.

GENERAL DEPENDENCE OF LOCALIZATION ON FRAMEWORK. The auto-kinetic movements are the most impressive demonstration of the existence and functional effectiveness of the general spatial framework, but the operation of this framework pervades our whole experience. A line may be projected on the vertical meridians of our eyes by a vertical line, when I stand in front of it and look straight ahead; or by a horizontal, as when it is on the sheet of paper on my desk upon which I am looking down, and as well by a line in any position between these two extremes. And, as a rule, I see the line vertical, horizontal, oblique, in accordance with reality. Of course we know that the *real* position of the line can have no direct effect upon its phenomenal position; we excluded this "first answer" to the question why things look as they do in Chapter III (pp. 77-80). We concentrate, at the moment, on the fact that the same local stimulation may give rise to a very great number of different localizations, and that, conversely, the same localizations may be produced by different stimulations; for I need only raise and turn my eyes, and the line on the paper in front of me will be projected on new parts of the retina and yet appear in the same location as before. And if I turn my head out of the vertical, the same objective lines which before were projected on vertical retinal lines will now be focussed on oblique retinal lines without ceasing to appear in space as they did before. Without discussing the manner in which the classical Hering theory accounted for it,[2] we shall use this effect for our theory of the framework.

At any one moment vertical lines on our retinae will give rise to phenomenal lines which are partly vertical, partly horizontal, and often enough partly oblique. Moreover, as we have already pointed out, quite frequently oblique lines on the retina produce the same results which under "normal" conditions arise from vertical ones. On the other hand, when a vertical line on the retina produces a vertical line in the behavioural environment, then a non-vertical one will not be seen as vertical, unless special factors are operative within the field part that contains this non-vertical line. Just so, and with the same proviso, if an oblique retinal line causes us to see a vertical one, then a vertical retinal line will cause us to see an oblique one. Therefore, although the direction of the retinal line is a factor that codetermines the direction of the behavioural lines, it is not a factor working by itself.

TWO PROBLEMS. We are now dealing with two problems, closely related to each other, and yet to be distinguished: (1) retinal lines of equal direction will *simultaneously* give rise to behavioural lines of different directions; (2) the same retinal lines will under different conditions, i.e., at different times, give rise to different behavioural lines.

Let us give examples for these two cases. For the first our variety of choice is so great that it is hard to choose. In front of me on my desk stand a number of books; their edges are vertical, and are, provided my head is held straight, projected on vertical retinal lines. In front of these books and pointing towards me, lies a pencil in such a position that when the edges of the books are projected on vertical retinal lines, it is too. For brevity's sake I omit my calendar

[2] See Chapter IX.

pad which might serve as an instance of the objective line neither horizontal nor vertical projected on a vertical retinal line.

We have already given an example of the second case. As soon as we tilt our heads, vertical lines are no longer projected on vertical retinal lines,[3] and yet the objects which looked vertical before will continue to do so, as long as we are not in a totally dark room in which a vertical luminous line is the only visible object.[4]

Another highly significant example we owe to Wertheimer (1912). A mirror can easily be tilted in such a way that the images of real vertical lines will be projected on oblique retinal lines. An observer looks at such a mirror through a tube which excludes from his vision all parts of the environment which would be visible beyond the mirror, and observes the room and what happens in it through the mirror. At first this room will be topsy-turvy. People will walk on a tilted floor, objects will drop to the floor in oblique lines. But after a short time this "mirror-room" will be all right again; the floor will be horizontal and the path of falling objects vertical.

THEORETICAL SIGNIFICANCE. What is the theoretical significance of these facts? Those of our first problem show clearly that the phenomenal direction to which a vertical line will give rise depends upon the total organization of the visual field. Our phenomenal space is filled with tri-dimensional objects and surfaces. Lines, under normal conditions, are not lines by themselves, but lines belonging to, or bounding, the surfaces of these things or those that confine our space. Therefore these lines will be determined in their direction and other aspects by the things or surfaces to which they belong. Otherwise expressed: it is an altogether futile task to build up perceptual space from points or lines, i.e., "space sensations"; again we find that visual space can only be understood as the product of field-organization.

GENERAL PRINCIPLE: THE MAIN DIRECTIONS OF THE FIELD CONSTITUTE THE FRAMEWORK. The examples given for our second problem lead us beyond this general statement and bear a direct reference to the framework. Why is it, so we must ask, that the mirror world rights itself? In the mirror world after it has righted itself the organiza-

[3] Despite the compensatory swivel movements of our eyes which are, as a rule, not sufficient to compensate the shift completely.

[4] This case, which is of particular interest to our theory of the framework, must be omitted here. The phenomenon occurring under these conditions is referred to as the Aubert phenomenon. G. E. Müller has devoted an elaborate study to it (1916) and I have interpreted it from my point of view in my article, 1922 (pp. 572-76).

tion is the same as in the real one, the same objects are being seen in the same relationships. One feature only has been altered, i.e., the relation between retinal and phenomenal lines. The principle of this change can be described thus: although the lines on the retina which correspond to objects seen as vertical are in the one case vertical, in the other oblique, yet the *main lines of organization* are in both cases seen as the *main directions of space*. These main directions are the vertical and the horizontal with its two main directions, which in a "normal position" are frontal parallel and sagittal. The horizontal ground plane and the vertical upon it, then, determine our framework. And no definite lines on the retina have the function of supplying us with this framework; rather is this the function of the main lines of the total organization. Thus the contours, with their one-sided function of shaping the things but not the spatial framework, have also a function for this latter by determining the main directions.

The answer to our question why the mirror world rights itself is implicit in our last conclusions. When we first look at the mirror the main lines of organization are not seen in the main directions of space; the floor is tilted, vertical objects are leaning over. This must be so, because at the moment we begin to see the mirror world we are still in our normal framework, in which vertical retinal lines produce vertical object-lines. Therefore, according to the previously derived relation (see p. 214), non-vertical retinal lines, which correspond to the vertical contours of objects reflected by the mirror, cannot appear vertical. But this old normal framework has no support in the mirror world and it cannot maintain itself without such support. Instead the new main lines of organization take over the rôle of creating the framework: the mirror world rights itself. The effect is in principle the same as that of the coloured homogeneous field which we discussed in Chapter IV. In either case the beginning of the new experience must be different from its later stages, in both cases we must consider the temporal course of stimulation as well as its spatial distribution.

LOCALIZATION OF THE EGO THROUGH CONSTITUTION OF FRAMEWORK. Another example, which I can only indicate briefly, will elucidate a similar point. Let us make two perspective drawings of a room from the same point. In one, we face one of the walls of the room, in the other we have turned a bit so that our face is no longer parallel to the wall and our eyes are directed towards another part of the wall. These two drawings will not be identical, and correspondingly our retinal images of the room, quite over and above the different parts visible, will not be identical. Yet we see the same room, i.e., our behavioural environment will be the same; but, as a datum of experience, our own position within this behavioural environment will be different. Again we have to transcend the environment and must include the Ego in a complete description. And we see now, what we had found before for non-visual ground, that the visual framework is a framework as much for our Egos as for the objects in the behavioural environment.

But our example deserves a more careful scrutiny. In either case we have, as the external conditions of our organized field, a certain distribution of light and colour on our retinae, different in the two cases. This difference might as well be produced by two rooms of *different shapes* both looked at while facing a main wall. The room that would, under these conditions, give the same projection as our ordinary room when we look at it from an oblique position would be a somewhat strange room. The question, then, is: Why do we, in reality, perceive an ordinary room with ourselves in a lop-sided position, and not this queer room with ourselves in a normal position?

Empiristic Explanation Again Excluded. Traditional psychology, and the layman who has imbibed more of it than he knows, would answer: Because, through experience, we know our room. Again we might raise the question how we succeeded in getting to know our room when our only visual source for attaining this knowledge is the retinal images? I do not want to extend this argument. The reader might test his own understanding of the anti-empiristic argument by developing it for himself, keeping in mind the continual movements of our heads and bodies, and asking himself the question why, from a purely empiristic point of view, the frontal parallel position should become the normal. Instead I shall adduce a few observations which are in strict contradiction to the empiristic explanation. We know that trees, telegraph poles, and houses stand vertical. If one travels on a mountain railway up a fairly steep slope one finds to one's great surprise on looking out of the window that in these strange parts of the world the trees grow at a fair angle against the vertical, and that in conformity with the trees, the people erected their telegraph poles and built their houses in the same curious fashion. In a recent paper (1932 a) I reported another particularly striking case: "On the west side of Lake Cayuga, a couple of hundred feet or so above its level, stands a public building on a wide lawn that slants slightly towards the lake. To everyone this building seems to be tilted in a direction away from the lake in a most striking manner."

APPLICATION OF THE GENERAL PRINCIPLE TO OUR VARIOUS EXAMPLES. *The Invariants.* Therefore we shall discard the empiristic theory as an ultimate explanation of our framework, without, however, raising the claim that experience can have no effect at all upon it. Such a claim would, in the present state of our knowledge, be unwarranted. Having rid ourselves of the empiristic bias we find in our last examples a very simple principle: such parts of the behavioural environment as become part of our general spatial framework assume one of the main spatial directions. Let us see what this principle means in our examples. When we look through the window of our mountain-railway carriage, this window becomes our spatial framework and appears, therefore, in normal, horizontal-vertical orientation. The contours of the objects seen through the window do not intersect the sash at right angles. Therefore, if the sash is seen as horizontal, these objects cannot be seen as vertical, but must appear leaning away from us on the ascent, and towards us on the descent. If Fig. 72 gives a somewhat exaggerated picture of the real positions of the window and a telegraph pole, then it shows at the same time why the telegraph pole cannot appear vertical when the window becomes the framework and thereby horizontally-vertically oriented. All one has to do is to turn this picture until the lower side of the window is horizontal; then of course the telegraph pole is tilted to the right as much as in our drawing the window is tilted to the left. The angle between the pole and the window sash, then, determines the *relative* localization of the two objects with regard to each other, whereas their absolute localization is determined by those parts of the field which form the spatial framework. If one sticks one's head out of the window, the telegraph pole will soon look vertical; when then, without losing sight of it, one withdraws the head, the telegraph pole will still appear vertical and the windows, the whole carriage, tilted. One factor in these two situations is *invariant,* the angle between ground and object.

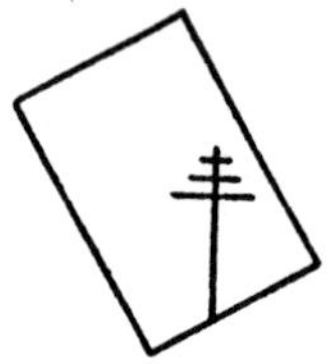

Fig. 72

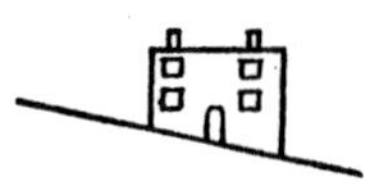

Fig. 73

It is easy to apply the same principle to the house on the western shores of Cayuga waters. The big lawn here provides the base, and therefore looks level. Consequently the house upon it must appear tilted. Again, one need only turn Fig. 73 until the ground line, representing the slightly sloping lawn, is horizontal, to see what happens.

We shall find the same principle, involving naturally other invariants, operative in the field of colour and of movement as well: relative properties of the stimulus distribution determining relative properties of the objects and events in the behavioural world, but the absolute properties of these latter depending upon a new factor, which in our case of the spatial framework is the stress of this framework towards the main directions of space.

THE SPECIAL CASE OF EGO LOCALIZATION. Our principle applies as well to our example of the room viewed when standing parallel or oblique to a wall. The case is more complicated than our last instances in so far as it involves more than directions. The two variables in this case are: shape of the room and position of the Ego with regard to it. When we face the room squarely, we perceive the proper room with its vertical and horizontal directions and ourselves in a normal position in it. We might, as far as the retinal stimulation goes, perceive a queerly shaped room with tilted sides and ourselves in an oblique position. If F stands for framework, and E for Ego, the index n for normal, and the index a for abnormal, we can represent all the different possibilities by the formula: $F_nE_n — F_aE_a$. Of course the first alternative is the one always realized: for that reason it seems to contain no problem. But once we have understood that there are numerous other possibilities, all described by F_aE_a, we see that this normal case needs an explanation as well as the abnormal ones. In this case the explanation is particularly simple: the framework is normal, and we know that a framework tends towards normality, and the position of the Ego is normal too, i.e., the "straight ahead" from the point of the Ego is perpendicular to one of the main planes of the framework. Two systems of direction, then, coincide in this case, the system imposed by the framework and the system depending on the Ego. A conflict between these two systems may greatly interfere with our direction of "straight ahead," for not only is this determined by the position of our Ego, it may as well be determined by the framework, being the sagittal direction of this framework rather than that of ourselves; as a matter of fact, even this latter determination is ambiguous, it may refer to our eye-, our head-, or our trunk-systems. G. E. Müller (1917) was the first to establish these different systems of localization. I shall adduce a very striking example of the conflict of the objective and the "egocentric" straight-ahead, an example which is the more important as it shows at the same time that the visual framework is not a framework for visual objects alone. My illustration is taken from acoustical experiments. The subject's task is to make a noise come from straight ahead. In order to understand this we must know what determines the localization of sound to the left or right. Since the original discovery by von Hornbostel and Wertheimer a great literature has grown up about the subject.[5] But the facts originally discovered remain unaffected. The left-right localization of sound depends upon the time difference with which the sound wave strikes the two ears, localization occurring towards the side whose ear is struck first, and the angle toward the median increasing, at least in a first approximation, proportionally with the amount of this precession. Consequently, a sound will be heard straight ahead when the time difference is 0, i.e., when the two ears are struck simultaneously. Knowing this, one can make a simple experiment. A constant or recurring noise is produced, and the sound is conducted to the two ears separately by a system of pipes, which contain, for each ear, a variable piece, like a trombone. As long as these two pipe systems are of equal length, the two ears of the observer will be stimulated simultaneously, and he will hear the noise straight ahead. If now the left trombone is pulled out, the sound will reach the left ear of the observer with a greater and greater delay compared to the right ear, and consequently the observer will hear the sound travel towards the right. And now comes our experiment: we set one of the trombones at a certain position so that our observer hears the sound at a certain angle; we then ask him to pull out the other trombone until he hears the sound again in the middle, i.e., straight ahead. This can be done with great accuracy. After some practice the average error of a good observer will not be more than one-half centimetre, i.e., he will pull out his trombone to a position on the average no more than half a centimetre in either direction from that of the other trombone. Let us pause for a moment to appraise this achievement. The velocity of sound in air is in round figures $330 \frac{\text{m.}}{\text{sec.}} = 33000 \frac{\text{cm.}}{\text{sec.}}$ The average error of ½ cm. means that when the observer hears the sound straight ahead the differences between the two paths may be ½ cm. What does this mean in terms of time?

$$c = \frac{s}{t},\ t = \frac{s}{c},\ t = \frac{.5}{33000}\ sec. = .015\sigma$$

This accuracy is amazing, but it depends upon one condition, viz., that the observers be seated squarely facing one of the walls of

[5] See von Hornbostel (1923 and 1930) and Banister.

the room. If they are not, their accuracy will suffer, in many cases even when they close their eyes during the observation. And the loss of objective accuracy is accompanied by a loss of subjective assurance. When, during my war work, I had acquired enormous practice by several thousands of such measurements, I was still unable, working with closed eyes, to find a good auditory "straight ahead" when my position in the room was not normal.

After this excursion let us return to our case F_nE_n. F_n is the most stable form of F, and therefore most easily produced, and under the conditions of our case F_n entails E_n. For the variables F and E are closely coupled together, in the same way in which the two directions of base and object were coupled together in the previous examples. We might say that in all possible organizations due to the respective stimulus distributions the relation between F and E is *invariant,* just as the angle between framework and object lines is invariant.

The Framework's Tendency Towards Normality. We turn now to the second case, our perception of the room when we are in a non-normal position in it. This time we need three formulae to describe all possible organizations: $F_nE_a — F_a E_a — F_aE_n$, of which the middle one comprises a great number of cases. Again F and E are coupled together, but of course, owing to the change of conditions, in a different manner from what they were before. Again the first formula is realized, the framework remains normal, and the Ego is turned. This is exactly comparable to the building on Lake Cayuga, where the framework became normal and the object upon it, the house, was tilted. If O stands for object, then this example would be described by the three formulae:

$$F_nO_a — F_aO_a — F_aO_n$$

the last one being the "true perception," the house appearing vertical and the ground sloping. Therefore the tendency towards normality is a tendency of the framework, and both the Ego and the objects within the framework are determined by the framework and its invariant connections with its content, viz., objects and Ego.

Normality and Frequency. We have so far used the term normal orientation in a descriptive and functional but not a statistical sense. The normal case for us was not the one most frequently realized. And yet it seems as though our normal orientation were also the most frequent orientation, since it is the one which we assume spontaneously; we have a tendency to put our chairs and couches parallel to a wall, and when we want to inspect anything we face it directly. But this statistical aspect of the normal, far from being the cause of its functional aspect, is its effect. Using the symbolism introduced above, we may say: $F_n E_n$ is of all possible organizations the stablest. And since such organization can generally be realized by movements of our body, such movements will take place if no other field forces are present to prevent them. Thus the normal becomes the most frequent because of its normality, but it does not become the normal because of its greatest frequency—an observation pertinent to many discussions of these two pairs of concepts, and absolutely fatal to the positivistic reduction of the normal, or the type, to the statistical average.

Constancy of the Framework. Constancy of Direction, Size, and Shape. We can describe the result of our last discussion in still another manner which will be elaborated in more detail in our chapter on Action. We found that the movements of our eyes, heads, and bodies, which change the retinal pattern, leave the framework intact. Therefore we may say: The framework is as constant as the conditions permit. This explains at the same time the relative constancy of direction, size, and shape of the objects which we perceive.

THE INVARIANTS OF CONSTANCY OF SIZE. We have discussed the dependence of the direction of lines and the size of objects and after-images on the framework to which they belong. We can, to make the point more clear, introduce again our principle of invariants. Remember the experiment of the perspective drawing of a tunnel. Let the after-image projected upon it be that of a line half as long as that of the near vertical edge of the tunnel. Its apparent size will then depend on two factors: its relation to the geometrical height of the tunnel at the point at which it is projected, and on the apparent size of the latter; the invariant being the relation between the two sizes. Thus, when the after-image is close to the front edge, it will appear about half that size; if it is near to a vertical line which appears further back and which is itself only half as long as the front edge, it will appear equal to it, because the retinal images are equal, and this equality is now the invariant; but since the latter vertical line appears to be approximately as long as the front edge, the after-image will also appear as large, i.e., it will now look twice as large as in the beginning.

THE INVARIANTS OF CONSTANCY OF SHAPE. The same point of view applies to shape. The details of the relation of shape to framework have not been worked out, but in accordance with the last discussion we can make the following deduction. If a square surface produces a square retinal image, and is seen as a square in a frontal parallel position, then a circular after-image projected upon it will also appear as a circle. But when now this square is turned, say, by 45 degrees around a vertical axis, it is projected on the retina as a trapezium, but is seen as a square in a non-normal position. Now the circular after-image projected upon it can no longer look like a circle. For if a trapezium looks like a square, a circle can no longer look like a circle, if we are permitted this somewhat elliptical formulation. Correspondingly, a real circle on the square will in this new position produce the retinal image of an ellipse, but will be seen as a circle, for when a certain trapezium looks like a square, a certain ellipse will look like a circle.[6] The principle is exactly the same as that in the preceding cases. And the invariants here are the relations between the different shapes. Since these relations may be much less simple than the size and direction relations, the invariances may be less complete. Many interesting problems await experimentation in this field. A very ingenious experiment which demonstrates the above relation beautifully has just been reported by Thouless. "A subject sits below the objective of a projection lantern. Facing him and normal to the line of vision is a square cardboard screen on which the image from the lantern is cast. If now the screen is tilted at an angle to the frontal-parallel plane of the observer, the retinal image of the picture will be unchanged . . . Phenomenally, however, the picture becomes distorted, being elongated laterally. The screen itself, although its retinal image is compressed laterally, is phenomenally very little different from a square" (1934). It must suffice at the present to have demonstrated the connection between the constancy of the framework and the constancies of size, direction, and shape. Again our explanation of these fundamental facts of perception is unempiristic.

Empiristic Explanations of These Constancies, and the Reason for Their Popularity. And yet these constancy phenomena seemed to cry for empiristic explanations. Here were the constant objects and the changing retinal images. As long as one did not look beyond the local retinal images one could not see how it was possible that different retinal images should give rise to identical shapes as pure sensory data. And therefore one had recourse to experience: for what we saw with these varying retinal images corresponded in the vast majority of cases, more or less, to reality, to reality which could not directly influence our sense organs so as to be seen correctly. Therefore the recourse to experience was inevitable. We have learned

[6] The connection between this trapezium and this ellipse may not be quite simple, since squares and ellipses show different degrees of constancy. See below.

that things are constant, have such and such properties, and therefore, not being interested in our sensations but in things, we unwittingly interpret our sensations in accordance with what we have learned about things. But the empiristic theory, which is so plausible only because of the constancy hypothesis which it silently implies, is as untenable here as it proved to be in the other fields in which we encountered it. We have already disproved it for the constancy of size by animal experiments (see Chapter III, pp. 88 f.); we produced a still stronger argument against it when we showed cases where our perception is in accordance with our laws of framework and invariance but contradicts an explanation in terms of experience and reality (the tilted telegraph poles and houses); and we shall give examples of the same kind, possibly still more striking, when we discuss colour constancy.

The refutation of the empiristic explanation does not prove ours to be right. But at least we can claim that our theory explains the cases which apparently fit the empiristic theory—veridical perceptions—and those which are in discord with it—illusory perceptions—by the same principles. And these principles are of an extreme simplicity: the establishment of a framework in the main directions of space by the main contours of the field, and an invariant relation between certain aspects of stimulation, our invariance principle taking the place of the old constancy hypothesis.

THEORY OF PERCEPTUAL CONSTANCIES

Constancy of Shape. Even so, our hypothesis is incomplete. It says that an effect *a* will occur *if* an effect *b* occurs, but it does not say under what conditions this second effect will be realized. More concretely, we do not yet know when a square retinal image gives rise to the perception of a square. We avoided this difficulty in our formulation by adding the second condition that the square retinal image was produced by a real square. But this was only a postponement of the real problem. True, under this condition a square retinal image will give rise to the perception of a square, while under other conditions it will not (a trapezium in a non-frontal-parallel position); but we want to know why. The case mentioned in this condition, viz., a square producing a square retinal image, is undoubtedly a unique case. It is so in many respects: the figure perceived is the simplest possible (square as opposed to trapezium), it is so in its orientation (frontal parallel), and besides, the perception is veridical; that is, one sees a square in agreement with both the distant and the proximal stimulus. It is natural to connect the cause of the uniqueness of this condition with one of these aspects, and one must in consequence choose between them. Quite naturally the choice falls upon the last, the veridical aspect. For a square which projects a much distorted picture on our retinas, even if it is not perceived in the shape corresponding to the retinal image, is not seen entirely as a square, but usually as a rectangle approximating a square more or less closely. Now in this case the form of the behavioural object coincides neither with the shape of the distant stimulus (square) nor the proximal (trapezium) but has an intermediate position. What surprised psychologists in this discovery was the fact that the perceived form was so much closer to the "real" than to the retinal one, and this fact was expressed in the statement that shape, like size and colour, shows the phenomenon of relative constancy, i.e., the different percepts produced by one and the same distant stimulus will vary much less than the corresponding proximal stimuli, and will stay closer to the percept produced under the unique condition of stimulation just discussed. Two concepts determine this interpretation, viz., the distant and the proximal stimulus: the percept depending upon the *proximal* stimulus approaches the properties of the *distant* one. In the realm of colour, where, as we know, the same phenomenon obtains, the term "transformation" has been introduced which implies that a process peripherally like the proximal stimulus is changed by central factors into a process more like the distant stimulus. Thouless calls this effect, equally apparent in the realms of shape, size, and colour, "phenomenal regression to the real object."

The Danger of the Traditional Formulation of the Problem. This interpretation of the effect was historically justified,[7] because it raised a very important problem. But it has its dangers when an explanation of the effect is attempted. This appears even in the definitions of the magnitude of this effect.

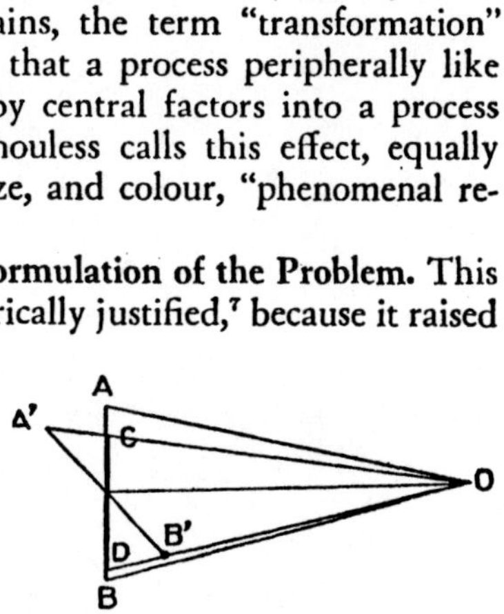

Fig. 74

To illustrate this we shall choose the example of ellipses, including the circle, rather than that of rectangles including the square, because the perspective is somewhat simpler in the former case. An observer at O looks at an ellipse with a horizontal axis AB = r (*"real"*) which is turned round a vertical axis passing through its centre so that the horizontal axis has the position A′B′. This hori-

[7] See our discussion of colour constancy, p. 241.

zontal axis, oblique to the observer, will produce the same retinal image as the frontal parallel line CD = p (*"projection"*), the heavy line of Fig. 74. The subject has to compare this ellipse with other ellipses in a frontal plane, all having the same vertical axis as the oblique one, but different horizontal ones, until he finds one among them that seems to him to have the same shape as the oblique one. The horizontal axis a of this frontal parallel ellipse would then also be the *"apparent"* horizontal axis of the oblique one. As a rule, and this has been found in many experiments by Thouless, Eissler, and Klimpfinger, a will be greater than p, but smaller than r, $p < a < r$. If a were equal to r, constancy would be complete, phenomenal regression to the real object total. If a were equal to p there would be no constancy or regression. The actual size of a is therefore used to measure the degree of constancy.

Brunswik's and Thouless's Measure of Constancy. Since the total range of constancy between 0 and totality lies between the limits $a = p$ and $a = r$, the difference $r - p$ is taken as the whole range, and the difference $a - p$ as the part of this range which characterizes the constancy achieved in the experiment. Thus the constancy itself is measured by $c = \frac{a-p}{r-p}$. If $a = r$, complete constancy, $c = 1$; if $a = p$, no constancy, $c = 0$. All degrees of constancy must therefore lie between 0 and 1, or, if one multiplies the right side of the equation by 100, so as to avoid decimals, $c = 100\frac{a-p}{r-p}$, the constancy ranges between 0 and 100.[8]

However convenient and useful for special purposes these measures may be, theoretically they do not seem to me to have any special significance,[9] because of their assumption of the range of possible constancies. Let us consider a simple example. Let us suppose the line A′B′ to represent the horizontal axis, 15 cm. in length, of an ellipse with a vertical axis of 20 cm., viewed from a distance of 450 cm. and at an angle of 45° towards the line of regard. Its retinal image is approximately equal to that of a frontal parallel ellipse

[8] This formula has the advantage of simplicity but also several disadvantages (see Brunswik [1933a] and Thouless). It is nevertheless frequently used by Brunswik's pupils, whereas Thouless uses exclusively a logarithmic formula, also employed by Brunswik, which is free of the drawbacks of the other formula, viz., $c' = \frac{\log a - \log p}{\log r - \log p}$. If $a = p$, no constancy, $c' = 0$, and if $a = r$, complete constancy, $c' = 1$.

[9] I forbear to discuss the theoretical justification which Brunswik gives of these measures (pp. 390 f.).

with an equal vertical axis and a horizontal axis of 10.7 cm., but it is also approximately equal to that of a circle (20 cm. diameter) at an angle of 15° 30′ to the line of regard. Now the two formulae consider only cases in which the horizontal axis *a* of the frontal parallel ellipse chosen as of equal shape is not shorter than 10.7 and not longer than 15 cm., i.e., they exclude all shapes which lie between the latter shape and the circle (horizontal axis = 20 cm.). *A priori* there is no reason why it should not appear equally easily as having a horizontal axis *a* between 15 and 20 cm. And as a matter of fact this happens. Eissler reports two cases for the very conditions which we have stated[10] and similar ones for other conditions.

A Flaw in This Measure. This seems at first not to impair the value of the measures, the constancy would simply assume values greater than 100 in Brunswik's formula and greater than 1 in the logarithmic measure. Thus one of the values Eissler adduces for our constellation is $c = 164$, and to this corresponds the logarithmic value $c' = 1.45$. And yet it comes as something of a shock to find values which are greater than complete constancy. The main point however is this: these measures were so useful because, by referring each result to a well-defined range, they yielded comparable figures for very diverse constellations, each having its own range defined in the same way. But the fact of more than complete constancy destroys this advantage. The range itself becomes a function of the constellation and is no longer $r - p$ for *all* constellations. Therefore the comparison of *c* quotients derived in the fields of form-, size-, and brightness-constancy, even if it leads to similar curves of development (Klimpfinger 1933 a), does not as yet seem to be a fully justified procedure.

The Problem Reformulated. If now we return to our main problem we find that the connection between this uniqueness of one set of conditions and its cognitive value should not be used in any sense as explanatory of the uniqueness. Rather, the cognitive value should be derived from uniqueness. More generally: the problem which has been called the constancy problem should be re-formulated in this way: What shape, size, brightness, will correspond to a certain local stimulus pattern under various total external and internal conditions? Once we have answered this question we shall know when to expect constancy, when not. Indeed some effects of non-constancy are just as striking as the effects of constancy which have been so much emphasized, particularly in the field of colour and brightness.

[10] Since Eissler reports only *c* values, I had to compute the *p* and *a* values myself from his data.

An Attempt at Its Solution. Let us see how far we can go towards the solution of the general problem with regard to shape. We begin by analyzing some examples. In the one discussed on pp. 226 f. a subject judged the shape of an ellipse turned through 45° from the frontal parallel plane equal to another ellipse which appeared in a frontal parallel plane, when the two axes of the former were 15 and 20 cm., those of the latter 17.75 and 20 respectively. In another example the ellipse is turned 60° from the frontal parallel, its horizontal axis and that of the frontal parallel ellipse judged equal to it being 40 and 35 cm. respectively (the vertical ones being always 20 cm.). Therefore in each case we find two different stimuli giving rise to the perception of equal shapes, and not only different distant but also different proximal stimuli. We called the length of the horizontal axis, as far as it determines the proximal stimulus, *p;* the length of the horizontal axis, measured absolutely, *r*. Now when the figure is in "normal" orientation (frontal parallel) $p = r$, but not when it is turned from the normal. I omit the formula which connects *p* with this angle, and shall list instead the *p* values for the two examples. The horizontal axis of the normally oriented ellipse which was judged as of equal shape to the turned one will again be called *a*, the angle through which the figure is turned δ.

TABLE 7

case	*r*	δ	*p*	*a*
I	15	45	10.7	17.75
II	40	60	20	35

In both cases the vertical axes were 20 cm. long. Therefore the two stimulus ellipses with equal vertical axes and horizontal axes 10.7 and 17.75 produced the same shape, and similarly the two stimulus ellipses with horizontal axes 20 and 35 produced the same perceived shape (though of course a different one from that produced by the first pair).

The Two Components: Shape and Orientation. Now we have stated it as a general rule that two proximal stimuli if more than liminally different cannot produce exactly the same effect. If this effect is equal in one respect it must differ in another. This other respect is easy to discover in our cases: the two ellipses which appeared of equal shape were seen in different *orientation*. The effect of the stimulus pattern has therefore at least two different aspects or components, viz., shape and orientation. This reminds us of the example of the mountain railway which we discussed some time ago (pp. 217 f.). There an angle between two lines, e.g., sash of the window and telegraph pole, gave rise to a perception in which we also distinguished two components, viz., the angle and the orientation. We found the former determined by the stimulus angle, but not the latter, and we called the former an invariant of the situation.

THE INVARIANT OF THE CASE. Our present case is palpably more complex, but we might try to look again for an invariant. If there were one, it would not be of such a simple kind, namely, one aspect, independently of the other, being in an invariant relation to a stimulus property. Rather the two aspects of the percept will be coupled together so that if one changes, the other changes also. In this respect shape is much more similar to size, where, normally, a relation of proportionality exists between perceived size and distance, so that if two equal retinal lines give rise to the perception of two behavioural lines of different length, these two lines appear at correspondingly different distances. Applied to shape this would mean: if two equal retinal shapes give rise to two different perceived shapes, they will at the same time produce the impression that these two shapes are differently oriented. The question is whether shape and orientation are as rigidly connected as size and distance.

CRITICISM OF THE EXPERIMENTAL EVIDENCE WHICH SEEMS TO CONTRADICT THE ASSUMPTION OF AN INVARIANT. According to Eissler such a connection does not exist, for he reports several cases where figures which were actually not normally oriented were seen in normal orientation and yet at the same time with a fair degree of constancy, and fewer cases of the opposite kind where the perceived orientation was non-normal and corresponded to the real orientation, and yet practically no constancy occurred (pp. 538 ff.). The first would mean that two different retinal figures produced percepts equal both in shape and orientation, the second that two practically equal stimuli[11] produced unequal percepts, different namely with regard to orientation.

Eissler's results gain some support from Klimpfinger (1933 a, p. 626 f.), who used a very similar procedure, and from Holaday, for constancy of size. All three authors interpret this paradoxical effect by saying that "cues" (*Umstandsdaten*) may be lost in the perception of objects without losing their effects, or that the functionally effective depth data need not become conscious as such, so that the

[11] If constancy is zero, the retinal image of the frontal parallel ellipse is equal to the retinal image of the turned ellipse.

"mediation of perceptual things" takes place on a level lower than that which carries conscious processes.

It would be dogmatic to deny that such an interpretation is possible. On the other hand, on the basis of the existing experimental material I am loth to accept it. It would invalidate one of our main axioms of perceptual organization, viz., that supraliminally different stimuli do not produce entirely equal *perceptual* effects, and would thereby make an intelligible theory of perception well-nigh impossible. Such radical theoretical conclusions seem to me unwarranted by the adduced evidence. The second case—oblique orientation or difference of distance being perceived without constancy of shape or size—can be dismissed at the outset, since the authors themselves call them rare (Eissler) and ambiguous (Holaday). The other case, viz., constancy of a relatively high degree without perception of non-normal orientation or depth difference, on which the preceding interpretation is based, is not sufficiently supported either. Eissler lists nineteen cases, and of these seven belong to a one-eyed subject, whose results differ in many ways from those of the normal subjects. Of the remaining twelve only one occurred under normal conditions, all the others under circumstances which interfered with clear spatial organization, e.g., monocular observation, regard fixated on a point between the two objects to be compared so that they were seen peripherally, looking through semi-closed lids, etc. The same is true of all examples given by Holaday.

Under these circumstances it seems to me justifiable not to abandon the fundamental axiom, but to seek the explanation of the paradoxical cases elsewhere. I can think of two possibilities. Either the two ellipses judged to be equal with regard to both shape and orientation differed in a *third* aspect, or the paradoxical effect is due to the serial character of presentation, trace aggregates influencing the results. A decision between the different hypotheses must await further experimentation. Such experimentation should, however, fill a gap in our knowledge: matchings of shape (and size) should be supplemented by matchings of orientation (and distance). Only when we possess these data shall we be able to see clearly what the relation of shape and orientation (or size and distance) is.

THE FRONTAL PARALLEL ORIENTATION A UNIQUE CASE. "NORMAL ORIENTATION." Such knowledge would be a prerequisite for a theory of the constancy of shape, but it would not in itself supply it. For a theory would have to answer the question when a circular retinal image will lead to the perception of a circle, when to that of a non-normally oriented ellipse, and *why* it has the two different effects in the two different cases. Such a theory might start from the case where a circular retinal image gives rise to the perception of a normally oriented circle. That this is a unique case we have stated before, and we can now choose among the various factors which contributed to its uniqueness. After having discarded the "veridicalness" of the percept as a factor which causes it, there remains the choice between the greatest simplicity of figure and orientation. Of these two the first is ruled out easily, for as a rule an ellipse presented in a frontal parallel position will appear as such and not as a circle non-normally oriented. This leaves us with the frontal parallel plane as a special case. Not only is this view accepted by Eissler (p. 540), it may also be deduced from our findings about the main directions of space. Dynamically this assumption would mean that a frontal parallel plane is well balanced within itself, so that special forces are required to dislocate it. In such a plane stimulus patterns would produce perceptual patterns according to the most simple laws, and indeed our study of perceptual forms was carried out under conditions where the figures appeared in the frontal parallel (or some other similarly unique) plane.

Shape in Non-normal Orientation the Product of Organization in a Field of Stress. To perceive a non-frontal parallel plane would then require special forces which would turn the plane from its normal position and which would be opposed by forces tending to pull it back into normal. Thus the stimulus pattern of the figure would lead to an organization in a field of stress, and therefore the product of this organization would be different from what it is when the field is free of stress, i.e., the frontal-parallel plane. In this situation the stimulus pattern introduces new forces which will combine with the forces of orientation responsible for the stress in the field, and the final organization will be that in which all these forces are best balanced.

Constancy Facts Deduced from This Hypothesis. Let us apply these ideas to the concrete case of Eissler's experiments, an ellipse turned round its vertical axis so that its retinal image is more slender (horizontal axis relatively shorter) than that of the same ellipse in a normal position. The result is that the ellipse appears turned and not as slender as it would if its retinal image were produced by a frontal parallel ellipse. Otherwise expressed, the forces in the plane of the ellipse must, owing to its being turned, be such as to extend it horizontally. These are not the only forces in the field, as we see when we consider the case of a rectangle turned in the same way. Not only does its retinal image become more slender with this change of orientation, but its shape is transformed from rectangularity to that of a trapezium. (See Fig. 75 a, b, which represent a normal and a non-normal view of a rectangle.) If, then, this retinal shape gives rise to the perception of a rectangle, forces must have been at work which have changed the converging lines into parallel ones. It would be premature to speculate more about the actual distribution of forces within the non-normally oriented plane without more specific data or a more concrete hypothesis about the event in the brain field which corresponds to the obliquely oriented figure.

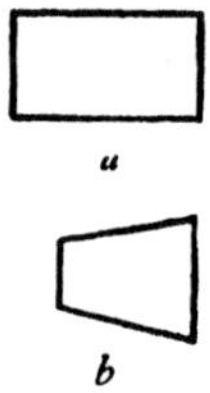

Fig. 75

Besides these forces in the field there are two other kinds of forces responsible for the perceived shape, viz., internal forces and those external forces which are produced by the proximal stimulation. We have studied them in the preceding chapters (pp. 138 ff.), where we have seen the great power of the latter. The fact that the stimulus forces are very strong means in our present context that a retinal shape will most easily produce that behavioural shape which corresponds to it, i.e., it will resist transformation. In other words, the forces within the field which tend to "distort" the retinal shape will have to contend with the forces imposed by that retinal shape. In our example: a slender retinal ellipse produces a behavioural shape in a field of stress which tends to make it less slender. Owing to the forces produced by the retinal pattern the perceived figure will not entirely yield to this stress, and therefore the perceived shape will be somewhere between the retinal and the "real" shape, unless the internal forces of organization complicate the situation. We consider, for instance, the real shape of a slender ellipse whose retinal image, owing to the orientation of the figure, is still more slender. Then, owing to the forces in the field produced by the non-normal orientation of the figure, the behavioural ellipse will be broadened, and if this broadening is sufficient it may make its shape sufficiently similar to a circle so that the internal forces of organization, which are in their most stable equilibrium in the circular shape, succeed in producing, or at least approximating, this simplest form.

A last deduction is possible: the final equilibrium will be an equilibrium for *all* participating forces. That means: perceived orientation and shape will depend upon each other: if a retinal shape resists distortion by the field forces it will thereby influence the apparent angle of orientation. It is therefore probable that the amount by which the figure appears turned from the normal decreases as the "constancy of shape" decreases, i.e., the more similar the perceived shape is to the retinal, the less similar to the real shape. That means, of course, that a certain combination of shape and orientation is invariant for a given retinal shape, as we had previously supposed.[12]

Experimental Verification. A number of our conclusions are confirmed by the experimental evidence. In the first place "constancy" is, as a rule, not perfect, "phenomenal regression not complete," as Thouless, Eissler, and Klimpfinger have found. In the second place, the constancy decreases with the angle of orientation (Eissler). This result is deducible from our hypothesis, for the more different the retinal image is from the "real" shape, the greater will be the forces required to produce a perceived shape equal to the real. If the stress in the field resulting from non-normal orientation increased in the same way as the force required to transform the retinal shape into the real, then constancy could not be a function of the angle. Now we do not know either of these two functions, but it is more than unlikely that they are the same. Let us begin with the latter, the dependency of the force necessary to transform the retinal shape into the real one upon the angle of orientation. According to our assumption a retinal shape sets up forces to produce a similar psychophysical shape. These forces come into conflict with the stress in the field when the plane in which the shape appears is non-normal. Owing to this stress the retinal shape is changed into another shape more like the real one. Now, the greater the difference between retinal and real shape, owing to the turning of the figure, the greater the force necessary to change the retinal shape into the real. It is, however, most unlikely that this relation is one of simple proportionality. Dynamically it is much more probable that this change becomes the more difficult the farther it has proceeded, just as it requires an increasing force to produce equal successive contractions of a spiral spring. Turn a figure with a horizontal axis h round its vertical axis first through a certain angle which reduces its horizontal axis by a certain amount m, and then through another angle which reduces its horizontal axis by another equal amount, so that this axis is now $h - 2m$. If it requires the force f to change the figure with the horizontal axis

[12] *Which* combination cannot be deduced, unless one either has the necessary empirical data or knows the different interacting forces. Furthermore, the invariant may depend upon total sets of conditions, and need not necessarily be the same under all circumstances.

$h - m$ into one with the horizontal axis h, then, according to our hypothesis, it will require more than $2f$ to transform the figure with the horizontal axis $h - 2m$ into one with the horizontal axis h. Now it seems very unlikely that the stress within the field due to the non-normal orientation should increase as rapidly with the angle as the force required to achieve perfect constancy. Therefore constancy should decrease with the angle, as it does.

I have used the term "transformation" without implying that at first a non-transformed shape is produced by peripheral stimulation to be later centrally transformed. I used the term to indicate an effect which would follow from one set of forces abstracted from their context, against the actual effect due to a combination of different sets of forces. The term transformation as here used means merely a double vectorial determination, to borrow a term from Kardos (p. 170).

Thirdly, the more the real figure is turned from the frontal-parallel position, the more does it appear to be non-normally oriented. Therefore the stress in the field toward transformation increases with the angle of orientation, and therefore the transformation, measured in absolute terms, should increase also. Such a measure is given by Eissler as $A = \frac{a-p}{p}$.[13] This value increases indeed with the angle of orientation, both in Eissler's and Thouless's (1931) experiments.[14] Lastly, the cases of "super-constancy" discussed on page 227 are perfectly compatible with our theory; they follow from it under special conditions, whereas I have found no other explanation of them elsewhere. Eissler's discussion of these cases, which I shall omit here, is also in perfect accord with our interpretation.

Much work has to be done to raise the rank of our explanation above that of a mere hypothesis. But that the true explanation will have to be on lines similar to my hypothesis seems to me certain. For "*knowledge*" of the real shape does not account for the effect, as Thouless (1931 a) has shown by special experiments. If I interpret this author correctly, he too believes that the true theory must be of the kind here presented. He rejects a "summative or integrative theory" and postulates a "response theory." On such a theory, "the ellipse seen with binocular observation of an inclined circle is

[13] One might just as well take $Q = \frac{a}{p}$, a measure which Katz used in his investigation of brightness constancy (Q-Quotient) in 1911 (see p. 242).

[14] Thouless does not use this measure, but since he reports the raw figures of his results, it is easy to calculate it, and this calculation confirms Eissler's results.

a fact of perception of the same order as the ellipse seen with monocular vision and elimination of distance cues" (1931 a, p. 26).

Constancy and Spatial Organization. In our theory the behavioural shape produced by a certain retinal image depends upon the spatial organization to which the retinal image gives rise. Constancy will therefore be the greater the more "adequate" the perceived orientation of the figure is, i.e., the more closely it approximates to the real orientation. All factors, therefore, which determine orientation must *pari passu* influence perceived shape. This conclusion, which is not specific to our theory but would be included in some form or other in any theory of constancy of shape, is amply confirmed by facts. Eissler has very systematically investigated a number of conditions which vary in respect to the general space-organizations which they produce, and has found a clear correlation between these conditions and shape constancy. Among them binocular parallax, retinal disparity, was found to be of particular importance, and good articulation of the central figures as well as of the surrounding, hardly less relevant. Furthermore he found that, as he puts it, different criteria of depth can be substituted for each other without essentially changing the effect. Schematically this means: of the three criteria *a, b* and *c, a* alone may be as effective as *a* and *b* combined, but *b* and *c* not much inferior to *a* and *b,* or *a* and *c,* in combination. The theoretical meaning of this result can be developed only by a discussion of the depth factors *per se,* a task which we shall undertake later after we have finished our discussion of the constancy problems.

Influence of Attitude. Constancy can be tremendously affected if the subjects' attitude is directed towards "projection" rather than towards real shapes, as shown for shape by Klimpfinger (1933), for size by Holaday. In neither case is the result a complete loss of constancy; the frontal parallel figure selected to look equal to a turned figure under "analytical" attitude, though much closer to the retinal image of the latter than under a normal attitude, still differed from it in the direction of being more similar to the "real" shape of the turned figure, and the same is true *mutatis mutandis* for size. It is, however, possible to vary the external conditions for normal observation in such a way that constancy is lower than under the analytic attitude and normal external conditions.

Constancy of Size. A few words must be added about the constancy of size, which we have already discussed in Chapter III (pp. 88 f. and 90 f.). Holaday, another of Brunswik's pupils, has done for this problem what Eissler and Klimpfinger have done for the constancy of shape, investigating a number of external and internal conditions which affect this constancy. These results are similar to those of the two other authors, as we have already mentioned with regard to the internal condition of analytical attitude. As regards the external conditions, constancy varies again directly with space organization, but disparity has a much weaker influence on size than on shape, a fact which is explained by both Eissler and Holaday by the circumstance that depth organization must be much finer for shape than for size constancy.

THE INVARIANT OF THIS CASE. The similarity between the results of Eissler and Holaday indicates a similarity in the underlying causes. For size as for shape *some* effect will be invariant for a given stimulus, and this effect will be some combination of size and distance. It has already been mentioned (p. 229) that some of Holaday's results seem to contradict such an assumption, but I have also indicated why I cannot consider these contradictory results as decisive. Again the form of this combination has to be worked out in future experiments, and it will prove to be dependent upon the direction in which the objects recede from the observer. This follows from our discussion of the zenith-horizon illusion in Chapter III (p. 94 f.).

NO UNIQUE SET OF CONDITIONS FOR SIZE. In one important respect, however, the theory of perceived size will have to be different from that of perceived shape: in the latter we found a unique case, the normally oriented, i.e., frontal-parallel plane. For size there exists no such unique case, no "normal" distance comparable to a normal orientation. On the one hand, the normal distance is different for different objects, e.g., for a printed page, a person, a house, a mountain, and on the other such normal distance is at best a rather wide range and not a well-defined point. But it seems likely that something else plays an analogous rôle in the field. Lauenstein (1934) [15] has made an observation according to which constancy is not so simple a function of distance as has so far been supposed, but holds for definite unified ranges, so that *within* two such ranges, which lie at different distances from the observer, constancy is approximately equally good, although compared with each other the nearer one has the greater degree of constancy. From this concept of range, which, as we shall see later, finds its counterpart in the realms of

[15] Lauenstein's observation was made from a hilltop: he saw in the surrounding distance numerous small mounds all approximately of the same size, which he supposed to be bushes. On descending he found them to be hayricks of 3-4 metres.

colour-constancy (Kardos), he concludes that the "real" (normal) behavioural size may appear within that range which includes the observer's behavioural Ego.

A Possible Theory of Perceived Size. A theory of perceived size may possibly be derived from the theory of perceived space indicated in the fourth chapter (p. 119). If articulated space tends to become as large as possible it requires forces to make an object appear near. This theory, which I have learned from a discussion with Köhler, suggests that the more energy is consumed in bringing the object near, the less is available for keeping it large. This indication must suffice with the addition that nearness need not be the only factor that determines size, other factors being possibly "clearness" articulation, surveyability. The facts of micropsia seem to support such a more general theory, facts whose importance for the theory of size were long ago recognized by Jaensch (1909), whose first publication on the subject was almost epoch-making.

H. FRANK'S EXPERIMENTS. A special form of Köhler's theory has been tested in his laboratory by H. Frank (1930). In ordinary experiments on size constancy the two objects to be compared with each other are alternately fixated, i.e., a far fixated object is compared with a near fixated object. Within a certain range size constancy is perfect, so that the *same* geographical object will look equal at, let us say, a distance of one and two metres, although the retinal image of the far object is only one fourth of the area of that of the near one. But in changing fixation from the near to the far object "the tension of the muscalature for accommodation and convergence is decreased. If, then, one assumes that the visual field would have to part with some of its energy for the purpose of 'near-innervation' and that this loss of energy leads to a relative shrinking of the fixated object . . . then decrease of the tension of the eye-muscles, accompanying 'far-innervation,' i.e., a smaller loss of energy by the visual field, would result in a relative enlargement of the fixated object which would more or less compensate (centrally) for the retinal diminution" (Frank, p. 136). Certain observations by Hering and others seemed to confirm such a view. Frank, however, performed quantitative experiments to subject it to a rigid test. A square fixated directly was (successively) compared with a square at the same objective distance observed while fixation was either nearer or further. It was found in agreement with Hering's observation that a square at a fixed distance appears larger when it is fixated than when it lies *behind* the fixation point, and smaller than when it lies in front of it. Moreover, the size of the non-fixated square varies with the distance of the fixation point from the observer more or less as accommodation and convergence do, except for the fact that this agreement is better for the near than for the far fixation point. Thus the original assumption seems to be proved apart from the unpredictable and unexplained asymmetry of fixation in front of and behind the square. But the effect is far too small to explain constancy of size. To give an example: a square with a side of 8 cm. at a distance of 200 cm. if observed with a fixation at 90 cm. (from the observer) appeared equal to a fixated square at 200 cm. with a side of 7.5 cm. In this range constancy is perfect, i.e., a fixated square of 8 cm. at 90 cm. looks equal to an equal square at 200 cm. Thus constancy is slightly reduced by change of fixation with changed accommodation and convergence. But the retinal image of a square at 90 cm. is more than twice as large linearly as that of an equal square at 200 cm. This means that the retinal image of an object 8 cm. in diameter at 200 cm. distance, which gives the same perceived size as that of an equally large object 90 cm. distant, has a "size effect" $^{200}/_{90}$ greater than the latter. If this were entirely due to the energy that goes into the greater strain of convergence and accommodation for the near one, then we could make the following deduction. If we fixate at 90 cm. looking at an object (8 cm. long) at 200 cm., the retinal image should, by virtue of the near accommodation and convergence, have a size effect only $^{90}/_{200}$ of that which it would have if it were fixated directly. Therefore an object at 200 cm., fixated directly, should be only $8 \times \frac{90}{200} = 3.6$ cm., whereas in Frank's experiment it had the size of 7.5 cm. For the assumption is tantamount to assuming that the energy that goes into accommodation and convergence compensates exactly for the gain in retinal image. Therefore a constant retinal image [16] should produce a perceived size directly proportional to the fixation distance. In our case the shrinkage should be from 8 to 3.6 cm., whereas in reality it is only from 8 to 7.5 cm. Therefore, even though the accommodation-fixation energy may contribute to the constancy effect, it is at best responsible only for a very small fraction of it.

DEVELOPMENT OF CONSTANCY. A last point before we turn to the discussion of colour constancy. In Vienna careful and elaborate studies have been made of the development of constancy during the life of the individual, first by Beyrl (see Chapter II, p. 92) in the field of size, then by Brunswik (1929) in the field of brightness, and lastly by Klimpfinger (1933) in the field of shape. All three studies seem to reveal the same progress of development; the curves in which constancy is plotted against age have a similar shape for all three fields. However, even if one disregards the criticism levelled in the preceding pages against the measure of constancy employed in the construction of the curves, one may doubt whether the similarity of the three curves is due to the fact that all represent *constancies,* or to another factor common to all three investigations. An examination of this possibility might even lead to the

[16] The change of size of the retinal image due to change of accommodation is negligibly small for this argument (see Frank, p. 141).

conviction that there is *no* development of constancy and that the age progress which the curves demonstrate must be laid to the account of an external factor. Katz (1929) was the first to make this point in a review of recent work done in the field of colour constancy. His student Burzlaff repeated the experiments of Brunswik and Beyrl, and amplified his investigation by varying the method by which constancy was tested. Whereas in all experiments of the Vienna school the method consisted in comparing one standard object (size, neutral shade, shape) with one comparison object, both being in the same field of vision, Burzlaff introduced other methods which have in common the feature that they employ a *number* of simultaneously presented objects either in place of the comparison object or in place of both standard and comparison object. Since the latter method differed most in its results from the method of paired comparison and was therefore used by him both for colour and size, I shall confine myself to it. In the size experiments two equal series of white cardboard cubes were used, one, the standard, arranged in random order as regards size, but in a frontal-parallel plane on a table 1 m. from the subject, the second, again in a frontal-parallel plane, but arranged in order of size on a table 4 m. distant. One of the near cubes was marked and the subject had to designate the one on the farther table that looked equal to it. The procedure for brightness constancy was *mutatis mutandis* the same, tableaus of different shades of grey taking the place of the different cubes. Under these conditions children at the age of four years, the youngest examined, showed complete constancy already. Katz and Burzlaff conclude from these experiments that constancy undergoes no development and that the results of the Vienna school are due to the method, which brings into play an extraneous factor. "One must be aware of the fact that wherever the phenomena are controlled by comparison, a complicating factor is introduced of whose effectiveness one has no adequate conception" (Burzlaff, p. 202).

Brunswik, in a note appended to Klimpfinger (1933 a, pp. 619 f.), disputes the justification of this criticism, although he accepts the results, which he has partly repeated, and does not doubt that similar results would be obtained in the field of shape. He argues that the failure to reveal any development of constancy is the fault of Burzlaff's method, which set too easy a task to the observers. One may, so he argues, lower the difficulty of the task to be accomplished by the subjects so as to destroy all differences between them. A teacher who wants to grade his pupils does not set them examination papers which they can all pass with grade A.

I find that this argument presupposes the existence of constancy as something absolute which can be submitted to tests of various degrees of difficulty, but is always the same constancy, just as in Brunswik's own analogy I can test the spelling ability of a boy by dictating to him texts of different degrees of difficulty. But such an analogy is entirely fictitious. It is the result of considering constancy phenomena as something in themselves rather than as heuristically valuable aspects of the process of perceptual organization. The Viennese experiments prove only that perceptual organization shows "greater constancy" for older children than for younger ones *under certain conditions;* otherwise expressed that these special conditions have a different effect at different ages. Nor is it difficult on the basis of the facts to discover these different effects. Paired comparison of two objects, particularly when they are spatially close to each other, may easily produce such a communication between them in the psychophysical field that they influence each other. If, on the other hand, each of the two objects is a member of a group, as in Burzlaff's serial method, then it will be much harder to isolate them from their proper surroundings and integrate them with a member of the other group. If, then, young children show a lower degree of constancy by the paired comparison method than older ones, one has to infer that for these younger children the excitations started by the two proximal stimulations are more interdependent than for the older ones, where this interdependence may vanish altogether. This conjecture is confirmed by experiments of H. Frank (1928). She found in comparing Beyrl's method with her own, in which the two objects to be compared were far wider apart, that the latter yielded far better constancy than the former, and that this superiority of the one method over the other was particularly marked for the younger children.

The similarity of the age curves for size-, colour-, and shape-constancy proves therefore probably no more than that progressively, and in the rhythm discovered by the Viennese, segregated field parts become more and more independent of each other. Since, however, constancy of any kind presupposes dynamic intercourse between the segregated object and the whole field, constancy itself should under favourable conditions appear from the start, since progress consists not in creating or increasing but in decreasing the mutual interdependence of field parts.

Whiteness and Colour Constancy. It is now time to take up the problem of the last constancy, that of colour and brightness.[17] The similarity of all constancy problems had, as we have seen, struck a number of investigators, notably Thouless and the Viennese. But the similarity, relevant though it is, must not blind us against the specific characteristics of each. Thus we saw that even size- and shape-constancy differ from each other in the dynamical factors which bring them about. And we shall find entirely new factors in the realm of colour and brightness. As a matter of fact we shall not find brightness constancy and colour constancy, in the narrower sense, entirely identical.

[17] There exist other constancies which we omit from our discussion. I mention only "intensity" constancy, according to which a soft near sound is not confused with a loud far one, and weight constancy, which appears, e.g., in the fact that we become aware of a "specific weight" as much as of an absolute one.

Brightness- and colour-constancy have been more extensively investigated than any of the others, although the first specific work in that field was not published till 1911, while Martius published his investigation of size constancy as early as 1889. That the problem emerged at last was due to the psychological insight of Hering, who discussed it in his last publication on vision (1920) [18] and introduced the name "memory colour." But the classical book in the field is Katz's (1911, 1930). Its importance at the time of its publication can hardly be overrated. I shall not go at length into the history of the various investigations, since Katz and Gelb have both given excellent surveys. In English there is the introductory chapter of MacLeod's monograph to be recommended as a good introduction.

THE DILEMMA OF OLDER THEORIES. The theory of brightness- and colour-constancy found itself suspended between two poles. On the one hand there were attempts to explain it by factors which in themselves had nothing to do with constancy, on the other hand, the result itself, i.e., constancy, entered the explanation. Both poles were already inherent in Hering's discussion, the first in his attempt to explain the facts by adaptation, pupillary reaction, and contrast (in Hering's sense), the second in his concept of *memory* colour. But all these principles were proved to be inessential by Katz and Jaensch. Constancy remained under conditions when Hering's external factors were ruled out, and memory in the ordinary sense could not explain the effect, since the experiments were performed not with well-known objects, the colour of which might be remembered by the observer, but with pieces of paper or colour wheels which as far as the subject knew might have any colour.

A STANDARD EXPERIMENT ON WHITENESS CONSTANCY. Thus, for instance, a light grey paper would be presented in a dark corner of the room and a colour wheel with black and white sectors near a window. The subject had to find a black-white mixture on the colour wheel which looked the same grey as the paper in the dark corner. Under such conditions, as Katz was the first to discover, complete equality is impossible. In one or more respects the disk near the light and the paper in the shade will always look different. However, the subjects can fulfil this task with reasonable assurance. When this is done the black-white mixture on the colour wheel, though darker than the paper in the corner,[19] sends much more light

[18] This is the date of the publication of the complete book. The first instalment which introduces the term "memory colour" appeared in 1908.

[19] This means: a paper next to the colour wheel which would look exactly like it would be a darker shade than the other paper.

into the observer's eye. This is easily proved by a method introduced by Katz. A screen with two holes is introduced between the observer and the two matched greys, so that one hole is filled by light coming from the paper, the other by light coming from the disk. If, before the introduction of this "reduction screen," the two appeared of equal grey, then through the reduction screen the hole filled by the colour wheel is much lighter. If one changes the mixture on the wheel so that the two holes look equal, and then removes the screen, the colour wheel will be almost black, much darker than the grey paper.

SEVERAL MEASURES OF CONSTANCY. By this method we can measure constancy in various ways. Let us suppose the light grey paper in the back part of the room was equivalent to a mixture of 300° white and 60° black, which value we will call *r;* the disk in front that looked equal to it without a screen contained a mixture of 200° white and 160° black, this value we call *a;* and the disk "reduction-equal" to the paper 20° white and 340° black, value *p*. We can say that whereas *r* characterizes the far paper as a distant stimulus, *p* characterizes it as a proximal stimulus, and *a* its effect under normal conditions (without reduction screen). Neglecting for simplicity's sake the black sector altogether[20] we can compute two quotients, Katz's H- and Q-quotients. In the first we divide value *a* by value *r,* in the second we divide value *a* by value *p*. Thus, in our example $H = \frac{200}{300} = .67$ and $Q = \frac{200}{20} = 10$. These values have certain drawbacks which Brunswik has pointed out. If constancy were complete, $H = 1$, but "no constancy" has no fixed H value; in our example it would be $\frac{20}{300}$, in other cases a different value. Conversely "no constancy" has a fixed Q value $= 1$, but the Q of complete constancy depends upon the prevailing conditions. It is for this reason that Brunswik introduced his value $c = 100 \frac{a-p}{r-p}$ (see p. 226). In our example $c = 100 \frac{200-20}{300-20} = 100 \frac{180}{280} = 64$. If $a = r$, complete constancy, $c = 100$; and if $a = p$, no constancy, $c = o$. Useful as the c value is, it is open to the objections which we have raised against it before (pp. 227 ff.).

[20] In reality one has of course to add the white value of the black sector, 360° of black being equal to about 6° of white.

Our example, which is typical of many real experiments, reveals another similarity between brightness constancy on the one hand, and size- and shape-constancy on the other. As a rule constancy is not perfect, the apparent whiteness of the comparison disk lies somewhere between the albedo of the standard disk and the amount of light it sends into our eyes. Returning to a terminology we introduced in Chapter IV we call the light that is reflected by a surface *i*, the light that is thrown upon it *I*, and the albedo of the surface *L*; then $i = LI$ (see p. 112). Two surfaces under different objective illumination would show perfect constancy if they look equal when $L_1 = L_2$, they would show no constancy if they look equal when $i_1 = i_2$, and therefore $\frac{L_1}{L_2} = \frac{I_2}{I_1}$ (since $i = L_1 I_1 = L_2 I_2$). In the ordinary case the relation of the two albedos is neither of these two, but somewhere between them; to use Thouless's terminology, regression is again incomplete.

The Different Components; Whiteness and Brightness. Furthermore, as already mentioned, a disk of a certain whiteness near the window will not look exactly like a disk of the same apparent whiteness in the shadow. Again the case is parallel to the two other constancies. A turned circle, even if it still looks circular, does not look entirely like a frontal parallel circle, because it will appear as a circle turned round an axis; nor will a stick of a certain size at distance *a* look exactly like a stick of the same apparent size at distance *b*; these two sticks, equal with regard to size, will appear different with regard to distance. What then is the aspect in which two greys which appear equal with regard to whiteness will appear different under the condition specified? The analogy with the two other cases indicates that such an aspect must appear. Katz's experiments long ago confirmed this conclusion. As a matter of fact there are more aspects of difference than one, in the first place the aspect which in conformity with Thouless I will call "brightness" and which Katz had called illumination, and in the second place an aspect which Katz called "pronouncedness" (*Ausgeprägtheit*). We shall disregard the latter and confine ourselves in our discussion to brightness and whiteness, a term which in conformity with Thouless we apply to that aspect which is a more or less permanent characteristic of an object, like "white," "light grey," "black." For the sake of consistency we must speak therefore of "whiteness constancy" instead of using the traditional term "brightness constancy."

THE INVARIANT OF WHITENESS CONSTANCY. With this terminology we can derive another result from the standard experiment. If we have set the colour wheel near the window so as to make it reduction-equal to the paper at the back of the room, i.e., when we are dealing with *r* and *p* values which correspond to the same amount of light *i*, though to different *L-I* combinations, then the disk looks much less white than the paper and at the same time much more bright. This suggests the possibility that a combination of whiteness and brightness, possibly their product, is an invariant for a given local stimulation under a definite set of total conditions. If two equal proximal stimulations produce two surfaces of different whiteness, then these surfaces will also have different brightnesses, the whiter one will be less, the blacker one more bright.[21]

AN ATTEMPT AT A THEORY OF WHITENESS CONSTANCY. How are whiteness and brightness produced? This is the question which a theory of vision has to answer. To discover a possible solution we begin by comparing whiteness constancy with that of size and shape. Since, however, the two latter are similar with regard to the point I wish to make, I shall for simplicity's sake confine myself to size. Then we can say: two equal proximal stimuli (sizes, light intensities) can give rise to two different perceived objects (large-small, white-black).

A PECULIARITY OF WHITENESS AS COMPARED TO SIZE AND SHAPE. The conditions under which this occurs are, however, not identical in the two fields. The effect in the field of size requires the production of differences of *distance,* and these cannot as a rule be produced by a mere difference or gradient between *sizes.* As optical illusions prove, one can indeed make two equal lines appear different by surrounding them with other lines, as in Fig. 76, but this effect is comparatively small when we compare it with analogous effects in the field of whiteness. For here it is actually possible to change the effect of a local stimulation from black to white by merely changing the gradient of intensities on the retina. To give an example from Hering (1920): in the evening, when our rooms are illuminated by lamps, the windows look black; but as soon as

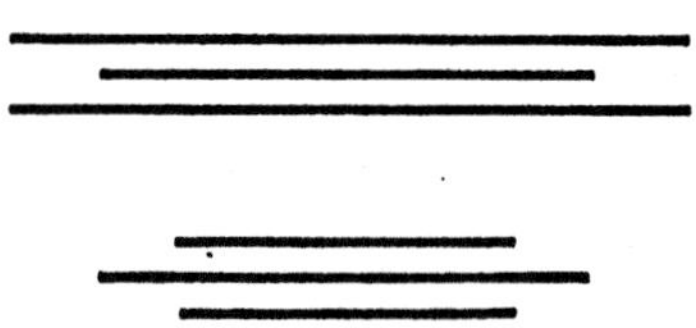

Fig. 76

[21] A striking example of this is given by one of Kardos's experiments where the same field-part becomes simultaneously darker and whiter without any change in the local proximal stimulation (p. 38).

we turn out the lights—thereby even diminishing the light that comes from the panes—they look quite light. The same effect can be demonstrated with Hering's hole method. A white screen with a hole is set in front of a fairly well illuminated white wall. At first the screen is totally dark, and then the hole looks brilliant white; thereupon the screen is illuminated by a very strong light with the result that the hole turns black. The same local radiation, coming through the hole from the white wall, thus produces either white or black according to its relation to the rest of the radiation. It looks white when it is on the top of the gradient, and black when it is at the bottom; the variation of the conditions is entirely confined to the intensity of radiation. The phenomena here described are, of course, adduced by Hering as instances of contrast. But since his contrast theory has to be abandoned, as we have shown before, the term contrast is no more than a name which we prefer to avoid since it implies an explanation not in terms of gradient, but in terms of absolute amounts of light (see Chapter IV, p. 134).[22]

Our theory of whiteness constancy will be based on this characteristic of colours, which is only a pronounced example of the general rule, which we found confirmed in so many passages, that perceived qualities depend upon stimulus gradients.

TWO OTHER FACTS FUNDAMENTAL FOR THE THEORY. Two more well-known facts must be added before we sketch a theory. The first is the range of albedos. The best white which we use in our laboratories reflects approximately only sixty times as much light as the best black, a very small ratio when we consider that full sunlight is many thousand times as strong as an artificial illumination sufficient for comfortable reading. The second fact is already implied in the first: we can produce all neutral shades from black to white by a mere change of albedo, i.e., by a change in the light-intensity from 1 to 60.

AN EXPERIMENT BY GELB. The theory which I have outlined in two brief publications (1932 b, 1934) starts from a very ingenious experiment described by Gelb (1930, p. 674). Somewhat simplified, it is like this: In a dark room a perfectly homogeneous black disk is rotated; this disk, and nothing else, is strongly illuminated by a projection lantern. Under these conditions the disk looks white and the room black. Then the experimenter holds a small piece of white paper close to and in front of the rotating disk so that it falls within

[22] I will only mention that I have given an experimental proof of the fact that "contrast" depends upon gradients and not upon absolute amounts of light (1923 a).

the cone of light. At the same moment the disk alters its appearance, and looks black.

EXPLANATION OF GELB'S EXPERIMENT. APPURTENANCE. How is this effect to be explained? We shall consider the stimulus gradients produced in these experiments and shall, for simplicity's sake, divide the whole field into three parts: the room A, the disk B, and the strip of paper C. At the beginning of the experiment the field is composed of two parts only, room and disk, of which the latter sends much more light into the observer's eyes than the former. Supposing the ratio of these intensities to lie around 60:1, the disk is at the top of the full gradient which leads from black to white, the room at the bottom. Consequently the room should look black, the disk white, which is in conformity with the facts. The white-looking disk is in reality black, but this fact is quite irrelevant for the explanation. A grey disk in a less strong cone of light would look exactly like the black disk in the stronger light. There is no question of constancy here. As soon as the strip of white paper is introduced a new situation arises; now we have three field parts, A, B, and C, such that in terms of intensity of stimulation per unit area A : B = B : C = 1 : 60. How should we on the basis of our assumption expect this configuration to look? B had to look white before the introduction of C, because it was at the top of a 60:1 gradient. After the introduction of C it retains this position, but at the same time it is at the bottom of the new 60: 1 gradient B C, and should, as such, look black. Therefore we can give no answer to our question without introducing a new assumption. This assumption is the following: a field part x is determined in its appearance by its "appurtenance" to other field parts. The more x belongs to the field part y, the more will its *whiteness* be determined by the gradient xy, and the less it belongs to the part z, the less will its whiteness depend on the gradient xz. This assumption is not entirely new inasmuch as we have encountered the factor of "appurtenance" or "belongingness" before, viz., in our discussion of the Wertheimer-Benary contrast experiment. Which field parts belong together, and how strong the degree of this belonging together is, depends upon factors of space organization. Clearly, two parts at the same apparent distance will, *ceteris paribus*, belong more closely together than field parts organized in different planes. Ultimately this organization depends of course on the proximal stimulus distribution on the two retinas.

We can now return to Gelb's experiment. Here C, the white strip of paper, belongs more closely to B, the black disk, than to the background A; B and C belong together and are set off against the background. Therefore B will now be primarily determined by the gradient B C and will therefore look black, as it actually does. A, on the other hand, is at the absolute bottom of all gradients. That it looks black is therefore natural. But this is not enough. It looked black before the introduction of C, the gradient A B being 1:60. By the introduction of C a new gradient A C, 1:3600, is created and the effect of this gradient cannot be the same as that of the much smaller one A B. The difference between A and C therefore cannot be one of whiteness alone, since the maximum of this difference was achieved by the gradient A B. Something new must happen: A must look different from C in a new dimension or aspect, and this dimension is the dimension of brightness. B and A look both black, but B looks as bright as the white C, while A looks very much *darker*.

This explanation of Gelb's experiment is also given by Kardos (p. 84 f.), whose theory seems to me in all essential respects to agree with the one here propounded. I see the particular importance of Kardos's contribution in his systematic formulation of the problem of appurtenance and in his many experiments, as striking as they are simple, to demonstrate the effectiveness of this factor. By changing conditions of appurtenance he succeeds by a number of different methods in changing the "effective gradient" and thereby the appearance of the field parts concerned. His experiments, which cannot be described here, prove beyond a doubt the functional reality of appurtenance and thereby the justification of the assumption which we had to introduce to explain Gelb's experiment.

APPLICATION OF THE THEORY TO OTHER CASES. We can now continue our theory. We consider once more our three surfaces A, B, and C, but suppose that now A and B belong together, being set off against C. Then A and B should look black and white as they do in the absence of C, and C must look white and extremely bright, probably luminous, a conclusion which is also reached by Kardos. If the conditions are less simple, so that B does not belong to a very much higher degree to either A (or C) than to C (or A), then the two gradients A B and B C will both have effects on C, so that it appears different from the two other surfaces both in whiteness *and* brightness, whereas in the simpler cases so far discussed it shared its whiteness with one and its brightness with the other (in Gelb's experiment B has the same brightness as C and, approximately, the same whiteness as A).

WHY THIS THEORY IS STILL INCOMPLETE. I am fully aware that the hypothesis developed in the last pages is far from being a complete theory of the facts usually called facts of brightness constancy. But it is at least a *real* theory, i.e., an explanation which deduces the observed effects from the only available causes, the proximal stimulation which gives rise to perceptual organization. A complete theory would have to answer, among others, the following questions: given two adjoining retinal areas of different stimulation, under what conditions will the corresponding parts of the behavioural (perceptual) field appear of different whiteness but equal brightness (or "illumination"), when of different brightness but equal whiteness? A complete answer to this question would probably supply the key to the complete theory of colour perception in the broadest sense.

SOME EXPERIMENTAL EVIDENCE. Since this answer is still lacking, we shall do well to give some experimental support to the hypothesis as developed here. It depends upon the truth of two propositions: (a) the qualities of perceived objects depend upon *gradients* of stimulation, (b) not all gradients are equally effective as regards the appearance of a particular field part; rather will the effectiveness of a gradient vary with the degree of appurtenance obtaining between the two terms of this gradient. Since proposition (b) has been proved by Kardos's new experiments, we concentrate on proposition (a).

OBJECTIVELY EQUAL INLYING FIELDS WITHIN OBJECTIVELY EQUAL SURROUNDING FIELDS OF DIFFERENT APPEARANCE. We begin with the following case. Let there be two large (surrounding) fields S_1 and S_2, each containing a small hole in its centre, the infields I_1 and I_2. Let the S_1 and S_2 be equal with regard to intensity of light reflected and similarly I_1 and I_2. Is the appearance of I_1 and I_2 under these conditions equal? The reader may at first think that this is a trivial question which must evidently be answered in the affirmative, since it seems to state nothing but the principle of Katz's reduction screen. But this impression would be hasty, for we know that two fields which reflect the same amount of light per unit area may look very different from each other, i.e., one white and dark, the other black and bright. When we use a reduction screen we naturally do it under conditions where S_1 and S_2, the surroundings of the two holes, are not only of equal objective intensity but also *look* equal. But supposing S_1 looks white, S_2 black, will I_1 look equal to I_2, or if it does not, in which direction will they differ from each other? One way of arguing would be this: Since S_1 looks whiter than S_2,

I_1 should, by contrast, look blacker than I_2. This prediction neglects the fact that the gradient S_1–I_1, expressed by the ratio $\frac{S_1}{I_1}$, is exactly the same as the gradient S_2–I_2, $\frac{S_2}{I_2}$, since physically $S_1 = S_2$ and $I_1 = I_2$. If then the appearance of the inlying fields depends upon the gradient which connects them with the surrounding fields, I_1 should look whiter than I_2. That this must be so will appear when we consider the case where the two inlying fields are physically almost of the same intensity as the two outlying fields so that they look almost equal to them. Then I_1, looking almost equal to S_1, must look white and I_2 correspondingly black.

Which expectation is correct? In actual fact does I_1 look whiter or blacker than I_2? The first experiments to answer this question were made, in a different context, by Harrower and me (II),[23] then independently in various forms by Gelb (1932), although in neither publication the theoretical problem was stated as in this text. Both experimenters obtained unequivocally the same result: I_1 looked whiter than I_2. Thus this experiment serves as a proof of our proposition that the appearance of a field part depends upon the gradient which connects it with other field parts.

As a matter of fact a much older experiment by Jaensch and Müller proves the same point. This experiment employs a method for measuring constancy introduced by Katz. A uniform background B (see Fig. 77) at right angles to the wall with the window W is set upon a table. On the same table and at right angles to the background is a screen S which casts a shadow on the right side of the table, leaving the left fully exposed to the light coming through the window. On either side of the background two disks are set up in such a way that they are reduction-equal, i.e., that the light reflected from the left one, d_1, is equal to that reflected from the right one, d_2. For that purpose d_1 must have a lower albedo than d_2, to compensate for the greater amount of light it receives. An observer sitting at O then sees a blacker disk on the left and a whiter one on the right. It was possible to explain this effect by the classical con-

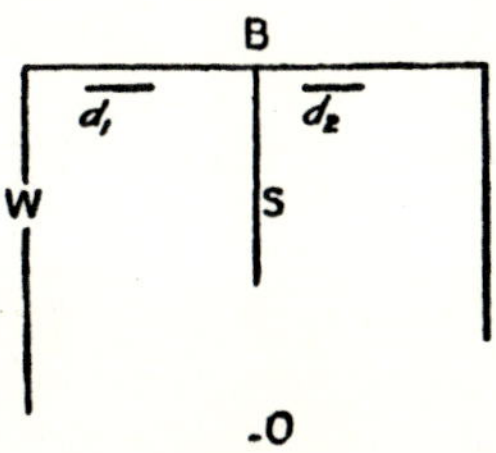

Fig. 77

[23] In our experiments, to be sure, the inlying fields were as a rule coloured and not neutral. But this does not affect the main issue.

trast theories, because the left half of B, surrounding d_1, receives, and therefore reflects, more light than the right half, which surrounds d_2. Therefore d_1 should be blackened by contrast more than d_2. In order to exclude this explanation Jaensch and Müller made the following modification. Instead of using a uniform background they used two different ones, a blacker one on the left side and a whiter one on the right. If then the radiation reaching the eyes from these two backgrounds is the same, we have conditions identical with those discussed above, viz., $S_1 = S_2$ and $I_1 = I_2$, except for the fact that I_1 and I_2 are no longer holes in screens but disks in front of screens. According to a pure contrast theory I_1 should now look exactly like I_2, constancy should have disappeared, whereas in reality they look about as different as they did in the original set-up with a uniform background.[24] This difference cannot therefore be explained by contrast. However, it follows directly from our proposition about the effect of gradients. Since under the conditions of Jaensch and Müller's experiment the two backgrounds look different, although they reflect the same amount of light, the disks which have equal gradients to their respective backgrounds must look different too. The argument is identical to the one given above for the two holes. It is also the same as an argument developed in our discussion of shape constancy (pp. 222 f.). It may be put in this form: if a certain radiation produces the impression of a light-grey object, then a slightly stronger radiation will produce the impression of a *white* object, but if the first radiation produces the perception of a black object, then the second slightly stronger one will lead to the appearance of a dark-grey object. In this formulation we explain the appearance of one object by the gradient of stimulation which connects it with another and by the appearance of the latter. This itself is not explained, just as we have not explained why in Jaensch and Müller's experiment the two backgrounds look different. The explanation must fall back on conditions beyond the four surfaces so far taken into consideration. It is an application of the general problem formulated on page 248.

Conclusions with Regard to the Concept of Phenomenal Regression. These experiments (Koffka-Harrower and Gelb on the one hand and Jaensch-Müller on the other) clearly belong together. In the last it is sensible to speak of constancy or phenomenal regression, for the *apparent* difference of the two disks d_1 and d_2 corre-

[24] In the experiment of Jaensch and Müller the white background in the shadow reflected actually more light than the black one in the light. Thereby the point made in the text is proved *a fortiori*.

sponds much more to their difference of albedo (what they are "really" like) than to their difference of stimulation, which in this case is zero. But in the two first experiments such a point of view is inapplicable, since the effect does not depend upon the albedo of the screen seen through the holes but merely upon the radiation which passes through the holes. Therefore I cannot agree with Thouless's contention that the term "phenomenal regression to the real object" should be substituted for the term "constancy" to designate this whole range of facts. Thouless (1934) has indeed given a very ingenious criticism of the term constancy, and has shown that in many cases it has no proper meaning, whereas his own term is still meaningful. But cases like those just discussed, which belong to the same province, prove that Thouless's term also fails to cover all facts.

MODIFICATION OF GELB'S ORIGINAL EXPERIMENT BY KOFFKA AND HARROWER. The experiments so far adduced were carried out without regard to that experiment of Gelb's which we used as a starting point for our theory (see pp. 245 f.). I shall now briefly report some unpublished experiments by Harrower and myself [25] which were undertaken with the express purpose of testing my explanation of Gelb's effect. In this experiment there were three field parts, A, B, and C, the dark room, the brightly illuminated black disk, and the equally brightly illuminated white strip of paper, such that the radiations were A:B = B:C = 1:60.[26] If C was omitted, B looked white; as soon as C was introduced B looked black and bright, and this change was explained by the fact that B was determined by the gradient BC. If this interpretation is right, then B will no longer appear black if the relation of C:B is smaller than 60:1, i.e., if one substitutes grey strips for the white one; the less white the strip, the less black should the black disk (B) appear, while the strip itself should still look white though less bright, owing to the fact that the relation C:A is still greater than 60:1. This expectation was confirmed, the apparent blackness of B, and thereby its constancy, was a direct function of the albedo of C, and that, both under the conditions of Gelb's original experiment and with hole colours, in which case A was a black unilluminated screen through a hole in which B and C were visible.

Using again a formulation previously employed, we can say: if

[25] I have briefly reported on these experiments in the two papers referred to on p. 245.

[26] Only the second ratio, B:C, was made exactly equal to 1:60. The other ratio was in reality greater.

a radiation 60*i* looks white, then radiation *i* looks black; if 30*i* looks white, *i* looks grey. Our formulation is in this case more adequate than in the former ones, because we understand why C (60*i*, 30*i*, etc.) looks white.

We also inverted Gelb's experiment. In general terms we have three surfaces, A, B, and C, such that now A:B = B:C = 60:1. A is a white background strongly illuminated, B a white disk in a deep shadow which coincides with its boundary, and C a black or grey strip close to the disk and in the shadow area. If, then, A and B are exposed alone A will look white, B black. Introducing C in such a way that B C belong together, B should turn white; again, if B:C were smaller than 60:1, B should change to a shade blacker than white.

With hole colours this prediction was confirmed, although it required stronger measures to insure the belonging together of B and C than in the original case. With a set-up corresponding to that of Gelb's we failed to obtain the effect, i.e., the introduction of the black strip did not change the appearance of the white disk strongly shadowed. I shall not try to explain this unexpected result, only adding that equal intensity gradients have different effects according to whether the part chiefly influenced is at the top or at the bottom of the gradients. As we know from other experiments, taking a middle grey as the centre, the black-white series is not functionally symmetrical.

FUNCTIONAL DIFFERENCES BETWEEN LIGHT BLACK AND DARK WHITE CORRESPONDING TO THE SAME STIMULUS INTENSITY. It remains to be seen how many facts can be explained by our theory, a task which transcends the limits of this chapter. We shall take up only one more point. At several places in our discussion of perception we have attempted to substantiate facts of pure phenomenology by functional facts. We shall do the same in this field. If two areas of the visual field corresponding to equal local stimulations *look* different, do they differ in any other property except their appearance? Three such effects have been discovered, the first by Gelb (1920) in his experiments with the two mentally blind patients reported in Chapter IV (p. 118). It will be remembered that these patients never saw surfaces, but that the colour of objects always had a certain thickness which was the greater the blacker the colour. These same patients possessed colour constancy. If, for example, the experiment described on page 249 (Fig. 77) was performed with them, the two disks d_1 and d_2 which reflected the same amount of light looked as different from each other as for normal persons. At the same time the rule for the "thickness" of colours still held: d_1, looking blacker, looked thicker than d_2. Thus, two surfaces of equal local stimulation not only looked different from each other, but at the same time and in accordance with their different appearance were differently organized (Gelb, 1920, p. 241).

The second experiment was performed by Mintz and myself. Gelb's result seemed to be explained if white was a harder colour than black, in the meaning explained in Chapter IV (p. 127); i.e., if it had stronger power of organization and cohesion. Under ordinary conditions this difference of hardness between white and black had been discovered by Harrower and myself; the question was whether it would also hold for black and white corresponding to the same local stimulation. We argued that if it did, a black field should offer less resistance to the introduction of a *coloured* figure than a white field produced by the same local stimulation; less colour should be needed in the first than in the second. Our experiments verified this deduction, thereby supplying another effect in which two such surfaces differ.

The third effect was discovered by Harrower and myself (II, p. 211 f.). The saturation of a coloured figure on a neutral ground is the greater the more similar the whiteness of the two; it reaches its maximum at the coincidence point, the point of whiteness equality. (See Ackermann, Eberhardt, G. E. Müller, 1930 II.) It was customary to define this effect in terms of brightness, but this definition disregarded the fact that one and the same radiation may produce different combinations of whiteness and brightness. All previous experiments on the dependence of the saturation, or the threshold, of a coloured figure on the brightness of the ground were performed when figure and background were in the same plane and subject to the same illumination, in which case the whiteness (brightness) of the background can only be varied by a variation of its albedo. Harrower and I, however, produced figures on neutral grounds by a method which separated the sources of light for figure and ground. Thus it was possible to compare two figures reflecting the same amount of coloured light on two backgrounds which, though they also reflected equal amounts of (neutral) light, looked different, e.g., the one black and light, the other white and dark. Not only then did the colours of the two figures, as already mentioned, look different from each other, but the maximum saturation was no longer obtained at the coincidence point. At the coincidence point blue will look more saturated on a black than on a reduction-equal white background, whereas yellow will look more saturated on the former than on the latter.

COLOUR CONSTANCY. We now turn to colour constancy in the narrower sense; just as the object colours do not follow the changes in the intensity of neutral illumination,[27] so do they fail to follow the changes of the *colour* of the illumination, although "colour constancy" is less perfect than "brightness constancy." Katz included the investigation of this set of phenomena in his first great book, and the constancy aspect has largely determined the research in this field. And yet, for the sake of the theory, it will be profitable to eliminate this aspect just as we eliminated it in the discussion of brightness constancy.

A FIRST EXPERIMENT. Let us perform the following experiment: Close to one wall of a room which is illuminated by coloured light we set a neutral disk d_1; not far from this disk the wall has an opening to another, normally illuminated, room, and behind this opening in the second room, shielded from the coloured illumination of the first, we set another neutral disk d_2. Then d_1 reflects the light of the coloured illumination, d_2 neutral light. Under these conditions d_1 looks more or less neutral, whereas d_2 appears in a colour complementary to the colour of the illumination, and that the more, the more saturated the colour of the illumination is, and the more nearly equal the luminosities of the two illuminations are. The two effects, neutral appearance of d_1 and coloured appearance of d_2, exemplify the same general effect, although d_1 shows constancy and d_2 does not. For d_1 and d_2, reflecting different kinds of light, cannot look equal. If d_1 reflecting coloured light looks neutral, d_2 reflecting neutral light must look coloured and that in such a way that its colour differs from neutral in the same direction and by the same amount as the neutral colour of d_1 differs from the colour of the illumination; i.e., the colour of d_2 must be complementary to the colour of the illumination. If one looks at the same two disks through the holes of a neutrally illuminated reduction screen, one hole being filled by d_1, the other by d_2, then d_1 will look coloured, in the hue of the illumination, and d_2 neutral.

AN ATTEMPT AT A THEORY OF COLOUR CONSTANCY—TWO PRINCIPLES. Jaensch was the first to perceive that the appearances of d_1 and d_2 belong together, and he used this insight for the development of a method for measuring transformation, but other psychologists failed

[27] We have only discussed neutral object colours. But chromatic colours follow the same laws; their introduction does not involve a new principle.

to see the significance of Jaensch's arguments.[28] And yet the connection between the appearance of d_1 and d_2 seems to me to contain the key to the theory of colour constancy, or expressed without this special bias, the theory of colour perception. In the first place it supplies us with an invariant, viz., the gradient between d_1 and d_2. Although the quantitative verification is still missing—and very difficult to obtain—we may assume that the stimulus gradient d_1–d_2 gives rise to an equal apparent colour gradient with and without reduction screen,[29] but this gradient alone does not determine the absolute position of this apparent gradient. If c_1 and c_2 are two different shades of the same stimulus colour, then two coloured behavioural fields of a fixed difference will correspond to these stimuli, and these two fields may have colours anywhere between a maximum saturation of the colour and the maximum saturation of the complementary. This whole manifold of colours may be considered as a fixed scale, on which the two colours produced by the two stimulations c_1 and c_2, keeping the same distance from each other, may slide, according to the general conditions. I have called this the principle of the shift of level.[30]

In this respect colour phenomena have a striking similarity to the phenomena of space-directions, where the angle between two lines is an invariant, whereas the absolute orientation of the perceived lines depends upon the general field conditions. The analogy goes even further. In our discussion of space directions we found that certain directions play a unique rôle, the horizontal and the vertical, and we found that the main lines of organization tend to become main lines of direction (see p. 216). In the field of spatial orientation we found a similar unique constellation, the frontal parallel plane, whereas in the fields of size and of neutral colours no such unique constellation exists. We find it again, however, when we consider all colour phenomena, the neutral and the chromatic, for here the *neutral* colours have a unique position. And it seems in good agreement with the facts to formulate a principle, which I have called the principle of the neutral level (1932 a): just as each individual spatial direction depends upon the general spatial framework, thus each individual perceived colour depends upon a colour framework or level. And just as the horizontal-vertical directions establish the

[28] I have gone into the history of this problem in my article (1932 a).

[29] In order for this to be true, certain conditions must be fulfilled. If, e.g., the light reflected by the reduction screen is very much stronger than the light coming through the holes, then both holes will look black, the gradient between them will be lost.

[30] This notion was first employed by Jaensch (1914).

spatial framework, the neutral colour serves as the colour level. How the level is established in each particular case depends upon the special conditions. In the field of colour these conditions are not as easy to formulate as in the field of direction; but bearing in mind the relation existing between framework and ground we can advance the hypothesis that the general background will determine the level and therefore appear as neutral as the conditions allow. With this principle and the principle of the shift of level we can explain the appearance of the two disks d_1 and d_2 if viewed with and without reduction screen. In the second case the background reflects the colour of the illumination; qua background it determines the colour level and therefore looks neutral. The disk d_1, reflecting the same kind of light, must therefore look neutral also, while the disk d_2, reflecting neutral light, must look complementarily coloured. With reduction screen, the screen, reflecting neutral light, is the background and therefore looks neutral; d_2, also reflecting neutral light, must look neutral also, while d_1, reflecting coloured light, the light of the illumination, must look coloured.

A GAP IN THIS THEORY. But although these principles allow us to deduce a great number of facts, they cannot, as yet, serve as a general theory. For the principle of the shift of level has so far been formulated only for two colours which can be represented on a straight line which connects two points of the colour circle and passes through its (neutral) centre (or for corresponding lines in the colour pyramid). But we do not yet know how the shift of level of one of two colours affects the other if it does not lie on such a line. To be concrete: supposing d_2 in our experiment to be green and the illumination of the first room to be yellow, then when viewed through a neutrally illuminated reduction screen d_1 looks yellow, d_2 green. If we remove the reduction screen, d_1 looks again neutral, but how will d_2 look? It should look as different from neutral as green looks different from yellow. The experimental solution of this problem is easy; it would lead to very interesting generalizations about the whole system of colours.

CONSTANCY OF COLOURED OBJECTS IN COLOURED ILLUMINATION. I believe that it is clear how our principles explain the constancy of neutrally coloured objects in coloured illumination. Do they also explain the constancy of coloured objects? Lest we ask too much of our hypothesis we must mention the fact, well enough known to ladies who will not choose dress material in artificial light, that colour constancy is far less perfect than brightness constancy, a fact emphasized by Bühler. Such imperfect constancy, decreasing with the saturation of the illumination colour, is indeed compatible with our hypothesis, and will be deducible from it in full detail once the general problem stated on the previous page is solved. Let us discuss only two examples. In the first place we choose a blue object under the yellow illumination of an ordinary bulb. We know that under such an illumination a neutral surface which reflects yellowish light will look neutral, and that consequently a surface reflecting neutral light will look bluish and a surface which reflects blue light more blue than under neutral illumination. Now our blue object illuminated by yellowish light reflects less blue light than when normally illuminated, as can be ascertained if one looks at it through a normally illuminated neutral reduction screen. This less blue light must now, however, produce a bluer colour than it would under neutral illumination. Therefore the illumination has two opposite effects. Physically it reduces the blue light coming from the object but psychophysically it enhances the blue-effect of this light. That these two effects of opposite sign are of exactly the same magnitude so as to cancel each other and produce perfect constancy is only one possibility out of a great multitude and will be realized only in a negligibly small number of cases. For the change of the light reflected from a body by a change of illumination depends upon the constitution of the light thrown upon it and the selectivity of its own surface. Two lights which look equal may have very different constitutions and two surfaces which appear equal may have very different selectivities.[31] Therefore two lights which appear of equal colour may yield very different radiations reflected from one and the same surface, and the same light may be reflected in a different composition from two surfaces which under neutral illumination look equal. Another consequence of this fact is that the relation between the stimulations coming from two surfaces will as a rule be changed when coloured illumination is substituted for neutral; and this means again that constancy must be incomplete, whereas a mere change of the *intensity* of illumination leaves these relations constant, thereby guaranteeing a much higher degree of (whiteness-) constancy.

As our second example we choose a monochromatic illumination. In this case, since there is only one kind of light to fall on the objects, there is only one kind to be reflected by them, the only

[31] The selectivity corresponds to the albedo in the field of neutral colours, but whereas the latter is one-dimensional, the former, according to the laws of colour mixture, is three-dimensional. This difference explains the greater complexity of colour- as compared to whiteness-constancy.

stimulus differences possible being differences of intensity; hence all objects should appear neutral, inasmuch as according to our principle of the neutral level, the whole visual field should look neutral, and therefore differences in intensity appear as differences in the black-white and the dark-bright dimension.

THE BEHAVIOURAL ILLUMINATION. An objection which might be raised against our theory will help us to introduce briefly a point which we have hitherto neglected, although it has played an important rôle in the theoretical discussions of colour constancy. We claim that a neutral surface under coloured illumination still looks neutral. Do we not thereby contradict our principle that two supraliminally different stimuli never produce exactly the same result? We would if we considered constancy of the neutral shade under coloured illumination as the full description of the facts. But we do not. Again there is a new aspect in which the neutrally and the chromatically illuminated neutral surfaces appear different from each other. In some cases this difference can be described by saying that the two surfaces, though of equal colours, appear under different illumination, illumination now being taken as a behavioural datum. In other cases such a description would be far too specific, and yet, some difference remains, although our language has no specific words to designate it. Put a pair of yellow glasses in front of your eyes—how the landscape becomes warm and radiant; replace them by blue glasses and observe how cold and dull everything now looks. I shall refrain from elaborating this point. In my article (1932 a) I have developed my theory so as to deal with the impression of illumination (pp. 349 f.).

SOME EXPERIMENTAL EVIDENCE. Consistent as the hypothesis so far developed appears, is it more than speculation? Is there any direct experiment to confirm it? When I first thought of the two principles of the shift of level and the neutral level, the following argument occurred to me. Supposing an area reflecting neutral light looks blue, because the surrounding area, reflecting yellow light, looks neutral, then the objectively neutral area should no longer look blue if the surrounding area looks yellow. If at the same time it was made objectively yellower, then the neutralization of the originally blue-appearing field would prove that its blueness was not due to contrast in the traditional meaning, since contrast in a surrounded field should increase if the saturation of the surrounding field increased. This argument led to a very simple experiment. In a room illuminated by diffuse daylight I. turned on an ordinary electric lamp which cast a shadow of a fixed object on a white sheet of paper. This shadow produces an area which reflects neutral light within a larger area which reflects yellowish light, composed of the diffuse daylight and the light of the lamp. If the intensity of the latter is properly adjusted to that of the former, the white paper looks white but the shadow is of a well saturated blue colour. This is nothing but the well-known method of producing coloured shadows, an effect which had always been explained by contrast,[32] although this explanation had neglected the fact that the non-shadowed area, although reflecting yellowish light, looked white. I now introduced the modification which at the same time made the surrounding field objectively yellower and subjectively yellow: I covered the white paper on which the blue shadow was cast by yellow paper (of relatively low saturation), leaving only the space of the shadow uncovered. Thereby I made the surrounding field reflect more yellow light than before, but left the shadowed area unaltered. The result was that the paper surrounding the shadow looked yellow while the shadow lost most or all of its (blue) colour. If I used a yellow paper of higher saturation, the effect was still stronger. Of course I varied the conditions so as to exclude a number of possible explanations, and used also other illumination colours than yellow. The result remained the same (see my article 1932 a, pp. 340 f.). Therefore, the fact that the shadow appeared blue under the original conditions, and neutral after this modification, proves that the appearance of the enclosed field does not depend, as contrast theories maintained, on its own radiation and the radiation of the surrounding field, i.e., on two factors which combine in a summative way, but on a gradient between enclosed and enclosing radiation and on the colour in which the latter appears. When, being objectively coloured, it appears neutral, then a neutral inlying field must appear in the complementary colour; when, however, it appears coloured, the inlying field will appear more or less neutral.[33]

Experiments like the one described last tend to make the problem of the relation between contrast and "transformation" a very pressing one. Naturally it has occupied all workers in the field from Katz to Kardos, and theories which separate the two effects completely from each other have been in conflict with others which explain either transformation by contrast, an attempt which, as pre-

[32] Except for Kroh, who saw that coloured shadows belong rather to the province of "transformation phenomena."

[33] For brevity's sake I have simplified the argument. The reader who discovers a gap in it may turn to my original publication, where the argument is given *in extenso* on page 342.

viously mentioned, was proved to be abortive, or contrast by transformation (Jaensch). I shall leave this problem open, because a number of crucial experiments are still lacking. That the two kinds of phenomena are totally different in their dynamics, I cannot, however, believe. If, as it is my conviction, so-called contrast effects depend also upon the gradient between stimulated areas, and if, as the Wertheimer-Benary experiment has shown, not all such gradients are of equal influence, but exert their effect according to "appurtenance," these contrast effects must be closely related to "constancy" effects. To return once more to the field of pure whiteness and brightness: we saw that two areas which appear in the same plane will determine each other primarily with regard to their whiteness, whereas areas organized in different planes will also mutually determine their brightness. The first influence may be identical with ordinary brightness contrast. This view gains support from an experiment by Wilhelm Wolff, who proved that two equal surfaces, reflecting the same amount of neutral light and appearing in the same frontal parallel plane, still look equal when one is in front of a dark, the other in front of a light-grey background (the backgrounds are both objectively and subjectively different), whereas the same two surfaces looked different from each other if *laid on* two backgrounds the albedos of which were as different from each other as the backgrounds in the first experiment were. This difference in their appearance is an ordinary case of contrast; but since, as far as infields and surrounding fields go, the retinal conditions are the same in the two sets of conditions, one of which only produced contrast effect, Wolff's experiment proves that contrast is not explained by retinal conditions alone, but depends on the spatial organization, and thereby on the appurtenance conditions, to which the retinal conditions give rise: it occurs when the two surfaces lie in the same plane, it fails to appear when they do not.[84]

TRANSPARENCY AND CONSTANCY. Before we leave the topic of colour constancy we will take up a problem closely related to it, because it will give us a new insight into the close dynamic connection which exists between space organization and colour. We have referred to this problem in our discussion of double representation (p. 181). The clearest case of this form of spatial organization is

[84] A recent experiment by Rubin (1934) shows that contrast may occur also under conditions similar to those of Wolff. This, however, does not at all contradict our theory, which considers *all* effective gradients and the degree of their effectiveness. Without further experimental analysis of Rubin's demonstration it seems unwise to offer a definite explanation. It will, I believe, have to be sought in conditions (and degrees) of appurtenance.

manifested when we see one surface through another. The conditions under which this phenomenon occurs have been most systematically investigated by Fuchs (1923), who demonstrated transparency to be dependent upon factors of spatial organization. One of the methods employed by Fuchs is the episcotister method. A large colour wheel with a coloured and an open sector revolves at some distance in front of a black screen. On this black screen there is a coloured figure. To choose a simple example: the episcotister is blue, the figure of a complementary yellow. If we observe this constellation through a reduction screen with two holes, so located that the observer sees the black background through one (and the open part of the colour wheel), and the yellow figure through the other, then the colour of the two holes will be determined by the Talbot law (see Chapter IV, pp. 127 f.), i.e., the one will be a highly saturated though somewhat dark blue, the other a mixture of blue and yellow.

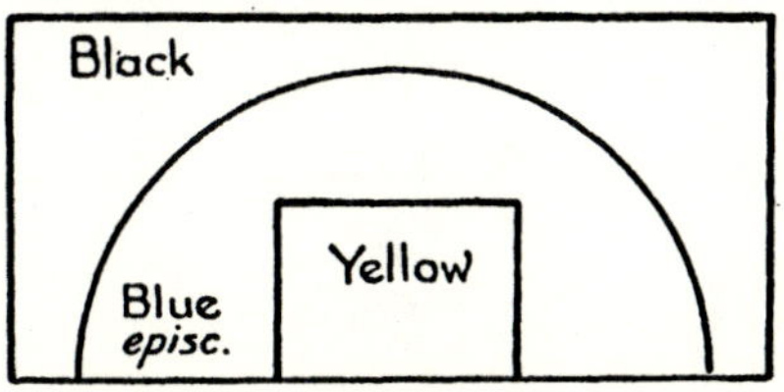

Fig. 78

By adjusting the sizes of the blue and the open sector properly this second hole can be made to appear grey (mixture of complementary colours). If we then remove the reduction screen, retaining only a screen which covers the motor and with it the lower half of the blue circle, the observer sees a yellow figure behind a transparent blue semicircle in front of the black background. Fig. 78 illustrates the set-up. To this perception there corresponds the following proximal stimulation: a black area, a blue area (mixture of blue and black) comprising the visible part of the colour wheel with the exception of the area where the figure lies behind it, and a neutral area (mixture of blue and yellow) where the colour wheel lies in front of the figure. Disregarding the black area, we find a discrepancy between stimulation and perceptual appearance. The area of the yellow figure is doubly represented; it appears on the one hand as a part of the uninterrupted *blue* transparent semicircle, on the other as a *yellow* figure, and yet on the retina it is neither blue nor yellow, but grey. As soon as this area loses its character of double representation, when seen through a reduction screen, it appears neutral. Therefore the colours seen one behind the other must be due to the double representation. At the same time, the colours perceived correspond to the "real" colours. The disk is actually blue, the figure actually yellow, although the retinal image which they produce in combination is neutral. This last fact, however, cannot enter the explanation, rather must the explanation be such that this correspondence of perceived and real colours follows from it. The explanation must, as we have already stated, start from the fact of double representation. There are many factors operative which produce this kind of organization—in the first place such figural factors as we discussed before, in the second place factors of spatial relief which make the figure belong to the plane of the background. Double representation means in our case that the semicircle is seen as one unitary figure. As such it has a tendency to appear in a uniform colour (see Chapter IV, p. 135). This seems to be prevented by the inhomogeneity of stimulation which occurs in its inside, where a neutral area interrupts a blue one. But *this* area is doubly represented, to it there correspond *two* surfaces, one behind the other. The one in front, belonging to the transparent semicircle, is under pressure to become blue. Everything would then be explained if we could make the assumption that if a neutral stimulation gives rise to the perception of two surfaces one of which is coloured, then the other one must be complementarily coloured. In other words we apply the laws of colour mixture to the splitting up of the effect of neutral stimulation. If $y + b = g$, then $g - b = y$ ($y =$ yellow, $b =$ blue, $g =$ grey). The figure, according to this explanation, would look yellow, not because it is really yellow, but because the neutral stimulation to which, under the condition of the experiment, it gives rise, is forced to produce two planes, one of which is blue.

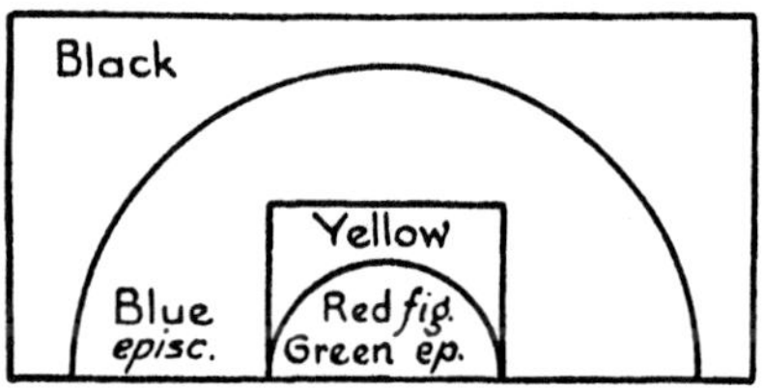

Fig. 79

The validity of this explanation was tested by Grace Heider in a number of experiments. According to the hypothesis the fact that the neutral stimulus area is in reality produced by mixture of blue and yellow light plays no part at all. All that is necessary is that double representation ensues, and that the front surface looks blue. Therefore the following modification of the experiment was introduced (see Fig. 79). The lower part of the figure was made red, and simultaneously the inner part of the episcotister semicircle green, colours and episcotister openings so arranged that through a reduction screen the red-green mixture at the bottom looked exactly like the yellow-blue mixture at the top. This modification of the stimulus conditions should have no effect upon the perception of the observer, and this was found to be true: the episcotister appeared blue, *the figure yellow,* over their entire surfaces; the differences in stimulation within each area were completely lost in the perceptual organization. The same result was also obtained when the smaller (green) episcotister and the lower (red) part of the figure were replaced by a colour wheel with black and white sectors which gave the same neutral colour as the outlying blue-yellow mixture.[35] Thus these experiments prove our hypothesis and demonstrate at the same time why on the one hand transparency is, as a rule, accompanied by colour constancy, on the other that this connection is not constitutive, since transparency may also lead to the opposite of constancy.

THE INTERPLAY OF SPACE AND COLOUR IN TRANSPARENCY. TUDOR-HART'S EXPERIMENTS. That transparency itself is a factor of spatial organization and requires that certain figural conditions be fulfilled we have emphasized when we introduced this topic (p. 181). The close interplay of colour and form in the spatial organization of transparency was demonstrated in special experiments by Tudor-Hart, who varied the colour and light determinants, leaving the figural factors intact. She found a close interdependence between the transparent surface and the surface seen through it. Of her various results I mention but a few.

1. "When an episcotister [the episcotister method described above being used for producing transparency] rotates in front of a background of similar colour and brightness,[36] whether there be, or no, a figure on this latter, the episcotister is invisible."

2. "If an episcotister rotates before a background of different brightness on which is a figure equal in brightness to the episcotister, the episcotister is visible in its entire area, even in front of the figure."

3. "Other things being equal the darker the episcotister the more transparent it is" (p. 277).

4. Other things being equal the brighter the background the more transparent the episcotister.

5. With episcotisters of a low degree of transparency, the transparency is not uniform but greater in front of the figure on the background than in the periphery.

[35] For brevity's sake I have described G. Heider's experiment in a form slightly different from the one it actually took. The result of the actual experiment, in which the yellow strip protruded beyond the outer edge of the blue episcotister, might be explained differently, but special experiments were made to exclude such an explanation. In order to omit these, I have chosen the presentation of the text.

[36] Tudor-Hart does not distinguish between whiteness and brightness, using the latter term exclusively. Both aspects must have played a rôle, predominantly that of whiteness.

6. Transparency varies in different aspects, depending upon different sets of conditions. Sharpness of figure, depending on the brightness difference between the background and the figure upon it, determines the clearness or "mistiness" of the figure, while the brightness of the background determines the "stuff" of the episcotister, it being the thicker, the more solid, the darker the background. Two equal episcotisters, one in front of a black, the other of a white background, "appeared so different in every way, that it seemed ridiculous to suppose that they were objectively the same" (p. 288).

Without going into a detailed analysis of these results I shall point out that they confirm the importance of gradients of stimulation for spatial organization, that they add proof to our theory of transparency, inasmuch as they add a new case of "splitting up," viz., the splitting up of a neutral colour into two equal neutral colours (result 2, where the grey area corresponding to the mixture of figure and episcotister which reflect the same radiation is seen in double representation as part of the transparent episcotister and as figure of the same brightness), and that they demonstrate the difference of hardness between white and black.

CHAPTER VII

THE ENVIRONMENTAL FIELD

Tri-Dimensional Space and Motion

The Interdependence of the Different Aspects of Visual Organization. Tri-dimensional Organization. Retinal Disparity. The Combination of the Different "Criteria of Depth." Anisotropy of Space. Perceived Motion. A General Principle of the Theory of Perceived Motion. Stroboscopic and Real Motion. Apparent Velocity. Brown's Experiments. Brown's Results and Korte's Laws. Motion and Time. Selection of Fusion. Conclusions as to the Nature of Behavioural Things. Summary

THE INTERDEPENDENCE OF THE DIFFERENT ASPECTS OF VISUAL ORGANIZATION

The discussion of the phenomena traditionally treated from the point of view of constancy of shape, size and colour (including transparency) should have demonstrated a general fact of fundamental importance for the understanding of perception: the different aspects of our visual world, size, shape, colour, orientation, and localization, are constituted in a thoroughgoing mutual interdependence. Psychology, when it began to tackle the problem of perception, did not recognize the complexity of its task. It was believed that different aspects of the visual world had different and independent origins which could be studied separately. At first a sense of colour and a sense of space were distinguished, to which later a sense of shape and possibly a sense of motion were added. Such a view errs by translating different problems into different realities. In truth, the colour which a local stimulation produces depends upon the general spatial organization, including size, shape, and orientation, that it calls forth. And this proposition remains true if one exchanges the positions of the different terms. To some extent this interconnectedness has been demonstrated in detail in the preceding discussion.

TRI-DIMENSIONAL ORGANIZATION

But one aspect, the importance of which has transpired in all constancy problems, has not received sufficient treatment. I mean tri-dimensional organization. To attempt a systematic presentation now would be impossible. Not only would it require at least a chapter as long as this, but also, and chiefly, the facts necessary for such a treatment are not yet available, since the great amount of excellent work done in this field was done under assumptions no longer tenable, while comparatively little work has as yet been done from the point of view of organization, though such work will not be long in forthcoming. Therefore in this context I shall take up only a very few points, notably the factor of retinal disparity and the problem of the combination of the so-called depth criteria.

Retinal Disparity. That tri-dimensional organization is not in itself the creation of retinal disparity we have emphasized sufficiently. That it plays a very important rôle in producing tri-dimensional organization need hardly be stated. What we shall try to do here is to show that retinal disparity is a factor of organization, depending upon organization. The traditional treatment of this factor consists in describing the facts without any attempt at going behind them. Corresponding points are defined as points which when simultaneously stimulated give rise to the perception of *one* object, or as points the stimulation of which gives rise to the perception of one and the same *direction*. Then the statement is added that if one and the same geographical point is projected on two non-corresponding retinal points it will appear double except when the amount of disparity is small: in that case the point will be seen as one, but either in front or behind the plane of the fixation point, the "nuclear plane," according to the direction of the disparity. I can omit the details, since they can be looked up in most textbooks. *Why* disparity has these effects is either not stated at all, often because it is assumed to be such an ultimate fact as that stimulation by long-waved light gives rise to the sensation of red, or is treated in such general terms—"utilization of a distance cue by the organism"—that the student is in reality no better off than in the first case.

Attempt at a Dynamical Theory of Disparity. It is clear that a psychology such as we are trying to develop cannot be satisfied with such a state of affairs. For this psychology the visual world is a product of organization in the psychophysical field, and it attempts to understand the process of this organization and the factors which determine it. The facts of retinal disparity, as usually stated, are facts of geometry. What we require are facts of dynamics. We want to know the *forces* which result from the geometry of disparity. Two first attempts have been made to discover the nature of these forces, one by Lewin and Sakuma, the other by myself (1930).

In the following discussion I shall more or less neglect the difficult, though significant and important, contribution by the first two authors and shall take up some of the points made in my article.

THE DEFINITION OF RETINAL CORRESPONDENCE AND DISPARITY. The first point concerns the very definition of correspondence and disparity. At first such a definition seems quite simple: one chooses a certain point in external space and sees on which points of the two retinae it is projected. If then the point is perceived as one and in the nuclear plane, then the two retinal points on which it is projected are corresponding or identical points; if the point appears double, or not in the nuclear plane, the points are disparate. Exploring the two retinae in this manner, one finds that its two centres are identical and, in a first approximation, also all points which have the same distance in the same direction from the two centres.[1] And thus one has reached a purely geometrical or anatomical definition of corresponding and disparate points, i.e., a purely geometrical method by which to assign to any one point on one retina the corresponding point on the other. And yet it is much more difficult to express the meaning of the co-ordination of two points as corresponding or disparate than it has so far appeared. Supposing I choose the point x_l on the left retina and find by the method just indicated the point x_r on the right retina which corresponds to it; how can I express the result of this process without using the word "corresponding"? I might say x_r which is as distant in the same direction from the right fovea as x_l is from the left has the property that when it is stimulated by the same external point as x_l, the owner of the two eyes will see one point in the nuclear plane. The trouble with this proposition is that it uses a point of external space as one of its terms, i.e., something which is external to the proximal stimulus and can therefore have no direct effect upon the process of vision. The eyes "cannot know" whether they are stimulated by the same external point or not; proximal stimulation of certain kinds will produce the perception of *one* point when in reality there are two (e.g., in the stereoscope), and this perception is as much the effect of correspondence as the seeing of one point when in reality there is only one. We must therefore try to eliminate the distant stimulus from our definition of correspondence and couch

[1] In reality conditions are much less simple, as the investigations of the line-horopter have shown. This complex field of research, the results of which are far from having found a satisfactory explanation, must be omitted from our discussion. The facts may be found in Witasek (1909). The simplified statement of the text is, however, sufficient for the following argument.

it entirely in terms of proximal stimulation. One might try to accomplish this by saying: when two corresponding points are stimulated *in the same manner,* then the result will be the perception of one point in the nuclear plane. Then *equality* of stimulation would be required for the definition of correspondence, i.e., something which transcends pure geometry.

What is true of corresponding points is equally true of disparate ones. To say that y_r is disparate to x_l means that when these two points are equally stimulated the result will *not* be the perception of *one* point in the *nuclear plane*—but either of two points, or of one point *not* in the nuclear plane.

THE DYNAMICS OF DISPARITY. This definition of correspondence and disparity, though by no means entirely adequate, covers a great many cases provided that "equality" is properly understood. For equality does *not* mean equality of radiation. Insert into the left half of the stereoscope a grey surface with a blue point on it and into the right an equal surface with a red point, these points being in approximately the same location on their respective surfaces, then *one* point, of inconstant colour, varying between red and blue, will be seen. This proves that, if we define equality of stimulation by equality of radiation, identical points may be *differently* stimulated and yet produce the normal result: *one* perceived point in the nuclear plane. In a second experiment both sides of the stereoscope are white and each has two black points on an imaginary horizontal line which halves these fields, but these points have a different distance from each other on the two sides (see Fig. 80). In that case

F_l P_l F_r P'_r

Fig. 80

only one pair of points, e.g., F_l and F_r, the fixated ones, can fall on identical points, whereas P_l and P'_r must be projected on disparate points. If this disparity is not too great, then the observer will perceive two points in all, each corresponding to a pair of stimulus points, and point P will lie to the right and behind point F because P_l and P'_r are disparate points. This case corresponds to our definition of disparity, for the two points P_l and P'_r are equal in colour, whereas the point P_r corresponding to P_l on the right side, located at the left of P'_r, provides a stimulation different from that supplied by P_l, and similarly P'_l corresponding to P'_r on the left side, reflects a different kind of light. But we have just seen from our first experiment that there are conditions where identical points, stimulated differently, produce the normal effect. Why, then, do they not do so here? The meaning of this question may become still clearer when we reformulate it. We throw two different patterns of stimulation upon the two retinae. To each point of the one retina there corresponds a point on the other retina; consequently it is perfectly correct to say: whatever these patterns are, they always stimulate the totality of identical points. This statement, though geometrically perfectly true, is entirely inadequate. It leaves no place for disparate points, which had to be introduced to explain the effects of all but the very simplest kinds of stimulation. Otherwise expressed, the effect of the stimulation by two retinal patterns will not, except in specially selected cases, correspond to the effect in our first experiment where two differently coloured points were projected on identical points on the two retinae, with the result that one point in a changing and intermediate colour was seen in the nuclear plane. Instead such stimulation will as a rule result in a depth relief, indicating that disparate points determine the effect. That means: which pairs of points, or lines, on the two retinae will co-operate in determining the perceptual organization depends upon the two retinal patterns. This is not a geometrical or anatomical but a dynamical fact. In each case there must exist real forces which lead to one kind of co-ordination rather than another. The immediate origin of these forces cannot lie in the retinal patterns themselves, since they are separate and therefore unable to interact. Interaction can take place only where the *processes* started in the two optical tracts by the retinal patterns converge in the brain. These processes will interact according to their structural properties; i.e., figure will interact with figure and ground with ground, and not *vice versa;* a unique point in a curve will interact with the corresponding unique point in the other curve, whether they are projected on identical retinal points or not, and so forth. In other words, the very concepts of corresponding and disparate points presuppose the concept of organization.

From this point of view we can look back on our first two stereoscopic experiments. In the first, a blue and a red point, one on each side of the stereoscope, will interact, each being the only figure in the field. As we shall see in the following chapter, the very fact that the eyes adjust themselves in such a way that these two points are projected on identical retinal points is explained by the same principle. In our second experiment the same argument applies only to one pair of points, F_l and F_r,[2] while the other two points cannot fall on identical retinal points if F_l and F_r do. They will, however, interact; being two figures in close proximity they will attract each other, their union being prohibited by the union of the two other points.[3] But there is no reason why P_l should interact with P_r which belongs to the background, or P'_r with P'_l. The question raised on page 269 has therefore been answered, and this answer has given us an insight into the dynamics of binocular vision. In the "combination zone," as I have called that part of the psychophysical field where the processes started in the two eyes combine, a stress results when the conditions are of that kind of which our second experiment with the two pairs of dots is the simplest example. We now introduce the assumption that, provided the disparity is not too great, this stress results in the unification of the two attracting points and at the same time in depth relief, one single point appearing either nearer or farther than the other. This hypothesis is consistent with our whole treatment of perceptual organization, since it attributes a definite effect to definite forces. It is incomplete because it cannot deduce why this stress, which according to its nature should lead to unification, produces depth relief. As a matter of fact one might argue that unification of the points P_l and P'_r cannot be of the same kind as that between F_l and F_r, since the latter reduces the stress in the field to a minimum while the former creates stress, and that the only possible difference between the two unifications in pure spatial terms is a difference in depth. Even so it remains unexplained why disparity of one kind or direction has the effect of pulling the unified area nearer while disparity of the opposite kind pushes it farther away, nor why this effect is more or less confined to cross disparity as opposed to longitudinal disparity. It seems to me highly probable that the explanation of these facts has to be found in the facts of the structure of the optical sector, i.e., in the permanent internal conditions as defined in Chapter III.

Some Experimental Evidence. I shall adduce three experiments in support of this hypothesis, the two first to demonstrate the selection of co-operating retinal areas by figural factors, the third to support the assumption that the depth effect is caused by stresses in the combination zone. The first experiment goes back to Helmholtz (III). The stereoscopic effect of two perspective drawings presented

[2] It would apply just as well to the other. In that case Fl and Fr would play the rôle ascribed in the text to Pl and P'r.

[3] See Chapter VIII, p. 315.

in a stereoscope is not changed if one of these is drawn black on white, the other white on black. To analyze this experiment, let us consider a corresponding corner of the two drawings which is not projected on identical retinal points. If the left corner be black, the corresponding point in the other eye is also stimulated by black, while the white corner stimulates a non-identical point in the other eye, whose identical point in the left eye is in its turn also stimulated by white. If P_l and P_r, G_l and G_r, are the two pairs of identical points concerned, then we have the following stimulation:

TABLE 8

	l	r
P	black	black
G	white	white

And yet not the identical and equally stimulated pairs P_l and P_r on the one hand and G_l and G_r on the other interact, but P_l with G_r, and G_l with P_r; the reason is that the two interacting points give rise to equal structural parts in the field organization.

The second experiment performed by myself (1930) is extremely simple, as illustrated by Fig. 81. The two pairs of lines, presented on different sides of a stereoscope, are so arranged that a point on the solid lines is fixated. The dotted lines are drawn in such a way that the dots on one side correspond to white interstices on the other, and on the left side the dotted lines are closer to the solid line than on the right. Geometrically to a dot on the left side there corresponds whiteness on the other; moreover, atomistically considered, there is no disparate point on the right side which receives the same stimulation as the point which is stimulated by a dot on the left. Let us call the point in the left eye which is stimulated by a dot p_l, the corresponding point in the right eye p_r, the point in the right eye which is stimulated by the interstice corresponding to the left dot g_r, and its identical point in the left eye g_l. Then the schema of stimulation is as follows:

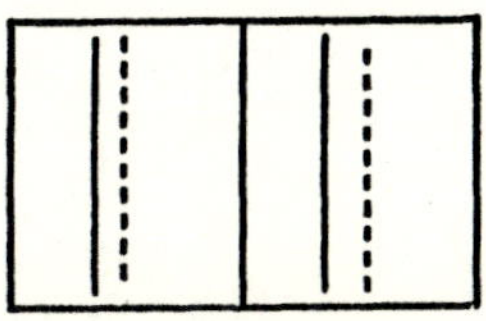

Fig. 81

TABLE 9

	l	r
p	black	white
g	white	white

Thus, considering first the different retinal points, there is not the slightest reason why p_l should co-operate with g_r rather than with p_r, both points being equally stimulated. And yet, if we want to formulate what happens, that is exactly what we must say; for the observer sees two lines in all, one corresponding to the two continuous lines of the stereoscope slide, the other to the two dotted lines, and the latter, though it need not even be continuous, lies like point P in Fig. 80 behind the other. In reality this experiment proves that interaction takes place not between points, but between the whole lines, i.e., between unitary processes started in each eye separately by the black dots. These lines interact with each other, since they are figures; disparate *points* come into play only because each point is a part of a larger whole. In these two experiments factors of organization have been proved to select which retinal areas will lead to interacting processes and which not; at the same time the difference between identical and disparate areas is considered to be anatomically conditioned; factors of organization decide whether anatomically identical or disparate parts interact. Lewin and Sakuma have tried to go one step further and to show that identity and disparity themselves may be determined by factors of organization (p. 334 f.). Since, however, I am not quite convinced that their proof is absolutely stringent, I omit a description of their ingenious experiments, satisfied with having mentioned this other more extreme possibility.

The third experiment, performed by Jaensch (1911), was made for the purpose of demonstrating that disparity *per se* does not produce depth. If three vertical threads are so arranged that two lie in a frontal parallel plane and the third between them and in front of their plane, the observer sees a wedge-like structure, with the edge pointing towards him, in conformity with the disparity of the retinal images. But when, as in Jaensch's experiment, these threads are luminous wires in an otherwise totally dark room, then the depth of this wedge is greatly reduced and may, if the centre thread does not stand out too far, disappear altogether, all three threads being seen in one plane. This fact lends support to our theory that depth effect is due to field stresses, in the following way. If the front thread is projected on identical points, then the two others are projected on disparate points, giving rise on the boundary of the combination zone to two pairs of "line processes" which do not exactly fit; but of these four processes the two left and the two right ones being in close proximity will strongly attract each other and each result in a single process. This is the repetition of the argument we have employed above in explaining our stereoscope experiment with two pairs of points. Why, then, does the wedge appear flat in a dark room? We explained the depth effect of disparity as due to stresses in the combination zone. Consequently, when no depth effect appears we must assume that this stress fails to be created. The reason for this is not difficult to discover. In the area prior to the combination zone two disparate lines have different distances from the identical lines, and the stress arises from the fact that by their fusion in the combination zone this difference is abolished. In a lighted room, each of the two disparately projected threads is in definite spatial relationship to a great number of objects, whereas in the dark room the only other object is the one identically projected line. In the lighted room fusion of the two pairs of disparate processes has to contend against stronger forces than in the dark room; otherwise expressed, the position of the lines in the pre-combination-zone area is more strongly determined when the room is lighted than when it is dark. Therefore in the former case the stress produced by the fusion must be greater than in the latter. Still, even when the disparate lines fuse without depth effect, there must be some stress. Since this does not become manifest in the orientation of the lines, it must reside in the surrounding field; it may be possible to put this hypothesis to a test by exploring the surrounding field.

The Combination of the Different "Criteria of Depth." At the end of Chapter IV we have already discussed the traditional view about the different depth criteria. We return to it from another point of view. Granted that depth is an aspect of spatial organization, and that the different depth criteria are factors which determine this organization, how are we to conceive of their co-operation? In the discussion of shape and size constancy we found depth-producing factors of various kinds to influence apparent shape and size (see p. 235), and we found facts which are hard to reconcile with a view in which the different factors combine according to a principle of algebraic addition. At first sight such a principle seems, however, to be required by our dynamic theory. If the different factors act as forces of organization, their resultant should be algebraically determined. There are, however, different possibilities, one of which we shall exemplify by the spring balance. If we put a weight of five pounds on the scale of such a balance, it will be lowered to a certain point, and when we add another pound the scale will be lowered further; similarly, if instead of adding a weight we exert a force equal to one pound in the direction of lifting the scale which carries five pounds, it will be raised to a position which it would assume if no such counterforce were present and the weight on the scale equalled four pounds. So far, then, the scale follows the law of algebraic addition. But now we pull the scale as far down as it will go and push it under a horizontal bar which holds it in this position. If then we put a weight on it the scale will not move and it will also remain immobile when we apply a force to lift it, provided this force is not so strong as to overcome the resistance of the bar. From this analogy we learn that the different factors may co-operate in such a way that one of them produces a maximum effect of great stability, so that other factors remain entirely ineffective. I do not consider this analogy an explanation, but a guiding principle for the study of the different depth factors. That this principle may be fruitful I infer from a significant experiment by Schriever, who subjected a number of depth criteria in isolation and combination to a careful investigation. A solid of the shape of a skewed H (see Fig. 82) suspended in front of a dark background was photographed from two different points, and the two photographs used as stereoscope slides. Thereby disparity, overlapping, and shadows were combined as depth factors. If in this experiment the two sides of the stereoscope were exchanged so that the object belonging to the right eye was seen by the left, and *vice versa,* the depth relief was *not* changed; some subjects mentioned only that space was now less impressive, although still of full plasticity, different from the depth of an ordinary perspective drawing. In this case, then, retinal disparity failed to produce any effect. Had it been effective, the whole depth relief would have been reversed, the beams of the H would have appeared as hollow angle-irons (L-irons). An explanation of this failure seems possible in the terms of our spring-balance analogy. The upper horizontal front bar is

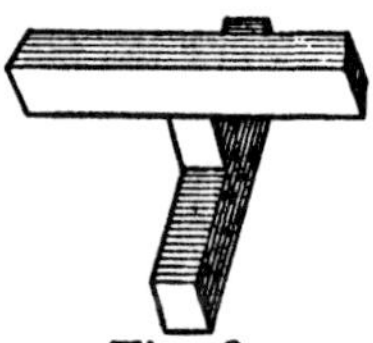

Fig. 82

seen as one thing, so is the lower horizontal bar which is being partly concealed by the former. To come forward this would have to go right through the upper bar, whereas the upper bar, as a solid thing, is impenetrable and therefore holds the lower one in its position, just as in our analogy the cross bar held the scale of the balance in position. True enough, this latter is a real, geographical, thing, whereas the former is a behavioural thing. But we have already seen that "thingness" is a property of many behavioural objects, and we assume that behavioural thingness is in many respects similar to geographical or physical thingness. This assumption, which we shall discuss in greater detail at the end of this chapter, explains several facts of perception.

ANISOTROPY OF SPACE

With these general remarks we shall close the discussion of the dynamics of space organization. Phenomenal, or behavioural, space has, however, a property which must be specially mentioned although we have encountered it in various places. Behavioural space is not Euclidean, or, otherwise expressed, it is anisotropic, it has different properties in different directions. Two aspects of this anisotropy have to be distinguished. On the one hand organization of figures and things creates stresses which are not restricted to the segregated units but affect the surrounding field to a larger or smaller extent. A number of well-known optical illusions, like the Jastrow and the Zöllner patterns, demonstrate this effect as I have pointed out in other places (1931, p. 1182, 1931 a, p. 1263 f.). On the other hand space as a framework is itself anisotropic and determines by its anisotropy the organization of figures and things within it. We have emphasized the fact that there are *main* directions, and that these main directions exert functional influences upon organization.[4]

Anisotropy of the Two First Dimensions. But even in its main directions space is not isotropic. The so-called overestimation of the vertical is a manifestation of the inequality of the horizontal and the vertical direction; it appears in the perception of every figure except the circle (see Koffka, 1931 a, p. 1228). Of other manifestations of this anisotropy which I have mentioned in one of my articles (1931 a) I shall refer here only to so-called γ motion. If a figure is exposed for a short time it appears with a motion of expansion and disappears with a motion of contraction (Kenkel); both these

[4] See, for instance, the discussion of orientation as a factor which influences the figure-ground organization, in Chapter V, p. 190 f.

motions arise from the dynamics of the figure organization as has been proved by Lindemann, Harrower (1929), and Newman. The direction of this motion is, however, indicative of spatial anisotropy. Lindemann and Newman found that the motion of a square is stronger in the horizontal than in the vertical axis. Lindemann found the same true of contour circles and ellipses.[5] Another anisotropy of the horizontal and vertical direction was discovered by J. F. Brown (1931 a). Of two equal motions, one in the vertical and one in the horizontal direction, the former appears to have the greater velocity. This effect shows the same direction as the overestimation of the vertical, but is quantitatively very much greater, 4–5% for the overestimation, and about 30% for the difference of velocity. Lastly, Oppenheimer has found the vertical to constitute the chief frame of reference for moving objects (see below).

Tri-dimensional Anisotropy. The anisotropy of visual space becomes, however, far more apparent when we consider, not a relatively small *surface*, but the whole space in its greatest possible extent. In the first place it appears that the third dimension is functionally different from the first two. The experimental data are not too numerous and are widely scattered among investigations of various kinds. Some data, like the Aubert-Foerster phenomenon whose great psychological significance was discovered by Jaensch (1909), are connected with the factors which determine apparent size, others were collected in the field of visual motion, others in experiments on patients with brain lesions.

I select a few results which demonstrate the facts of anisotropy particularly well.

(1) Loss of Surface Colours. I recall Gelb's two patients with loss of surface colours discussed in Chapter IV. We saw that for them the colour of a surface segregated from the background spread in all directions, but that this spreading was very much greater in the third dimension than in the other two. The explanation which we gave there (p. 118) can be expressed in terms of anisotropy. The patients look, for example, at a black square on a white background. Then the retinal distribution is the first cause of the perceptual organization; the gradient in the field creates not only the segregation of the figure from the ground, but also its localization in one plane. Now, for these patients this localization is not perfect; the white

[5] Newman, who used only surface figures, found no such asymmetry in a circle and in a star, probably because a surface circle is too strong a figure to yield to the forces of anisotropy, just as the circle, when permanently exposed, is the only figure which does not show the overestimation of the vertical. I hope soon to have experimental evidence whether this interpretation is correct.

background has a certain degree of "thickness," the black figure a much greater one and the latter also extends slightly beyond its objective boundaries. Thus the retinal conditions are more effective in producing forces of cohesion in the first two dimensions than in the third; the three dimensions cannot, therefore, be equivalent.

(2) Motion in the Third Dimension. Another experiment, described in the second chapter, seems to point in a similar direction, I mean the experiment with the iris diaphragm through which one sees a lighted surface in a totally dark room. If the diaphragm is opened the white circle seems to approach, when it is closed to recede—these results being more frequent than a perceived expansion and contraction without approach and recession. In this case a change of the retinal image in the first two dimensions gives rise to a behavioural change in the third, an indication that such changes are more easily produced, that the third dimension is not equivalent to the two others.

This interpretation is corroborated by experiments on visual motion by von Schiller which we shall discuss later. At this point it suffices to quote the author's statement that a stroboscopic motion in the third dimension seems to be generally preferred to motions in the two others (p. 208).

(3) Nearness and Clearness. The third dimension manifests an anisotropy itself inasmuch as organization differs with the distance of the appearing object. We know already that the same retinal image gives rise to a smaller *behavioural size* when the object is seen nearer than when it is seen farther (a fact which underlies constancy of size). At the same time the object is seen more *clearly* and appears often "brighter," more highly illuminated. The connection between apparent size on the one hand and clearness and brightness on the other is particularly apparent in micropsia, produced most easily by holding a concave lens of low refracting power before the eye, which produces only a small reduction of the retinal image quite out of proportion to the observed shrinkage of the perceived object. Jaensch called this effect the Koster-phenomenon. Sinemus has recently shown that micropsia changes both whiteness (or more generally, object colour) and brightness, these changes depending upon the intensity of the objective illumination. As far as I can see, the relation of these facts to apparent distance has not been mentioned by these authors. And yet a simple observation, familiar to most theatre-goers, seems to me to establish it without a doubt. An ordinary opera glass magnifies 2½ to 3 times linearly. Yet the actors on the stage seem hardly taller when seen through glasses

than with the unaided eye. One can convince oneself of this fact if one holds the glasses in such a way that the left glass is in front of the right eye while the left eye remains naked, and turns the glass in such a way that the two pictures of the same external object, the normal and the enlarged one, appear side by side. Then one becomes aware of the tremendous difference in size between them, whereas when one returns to the normal use of the glasses, the object appears much smaller than the enlarged picture. At the same time the object seen through the glasses appears *clearer and nearer*. The enlargement of the retinal image has, therefore, three different effects on the behavioural object: (a) it enlarges it slightly, the least pronounced effect; (b) it makes it clearer, and (c) it brings it nearer. Effect (a) proves that, paradoxical as it may sound, the use of an opera glass produces micropsia—the paradox disappears when we compare not the size of the object seen with and without glasses, but the perceived sizes with the respective retinal images. In this case, then, and probably in all others as well, greater nearness is coupled with greater clearness.

I believe that the Aubert-Foerster phenomenon is an indication of the same anisotropy of space. Since, however, as Freeman has shown, the conditions for its arousal are not so simple as Jaensch originally believed, I shall omit a detailed discussion and only mention that the Aubert-Foerster phenomenon manifests a dependence of visual acuity upon perceived distance, in the sense that the acuity, measured in visual angles, is greater at small than at great distances.

(4) ZENITH-HORIZON ILLUSION. Another anisotropy is demonstrated by the zenith-horizon illusion (see Chapter III). We can formulate it in this way. We describe a number of circles with different radii in the median plane of an observer with the midpoint between his two eyes as the centre, and attach to them equal disks at the end of a horizontal and a vertical radius, h_1, h_2, h_3 . . . and v_1, v_2, v_3 . . . (in other words we are using imaginary perimeters with ever-increasing radii), and we compare first the appearance of h and v on the same circle, then the relation between an h_k and v_k with that between an h_n and a v_n. Then we find that on a near circle the behavioural h_n and v_n will be equal, but that with increasing distance the h will look increasingly larger than the corresponding v. This is nothing but the statement of greater constancy of size in the horizontal than in the vertical dimension expressed in terms of anisotropy of space. As we have seen in our previous discussion in Chapter III, disks attached at positions intermediate between h and v would appear in an intermediate size,

showing that the anisotropy pervades the whole space. This anisotropy pertains not only to apparent size but also to apparent distance—the shape of the sky is not spherical, but flattened; but the quantitative aspect of the distance anisotropy has not been as well worked out as that of the size aspect.

ANISOTROPY AND LOCOMOTION. VON ALLESCH'S EXPERIMENTS. It is plausible to connect this anisotropy with the fact that we live on the ground and move predominantly horizontally across it. If this connection, not to be interpreted empiristically, but as an effect of the structure of the total nervous system, is valid, then the space of animals with different locomotion should be different. This argument was developed by von Allesch, who put it to an experimental test by comparing several space functions of human subjects with those of an animal that lives in trees and whose locomotion consists in climbing and leaping. If spatial asymmetry is connected with the direction of locomotion, then one might expect that for such an animal the vertical would be favoured over the horizontal, that to it the moon would appear larger at the zenith than at the horizon. Von Allesch chose as his subject a lemur. He did not test a function which would allow us to verify the last conclusion directly, but two other functions, viz., discrimination of distance and discrimination of size, and found that whereas for men the thresholds were finer when tested with objects straight ahead than with objects straight above, the opposite was true of his test animal. Perhaps one such experiment is not quite sufficient to prove so radical an assumption. Nevertheless, the experiment seems significant enough to lend it a considerable degree of probability. It is to be hoped that new experiments will decide this highly important issue.

(5) ANISOTROPY AND CONSTANCY. Anisotropy of perceptual space must be in close relationship with constancy of size and shape, and thereby with the constancy of *things*. The relation to constancy of size has already been mentioned. I add a few words about shape. Remembering our discussion of turned figures (ellipses, rectangles) we can now say: a retinal line will appear the shorter the more it appears in a plane normal to the line of regard, i.e., the more its whole length appears to be equidistant from the observer. The stresses which we made responsible for this effect can easily be interpreted as constituting the anisotropy of psychophysical space. Inasmuch as this anisotropy leads to a truer cognition of reality and thereby to a more adjusted behaviour than an isotropic space would, one might try to connect it with its biological usefulness. Such speculations seem to me, however, spurious as long as one has no

conception of the causal connection between the two terms. Usefulness in itself is not a cause. A genetic explanation, which could attribute to individual experiences at best a very minor rôle, would have to take account of the fact that the anisotropy of perceptual space achieves its cognitive result by cancelling, more or less, the effect of perspective in real space.

PERCEIVED MOTION

The behavioural world has been treated so far as though it were produced by unchanging stimulation, and contained, correspondingly, only objects at rest. This implicit assumption restricts our field of study to unique cases which are realized only under very special conditions. As a rule, moving objects are in our field; at this moment in my own field there is my pen which is moved across the page by my fingers; now a buzzing fly passes through my field of vision, and as soon as a visitor enters my office, he is never so rigidly calm as to produce an unchanging retinal image; but even if being alone I lean back in my chair and begin to think out the solution of a problem, my eyes are not kept steady but will change their line of regard from one object to another, thereby producing a change of the retinal patterns. In the first cases, real moving objects present in the field, the shift of the retinal pattern leads to behavioural motion of objects, whether I fixate a non-moving object or follow a moving one with my regard; in the second case, when my eyes roam over stationary objects, such a shift will *not* have this result. Although the two facts belong closely together, the second one will be fully discussed in Chapter IX, after we have introduced the Ego. Here we concentrate mainly on the first, even if we cannot entirely avoid referring to the second. Thus we turn now to the theory of perceived motion. It is a well-known fact that a paper on visual motion was the beginning of Gestalt psychology. Wertheimer (1912) utilized the results of his classical study to formulate briefly a number of new principles constitutive for every kind of psychological theory. Even though we have developed these principles in other fields and with the help of other facts, it might be tempting to introduce the discussion of our present topic with Wertheimer's paper and then follow the history of psychological progress in this field. I shall, however, choose a different mode of procedure and present facts and theories systematically according to all the knowledge now available, and shall in this attempt concentrate more on the later than on the earlier publications. The earlier ones are today fairly well known; they are, and they had to be, full of experiments which refuted theories accepted at the time they were written, but which today can be considered dead. Since I have treated the subject so often (1919, 1931), most explicitly in 1931 (an article which contains a great mass of detail which will be omitted here), a similar procedure would be mere repetition.

Wertheimer's paper and a number of publications which followed it dealt chiefly or exclusively with stroboscopic motion, i.e., the case where perceived motion is produced by stationary objects. Since it has been proved beyond a doubt (Wertheimer, Cermak and Koffka, Duncker 1929, Brown 1931, van der Waals and Roelofs 1933) that as far as psychophysical dynamics are concerned there is no difference between stroboscopic and "real" motion,[6] i.e., perceived motion produced by actually moving objects, it seems more adequate to begin with the latter case, which is the more usual.

A General Principle of the Theory of Perceived Motion. We begin with a very general statement formulated explicitly by Köhler (1933, p. 356). The physiological correlate of perceived motion[7] must be a real process of change within the total physiological process patterns. Supposing that the perceptual field were totally homogeneous except for one point moving through it, then the motion of this point would *not* lead to such a change as we have postulated, since in the totally homogeneous field it would be exposed to the *same* stresses everywhere, all positions being dynamically indistinguishable from each other. Under such conditions no motion would be perceived, and although this condition is unrealizable its discussion elucidates the significance of the conditions which are realized.[8] Our perceptual field is in this sense never entirely homogeneous. Even in complete darkness it has an above and below, right and left, near and far; and a point passing through it if it changes its distance from the fovea, apart from changing its position with regard to these three determinations, passes at the same time through regions of different functional properties. Inhomogeneity of the total field and a displacement of a point within such an inhomogeneous field are therefore two necessary conditions for the arousal of the psychophysical process of motion. For in an inhomogeneous field the motion of an object changes its dynamic condition with regard to the total physiological process pattern. From this we

[6] This proof was once of great theoretical significance. We shall occasionally mention one or two points.

[7] Although we shall largely confine ourselves to visual motion, tactual and acoustic motion are essentially of the same kind (see my article 1931).

[8] Similarly Newton's first law of motion treats an unrealizable case and has nevertheless been of great significance.

can deduce that more inhomogeneous fields are more favourable for the arousal of perceived motion than less inhomogeneous ones, a deduction amply confirmed by facts. All movement thresholds are higher in relatively homogeneous fields than in inhomogeneous ones (see my article 1931, p. 1194 f.), and the apparent velocity of objects moving objectively with the same velocity is greater for those which move in inhomogeneous than for those which move in relatively homogeneous fields (Brown 1931, p. 218). These two facts are closely interrelated, as Brown (1931 b) has proved.

Our conclusion that perceived motion in the visual field presupposes displacement of objects relative to the rest of the field also fits the facts from which we started our discussion. If objects move in the geographical environment, then their retinal images are displaced with regard to other objects whether we fixate them or an object at rest, while movement of our eyes across stationary objects leaves their relation to the objects surrounding them intact. True enough, eye-movements also produce a shift of pattern on the retina, and therefore must have some effect of perceived motion, but this motion should not belong to the field objects. We shall see later that the perception of our eyes, or even of "ourselves," as moving is the result of this shift (Duncker).

Duncker's Experiments. Such a view of the origin of the perception of motion must lead to very definite experiments. The excellent work done by Duncker (1929) was entirely determined by it. Supposing the field is homogeneously dark and contains only two light objects, one of which is in objective motion while the other one is at rest. Then, if the velocity of the motion is not great, the chief determining factor will be the relative displacement of the two objects. This, according to our theory, must lead to perceived motion, but our theory does not permit us to deduce which of these objects will be the carrier of the motion, as long as their relative displacement and no other factor becomes effective. But our theoretical equipment contains other concepts which suggest a solution of this problem.

Systems of Reference. We fall back on our distinction of things and framework and our knowledge that the framework is more stable than the things within it. If we apply this to the case of motion we must deduce the following proposition: if one of the two field objects has the function of framework for the other, then it will be seen at rest and the other as moving no matter which of the two moves in reality. If on the other hand the two objects are both things, then under symmetrical conditions (fixation between them or freely wandering regard) they should both move in opposite directions.

Both these deductions were confirmed in Duncker's experiments. He also found, what Thelin had discovered before him, that fixation of one of the two equivalent objects tended to make it the carrier of motion, whether it moved objectively or not, a fact which he tentatively explains by the thing-framework, or figure-ground, distinction, the fixated point keeping its figure character, whereas non-fixated ones become part of the ground. Duncker's findings have been corroborated and amplified by an investigation of Oppenheimer's which is just about to appear. Of her results I will only mention two: (1) the relative intensity of the objects plays a rôle, the stronger one tending to become the frame of reference for the weaker; therefore, *ceteris paribus,* the stronger one will be at rest, the weaker one in motion; (2) the shape of the objects determines the apparent motion in this way: if the relative displacement between the two objects occurs in such a manner that its direction coincides with one of the main directions of one object, but not with that of the other, the former will tend to be seen as moving further than the latter. The relative displacement does not, therefore, determine the motion carrier, but under these conditions it determines the *amount* of motion. This is an invariant, no matter whether one point is seen in motion, or both. As a matter of fact it was Duncker who introduced the concept of invariants (though he did not use the term), which has been so fruitful in our discussion of perceptual organization. The invariance of the amplitude of motion holds, if only two objects take part in it, whether they are equivalent to each other or whether one is the framework of the other. As soon as a third object enters, this invariance may no longer hold. If *a* is the framework of *b,* and *b* the framework of *c,* and objectively *b* is moved, then two different kinds of relative displacement take place; *b* changes its place in its own framework *a,* and *c* changes its place in its framework *b.* The sum of the two perceived motions resulting from these conditions will be greater than the perceived motion resulting if *b* is moved exactly as before but either object *a* or object *c* is removed. Duncker has discussed the possible relationships between a third object and the two other ones and has demonstrated experimentally that the effects on perceived motion depend upon the kind and degree of appurtenance between them. Plurality of frameworks, or systems of reference, has still another important effect, first recognized by Rubin (1927). His ingenious and elegant experiments were supplemented by Duncker.

I shall discuss only a very simple case which is unique because of its familiarity. Continually we see wheels rolling over the ground, and perceive simultaneously two motions, a circular and a rectilinear translatory one. In reality each point of the wheel, with the exception of the centre, describes cycloids, whose shape is entirely different from that of the circle; the centre alone performs a pure translatory motion. But the points of the wheel have the centre as their point of reference, while the centre itself is referred to the general spatial framework, or, when the room is in darkness, to the observer himself (see the next paragraph). The double motion which is actually perceived is the result of this separation of systems of reference. If only one point of the wheel (not the centre) is visible during its rotation, then motion on a cycloidal curve is perceived. If the centre is added (Duncker) the phenomenon changes at once, different phenomena emerge, partly depending upon the velocity of the wheel motion, all of which have the common feature that the peripheral point describes a rotatory motion. If instead of adding the centre one adds a point on the same concentric circle as the first point, then, to judge from one of Rubin's experiments performed with a somewhat different motion pattern, one can see two such cycloidal motions. If one increases the number of such points, one soon reaches the normal wheel effect, i.e., one sees all points rotating round an invisible centre, and at the same time a translatory motion.

THE EGO AS A FIELD OBJECT. A possible objection which may have occurred to the reader will lead us to a very important generalization. We have chosen as the simplest case that in which *two* objects are in the field. But it is perfectly possible to see also *one* point in motion. Does this not conflict with our theory? It would if we confined our consideration to the "surrounding field," but such a restriction would be inadequate; we have seen in various places that field processes cannot be treated exhaustively without including the Ego. How the Ego fits into our theory will be discussed in the next two chapters; at this point in our discussion we have to regard it as a field object in its own right. Then motion of one point is displacement of two objects with regard to each other, viz., the point and the Ego. In reality, therefore, we deal with three objects when we have two points in the field. Duncker, however, succeeded in excluding the influence of the Ego by working with such slow velocities and small excursions that they were subliminal with regard to the Ego, or only just supraliminal. If they are subliminal, only the relative displacement of the two points becomes effective; if they are slightly supraliminal, a new effect appears. The Ego as a third object may be so strongly coupled to one of the two points that it takes part in its motion. This coupling is achieved by fixation. A fixated object does not change its relation to the ocular system of the Ego, whether it is objectively moving or at rest. Therefore, in the experiments with the points, the subjects fixating the objectively stationary point saw it in motion and experienced at the same time *movement of their own eyes* (Duncker, p. 201). If one of the two objects is a rectangle enclosing the other, a point, and if then the non-moving point is fixated, then "the impression of one's self being at rest is lost; the space level becomes unstable, even vertigo may ensue, one feels one's own body, rigidly connected with the point, glide along the (phenomenally more or less stationary) rectangle" (Duncker, p. 206).

The Ego, therefore, behaves like any other field object, a claim which can be confirmed by two common observations: the moon seems to be floating through the drifting clouds, and *we* seem to move up a river when, standing on a bridge, we fixate one of its pillars at the edge of the water. The reason is the same in both cases, the enclosed object carries the motion, and the Ego in the second example takes part in its motion because through fixation it is firmly coupled with it.

Identity. Fusion of Processes. It is time to state an aspect of our theory which so far has been concealed. We explained the perception of motion as due to dislocation in the process pattern. If an object is seen in motion, we assume that the process distribution which corresponds to its perception is displaced with regard to other process distributions. This implies that during the course of the perceived motion the process distribution corresponding to an object remains *dynamically identical,* even though it shifts within the field of other process distributions. Since we have so far treated unification and segregation only in stationary fields, i.e., without regard to time, the identity in time of a process changing its place is a new problem, full of significant ramifications, as we shall see later. We can state this problem in this way: if a point of light moves across the retina, constantly new cones are being stimulated, continually new processes therefore sent up into the centre. The cones are separate structures spread out in a fine mosaic with variable density across the retina; therefore a continuously moving point of light gives rise to a discrete and finite number of nervous excitations, according to the number of cones it passes. Somewhere these *successive discrete* excitations must become *one continuous* process if displacement of an object is to occur; i.e., the excitations started in the cones cannot remain separate from each other but must become *fused*. Since in our case they are equal in quality and in very close proximity these nervous processes will attract each other with great force so that their final fusion is deducible from our premises.

We may, however, try to alter these conditions and see what effects such alterations will have on fusion of processes. The first factor to be changed is the distance between processes. Let A and Z in Fig. 83 represent the two terminal cones stimulated by a light point moving from left to right, and the dots between them, i_1 i_2 . . . , all the intermediate cones.

. . . .
A i_1 i_2 . . . Z

Fig. 83

Then the peripheral (retinal) events which eventually give rise to the process of perceived motion can be described in this way. First, for a very short time (e_A), A will be stimulated; then follows a very short interval (p_{A-i_1}), without any stimulation; then stimulation of i_1, followed by another dead interval, and so forth. According to our theory the excitation started at i_1 fuses with that started in A, and so forth. Let us now stimulate first A for a certain amount of time e_A, then leave a dead interval p_{A-Z}, such that the sum of e_A and p_{A-Z} is as long as the time it would take the light point to pass with a moderate velocity from A to Z, and then stimulate point Z. Will the excitation at Z still fuse with that started at A? This argument has led us from the perception of ordinary, to that of stroboscopic, motion. For in the simplest kind of stroboscopic experiment we expose first an object at a place A and then, after an interval, another object at Z, and thus stimulate successively for short periods only two points, which are much further apart than two adjoining cones.

Stroboscopic and Real Motion. Historically it is interesting that this theory of perceived motion was first developed for stroboscopic motion (Hartmann, Köhler 1923 a),[9] and a special investigation was carried out by Scholz to prove it in this field. The fusion between the two successive processes must result from a force of attraction between them. The reality of this force was demonstrated

[9] Van der Waals and Roelofs reject this theory (1930); but I find that their own, apart from using a much more conservative system of concepts, contains the same or at least a very similar idea, viz., that the localization of the second object changes continually during the perception of motion. That the relative phase of the two fusing excitations (whether they are still in the state of arousal, stationary, or falling off) is an important factor on which fusion depends, is not either a specific characteristic of van der Waals' and Roelofs' theory, but was specifically stated in Köhler's theoretical sketch.

by the fact that two stroboscopically exposed lines appear at a shorter distance from each other than two permanently exposed ones, and that the amount of contraction of their distance reaches its maximum when they are seen in optimal motion.

The problem of stroboscopic motion consists, according to this theory, in establishing the conditions under which fusion between the two (or more) separate excitations takes place, or when attraction, though not strong enough to result in fusion, affects the attracted processes sufficiently to displace them, with the phenomenal result that both or either are seen to move over part of the way (Wertheimer's dual and singular partial motion). Formulated in this way the problem of stroboscopic motion is no different from that of real motion, where, as we have seen, processes separately started must fuse also. But because in real motion the spatial distance between the interacting processes is so small as to produce very strong forces of attraction so that other factors are small compared to them and therefore hard to demonstrate, such other factors play a much more important rôle in stroboscopic motion, where, owing to the greater distance between the processes, the forces are much weaker. Of such other factors I mention the temporal determinants, i.e., the exposure times and intervals, the intensities (or, better, the gradients between figures and background), the distance between the exposed objects, their size, and shape. We shall discuss most of them by and by.

Meanwhile we return to the theory. That stroboscopic and "real" motion are essentially alike is a strong point in its favour. To explain the "induced" motion of an object at rest through relative displacement with regard to another, introduces no new difficulty.[10] But one addition must still be made. Duncker has produced such induced motion also by exposing the inducing object successively in two different positions, the induced one simultaneously in two equal positions (p. 224 f.; see Fig. 84, where the two successive exposures are represented one below the other, while in reality they were so arranged that the two points coincided). Under special conditions an enclosing object in stroboscopic displacement may appear practically stationary while the enclosed one, successively exposed in the same place, carries the entire motion. In this case the fusion of two spatially distant excitations does not result in motion, while the fusion of two spatially

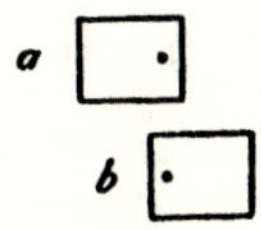

Fig. 84

[10] I shall omit the problem of the temporal unity of a continuously exposed object, since it finds its treatment in a later chapter (Chapter X, pp. 439 and 446 f.).

identical ones does. This, however, is no difficulty, since according to our most general principle motion depends upon *relative* displacement between two, or more, field objects, without any limitations how these field objects have become organized. Duncker's last-mentioned experiment serves as a demonstration that real and stroboscopic motion are essentially alike.

Apparent Velocity. Brown's Experiments. Let us now become more concrete and investigate not motion *per se,* but motion in its concrete fulness. Motion has direction and velocity, both in mechanics and in experience. If we think of perception of real motion, there seems at first to be no problem; one expects the apparent velocity to be equal to, or to be in simple dependence upon, the real velocity, within the psychologically possible limits, i.e., between the lower and the upper threshold. The brilliant investigations of J. F. Brown have, however, demonstrated how erroneous such a view would be. We disregard for the moment the difficulty which arises from the question *which* real velocity we should choose as our standard, the velocity of the object itself, the distant stimulus, or that of its retinal image, the proximal stimulus, pointing out at the moment merely that these two are in close correspondence only when the distant stimuli are at the same distance from the observer; for the retinal velocity corresponding to one and the same distant velocity varies inversely with the distance. But quite apart from this problem Brown has shown that the apparent velocity of an object seen in motion depends upon the field and the object itself, viz., its size and orientation, and, as previously mentioned, on the direction of the motion (1928, 1931). In his experiments two velocities had to be matched. Behind two diaphragm apertures figures were seen in motion, the motion being produced by two rotating drums over which rolls of white paper with figures upon them were stretched, so as to form endless bands. During each experiment the velocity of the standard band was kept constant while that of the variable was changed until the observer judged the two velocities to be equal. The relation of the two objective velocities which *appeared* equal was then a measure of the relation between objective and subjective velocity.

To give a concrete idea of the procedure I will describe one experiment in detail. Both standard and variable were at the same distance, the fields were homogeneous except for band and figures (dark room, the rotating band illuminated from behind); the diaphragm aperture of the standard S was 15×5 sq. cm., that of the variable B 7.5×2.5 sq. cm.; the figures on S were circles of 1.6 cm.

diameter following each other at 4 cm. intervals, on B circles of .8 cm. diameter, following each other at 2 cm. intervals. In short the dimensions of B were exactly half those of S. The velocity in S, V_S, was 10 $\frac{\text{cm.}}{\text{sec.}}$, and the average velocity on B, V_B (7 subjects), which appeared equal to V_S, was 5.25$\frac{\text{cm.}}{\text{sec.}}$, $\frac{V_S}{V_B} = 1.9$, or approximately $= 2$. This means: if in a homogeneous field one pattern is in all linear dimensions twice as large as another, then the objects moving within this pattern will appear to have the same velocity if objectively their velocity is (approximately) twice as great as in the smaller. From this we may infer that if the objective velocities are equal, the objects in the smaller pattern will appear to move twice as fast as in the larger. This result was confirmed with various velocities, with various size relations, and with a number of controls. The result of all these experiments could rightly be summarized by Brown in the following sentence: "If in a homogeneous field one transposes a moving field in all its linear dimensions one must transpose the stimulus velocity by a like amount in order that phenomenal identity of velocity result. As the linear dimensions of one field are changed from one to ten, the V_S/V_B quotient tends to change from one to ten" (1931, p. 226).

That the fields must be homogeneous for this result to be true, we understand easily from our theory. If the fields are inhomogeneous, the diaphragms covered with patterned papers, then the displacements in the two fields are no longer restricted to the frames of the apertures which differ in size, but refer also to those inhomogeneities which are similar in the S and B patterns. Consequently the difference between these should be reduced, and this is the case as proved by Brown (that the inhomogeneity increases the apparent velocity has already been mentioned; see p. 282).

If only some of the dimensions are changed, and the others kept constant, the corresponding change in velocity has to be smaller than when all are changed. This was proved for changes of length of aperture, breadth of aperture, and size of objects in a number of different combinations. I shall give only two examples: with figures constant, but aperture in S linearly twice as large as in B, the quotient $\frac{V_S}{V_B}$ was 1.38, whereas it is 2, if the figures are transposed too. If the diaphragms are equal and the figures of different size, the larger ones have to be moved faster than the smaller ones to appear equal. This means: under equal stimulus conditions large objects move (phenomenally) more slowly than small ones.

If the fields are exactly alike except for amount of illumination, then the objects in the brighter field must move objectively faster than those in the darker to appear at equal velocity. "Increase of phenomenal brightness decreases phenomenal speed" (1931, p. 223).

Lastly, lines oriented in the direction of the motion are phenomenally faster than lines at right angles to it.[11]

The Deducibility of Brown's Results from General Principles. Velocity has thereby been proved to be a field-conditioned phenomenon. To deduce all of Brown's results from general principles is at the moment impossible. A few hints may, however, be in place. The dependence of apparent velocity on the dimensions might be deducible from the principle of displacement if it could be formulated more concretely, so as to make quantitative predictions possible. At present we do not know how to quantify displacement.

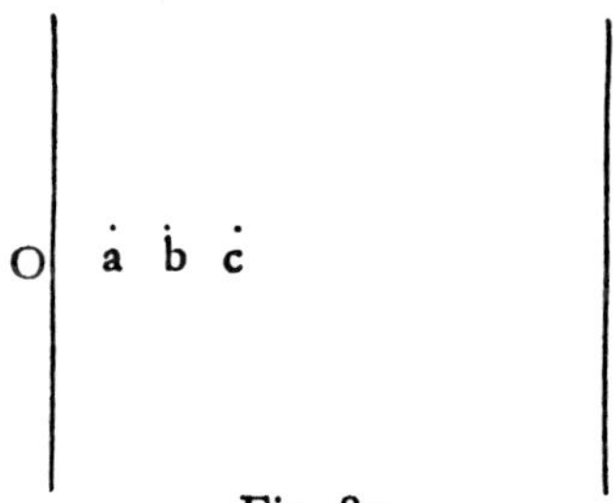

Fig. 85

A simple example will explain what I mean (see Fig. 85). A point moves with uniform velocity between two terminal lines, starting at the time t_0 from the left line at O, reaching at the time t_1 point *a*, and so forth, till it passes into the right line. During the first time interval, t_1–t_0, the distance between the point and the left line has changed from nothing to O*a*, during the next interval, t_2–t_1, it changes from O*a* to O*b* and so forth, all increments during equal intervals being equal. But are these equal increments of distance equally effective for the arousal of perceived motion, or will the increment be the more effective the smaller the pre-existing distance is, perhaps in the form that not equal increments are equally effective but equal quotients of increment over pre-existing distance, according to a logarithmic law? In that case, the farther the point had moved from O the less effective would a further displacement from O become, while simultaneously its displacement with regard to the right line would become increasingly more effective, these two changes combining in such a way that in the centre of the path the same objective displacement would have the least

[11] Confirmed *mutatis mutandis* by Oppenheimer.

effect on motion. It is unlikely that quantitatively this assumption is right, but equally unlikely that absolutely equal increments should have equal effects. Brown himself reports that in threshold experiments motion appears first near the edges of the diaphragm aperture and only later in the centre (1931 b). Qualitatively such a consideration leads to the inference that smaller fields must have greater velocities than larger ones, but as long as our knowledge goes no further than at present, we can do no more than point at the possibility of such a relation being responsible for Brown's law of transposition. Under these conditions it is also premature to speculate whether the effect exercised on apparent velocity by the size of the moving object is altogether of the same kind as that of the size of the aperture, or whether size or bulk would lend to the moving object an inertia which by itself would make the bigger object move more slowly. The fact that lines oriented in the direction of the motion move faster than those at right angles to it suggests at least the possibility of such more strictly "dynamic" interpretation, which gains added weight from the fact that in stroboscopic experiments DeSilva found wider lines to move definitely more slowly than thinner ones, and that the motion of the latter was smoother under conditions where mere size and distance relationship seem to have played no rôle.

The brightness effect, lastly, becomes intelligible, if we interpret brightness as figure-ground gradient, and thereby as stronger articulation of the figure, in accordance with Brown's apparatus and the description he gives of the effect of a strong darkening of the field, where the figure contours became blurred (1931, p. 223). We might then conclude that the more pronounced its figure character, the smaller the motility of an object.

These suggestions, all in need and capable of experimental verification, must suffice. They reveal at least the great theoretical possibilities of Brown's results.

Brown's Results and Korte's Laws. We shall now derive some other consequences from them, viz., with regard to stroboscopic motion. Stroboscopic motion has phenomenally a velocity just as any phenomenal motion, although there is no physical velocity corresponding to it, since physically there is no motion. But we can define the objective stroboscopic velocity by the following consideration. In stroboscopic presentation a point appears at A at the moment t_1 for a certain time (e_1), and after an interval p another point at B at the moment t_2. We can then say that the objective stroboscopic velocity is the velocity which the point would have if it actually travelled from A to B between the moments t_1 and t_2. Designating objective stroboscopic velocity by $\bar{V}$, we therefore define $\bar{V} = \frac{AB}{t_2 - t_1}$, or since $t_2 - t_1 = e_1 + p$, $\bar{V} = \frac{AB}{e_1 + p}$. Finally, designating the distance AB by s, and $e_1 + p$ by t, we have $\bar{V} = \frac{s}{t}$.[12]

Let us now suppose that we have succeeded in producing good stroboscopic motion of a line across a certain distance s. We then increase the intensity of the two successively exposed lines. Then, on the basis of Brown's results, we can predict what will happen. Since phenomenal motion is slower in a brighter field than in a darker, the two brighter lines will appear to move more slowly, and in order to make them move as fast as the darker lines we have to increase their objective stroboscopic velocity $\bar{V}$. This can be done by either increasing the numerator s, or decreasing the denominator t of the quotient $\frac{s}{t}$ by which $\bar{V}$ is defined. In reality, stroboscopic motion, provided s is not small, is very sensitive to changes of distance, time, and intensity; it responds to such changes by more than mere changes of velocity. If t becomes too great or too small, no stroboscopic motion is seen; in the first case the two objects appear as two in *succession*, in the second as two in *simultaneity*. Between these two stages of succession and simultaneity lies the stage of optimal motion, surrounded on either side by intermediate stages (Wertheimer, 1912), the details of which we omit, except that here differences in velocity become apparent. We can now formulate our deduction for the case of altered intensity in this way: if we increase the intensity of a pair of lines exposed in such a way that the stage of optimal motion is produced, then the phenomenon will be changed towards the stage of succession, and it can be re-established either by increasing the distance between the two objects or by decreasing the time elapsing between the moments the first and the second are exposed. That this is actually true was demonstrated twenty years ago by Korte, whose two first laws say just this.

Korte's third law deals with the relation between distance and temporal distribution of the two objects. Confining ourselves to the relation between s and t, we see that if again we start from the condition of optimal motion and increase s, we thereby, by defini-

[12] Probably this is not quite correct, since the time during which the point is exposed at B, e_2, is also of influence. But as a first approximation this definition will serve.

tion, increase the stroboscopic velocity $\bar{V} = \frac{s}{t}$. If perceived velocity were a linear function of stroboscopic velocity, we should have to increase *t* in the same proportion as *s* in order to maintain the same apparent velocity; in short, a change of *s* demands a proportional change of *t*, if stroboscopic and phenomenal velocities stand in the simple relation indicated. Korte's third law simply states that an increase in *s* or *t* can be compensated by an increase in *t* or *s*, without regard to the quantitative relationship. This law has puzzled psychologists more than the others, and I must admit that when Korte and I discovered it, I was surprised myself; at the time of Korte's work one was still inclined to think as follows: if one separates the two successively exposed objects more and more, either spatially or temporally, one makes their unification more and more difficult. Therefore increase of distance should be compensated by decrease of time interval, and *vice versa*.

The facts belying this deduction disproved that whole way of thinking and for that reason, if for no other, I still think that the discovery of the Korte laws was valuable. Not till I read Brown's papers did I see the connection presented in the text. What is surprising in this Korte law is not the fact that *s* and *t* vary directly with each other, but a fact already contained in Korte's tables but unnoticed by him (and me) which became apparent in experiments performed under very different conditions by Cermak and myself, viz., that the direct function between *s* and *t* is not one of proportionality, but that *t* increases more slowly than *s*. The following table taken from Korte contains the *t*-values for optimal motion at three different distances, in $\sigma = 1/1000$ sec.

TABLE 10
(from Korte, p. 264)

distance in cm.	*t* for optimal motion in σ
2	183
3	219
6	256

One sees: when the distance is trebled, t is only lengthened in the proportion of 1.4:1. Or if we calculate the stroboscopic velocities at 2 and 6 cm. distance, $\bar{V}_2$ and $\bar{V}_6$, we find their relation

$$\frac{\bar{V}_6}{\bar{V}_2}=\frac{\frac{6}{256}}{\frac{2}{183}}=2.1, \text{ whereas } \frac{s_6}{s_2}=3.$$

If instead we choose the values for 3 and 6 cm., we obtain $\frac{\bar{V}_6}{\bar{V}_3}=1.7$, and $\frac{s_6}{s_3}=2$; in both cases the ratio of velocities is smaller than that of the distances. With these values we compare a value from Brown quoted above (p. 289), the relation of the real velocities $\frac{V_S}{V_B}$ where field S was linearly twice as large as B (in length and width), and the figures identical. Here to a relation of linear field dimensions $\frac{F_S}{F_B}=2$ there corresponds a quotient $\frac{V_S}{V_B}=1.38$. Just as in Korte's experiments the quotient of the stroboscopic velocities is smaller than that of the distances, so in Brown's the quotient of the real velocities is smaller than the quotient of the field dimensions.[13]

We formulated Brown's result by saying that the apparent velocity is the smaller, the greater the field, and we can apply this same formulation to Korte's identical result: increase of the distance through which a stroboscopically moved object passes decreases its phenomenal velocity. When, therefore, we change a constellation which yields optimal stroboscopic motion by increasing s, we produce two opposite effects. On the one hand, on purely kinematic grounds, we increase the stroboscopic velocity $\bar{V}$, on the other hand we reduce the effect of $\bar{V}$ on the perceived velocity, because larger fields have slower apparent velocity. Ordinarily the second effect is not so strong as the first, and therefore, in order to compensate for an increase of s, we have to increase t also, though to a lower degree. Only in those cases where Brown's compensation law holds will the two effects cancel.

[13] The figures are not strictly comparable, because the difference between the two constellations is greater for Brown than for Korte, since Brown changed not only the length of the field and thereby the distance traversed by the moving object, as Korte did, but also the width of the field. That the width of the field has an influence by itself was proved by Brown. Unfortunately for our comparison he reports no experiment in which the *length* of the field was the only difference between S and B.

If all linear dimensions in two fields are f and nf respectively, then equivalent stroboscopic velocities $\bar{V}_{ns}$ and $\bar{V}_s$ must be in the relation $\frac{\bar{V}_{ns}}{\bar{V}_s} = n$. Therefore, if we call t_1 and t_2 the respective times in the two fields, $\frac{\frac{ns}{t_1}}{\frac{s}{t_2}} = n$, $t_1 = t_2$. In this case, and in this case only, the third Korte law cannot hold any more, not because this case is an exception, but because it is the limiting case in which two effects exactly cancel each other. This deduction is fully confirmed by Brown, who finds that when all linear dimensions of a field are changed in the same proportion the stroboscopic velocity must be changed in the same proportion, i.e., t must remain constant although s changes.[14]

The Korte laws were purely empirical generalizations when they were discovered and they retained that rank till Brown published his results. They were confirmed by some authors under some conditions, whereas other authors, working under other conditions, failed to verify them. Moreover, Cermak and I had added a new law, the zone law, which restricted the validity of the Korte laws in a certain manner. This law says that when t (and s) are made increasingly smaller the range (zone) of s-t combinations which produces optimal motion becomes increasingly larger, so that within this range the Korte laws no longer hold. The zone law is undoubtedly true, but I do not believe any more that it necessarily restricts the validity of the Korte laws. Cermak's and my test was optimal motion vs. disintegration, but we did not observe the apparent velocities. If they are taken into consideration, then the Korte laws will probably hold also within the "zones." I also believe that the same consideration would reconcile the conflicting results of different investigators.

Even as pure empirical generalizations the Korte laws had their value. Apart from the contribution they made to the theory of stroboscopic motion (see above, p. 293), they were used by Cermak and me to prove the dynamic similarity of perceived stroboscopic and real motion, by arguments and experiments to be omitted here,

[14] It is only fair to mention that my deduction did not precede Brown's result, but was caused by it. Brown himself has not seen the connection between his findings and Korte's laws as indicated in the text. I may add that several details remain as yet unexplained, for instance, the different effect which a change of either of the two components of t, viz., e_1 and p_1, exerts on stroboscopic motion.

and to recognize the connection between motion and (flicker-) fusion phenomena which has been directly confirmed by Brown (1931 b), and in a somewhat different context by Metzger (1926). The connection now established between them and Brown's laws lifts them above the rank of mere empirical generalizations and proves that they are the expression of essential facts of perceptual organization. In themselves they are no real laws, and should more properly be named the Korte rules, but they follow from fundamental laws which are not yet totally recognized. The logical consistency between the results of Korte, Cermak and myself, and Brown, obtained at widely different times with widely different methods, is indeed a strong argument in favour of the significance of these results and deductions.

Motion and Time. Brown's ingenuity of theoretical deduction and experimentation has carried our knowledge of the motion processes still a step further. We have discussed phenomenal velocity and phenomenal distance, but not phenomenal time. And yet the very definition of velocity is impossible without time. In kinematics velocity is defined as $\frac{dS}{dT}$, which for uniform velocity is equivalent to $\frac{S}{T}$. Is it possible to transfer this definition to behavioural, or experienced, velocity, defining $v = \frac{s}{t}$, where the small letters mean phenomenal velocity, distance, and time? Brown not only introduces this hypothesis but proves it by beautiful experiments (1931 a). The implications of this assumption are indeed astounding. Supposing we have two equal fields differently illuminated. Then we know that the apparent velocity in the brighter one, v_b, is slower than that in the darker one, v_d, if the objective velocities are equal. Brightness differences, at least such as employed by Brown, do not influence the apparent sizes. We can therefore write $v_d > v_b, \left.\frac{s}{t}\right]_d > \left.\frac{s}{t}\right]_b$. Since the two numerators in this inequation are equal, the denominators cannot be equal also, but t_d must be smaller than t_b, and since objectively $T_d = T_b$, time must flow faster in the darker than in the brighter field. This conclusion is as inevitable as it is surprising. That it makes the experience of time a new field-conditioned property is not so astonishing in itself; the striking fact is that experienced time should be influenced by field factors which apparently have nothing to do with time. Brown was not satisfied with the logic of his argument but subjected it to an experimental test. In these experiments the observers had to compare the *duration* of a seen motion with that of a time interval marked by two, visual or acoustic, signals. This latter interval was kept constant, and the speed of the observed motion was changed until its duration seemed equal to it. If the apparent durations of two motion constellations are both equal to the standard duration, then their apparent velocities must be equal too. But we know from previous experiments that the real velocity in a brighter field must be greater than in a darker for these velocities to appear equal. In one particular constellation the relation $\frac{V_b}{V_d}$ was found to be 1.23.

$$\frac{V_b}{V_d} = \frac{\frac{S_b}{T_b}}{\frac{S_d}{T_d}}, \text{ and since } S_b = S_d, \ \frac{V_b}{V_d} = \frac{T_d}{T_b} = 1.23.$$

If therefore we know either T_d or T_b, we can predict the other. To appear of equal duration with the interval marked by the signals the duration of the motion in the brighter field (T_b) had to be 1.45 sec. (average of five subjects). From our last equation we deduce $T_d = 1.23\ T_b = 1.23 \times 1.45$ sec. $= 1.78$ sec. The average measured value of five subjects for T_b was 1.78 sec., a perfect confirmation of the prediction.

By the same method Brown has tested his time hypothesis for various other constellations, complete and partial transpositions of the field dimensions, and more and less homogeneous fields. Always the results confirmed the prediction, even when the determination of the $\frac{V_S}{V_B}$ quotient, on which the prediction was based, was made by other observers than those who confirmed the prediction by comparing two durations.[15] There can be no doubt that the experiments are sufficient to prove the general assumption, so that we can consider it as valid also in those cases for which it has not been proved by special experiments. If we include all constellations for which the phenomenal velocities were investigated, we can say: time flows faster in smaller, darker, and nearer fields, and the more vertical, the less horizontal, the motion is; furthermore the law of complete transposition of velocities was paralleled by complete transposition of durations.

[15] Not in all cases are the phenomenal distances equal when the real distances are. If in these cases one allows for this discrepancy, the confirmation is again complete.

These deductions and experiments of Brown's open up a wide field of research and speculation. The problem of the physiological correlate of our experience of time has recently been discussed by Boring (1933), who is fully aware of its difficulties and of the fact that this physiological correlate must be a process or an aspect of a process. Köhler's argument with regard to motion (and localization; see p. 281) finds its application equally in the field of time. In Chapter X certain hypotheses will be developed which are related to this problem. Here we only point out that if perceived time corresponds to a process or an aspect of a process, then the nature of the processes occurring in a field, and not only the other characteristics of the field, will determine the duration of events within it. This complication has not yet been investigated, although Brown mentions the fact, also confirmed in his experiments, that "filled" time is phenomenally longer than "unfilled" time. Future research may discover fundamental interdependencies between phenomenal space and time, an interdependence which has been demonstrated in similar experiments by Benussi (1913, pp. 285 f.) and Gelb (1914) and more thoroughly investigated by Helson and King, investigations which must be omitted here.

Selection of Fusion. We now turn to a last aspect of the problem of perceived motion, taking up a question formulated on page 287. Our explanation of motion, real as well as stroboscopic, contained as a part-hypothesis the fusion of peripherally separate processes. We now investigate factors which determine this fusion different from those so far discussed. If in stroboscopic motion only two objects are exposed, fusion, if it takes place at all, can occur only between the organized processes which correspond to these two objects. But if each of the two successive exposures contains more than one object, then indeed the question arises which object of the first exposure will fuse with which of the second exposure, i.e., what kind of motion will be perceived. The same principle applies to real motion. If only one object moves through the field, then again there is no problem: the processes aroused in the retina by successive stimulations of ever-different cone-aggregates will fuse with each other. But if two equal objects move through the field in different directions so that they pass simultaneously through the same point, then the problem of *selection* arises again. Three investigations have dealt with this problem, the first two, by Ternus and von Schiller, with stroboscopic, the last, by Metzger (1934), with real motion.

Ternus's Experiments. To introduce Ternus's problem we compare two simple stroboscopic experiments. In both of them each exposure consists of two points such that one of them, *a*, appears at the same place, in both exposures, while the other has different places, *b* and *c*. The first exposure, therefore, is in both cases *a b*, in the second *a c*. The only difference between the two exposures lies in the arrangement of the three dots, as illustrated in Fig. 86 A and

Fig. 86

B, where • signified the first, o the second exposure, therefore ⊙ the fact that a point is exposed twice in the same position. In A one sees point *a* at rest, and the other point moving from position *b* to position *c*. In B, on the other hand, no point is seen at rest, but two points in motion, one moving from *b* to *a*, the other from *a* to *c*. Thus in the first case fusion takes place between two excitations which occur at the same place (*a*), and between two others which occur at different places, while in B processes which occur at the same place (*a*) do *not* fuse, instead of which a_1 fuses with c_2, and a_2 with b_1. Therefore fusion must depend upon other factors than mere spatial proximity (spatial identity being considered as the case of the greatest possible proximity). What are these other factors? "Phenomenal identity is primarily determined by gestalt-identity, by gestalt-homology of parts, i.e., by whole characters and not by piecewise relationships" (Ternus, p. 101). Let us explain the meaning of this proposition by reference to our two experiments. In the first, A, *a* appears as a rule as the fulcrum of a pendulum; therefore a_1 and a_2 are gestalt-homologous, and similarly *b* and *c* are homologous, because they are the terminal points of the pendulum's arm. In B, on the other hand, a_1 is the right point of a pair, a_2 the left point, a_1 and a_2 are therefore not homologous, but a_1 is homologous with c_2 and a_2 with b_1. When a_2 arises in the first experiment, it *selects* the process a_1, occurring at the same place, for fusion, but when a_2 arises in the second experiment, it does not select the "syntopic" process a_1, but the homologous process b_1.

Homology of parts, which may also be qualitative instead of spatial homology, does not, however, exhaust the meaning of Ternus's generalization. Other factors of organization enter. From the great variety of cases studied by Ternus, I shall report only one more, illustrated by Fig. 87 A and B. In Fig. 87 A fusion occurs against identical location of points *d e f*, while in B these identical points fuse, and c_1 with g_2, b_1 with h_2, and a_1 with i_2. In A one sees a curved line moving as a whole and in its own curve to the right, in B a stationary horizontal arm (*d, e, f*) and an oblique arm which jumps from one position to the other. As far as homology of points is concerned, the two patterns are practically equivalent; in the first exposure the left terminal point is *a*, in the second *d*, and so forth. But in other respects the two patterns are different. Whereas the six simultaneously visible points are uniformly integrated in A, they have two unique points in B, viz., *d* and *f*, where the figure is clearly articulated and can therefore break in two. At the same time, and because of these characteristics, the six dots in A can move from their first to their second position without a change in the shape of the whole curve, whereas the broken lines in B can do so only by temporary distortions. Therefore unitary motion with selection against spatial identity occurs in A and not in B, where the whole figure splits up into two parts.

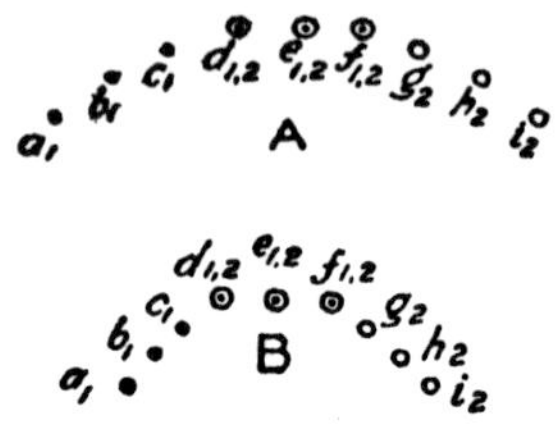

Fig. 87

Von Schiller's Experiments. Von Schiller experimented on the problem of selection without the distinction of spatially identical and different exposures. He starts from the fact that many stimulus constellations are highly ambiguous with regard to the ensuing motion. Thus Fig. 88 leads equally well to a clockwise as to a counter-clockwise rotation of the two vertical points. Such ambiguity has led several authors up to the present to conclude that visual motion, being at bottom arbitrary and unpredictable, is an affair of mental sets or attitudes, the stimulus pattern being of secondary importance. Von Schiller, by using potentially ambiguous patterns, disproves such a view, demonstrating that factors of organization determine the selection. Starting from a pattern like that of Fig. 88 he introduced all sorts

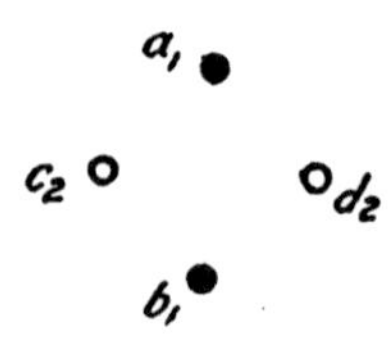

Fig. 88

of modifications by which he varied the distance, the quality and the shape of the exposed figures, and the pattern of the whole arrangement. He found the same laws operative for selection of stroboscopic motion that Wertheimer discovered for the organization of stationary forms. Thus he demonstrated the factors of proximity and equality, and showed at the same time that difference in brightness is more effective than difference in colour, a result which adds new weight to our finding that brightness differences have a stronger organizing power than mere colour differences. The factor of equality has, in these experiments, a very special aspect. Supposing in Fig. 88 the dots a_1 and d_2 to be dark blue, b_1 and c_2 light red. Then, if the motion follows the factor of equality, the blue point remains blue and the red red during the motion, whereas if stroboscopic motion were to occur in the counter-clockwise direction, the blue point would become red, the red one blue. This would involve a *change* of the total figure, and figures resist such changes. Therefore equality may produce a motion contrary to the factor of proximity, and this motion will be the stronger, the greater the number of aspects of equality (colour, brightness, size, and shape) that are employed. In extreme cases the direction may follow equality even when the lines of the cross intersect each other at an angle of 15°, so that the motion takes place through an angle of 75°, the enormous superiority of the smaller angle being over-compensated by the equality factors. This resistance against change, together with the factor of the shortest path, results under proper conditions in tri-dimensional motion. If one exposes alternately the two forms of Fig. 89, then the motion most frequently perceived is that of a rotation round the horizontal axis of symmetry through the third dimension, less frequently a motion in the plane of the figure round a vertical axis, and quite rarely a down-up-down motion with distortion of the forms during the motion (Steinig, von Schiller). A last general law relates to the ensuing path; the tendency to make the total path (of all moving parts) as simple and well shaped as possible could be demonstrated in cases where this factor conflicted with equality factors.

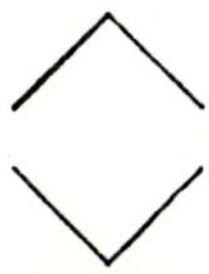

Fig. 89

METZGER'S EXPERIMENTS. Metzger's beautiful systematic investigation, to which we cannot do full justice in this short summary, examines the case of two or more moving objects passing simultaneously through the same point. In the vast majority of his experiments the moving objects were vertical shadows which moved horizontally back and forth through a certain distance, produced by vertical rods planted in a rotating disk. By varying the angle between the rods and their distance from the centre of the disk he varied the phase and velocities of the moving shadows. The problem can best be stated with the help of Fig. 90, in which the abscissa is to represent spatial distance, the ordinate, read downwards, to represent time. This figure then represents two points, the one moving from left to right with uniform velocity, the other from right to left with the same velocity, both meeting in the middle of their track *o*. When the two points pass through *o*, only one retinal point (in each eye) is stimulated; before and afterwards two points are.

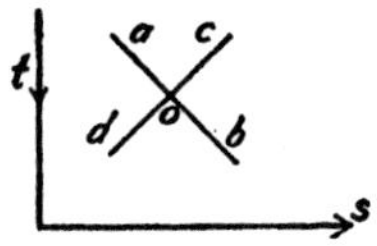

Fig. 90

It is therefore not a matter of course that the observer should perceive rectilinear motion of two points. When we look at this figure as a spatial pattern, we shall indeed at first sight see two lines crossing each other; *a* and *b*, *c* and *d*, will belong together. It is not impossible, however, to see two right angles touching each other in their vertices, so that *a* belongs with *d*, and *b* with *c* (the other combination, *a c*, *b d*, can be disregarded, since it can have no parallel in motion where only successive parts of the track can form part of one whole track). What is true of our simultaneous perception of this spatial pattern is equally possible for the perception of motion: the retinal geometry contains no factor which excludes that *a d* is one track and *c b* the other. But in motion there are still more possibilities. Since at *o* only one point is stimulated, this pattern of stimulation would also be compatible with both or either of the two points disappearing at *o* and two new points emerging from it. Are there any laws which determine what will really happen?

The main results of Metzger's experiment can be formulated in this way: if one represents the motion produced by diagrams of the kind of Fig. 90, then the spatial pattern which emerges or dominates when we look at the figure is as a rule the same as the motion pattern which emerges or dominates when we look at the moving shadows. And this means: the laws of successive organization, the laws which determine the selection of fusing objects, are the same laws that govern the organization of spatial patterns. Metzger states these correspondences explicitly. We shall only mention that to the factor of good continuation in purely spatial organization there corresponds the factor of the smooth curve of motion and of continuous velocity in spatio-temporal organization.

It is clear that conditions may be such that different factors favour different integrations. The greater the conflict between these objective factors, the greater the ambiguity, and the greater therefore the influence of subjective factors like set and attitude. This result, common to the investigations of Ternus, von Schiller, and Metzger, shows how completely false is a view that regards subjective factors as primary in the arousal of processes of motion (see p. 300). One argument of Metzger's strikingly demonstrates the absurdity of such a view. The number of possible tracks of motion increases tremendously with the number of objects and the number of periods of rotation. Thus ten rods on his disk give in one half-revolution as a minimum 3,628,800 possibilities and as a maximum 35,184,372,088,832, according to the arrangement of the rods on the disk. For one whole revolution the maximum is of the order of magnitude of 1.2×10^{27}. Metzger's subjects observed occasionally groups of more than ten members during a great number of revolutions, and yet could realize at the utmost only a handful of different tracks.

Space and the Sense Modalities. After we have learned from the last investigation the great power of Wertheimer's laws of organization, we derive a new insight into the nature of perceived space from an investigation by Galli. In stroboscopic motion one process fuses with another process, and that even when the two processes are different in respect of colour, size, and shape. But in all experiments so far reported the different objects stroboscopically presented belonged to the same sense modality, they were all visual objects (that they may both be acoustic or tactual has been previously mentioned). But what will happen if two objects successively presented belong to different sense modalities, if, e.g., a light and sound, or a light and contact, are combined? If visual, tactual, and acoustic space were three different spaces, related to each other merely by experience, such presentation should lead to no impression of motion, since according to our theory this impression implies that one and the same psychophysical process travels through (one and the same) space. If, therefore, stroboscopic motion can be produced by impressions of different sense modalities, we must, in accordance with our theory, conclude that perceptual space is *one* and that it can be filled with objects of different sense modalities. The experiment has clearly decided in favour of the second alternative. Galli could produce stroboscopic motion by combining two or three stimuli belonging to the modalities of sight, hearing and touch. The subjects experienced again and again the motion of *one* moving object which "affected them" in different ways. These experiments throw a new light on the dynamics of motion and on the structure of perceptual space.

CONCLUSIONS AS TO THE NATURE OF BEHAVIOURAL THINGS

Before we close this chapter we shall evaluate its results for the problem of thingness. All through our discussion of the perceptual field the distinction of things and framework has proved to be essential. In Chapter III we established three main characteristics of things, viz., shaped boundedness, dynamic properties, and constancy. The first of these has been treated sufficiently in the fourth chapter, so that we need not amplify this point. This chapter has, however, brought together a great deal of knowledge about the two other characteristics. As a matter of fact these two are closely connected with each other and will be treated in conjunction. From the point of view of these aspects one is tempted to hazard the following broad generalization of the bulk of our previous discussion: the response to a change of stimulation will be such that things retain their properties as much as possible. In the field of motion we found the principle operative; such fusions of processes and such paths were preferred as kept the things as intact as conditions permitted. One aspect of this is the stability of things while we move our eyes, for in this case the shape of the retinal images is constantly changed, and yet the things do not change their shape. The same effects are demonstrated by constancy of shape and size. Turn an object and thereby change its retinal image, the shape of the perceived thing will remain relatively unaltered, the change of the retinal image resulting in change of orientation. The application to size and distance is simple. And even brightness and colour constancy fall under the same general rule: change of objective illumination produces primarily a change in perceived illumination (or brightness) but not in the colour properties of the perceived things.

Constancy of shape and size is coupled with motility either of the things or the observer. The fact that things can move phenomenally, and that the Ego of the observer is in this respect a thing, makes it possible that they retain their shape when their retinal images change. Conversely, motion is only possible because in the change of retinal patterns constant perceptual things are produced. Both propositions are different aspects of one and the same fact of organization. A thing is a particularly well integrated part of the total field. The stronger its integration, the stronger the forces which hold it together, the more constant will it be in changes of stimulation, a conclusion which seems well supported by facts.[16]

Constancy as used in the preceding argument has not quite the same meaning as in our discussion of the different "constancies." Then we referred to appearances of the same thing at different moments of time which could be separated by arbitrarily long intervals. Now we mean chiefly those cases in which during a continuous change of stimulation the things maintain their properties. Nevertheless the two aspects must be related, although this relation is as yet by no means clear; moreover it involves memory, which we have so far excluded from our discussion. In later chapters the problem of things persisting through time will therefore be taken up again.

As *things,* phenomenal objects have definite properties. Apart from their resistance to distortion we have encountered their impenetrability (p. 275), and their inertia, according to which bigger objects move more slowly than smaller ones (p. 291). This correspondence between phenomenal and real things is, according to our theory, not primarily a matter of experience—although we do not deny that experience may influence thing properties—but the direct result of organization. Psychophysically, the process distributions which correspond to perceived things must in several respects be similar to physical things, and therefore we must, on the basis of isomorphism, conclude that behavioural things have autochthonously characteristics similar to real things. Here, as in so many other fields, a purely empiristic theory is bound to run in a vicious circle. Our theory avoids not only this but at the same time a Kantian apriorism.

SUMMARY

In these last chapters we have tried to fill in the frame provided by our final answer to the question: Why do things look as they do? We have studied organization in a great variety of aspects and have reached a consistent, though surely as yet very incomplete, theory of perception. At the same time we have tried to give a picture of what we mean by organization, an insight into the aims and method of our theoretical approach. In this respect these chapters should serve as an introduction to the following ones in which the scope of our investigation will be broadened. But in the wider scope of our future investigations we shall be guided by the same methodological principles and shall find the great power of the laws of organization which we established in our discussion.

16 Compare, for instance, one of Beyrl's results reported in Chapter III, pp. 93 f.

CHAPTER VIII

ACTION

Reflexes; The Ego; The Executive

The Results of Behaviour. The Problem of Behaviour. Humphrey's General Principle: Conservation and Development. Reflexes. The Ego. The Ego as a Field Object. The Problem of Its Segregation. A Case of a Behavioural World Without an Ego. What Are the Conditions for an Experience to Be Incorporated in the Ego? The Complexity of the Ego. The Executive. The Control of the Executive. Three Cases. The Demand Characters. An Excursion into Aesthetics. Dynamic Relations Between Objects and Ego. Objects Determining Our Behaviour. Physiognomic Characters. The Actual Control of the Executive. General Principle of Action

THE RESULTS OF BEHAVIOUR

Psychology is concerned with behaviour, and behaviour is, of all natural events, one of the most interesting. Let us compare the earth as it was before life appeared on it with what it is now, to give substance to this claim of ours. Then we would have to compare a "pure" landscape such as we may now find in polar regions or on the top of the highest mountains with our big cities, our villages, our harbours, and our tilled fields. As a purely geographical event the change is stupendous. Ore has been dug out of the bowels of the earth, has been purified, made into iron and steel, and these are now girding the globe in railway tracks, supporting the huge buildings of our cities, racing over oceans, and working for us day and night in our various machines. Similarly the coal deposits have been opened up and millions and millions of tons of coal are being consumed to make our engines go and to protect us against the harshness of our climate. Rivers have been deflected, valleys have been flooded, the rank growth of vegetation has been forced to give way to a regular alternation of crops of a few plants necessary for the support of men. Cities have sprung up, each of them being a system of such a complex structure and of such order as never existed before man appeared and had time to develop his civilization. And the strangest things happen in these cities: there are buildings, filled every night with crowds of people who watch in semi-darkness a white screen and listen to sounds produced by an intricate machinery, there are other buildings in which men flock to stare at pieces of canvas covered with paints, and still other ones where men sit quietly turning over the leaves of curious objects called books, books which need other men and big machines to be produced. And then there are funny strips of paper called money, which pass from person to person, are kept in great numbers in other kinds of buildings called banks, and which govern the behaviour of the buzzing millions and millions of men. I could go on indefinitely describing mere geographical differences between the world devoid of life and the world as it is today; and all these momentous changes are due to behaviour.

No wonder, then, that we, the *behaving* agents, are interested in this our own behaviour, our interest in behaviour being itself behaviour. But great as this interest is, and essential as I deem it for the future of our civilization, historically it appears late, and is secondary. The particular behaviour which is "interest in behaviour" is necessarily posterior to behaviour which is "interest in the world." At first we are concerned with getting food and shelter and warmth, only then with ourselves, as the providers of these necessities, and our activities in this labour.

THE PROBLEM OF BEHAVIOUR

I shall not develop this historical theme. Rather, I shall begin with the problem as it faces us today. We see what behaviour has done and we want to explain it; for by now we have developed a particular type of behaviour, called science, which turns back on itself and tries in this enterprise to follow the methods which it has developed in other fields.

Can Its Solution Proceed Unconcerned with Its Orderly and Meaningful Results? But if we want to explain behaviour, behaviour which has been such a powerful agent in the world, can we ever hope to succeed if, right at the outset, we forget what behaviour has accomplished? That is to say, must we not, in order to explain behaviour, first gain some knowledge about those universal aspects of behaviour which have been responsible for its success? Will it do to introduce explanatory principles indifferent to the results of behaviour, principles which would explain as well, or better, utter chaos, when in reality we have civilization, chaotic as this civilization may appear at the moment if measured in terms of civilization? Can we use principles which by themselves would make the probability of any kind of civilization, nay, of any survival of men and animals, infinitely small, calling the fact that this improbability has come to be realized by the name of chance? Or would not such an explanation be ultimately the abandonment of any explanation? Provided we knew what happened in every nerve, every muscle, every separate part of our organism during our behaviour acts, would that explain our railway systems, our literature, art and music, and our science? These processes would be exactly the same if a man transported a stone from a place A to a place B whether this was a mere transportation or a part in the great activity of building a pyramid or a Gothic cathedral. Man's behaviour, however, has been very definitely of the type of building rather than of mere transporting. Can, then, any attempt at an explanation of behaviour hope to succeed which excludes this fact from its fundamental principles? Otherwise expressed, in terms introduced in our first chapter, can a science of behaviour even begin without the categories of order and meaning?

Mechanism Leads to Vitalism. Any attempt to proceed in such a way will find, sooner or later, that it can never accomplish its task—that behaviour as the agency that created civilization, behaviour even that preserves the individual for a definite span of time in the ever-changing environment, remains the same X in the equation that we started with. And therefore any such attempt has always led to a dead wall. The human mind, unwilling to be stopped by such an obstacle, has built itself ladders to climb across it; i.e., it has introduced a new principle, totally alien to and different from the principles which kept it from its goal. The dualisms, or pluralisms, which we introduced in the first chapter, have been the necessary results of all such attempts. Since mechanistic theories, to call them by the name which they gave themselves, always failed to explain why behaviour is orderly rather than chaotic, these theories were supplemented by *vitalism,* which attributed order and meaning to a new agent, inherently endowed with order and meaning and capable of imposing them on mechanistic nature. At the very beginning we refused to accept such a solution, and later on we showed how order and meaning can be kept in the theoretical system without such a *deus ex machina.* This was done in the field of perception.

Humphrey's General Principle: Conservation and Development. Our first aim must therefore be to achieve the same end in the field of behaviour. "*The organism may be said to behave as an intricate system of material processes, tending actively to maintain a complex pattern under constantly changing conditions*" (Humphrey, p. 41).

This proposition, amply developed by its author, gives us such a first principle. It claims that the organism is a peculiar kind of system, a kind, however, which may also be found in the inorganic world, and which is so constituted that all its reactions have a conservative tendency. We may also say: if we consider the organism and its (geographical) environment as one system, then any disturbance of the equilibrium of this system will end in the re-establishment of an equilibrium which is also an equilibrium for the organism alone;[1] the equilibrium of the organism, then, is a stable equilibrium inasmuch as it re-establishes itself after a disturbance. Of course this is not strictly true; the new equilibrium of a living organism will never be quite the same as the old. Thus, what actually happens is not a mere conservation of pattern, but its development. The system is conservative and evolving at the same time. Were it not conservative, were it to become perpetually different at successive instants, it would never be the same organism long enough for us to call it so. Were it only conservative so as to revert always to exactly the same condition, it would not be an organism. "Objectively considered organic identity is then rather far removed from the continued identity of an inert thing. . . . Not identity of matter, nor identity of form, gives it, but a spatio-temporal unity of developing and changing form; we may say that the gradually changing pattern of any organic system is a single long event, conditioned by external change, at the same time regulated from within, and taking place, as do all events in our experience, in four dimensions, three of space and one of time" (Humphrey, pp. 54-5). Humphrey has investigated what properties of systems make such behaviour possible. Instead of following him in his very general approach, which encompasses parts of physics and chemistry, physiology and psychology, we shall stick to specific psychological problems and see how his general principle is borne out there.

One more word before we begin. The general principle which we took over from Humphrey seems at first sight far removed from the kind of principle we wanted, a principle, namely, which would envisage at the outset the orderly and meaningful results of behaviour. What has Humphrey's principle to do with civilization? That it cannot be sufficient is obvious. It applies to animals as well as to men, but animals have not produced a civilization. Granting this, acknowledging that we have to do more, we can still see that the principle at least starts us on the right road towards finding this needed more. For in the first place it excludes chaos as the result of behaviour, and in the second, by taking into account the develop-

[1] The reader is referred back to our definition of behaviour in Chapter II, p. 32.

ment of the system, it leaves a place for such behaviour results as we call civilization. In that sense it fulfils the demand which we made. It will be our task to fill in the gaps and to show what are the distinguishing characteristics that lead human behaviour so far beyond the results achieved by animals. But in outline even this answer may be anticipated: the new equilibria which organic systems establish depend upon the disturbances to which the old ones are exposed. Therefore we might expect the possibility of disturbances and thereby the possibility of equilibria to be enormously increased in the phylogenetic series and most particularly in the step from the subhuman to the human.

REFLEXES

Traditional Theory. The traditional theory of action begins with the so-called reflexes, i.e., with relatively isolated movements elicited by relatively isolated stimuli; the knee jerk and the contraction and dilation of the pupil may serve as examples. Traditional theory uses these reflexes in two ways: first it makes an extremely simple hypothesis about their occurrence, an hypothesis based on certain anatomical findings, and secondly it postulates these simple reflexes as the elements out of which by mere combination all our actions have been developed. In both respects the reflex theory is the direct counterpart of the sensation theory which we discussed in our third chapter, and in both respects it is equally unsatisfactory. Since I have discussed this theory at great length in an earlier book (1928, Chap. III, §§ 4 and 5), and since it is rapidly disappearing from the system of psychology, if not from the text books, I shall be very brief here. A reflex as a process found its explanation in a structure, the so-called reflex-arc, consisting of an afferent neurone, an efferent neurone, and ordinarily one or more intermediate connecting neurones. Excitation started at one end would travel over the whole arc, the stimulus would elicit the response. It is obvious that this theory is of the type which, a short time ago, we characterized as not very likely to give a satisfactory explanation of behaviour; for this theory lacks any principle from which the orderliness and meaningfulness of behaviour could follow. The organism being endowed with an enormous number of reflex arcs, a great many of which are being stimulated at the same time, how does it happen that the resulting behaviour is orderly, that it conserves the system, instead of changing it by every reaction? Moreover, one pattern of stimulation follows upon another, and in this sequence a great deal is perfectly haphazard; and yet behaviour is not haphazard, but purposive, goal-directed, i.e., orderly and meaningful.

Eye-movements. Let us then discuss a whole set of reflexes whose rôle in the total behaviour of the organism is patent, our eye-movements. Each eye has six external muscles attached to the bulb which can move it in its orbit, these six pairs of muscles being innervated by three different cranial nerves originating in a number of different cortical centres. Besides, each eye has the internal ciliary muscle[2] which controls accommodation. Thus, anatomically, the complexity of the oculomotor system is enormous. This system produces three distinguishable kinds of movements: (1) accommodation, (2) fixation and pursuit, (3) convergence.

Accommodation. We have already discussed the first rather amply (Chapter IV, pp. 74 and 119 f.). Accommodation means the creation of the best possible conditions for clear organization. Equilibrium is achieved when articulation is clear, i.e., when the sensory processes have attained a maximum property. If no clear articulation is possible, as when we look at a screen with a badly focussed picture upon it, the oculomotor system is under constant stress, our eyes begin to ache. Accommodation has all the characteristics of a true reflex, it is automatic and occurs "unconsciously," we have no notion of its taking place. But in terms of the stimulus arc theory: What is the stimulus for accommodation? The same retinal elements that were stimulated before accommodation took place are still stimulated afterwards, though somewhat differently. But there is no systematic way of describing this difference except by referring it to its success, the ensuing organization of visual processes. Thus this first example shows the helplessness of the pure reflex arc theory and gives at the same time an indication of a true theory: the reflex as a part event in a larger process of good organization.

Fixation and Pursuit. Although we have not discussed the second function of the oculomotor system, fixation and pursuit, directly, we have used it as an example when we derived the figure-function of the retinal centre. We connected it then with the fact that if the visual organization was a figure on a homogeneous ground, the eyes would move in such a way as to create the conditions for this figure to be as much figured as possible by making it the enclosed part, i.e., by shifting it on to the centre, by fixating it. We might add that under such simple conditions the balance of the whole field would be most stable if the figure were in the centre, since this is the condition

[2] We exclude from our discussion the sphincter pupillae, which regulates the width of the pupil.

of greatest symmetry. Our explanation of fixation in this simple case, then, is exactly the same as our explanation of accommodation: a movement of the receptor organ occurring in such a way that the organization resulting from the stimulation of the receptor is as good as possible.

Let us compare this explanation with the current one. "When carefully examined, these processes reveal a complicated and finely differentiated system of interconnections between the impression of light upon separate points of the retina and the specialized impulses of eye-movements. Strictly speaking, a different movement must arise from every retinal point; therefore every fibre of the optic nerve must have a different central connection with the motor nerves which innervate eye-movements" (Bühler, 1924, pp. 103 f.). I have argued against this explanation on several grounds (1928, pp. 78 f.). In the first place it has to be remembered that from each retina there issue about one million sensory fibres, so that all in all two million of such separate connections must exist. We should not, however, be frightened by mere numbers. What should give us pause is the much more startling fact that all these two million connections must be arranged in such a way that by their mere arrangement they give rise to the orderly result of fixation. The observed fact is, e.g., that wherever in a dark room a point of light appears, it will be fixated; otherwise expressed: the end state, projection of the solitary point on the fovea, will be reached whatever the initial state, i.e., wherever this point of light was originally projected. Who or what produced this arrangement? It was this difficulty that led men like Helmholtz to have recourse to an empiristic theory even for eye-movements, a theory which is as futile here as in other fields and as little in accord with the observed facts. Yet a rejection of the empiristic explanation does not improve the case for the nativistic one. Our concise formulation of the actual event, independence of the final state from the initial one,[8] points directly to a different kind of explanation, for the feature is common to a great number of purely physical events which occur without any such system of special connections as was assumed in the nativistic theory of fixation movements. A swinging weight suspended by a string will eventually come to rest in the same position no matter in what direction or how far it had been swung out, because in this position the actual forces, gravitation on the one hand and the elasticity of the string on the other, are in perfect equilibrium.

[8] See Köhler, 1927a, and Humphrey.

In the second place I have argued that the case as presented by Bühler is oversimplified. For although the end result is independent of the initial position of the eyes, the actual movements by which this end result is achieved are not. Therefore, instead of the two million connections which we found it necessary to assume before, we have to postulate many times two million such connections; if the first system possessed in itself a negligibly small probability, this probability is still indefinitely diminished. In the third place I referred to some transplantation experiments by Marina which refute this theory directly, and which I shall omit here. Instead I shall offer a fourth argument, viz., that the theory involves the experience error, that without it it cannot produce a stimulus for the response; in short I shall show that in this respect fixation and pursuit are similar to accommodation.

In the experiment so far described, a single point of light in a dark room, no difficulty seems to appear. But as far as fixation goes this case is no different from the opposite one: a homogeneous light field with a black spot emerging somewhere. In ordinary life conditions are much more complex. If we disregard for the moment the influence exerted on fixation by our attitudes and interests there is still the case of our eyes roaming around and coming to rest now on this object, now on that, but not, as a rule, on the intervening space. Then there are the pursuit movements in which our gaze follows a moving object, and lastly there is the fact that we turn our eyes also in the direction of a sound which suddenly breaks in upon us, a reaction which Löwenfeld found to be typical for the infant at three months.

What inferences can we draw from these four instances? If a dark point on a light background has the same effect as a light point on a dark background, then the stimulus as a physical event is no longer defined. In this case the whole retina is stimulated except for the one point which elicits the reaction. It is therefore in either case not a point stimulus that starts the reflex movement, but a stimulus inhomogeneity, and the movement takes place in such a way that this stimulus inhomogeneity is brought into the centre of the retina. Formulated in this way the fact of fixation no longer indicates anything like that complex system of neural connections which the nativistic theory assumes. For the cause of the whole process is no longer located in one retinal point, the peripheral starting point of the reflex, but resides in the total retina, or a part sufficiently large to give rise to inhomogeneous stimulation. Now we know that such inhomogeneous stimulation will give rise to a segregated figure, and we understand the whole process as a process of articulation and balancing of the visual field.

The fact that our roaming eyes are directed by contours and come to rest on things (not on the background) emphasizes the same point. The whole retina is again stimulated, each point is connected with a different eye-movement; why then are certain parts of the stimulus pattern carried into the fovea and not others? Unanswerable from the point of view of a mechanistic or machine-like reflex theory, which again cannot assign the proper stimulus to this effect, and easily explicable when the eye-movements are considered in conjunction with the total process of field organization. I need not repeat the argument for the pursuit movement, and turn now to the fixation of a sound. The function of this response is essentially the same as that of all the other fixations, viz., to bring the momentarily outstanding figure into the centre of the field. The only new fact added by this case is that this figure may be an auditory as well as a visual one. Thus this case involves no new principle from our point of view. But what about the reflex theory of eye-movement? What is here the initial peripheral end of the arc?

CONVERGENCE. We turn now to the last oculomotor function, convergence. This is a binocular function *par excellence,* for it guarantees that at any one moment as many points of external space as possible will be projected on corresponding points on the two retinae. No doubt, there exists an anatomical substratum for this function; as Hering, who compared the two eyes to a team of horses guided by the same rein, pointed out long ago (1868, p. 3), the two eyes will move together also if one of them is excluded from the act of vision. But we have learned that the existence of an anatomical structure may be primarily the effect of a function, which in its turn it influences only secondarily. That this must be the true state of affairs in our case is amply proven by the ease with which the normal co-operation of the eyes can be altered provided such alteration serves the end of vision. Hold a prism of not too great a refracting power in front of one of your eyes; you will not see things double. Let us assume that the eyes remained in their position when this deflecting device was introduced; then the same external points would no longer be projected on corresponding points of the two eyes, since everything would remain unchanged in the unobstructed eye, while the retinal pattern would be shifted on the other. Therefore we should see everything doubled, and the fact that we do not, proves that eye-movements have taken place so as to re-establish the old condition in which a maximum of points of external space was projected on corresponding points.

Therefore, although an anatomical structure for convergence exists, we must seek our explanation of convergence elsewhere. We use a case of eye-movements about which Köhler has made a great number of as yet unpublished experiments to prove his theory, which will underlie the new discussion as it did the preceding one.[4] We start with a fact known from our study of spatial organization, the law of proximity. Two similar objects in our field of vision will attract each other with a force decreasing with the distance between them. When ordinarily we look at two parallel lines fairly close to each other this force will have no measurable effect of displacing them.[5] But distribute these lines over the two eyes by means of a stereoscope or haploscope, and the effect of this force will at once become apparent. *One* line only will be seen, the eyes moving automatically in such a way as to bring the two lines on corresponding lines in the two eyes. The same principle explains why ordinarily we do not see things doubled. Let us consider a case of ordinary fixation, our fixation point being the centre of a vertical line. Any slight oscillation in the state of convergence would produce a slight disparity of the two lines and thereby a slight doubling. But at once forces of attraction would arise which because of the very small distance would be very strong and would, therefore, at once innervate the eye muscles in such a way that the lines would be pulled together again, that perfect convergence would be re-established. Thus our explanation of the lack of double images becomes dynamic. We can grant the existence of an anatomical structure which facilitates normal co-ordination of the two eyes—a structure which will have been built up by the function in the general manner which we described above in discussing the structural difference of centre and periphery of the retina (p. 207), but we cannot admit that such a structure would be perfect enough to exclude any double images without special forces. No fixation is perfect, slight tremor movements occurring during all continued fixation. This again is understandable, since a slight displacement on the retina identical in both eyes changes the field organization in a negligibly small degree. On the other hand, with the fixation "mechanism" not perfect, how can we assume a perfect convergence

[4] See Köhler, 1925b.

[5] As far as I am aware, no attempt has yet been made to measure such an effect. It does not, however, seem quite impossible to do so. That, however, under conditions of short successive exposure such alteration occurs as may reduce the distance to less than half its normal size has been proved by Scholz (see above, pp. 286 f.).

mechanism? But we must not overlook the difference between the two cases, for here the slightest deviation from perfection will arouse strong forces which at once push the system back into a normal position. Thus convergence is a beautiful example of Humphrey's conservative tendency, of the stability of organic equilibria.

Let us summarize our position. The traditional nativistic theory was unable to cope with accommodation, and in order to explain fixation it had to assume an enormously complex structure, working with an unheard-of perfection in an orderly manner, the order being due to the structure, and therefore no "real" order but only accidental order.[6] Our theory has to make one assumption only, viz., that the condition of the perceptual field may, by starting and "steering" it, influence the oculomotor system. This assumption is inherent in the traditional theory in the concept of the reflex arc, the centripetal excitation arousing a centrifugal one. Our assumption is more general and at the same time a much more powerful theoretical tool. For from this assumption all the rest follows: if communication between the sensory and the motor system exists —and this existence is not in doubt—then these two systems become part-systems of a larger system, the final equilibrium being an equilibrium of this larger system. The best equilibrium would, therefore, be that in which not only the larger system would be balanced, but also each of the two part systems by itself. Since the equilibrium of the oculomotor system, due chiefly to the arrangements of the eye muscles and the strains resulting therefrom, seems to be accomplished when the eyes are slightly divergent, such perfect equilibrium can never be accomplished so long as visual perception occurs. Consequently each actual equilibrium obtained during vision is an equilibrium against the motor system. However, over a wide range of positions the strains in the oculomotor system are very small, so that the forces originating in the sensory system determine the final equilibrium. Only with extreme positions of the eyes will the stresses in the oculomotor system assume high values, and then they have to be considered as determining factors in the final balance. If we try to fixate a point to our extreme left or right, it will quickly split up into double images, the forces of attraction in the sensory field being no longer strong enough to overcome the opposed forces of the oculomotor system.

Eye-movements, considered as typical reflexes, thus find their ex-

[6] The reader should turn back to our discussion of physiological patterns, Chapter II, pp. 58 f., where the same issue, real vs. purely geometrical, was raised.

planation, not in facts of anatomical structure, but in facts of systemic equilibria produced by processes of organization.

Reflexes as Special Cases of Humphrey's Principle. We can see now how hopelessly wrong the attempt was to explain behaviour by the combination of reflexes of the reflex-arc theory type. Instead we shall derive from our discussion the clue that behaviour must be explained in harmony with Humphrey's principles, as a process of the establishment of equilibrium.

THE "TOTALLY-UNCONSCIOUS" REFLEXES. We shall now briefly discuss the reflexes which have no conscious counterpart whatsoever, like most of our tonic reflexes which regulate incessantly the tone of our entire musculature and thereby preserve our poise and balance. Are they to be explained according to our conception or do they at least fall under the old reflex-arc scheme? I have no doubt that the first is true, and that the equilibrium they serve to maintain is an equilibrium of organization in lower brain centres and the spinal cord. The simplicity and rigidity which under certain conditions distinguish such reflexes must be due to the fact that under these conditions the sub-system whose equilibrium is disturbed and re-established is comparatively small and relatively well isolated from the rest. When we extended our psychophysical field beyond the confines of the behavioural environment (see Chapter II, p. 50) the reflexes were among our reasons for doing so. It is not the purpose of this book to follow up this idea, but this remark was necessary lest the reader should think it possible that at least for some reflexes the traditional theory were tenable. The reader more specifically interested in this problem may turn to Goldstein's papers on the subject.

REFLEXES AND ORGANIZATIONS AS "SILENT" AND "NON-SILENT." Another point is more important in our context. We have, as a rule, no direct knowledge of the dynamics of our eye-movements. Of the movements of accommodation and convergence this is completely true, while we frequently know that our eyes have wandered, resting first on this, then on that object. But even here our awareness of our eye-movements, or, otherwise expressed, the eye-movements in our behavioural world—where of course they belong to the behavioural Ego and not to the behavioural environment—may be very different from the real eye-movements. Before psychologists became interested in the subject, nobody knew, e.g., what kind of eye-movements we execute when we read. It was thought, because that was what everybody who is aware of his eye-movements while reading experiences, that the eyes moved continuously over the line, while we now know that the eyes are at rest most of the time, making no more than three or four fast sweeps while a line of print is read. But more often than not we are not aware of these movements at all. When we are not, the whole interplay of forces described in the preceding discussion has no counterpart in experience, just as the interplay of forces that produces sensory organization remains almost entirely outside experience (which contains only the result of these dynamics). Köhler, who was the first to emphasize this aspect of sensory organization, called it "silent organization" (1929, p. 371). The silence then refers also to the movements which contribute to this organization.

Our fixation and pursuit movements, however, are, as we have mentioned, not always silent. But the fact that their experience is by no means always veridical is significant. We add to the instance of the eye-movements during reading, two other cases: it has happened in many experimental investigations that the subjects, instructed to fixate a certain object during a definite interval, reported that their eyes had remained perfectly steady, while objective records show that the eyes had made distinct, sometimes quite considerable, movements; on the other hand a subject who follows the contours of an after-image figure, without moving his eyes, has the distinct impression that his eyes have taken part in the exploration (Rubin). Thus the experience of eye-movements is in such cases not due to any separate sensations from the bulbs or muscles of the eyes, but a result of the total field organization, just as perceived motion of an object may not be due to the real movement of the object as in induced movement.

In one respect, however, fixation really goes beyond these limits: it happens that we feel our eyes riveted to a certain object, that we cannot avert them and that when, with great power of will, we have looked elsewhere, we find an almost irresistible compulsion to turn our eyes back to this fascinating object. Here the force which controls our fixation is revealed in experience, here the motor side of our act of vision is no longer "silent." But in these cases the eyes are not merely indifferent receptor organs which work for us without telling us of their work; in such cases the eyes are very definitely parts of our Ego, and not only the eyes, our whole Ego is in such cases pulled in the direction of the attracting object. Therefore this case leads us beyond such cases of action as happen without participation of the Ego.

We have just dealt with the second point of our program, developed at the end of the second chapter, and must now turn to the third, take a new step, long deferred and often anticipated, and introduce the Ego. The stage is set, enter the hero of the play.

THE EGO

But how is he to introduce himself? What are his opening lines to be? Many modern psychological text books, if not the majority of them, are surprisingly reticent about this question. As a matter of fact, they give you to understand that psychology has nothing to do with the Ego or the Self, that the Self has to disappear from psychology as completely as the soul. The lonely voice of Miss Calkins, who waged a gallant fight for a Self-psychology, remained unheeded, nor did the way in which McDougall treated the Self in his system influence the current of psychological theory. Too much philosophical speculation had clustered round the Self-concept to make it acceptable to scientific-minded psychologists. They wanted facts, observable data, and so they turned their trained introspection on the alleged self and found either nothing or kinaesthetic sensations or feelings, but no special element, the Self. This is not surprising; for because of their systematic preconceptions they had to use a mental microscope in their search for an empirical foundation of the Self. But one will never discover that such things as faces exist if one looks through a microscope.

The same psychologists who treated the Ego in this manner and saw it disappear from psychology treated shapes, things, motions, no better. If motion is nothing but a "grey flash" the Ego may well be nothing but "kinaesthetic sensations from the lower trunk or from parts of the body in strained position" (Titchener, 1911, p. 547). Since we have established the reality of shapes, things, and motions, we shall have much less difficulty in establishing the reality of the Ego.

Indeed, it has proved impossible to discuss the behavioural environment without including the Ego. On the one hand we found the environment itself dependent upon the Ego, its attention and attitudes. On the other hand we found the orientation of the Ego established *pari passu* with the organization of the spatial framework. Both these groups of facts will be utilized as clues for our introduction of the Ego, but we deal first with the second, localization, orientation and motion of the Ego, since it is in a direct line with our preceding discussion.

The Ego as a Field Object. The Problem of Its Segregation. For in these last respects the Ego seems to behave like any other segregated object in the field. Is there then any justification for treating the Ego in this way? Our first question should be: What are the segregating forces? I do not think that this question has as yet been formulated, and therefore any answer to be given in the following paragraphs must needs be provisional and incomplete. But if the Ego, in however many respects it may differ from the other field objects, is to be treated as an object in the field, we must know at least that there are possible factors which may produce its segregation. We have advisedly used the term "Ego" without a proper definition, for no such definition could at the start of our discussion be adequate; the Ego cannot even be said to be constant, to be confined within unchanging limits. A possible test of such limits is an exploration of the means by which an Ego may be touched, insulted or elated. Imagine a sensitive person in the society of a vulgar and boisterous crowd. His Ego will shrink as a means of protection from their crude outbreaks of emotion. He will, to use popular parlance, which is probably nearer the truth than we ordinarily think, withdraw into his shell. To go further, there is the martyr at the stake; the shell into which he has withdrawn excludes even his body, whose mutilations cannot affect his Ego any more. That, on the other hand, under more normal conditions our body belongs to our Ego seems obvious. It is I who drove the ball into the corner of my opponent's court just clearing the net, I who sprinted the 100 yards, I who climbed the difficult "chimney," this "I" not being a spiritual point somewhere but something of which my body, which after all did all these things, forms an integral part.

Or look at the other side of the picture: deformities, moles, false teeth, the falling out of our hair, all these things we try to conceal as best we can; and there is nothing that hurts Miss N's Ego more than Mr. M's remark that she is not half so good-looking as her friend.

But the skin need by no means be the boundary surface of the Ego. Miss N would feel almost as insulted if the gentleman had said that her friend was so much better dressed than she. Indeed our clothes, which, as Flügel remarks, form an intermediate layer between ourselves and the outside world, may easily become a true part of our Ego. In the perfect dandy they have even reached the centre of his self.

The confines may be still wider. Mrs. P will think Miss Q an odious person and a bad teacher because Miss Q finds Mrs. P's little boy a lazy and stupid brat. Her Ego has been touched through her child, just because her child belongs to her Ego. This is a grim truth, a truth which lies at the bottom of many a struggle that often enough has a tragic quality, the struggle of the young to free themselves from the parents. But even the family is not the limit; you can rouse violent emotions in a good citizen by attacking the Republican or the Tory party. We need not continue. The limits of the Ego will vary from case to case, and with the same person in different situations. There are conditions which will contract the boundaries of the Ego, like a great sorrow, a cruel disappointment, and there are others which will expand it, until it may embrace practically the whole world, as in states of true ecstasy.

But this inconstant boundary is not a feature entirely peculiar to the Ego, without any counterpart in the external (behavioural) world. Here is a billiard ball, a thing in itself. But now we see the whole billiard table, of which the ball is only one item; and now we watch the progress of the game, and here the whole table has become part of a greater unit, the game. The expansion is not a continuous process, but goes by leaps and bounds prescribed by the boundaries of higher units. Just so with the Ego. From our skin to our clothes, from them to our families, and so forth. This remark was not added to minimize the specific character of the Ego, but to allay the criticism that the inconstancy of boundary by itself proved futile our attempt to treat the Ego as an object in the field.

Granted, then, that the boundary of the Ego is variable, it is still in each case a boundary, and our question remains, What forces produce it?

First Step Towards the Solution of Our Problem. This question, although not formulated in general terms, has been given a partial answer by Köhler as far as the bodily Ego or at least the visible bodily Ego is concerned (1929, pp. 224 f.). I sit at my desk writing this book. The top of the desk, my writing pad, my pen, are distinct, well-segregated units in my behavioural environment. Where is my pen? It is held by my hand, my hand being exactly such a unit in my field as pen and pad and desk top. The forces which segregate my hand from the pen are of the same kind as those which segregate pad and desk top, those forces which we have amply discussed in our fourth chapter. The same is of course true of the other parts of my body that I see. They are segregated and unified in my visual field exactly as any part of the visual behavioural environment.

A Second Step: Why Does My Visually Segregated Hand Appear as "My" Hand? But there remains this question: Why do I see this hand as my hand, this arm as my arm, and so forth, and not merely as a familiar hand and arm, or Koffka's hand and arm, just as I see X's and Y's hand and arm? There is sufficient evidence to believe that infants see parts of their bodies as external objects. Another argument of Köhler's which I have heard him use in discussion takes us a bit nearer to the answer of this question, which is a psychological question *par excellence,* although it is not even mentioned in our standard psychological texts. It starts with the behavioural environment: yonder is the wall of the room; in front of it is a desk; on that desk are various objects, nearer and nearer; there are other walls to the right and the left, and other objects between me and these walls; but space is not only in front and at the sides, space is also, though less articulated, less clearly defined, behind. That this last statement is true, though again not mentioned in psychological text books, can easily be demonstrated. Suppose in lecturing I was standing on a platform behind which the floor dropped for thousands of feet. The platform might be wide enough for me to walk along it comfortably, but would I behave on that platform as I would on an ordinary one? Certainly not. The fact that behind me there was empty space, dangerous empty space, would determine my actions at every moment. Therefore my normal activity on the platform is equally determined by the normal "behind"; but that implies that the behind exists, that behavioural space does not confront me but encloses me. Now then, Köhler's argument continues, what is there between the last thing just in front and the behind? Is space absolutely empty there? The answer is: Certainly not; here, between the "in front" and the "behind," is that part of the behavioural world which I call my Ego. It has a very definite place in that world, and well-defined, if variable, boundaries. From this argument we can take the following answer to our question: "in front," "to the left and right," "behind," and "above and below" are characteristics of space which it possesses with regard to an object which serves as the origin of the system of spatial co-ordinates. This object, then, is functionally different from all others, inasmuch as it determines fundamental space aspects. Therefore, we should expect this object to have properties different from all others. And thus we have gained a first clue in our search; for the object which we call Ego is in one decisive respect different from all other objects, just as the term Ego implies a difference between the object so designated and all other objects. This is a first clue, no more. Only one side, and a relatively superficial one, of the Ego can be the result of its rôle in space organization. But with all this restriction we have got something to build upon, and we can now give a first answer to the question why my hand, although it be organized by the same factors as a pen, a box, or another hand, appears as "my hand." It must, if it belongs to that nuclear object which determines the "in front," "behind," "left and right."

A Last Step: Laws of Organization Applied. We are still far removed from a complete theory of the Ego, we have not even answered our first question yet as to the forces which segregate this unit in the total field. But we have demonstrated that for mere reasons of organization this unit must be of a peculiar kind. We must now return to our question. In accordance with the principles we have introduced in the beginning of the fourth chapter, there could be no segregation in an entirely homogeneous field. There we considered purely visual fields, and saw what they will be like when they are completely homogeneous. But then we still had the Ego; that is to say, we did not investigate those conditions under which the total field is totally homogeneous. I doubt whether it will ever be possible to produce such conditions in the laboratory, for they are, of course, totally unnatural. But they do occur.

A CASE OF A BEHAVIOURAL WORLD WITHOUT AN EGO. I know of an extremely good example, the report of a famous mountain climber who woke from a deep swoon low down in a crevasse. The essay was written in 1893, I suppose soon after the experience, although the author does not state this point explicitly. Professor Eugen Guido Lammer, a teacher in Vienna, had made all by himself the first ascent of the Thurwieserspitze by the north face, a sheer cliff of ice, and had returned over the west ridge to the glacier below. The further descent led him through one of the worst glaciers in the Eastern Alps, a glacier torn by a labyrinth of crevasses covered by snow, which he crossed during the hottest hours of the day when the snow, which in the morning had been hard and safe to tread upon, had become softened by the heat of the sun. He had almost come across this glacier when a snow bridge on which he had stepped unawares gave way, and he fell into the chasm, hitting the side walls of the crevasse several times and losing consciousness. I now translate his description as literally as I can: ". . . fog . . . darkness . . . fog . . . whirring . . . grey veil with a small lighter spot . . . fog . . . faint dawn . . . a soft humming . . . dull discomfort . . . fog . . . something has happened to somebody . . . gloomy fog, and always that lighter point . . . a shivering shudder: something clammy . . . fog . . . how was it? . . . an effort at thinking . . . ah, still fog; but besides that light point there outside, there emerges a second point inside: right, that is *I!* . . . fog, dull ringing sound, frost . . . a dream? . . . Yes, indeed, a wild, wild, wild dream!—It has dreamed—no, rather *I* have dreamed . . ." [7] I shall not continue the quotation to the end, the full awareness of the situation, nor relate how by his own efforts the heroic climber succeeded in freeing himself. The part so far quoted is sufficient for our discussion. It shows, provided the description is correct, and its vividness and impressiveness makes it very likely to be so, that phenomenally quite a long period of time passed without an Ego, a period which began with as complete a homogeneity as we can imagine. The Ego did not even emerge with the first articulation of the field, the light point, not even with the first feeling of discomfort, and apparently not even with the first conscious thought, though it was this which led very soon to the momentary establishment of the Self, which was, however, as yet quite unstable; it disappeared again and re-emerged with greater stability and better organization, the experience appearing as a dream.

Conclusions from This Case. Interesting as this last turn is, we shall not discuss it here, but shall, instead, draw our conclusions: the Ego, just as any other field object, does not become segregated before the field possesses a sufficient amount of inhomogeneity. Let us try to collect the different constituents of the field at the moment when the Ego emerged: there are visual data, dark fog with a lighter point in it, auditory data, a soft humming, coenaesthetic data, the dull discomfort, the shivering, which also indicates temperature-sense data, and finally thought. All these data appear in the same field, phenomenally and physiologically, i.e., in accordance with the principle of isomorphism we assume that all these processes, started from the various parts of the body, occur in the same brain field. This is nothing new, since we have shown before that one and the same space contains objects of different sensory qualities. At first these various processes are spread more or less indiscriminately over the entire field. And then organization takes place, the field becomes bipolar, the visual figure, the light spot, becoming the one pole (objectively the light spot was produced by the light coming through a hole in a snow bridge halfway down the crevasse which Lammer's falling body had opened), and the Ego the other. We may assume that this point forming the core of the Self will have attracted to it the somatic data, while the auditory and visual data will have remained with the external pole. How this point-core

[7] I have been told that the experience on returning to consciousness after "laughing gas" is similar to this.

itself was formed we do not know. It must have had a great deal to do with the victim's earlier Ego, his wishes, fears, determinations, which are now brought into play. I am certain that an infant would never experience a Self under such conditions; as a matter of fact an infant will lead his life for a fairly long time without an Ego organization, and a still longer period with a very fluctuating and unstable one.

But if we disregard the person's history there is enough left to make us understand the segregation of the Self, for there are on the one hand the visual and auditory, on the other the somatic data, including the general feeling of the cold. It looks as though these latter had something in common which differentiated them from the others so that they formed a unit by themselves whose place in the total field would be determ ned by these others. We would then assume that with no other than purely visual homogeneous stimulation the field would be nothing but fog, fog without anything in it, not even a hole in the place where the Ego afterwards appears. As long as there is nothing to break the homogeneity of stimulation, there should be nothing to interrupt the fog which would constitute the whole behavioural field. The segregation, then, produced by inhomogeneity, would be due to the law of similarity, equal processes consolidating themselves and segregating themselves from others. The well-known fact that the data of the lower senses are much less different from each other than those of the higher ones tends to support our view, which would lead to the conclusion that at an early evolutionary stage, ere the different senses became separated, no Ego-world articulation will occur, a conclusion unfortunately not amenable to proof.

However, where such differences of sensory process occur, Ego organization becomes possible, the boundary surface between these different excitations may become the boundary "membrane" which holds the Ego system together and separates it from the rest of the field. Whether this first attempt at a solution is right or wrong I cannot say; but that *some* solution on such or similar lines must be true, unless our whole theory is wrong, seems to me obvious.

OTHER HYPOTHESES: CERTAIN EXPERIENCES BY THEMSELVES EGO-RELATED. In order to make more explicit what this hypothesis means I shall compare it with other possible hypotheses. One might say that there are certain processes, or experiences, which are by their very nature Ego-experiences, that they, by themselves, quite apart from any organization, constitute the Ego. Such experiences might be; pleasure and pain, the emotions, needs, wishes, and desires and our thoughts. But for most, if not for all of them, we can show that they can belong to parts of the environmental field as well as to our Ego. Let us begin with the emotions, which have been adduced so often in the past as examples *par excellence* for "subjective," i.e., Ego-related, experiences. And yet we may see a gloomy landscape, even when we ourselves are perfectly cheerful; may not a poplar look proud, a young birch shy, and has not Wordsworth immortalized the glee of the daffodils! Traditional psychology will retort: it is you who have projected these feelings into those objects of nature; you cannot seriously uphold that a landscape is really sad, that the daffodils are really gleeful. You yourself endow these objects with your own emotions by the process called empathy. The plausibility of this objection rests on two assumptions, the one palpably false, the other turning the argument into a vicious circle. The first is the assumption that when we ascribe sadness to a landscape we mean the geographical landscape. This of course would be absurd, but equally absurd is this interpretation of our opinion. Sadness and glee, and the other characteristics we have employed, apply in these descriptions primarily to the *behavioural* objects, and not to the geographical ones. And that these characteristics are characteristics of behavioural objects is explicitly admitted by our opponents who try to explain how they have come to be such, viz., by projection, empathy. The second assumption is that emotions are really subjective. Since, so the argument runs if made explicit, external objects appear to be endowed with emotions which, according to the assumption just stated, are purely subjective states, we must have projected these emotions into the objects. The cogency of this inference rests, of course, on the *assumption* of the subjectivity of the emotions, and therefore empathy does not *prove* this subjectivity. Rather, only when we make this assumption are we forced to *postulate* empathy, a process not directly verifiable, to doubt the truth of our first description, and replace it by the other one—the landscape is not really sad, but I project *my* sadness into it. But no proof is given for this assumption, whereas the fact mentioned above, that our own emotion of the moment may be different from, even in contrast with, the emotional characters of the objects we perceive, puts the empathy theory in a difficult position. But do we not experience emotions as processes of our Egos? Certainly we do; it was never claimed that emotions were always characters of external behavioural objects. But as little was it claimed that they were *always* Ego-related, and the fact that they are in some, or in a great many, cases nowise proves that they are so in all. Therefore it seems much more natural to say that emotions may be carried by (behavioural) objects as well as by myself, that they may enter other organized units in the field as well as that unit which we call the Ego. I should even be inclined to think that a field which contains no Ego organization may be highly emotional, and I believe that Dr. Lammer's extraordinary experience was emotionally tinged, if not charged, before his self-consciousness appeared.

What about wishes, needs, desires? As far as I see, the answer will be the same. We see the "greed" in that face over there, but do not experience it as our own desire, and we may admire the stern resolve shining through the eyes of our friend when we ourselves cannot make up our minds what to do. Even inanimate objects may appear with needs, like the melody before it is finished, or when it is broken off before its end, or an incomplete figure pattern.

What about our thoughts? Can thoughts be experienced outside of my Ego? The fact that we may see a man sunk in thought is not a case in point, for we do not know what his thoughts are. But there are other cases which prove that thoughts also may belong to external objects, which, for all normal persons, will be other persons. Many people have had dreams like or similar to the following: they are taking an oral examination with a group of colleagues; the examiner asks them a question which they are unable to answer, whereupon the examiner turns to the next candidate, who promptly supplies the correct answer. In this dream occur two thoughts and both in minds which are not the dreamer's Ego, although they are in his dream. The question is asked by the examiner, and the right answer is given by a student, while the Ego of the dreamer was unable to produce it. The answer then occurs in the dreamer's field, but not in that part of it which makes up his Ego. I have no evidence, but I believe that in the work of playwrights and novelists the same thing will occur. The author will get directly thoughts and speeches as thoughts and speeches of the "children of his mind," but not as his own thoughts and speeches.

There remain pleasure and pain. From Lammer's report we know that discomfort may be experienced without an Ego and therefore there is no reason to exclude the assumption that mild pleasure might be experienced in the same way. We may come pretty near to it when sleepily basking in the sun or drowsing in our hot bath. Intense pain, however, seems always an affair of the Ego. If it is, it proves no more than that an Ego must be there in order that severe pain be experienced. That of all experiences pain alone should be by and of itself the carrier of the Ego is too improbable to be believed without direct proof, although pain, or rather such excitation as will ordinarily lead to pain, may under given conditions contribute greatly to the organization of the Ego.

WHAT ARE THE CONDITIONS FOR AN EXPERIENCE TO BE INCORPORATED IN THE EGO? We conclude from this discussion that no process by itself and in isolation has an Ego-character, that it has to be incorporated in the Ego system to acquire it and that certain such processes are more than others fit to become so incorporated. But in each particular case the question remains: Why does this process at this moment belong to the Ego and not to an external object, a question which is closely connected with the other one: Which are the forces that at this moment keep the Ego segregated? We have guessed before at some of the forces which may be primarily responsible for this segregation. But we also mentioned that the Ego problem cannot be properly treated in the three dimensions of space alone, that without taking time into consideration we shall miss some of its main aspects, an idea which will be elaborated presently.

AN ANSWER TO OUR QUESTIONS. But let us return to our questions. Even though we have, at the moment, no real knowledge of the forces which keep the Ego unified and segregated from the rest, we must assume the Ego to be a particular field part in constant interaction with the rest of the field. And we can now turn to the other question—why certain processes are incorporated in this subsystem and others not. That not all processes occurring at a particular moment can form part of the Ego is a simple conclusion from our theory: no Ego would exist, as a special system, unless it segregated itself from other systems.

THE DIFFERENT SENSE DATA AND THE EGO. That visual data, apart from those of our own body, will remain outside the Ego derives directly from the nature of visual experience with its rich articulation into a great number of separate objects. If vision supplies us with many objects spatially distributed and clearly articulated, then vision must supply us mainly with non-Ego things. What then about the visible parts of our body, why are they drawn into the Ego? The answer can only be given in outline, but this outline is fairly clear. For we have knowledge of our limbs not only from vision but also from those other sources which give us notice about the non-visible parts of our body. These processes, aroused in the entero- and proprio-ceptors, form probably, as we have explained, the first material for the organization of the Ego. If, then, the place of the visual body data coincides with the place of the other data belonging to the same part of the body ("coincides," of course, in behavioural space), then we should be able to apply our law of proximity to explain why the visual data are experienced with the Ego character, "my hand," "my leg," etc. For the local kinaesthetic processes, since in their entirety they help to organize the Ego, are not independent local events, but part events in a larger system of events. If then a visual datum is welded together with a kinaesthetic one, it must also of necessity become a part in a greater whole, i.e., it must be incorporated in the Ego system. This welding together seems, as previously mentioned, not to occur right at the beginning of life, since the distinction between the infant's own body and other objects does not seem to become perfectly clear till well on in the second year.

While we found it a problem to explain why I see this hand before me as "my" hand and not just as a hand, psychology for a long time was occupied with the opposite problem: Why do I see things outside and not within me? That this problem originated in a bad confusion of the Ego as a datum of experience and the body as a part of the real world, and that it disappears as soon as this confusion is cleared up, has been beautifully demonstrated in Köhler's "Gestalt Psychology" and need therefore not be repeated here. Besides, the reader should be able to supply the argument himself.

EMOTIONS AND THOUGHTS. The localization of emotions does not seem any more difficult (barring the problem of the nature of the emotions themselves, which we shall take up later). But if we grant that emotions are processes with certain peculiarities, then their localizations in the Ego or external objects will depend on questions of proximity. When I see a rearing horse and hear its wild neighings, then the emotion carried by these processes will be incorporated in the horse. Conversely there must be special factors which will make the emotion appear as my own emotion, factors which must have the same relation to the Ego system that the rearing and neighing had to the horse system. To say more at the moment would be mere speculation. What holds for the emotions is true for the thoughts, except that we have still fewer concrete data to support our explanation with. We shall leave this to the future, satisfied that we have posed a problem and indicated possibilities of its solution.

THE NEEDS. CONSTANCY OF THE EGO DESPITE ITS LAPSE FROM THE BEHAVIOURAL WORLD. We could say the same about the needs, but they necessarily introduce a new and very important point. Emotions and thoughts are processes which, though they leave their traces in the organism, no longer exist after they have happened. But needs are, as we shall discuss more fully, states of tension which persist until they are relieved. Our most general aims are therefore permanent, tensions which last through great parts of our lives. These needs being our needs, they belong, of course, to the Ego system. Now we have discussed at least one case in which the behavioural field contained no Ego at all. Must we, then, assume that the Ego system had disappeared completely for the time being? Such an assumption would not be reconcilable with the facts, for the needs of the person survived that accident. Not only was he the same kind of person afterwards as before, with the same interests and ideals; he himself believes that his behaviour during his escape from the icy chasm was largely due to needs set up in his previous life. I translate again: "In retrospect it seems to me as though during this whole ascent my consciousness had never become fully clear. The purposiveness of my actions resembled more or less that of a somnambulist in the gutter on a roof; like a clockwork my brain did what for years I had planned to do. I cannot recommend warmly enough that one acquire the habit of dreaming through *all* possibilities in imagination. Although it makes one more cowardly, it also accounts for the flash-like 'presence of mind' which has often saved me" (l. c., p. 71). Our conclusion is clear: the disappearance of the Ego from the behavioural world does not mean for the normal adult an annihilation of the Ego. It survives as a part of the psychophysical field even when it is not represented in consciousness, and that forces us to the conclusion that normally, when the Ego exists in our behavioural world, this phenomenal, or conscious, Ego is not the whole Ego. It is probable that the Ego is first formed in organization which proceeds on the conscious level. But after it has been formed it becomes more and more stable, more and more independent of momentary conditions of organization, so that eventually it is a permanent segregated part of our total psychophysical field. This is, as I see it, the true justification of the various psychoanalytic theories which investigate the particular properties of this permanent Ego, the strains and stresses within it. The psychoanalytic terminology is, at least, misleading. The psychoanalysts' use of the term unconscious was unfortunate. We have briefly referred to it in our second chapter (p. 50 f.), where we said that the reason for this terminology would disappear if we treated the phenomena so designated as field events. Our Ego concept has fulfilled this promise. The Ego being a sub-system in a larger field, its states are field events even when this field is not the behavioural field, when it is not conscious. The emphasis on the "unconscious" seems to me to indicate, paradoxical as it may sound, an over-estimation of the conscious.[8] The term unconscious makes the conscious the reference point for all mental activity. The unconscious events are treated as though they were conscious. From the point of view here defended the mental or, if you like, the behaviour aspect transcends the phenomenal, the conscious, the latter being always but a small fragment of a much larger field event.

But rightly interpreted the principles of psychoanalysis cannot be dismissed by a shrug of the shoulder, much as the special claims of any psychoanalytic school may be open to just and severe criticism. The development of psychoanalysis has been influenced by the two poles which have affected the whole of psychology, the pole of mechanism, which was paramount in Freud's earlier work, and the pole of vitalism, vitalism even with a mystical tinge, which became so prominent in the later development, particularly in the hands of Jung. Psychoanalysis will, I dare to predict, enter a new and healthier state of development when it frees itself of the mechanistic and the vitalistic biases.

TWO CONSEQUENCES: (1) THE EGO AS CONSTANT AND DEVELOPING IN TIME; FOUNDATION OF A THEORY OF PERSONALITY. In a science which for such a long time has done all it could to disparage the idea of an Ego it is not easy to appraise justly the importance of our concept of the enduring Ego system. It may exert a far greater influence on the whole body of psychology than we can see at present. At the moment I shall only mention two consequences which it entails. In the first place it gives us a real basis for the scientific understanding of the development of a personality. For in all changes of the behavioural field the Ego remains as a segregated part. The segregation will not proceed along the same boundary lines all the time, it will not invariably be of the same strength, and the relative importance of the Ego in the field will change. Still the Ego within the total field seems comparable to the physical organism in its geographical environment. Both are strongly organized stable subsystems within a larger system, and just as in all changes the organism maintains its identity and thereby produces its growth and development, so will the Ego grow and develop by maintaining itself in the flux of the behavioural environment, or more generally of the psychophysical field. And the study of action as conduct is just the study of the continuous process of balancing the Ego subsystem in the total field, so that it may be possible to apply the

[8] See my article 1927.

principle of organic behaviour, which we have taken over from Humphrey, to the Ego. Now, the Ego in maintaining its identity in the stream of varying conditions must develop in accordance with the disturbances to which it is exposed and to the kind of Ego it is. It is in that respect not different from any real organism in any real environment. That the disturbances will vary enormously from case to case is so obvious as to need no further mention. But the Egos themselves, in their first formation, and owing to the nature of the individual psychophysical make-up, will perhaps not be less different. We shall go into the details of these differences later. Here we emphasize the point that mental development, as any other development, is not a mere chance affair, much as chance may affect it. The stable organization of the Ego system prevents it from being changed by every new influx. The term stability has, moreover, to be rightly interpreted. At no moment, even apart from external influences, can we regard the Ego to be completely balanced, completely at rest; the Ego in itself is fundamentally temporal, it is not a time-independent state. It is always going somewhere, and the stability of the Ego must, therefore, always be seen in relation to the direction in which it is moving. The law of good continuation which we discovered as a factor of space organization will find its application in this most vital problem of all psychology. Future work will, it is hoped, establish the workings of this principle. Its mere formulation is a step in breaking down the artificially erected barriers between scientific and understanding psychology, for it supplies to the study of personality what the "understanding psychologists" missed in the scientific body of psychology. Also the old problem of heredity and environment, of nature and nurture, will gain a new aspect from this side of our Ego-concept (Koffka, 1932).

(2) Mental Permanence Different from Memory. In the second place our Ego gives us "mental" permanence and continuity, which is different from memory as usually understood. After having abandoned the soul, psychology was left with the fleeting processes of each moment, with the stream of consciousness, although often enough psychologists treated ideas or images most inconsistently as actually persisting objects. The only factor to account for the consistency of mind was memory, a concept much more widely employed than clearly defined in much psychological writing. We shall treat memory later; we must only emphasize here that the persistence of the Ego is in our theory not a matter of memory, but of a direct persistence through time. Identity in time, persistence through time, may have different forms. A discussion of this point

would fall outside the scope of this book,[9] but two extreme cases may be mentioned: the persistence of a diamond, which is characterized by the fact that the same material which made it up yesterday makes it up today and will make it up tomorrow; and the persistence of an organism from conception to death, where the material of which it is composed changes constantly, and where even the form in which the material is organized is not constant. The second persistence can be called memory as little as the other. And therefore the persistence of the Ego, which must resemble the persistence of the organism, cannot be called memory either. On the other hand, as we shall see later, it is this persistence of the Ego which makes memory in some of its aspects possible. But if the Ego survives as a separate system, even when it disappears from consciousness or when consciousness disappears completely, it must survive in an environment from which it is segregated. Therefore the conclusion we have just drawn for the Ego applies also, in principle, to the behavioural environment. If the Ego persists as an actuality and not as mere potentiality, the same must be true of the behavioural world in which the Ego exists. And this conclusion must affect our whole theory of memory, as we shall see in a later chapter.

The Complexity of the Ego. We return to a more detailed study of the Ego as it is constituted at a given time. We have seen that its boundaries are variable, and that very fact implies that the Ego, unless it has shrunk to its minimum size, is complex, consists of a variety of parts which must be considered as sub-systems. Our modern psychology owes this conception of the complex character of the Ego to Lewin (1926). Its empirical foundation lies in facts of mental dynamics, in the realm of action. All action as a change of the pre-existing state requires forces to set it going, and so the question as to the nature of these forces has to be raised.

THE CAUSES OF ACTION. I write a letter to an absent friend. What makes me do so? The answer which during the last twenty years has been given to this and all questions of a similar kind by the behaviourists and those many other psychologists who fell under the sway of behaviourism, was: Writing, since it is a response, must have been evoked by a stimulus, just as the knee jerk occurs as a response when the tendon below the patella is stimulated by a tap. The stimulus-response concept had fascinated psychologists, particularly in America, and it was hard to argue against it, because

[9] But see Lewin 1922 a, and Humphrey.

any cause for an action which one demonstrated was at once downed by the question: Isn't that a stimulus, and how can any response take place without a stimulus? Therefore, if I said now that my writing of this letter was caused by my wish to do so, they might retort that the wish was the stimulus. But then they would be playing with words, and in this game the word stimulus would have lost all its original meaning by which it was to be an affection of a sense organ by an external agency. And such an external agency, such a stimulus in the legitimate sense, cannot be adduced to account for my action. The sight of neither pen nor paper is necessary to set my wish into execution. If I want to write and have no material at hand for carrying out my wish, I run over to the stationer's and buy it. If that is out of the question, I write a letter "in my mind." And when I have finally posted my letter, I may see pens and sheets of paper without beginning to write again. The writing of the letter must then be due to forces which disappear through the act of writing, to tensions which are being relieved by my writing. These tensions must be tensions within the Ego system, and action appears as a means of relieving these tensions.

THE COMPLEXITY OF THE EGO-STRUCTURE. ZEIGARNIK'S EXPERIMENTS. Now such a simple reflection leads at once to the conclusion that the Ego must be complex. Let us explore this complexity by considering one of the finest pieces of experimental work so far issued from Lewin's school, an investigation of remembering by Mrs. Zeigarnik. Since this investigation is as remarkable for its results as for its flawless technique, which proves that real experiments can be made in fields so much closer to the true psychological problems than any we have reported yet, I shall go somewhat into the detail of this study. The procedure of the experiment was to present the subjects during one sitting with a number of tasks (in one series twenty-two), half of which they were allowed to finish, while they were interrupted in the other half by the presentation of a new task at a time when they were well on the way to a solution. The subjects did not know beforehand whether they would be allowed to complete the tasks or not; they had no idea that interruption qua interruption was one of the principal features of the experiment. At the end of the hour the experimenter asked the subjects to tell her what they had been doing during the hour. Since after each task all materials had been put into a drawer "for the sake of keeping the table tidy," nothing in the situation had any direct connection with the diverse tasks. The subjects then enumerated a number of tasks, varying (for thirty-two subjects) between seven and nineteen, with an average of 11.1 = 50%; in another series with twenty different tasks (and fourteen subjects) between seven and sixteen, with an average of 10, again 50%. The experimenter then classified these tasks with regard to their completeness and incompleteness and thereby discovered whether either of these classes was favoured by recall. Since naturally some tasks will *per se* be better remembered than others, the total number of subjects was always divided into two groups, which received the same tasks but were treated differently with regard to completion; the tasks completed by one group were interrupted for the other. The relation of the remembered incomplete to the remembered complete tasks, $\frac{RI}{RC} = P$, is a numerical expression for any such preference. If $P = 1$, there is no difference between them; if $P > 1$, the incompleted ones are more frequently remembered; if $P < 1$, the completed ones are preferred.

THE SUPERIORITY OF THE INCOMPLETED TASKS. In the first series of thirty-two subjects P was equal to 1.9, in the second series with fourteen subjects $P = 2.0$. That is, the incompleted tasks were remembered about twice as often as the finished ones. The tasks were of all kinds and difficulties; they involved drawing, e.g., the continuation of a honeycomb pattern, other kinds of manual skill, like the stringing of beads or the punching of holes, ingenuity in combination, as in a jig-saw puzzle, certain memory tests, like the task of finding a German philosopher, actor, and city all beginning with the same designated letter. The result varied from task to task; some tasks (four in the first series) had P quotients greater than 3, and for three P was < 1. We disregard for the moment the influence of the task, and turn to the explanation of this perfectly clear result which was amply confirmed in group experiments, where P for forty-nine students turned out to be $=1.9$, and for forty-five children from elementary schools between thirteen and fourteen years of age $=2.1$.

TWO POSSIBLE EXPLANATIONS OF THIS SUPERIORITY REFUTED. A first explanation may be based on the emotional shock produced by the interruption. The emotional tone which the interrupted tasks received because of the interruption might be responsible for their better recall, in conformity with the view that an affective tone is favourable for memory.

This assumption was tested by the following method. Certain tasks must be interrupted, so as to be endowed with the emotional shock, but then again given for completion. The new presentation should for two reasons increase their recall value: on the one hand they would receive a second emotional tone by being presented for the second time, on the other the repetition of the same task should add to its memory value.

Two series were performed with this method. In the first, twelve subjects were given eighteen tasks, half of which were interrupted and not resumed while the other half was first interrupted and then completed. In the second series twelve other subjects were again given eighteen tasks, but there were now three kinds, the totally incompleted ones, the totally completed ones, and those that were first interrupted and then completed. In both series each task was as often of one kind as of the other. The first series yields again only one quotient, the incomplete over the interrupted-completed, $\frac{RI}{R(I\text{-}C)} = P'$, the second series this and the old P quotient.

The P′ quotient of the first of these two series was 1.85, i.e., exactly the same as the old P quotient, creating a strong presumption in favour of the conclusion that the tasks first interrupted and then completed are perfectly equivalent to those which are completed straight away. This conclusion is confirmed by the comparison of the P and P′ ratio of the second series, the former being 1.94, the latter 1.9, and the correlation between the two quotients for the different subjects being .8. The original assumption has thus been disproved. The tasks never completed are better remembered than those completed, whether the latter are temporarily interrupted or not. The emotional shock of the interruption can therefore not be the cause of the better recall of the incompleted tasks.

Another possible explanation of the superiority of the incompleted tasks would be that the subjects thought that they might be asked to finish the interrupted task later. Aall had proved that when subjects had been told before learning that they would be required to remember material for a long time, they remembered it better than when they had been given the instruction to learn for immediate recall. Although the situation in Zeigarnik's experiments was different from that in Aall's, a similar factor might have played a decisive rôle. This was tested by two new series, each with twelve subjects; in the first of these the subjects were told, when they were interrupted in a task, that the task would be completed later, in the second the interruption was characterized by the experimenter as final. If this explanation were right, the superiority of the incompleted tasks should be greater in the first of these two series than in the second. As a matter of fact P was in the first series 1.7, and in the second 1.8. Even though the difference is probably not significant, the assumption on which we started is disproved.

THE TRUE THEORY: THE TENSIONS AT THE MOMENT OF RECALL. Therefore the explanation has to be sought in the conditions which obtain at the moment of recall. It is here that the theory of systems under tension enters. The question of the experimenter, "What have you been doing this hour?" sets up a tension in the subject which is relieved by the actual recall. Similarly each task had set up a tension which was only relieved when the task was actually executed but remained unrelieved for the interrupted tasks. Therefore, at the moment of recall there exist two vectors deriving from these two tensions; the first is directed towards the recall of all tasks which had engaged the subject during the hour, the second one directed towards the completion of the unfinished ones. The result of the experiment indicates that the latter become effective also for recall, making the unfinished tasks more readily available. On the other hand it follows that the actual relation of remembered incomplete and complete tasks must depend upon the relative strength of these two vectors. Zeigarnik shows in a very thorough discussion of her results that these two assumptions are justified. The existence of the stresses towards completion is evidenced by the resistance which the subjects offered to the interruption and by the tendency to resume the tasks after the other work was finished. This last tendency was made the object of a special study by Miss Ovsiankina, which can only be mentioned here. Characteristically this tendency was much stronger with children than with adults, the former taking these tasks much more seriously than the latter. For days afterwards children would ask to be allowed to finish the incomplete tasks, while they never asked for the repetition of a completed task, however interesting it might have been. In conformity with this stronger stress towards resumption the children also had a higher P quotient, 2.5 as compared to 1.9.

The influence of the tension towards recall can be studied by a comparison of the different subjects. Some took the recall as a new task, comparable to the others, or even thought it was the main part of the experiment, which then appeared to them as a memory test; others, on the contrary, did not link the experimenter's question up with the experiment proper but treated the recall as an informal report, a social action. P for the former was 1.5, for the latter 2.8, the former remembering chiefly *more* finished tasks than the latter and thereby lowering their P quotient.

The same instruction, therefore, does not in the least guarantee that the subjects undertake the same tasks; only individual analysis, not a statistical treatment, can reveal such differences and their dynamic effects. The same is true of the effect of the interruption. Interruption of a task which has been completed subjectively though not objectively will have the effect of completion; the subject, really, though not in actual fact, having solved his problem, will have relieved his tension. Conversely, objective completion need not always coincide with subjective completion; the subject may feel that his success was more or less a chance affair, that he has not really mastered the task, and would not be able readily to accomplish it a second time. Such cases of objectively completed tasks are dynamically cases of incompleted ones. Individual analysis of P quotients bears out these arguments.

Lastly, the acceptance of a task itself will be different for different individuals. We have already seen that to the children these tasks meant more than to the adults, but it is possible to rob the task completely of its individual task character by making each individual task a mere specification of the general task, viz., behave as a good subject, do what the experimenter tells you. For such a subject there can be no incompleted task, because the interruption is to him as much a fulfilment of his general task as a real completion. This deduction was specially tested by a group of 10 high school children who had been told by their teacher that they should go to the psychological laboratory to see what such a place was like. They were not interested in the tasks themselves, only in the fact that in a psychological laboratory such tasks were being used. The result was that their average P quotient was 1.03, varying between 1.5 and .8, whereas the variation in the very first series with average P value of 1.9 had been from 6.0 to .75! Thus incompletion qua mere objective lack of completion does not exert any favourable influence on recall at all; only such incompletion does as sets up real tensions.

COMPLEX NATURE OF EGO: THE DIFFERENT SUB-SYSTEMS. And now we can at last use these experiments to prove the complex nature of the Ego, by stating explicitly what has been implicit in this whole discussion. We spoke of tensions set up by each task and retained by the incompleted ones. That means, of course, that each of these incompleted tasks must have been a sub-system, relatively independent of the other sub-systems. Without this degree of independence the discharge of tensions would have cleared the whole system. The fact, on the other hand, that the incompleted tasks were better remembered proves that they really belonged to separate systems. But this deduction was again submitted to new experimental tests. The whole experiment was so conducted that isolation of the different tasks was made more difficult or entirely prevented. The procedure was very simple. At the beginning of the hour the subjects were told all the tasks which they were to undertake during the hour. In this way their task became: all these things I shall have to do, whereas in the other experiments each individual problem had been a task by itself. The eight subjects who worked with this new instruction gave a P quotient of .97, with a variation between 1.25 and .75; that is, in the averages there was no difference between the completed and the incompleted tasks, owing to the fact that at the end of the hour the total task, viz., working at the previously known number of different problems, had been finished.

FATIGUE PREVENTS THE ESTABLISHMENT OF WELL-INSULATED SUB-SYSTEMS. The establishment of separate systems under tension can also be prevented by other means. If the subject is tired at the time of working on the tasks,[10] the P quotient is <1, the average P of ten subjects being .74, with a variation between 1.2 and .5. Of these ten subjects five had six months previously taken part in the regular experiment. Their average P at that time had been 2.18, while it was now .79, the fact of the repetition itself being without any influence, as other experiments proved. During fatigue, then, insulated sub-systems which can preserve their tensions are not so easily produced—it would be premature to say that they cannot be produced at all, since for adult persons these tasks involve relatively irrelevant problems, which should not be taken as typical of all possible tensions; the explanation is that in fatigue the system is less solid, less able to establish strong insulating walls between different parts.

The same result, $P = .78$, was obtained with excited subjects; in this case the variable extra tensions which caused the excitement prevented the establishment of the small sub-systems.

THE COMPLETED TASKS MORE STABLE THAN THE INCOMPLETED ONES. Why, however, is in these cases $P < 1$ and not $= 1$? The answer given to this question by Zeigarnik is the more interesting since we shall learn later of entirely different experiments by M. R. Harrower which prove the same principle. The answer is this: a completed task is a closed whole and therefore leaves a trace of a well organized and stable nature, while the traces left by the incompleted tasks,

[10] Special experiments with a separation between the work on the problems and the recall showed that fatigue at the time of remembering had no such effect.

now that they do not have the tension towards completion, lack this stability which derives from complete closure. Being less stable these traces are less likely to survive, and less powerful in determining future recall. Zeigarnik points out that this argument adds new weight to her main result, the superiority of the incompleted tasks for recall, inasmuch as it proves "that the dynamic tensions of the respective quasi-needs is in our experiments of incomparably greater importance for recall than the stable closure of the completed form" (p. 69). However, in consideration of Harrower's later experiments, briefly referred to, a slightly different interpretation seems equally possible if not more plausible. The very tensions which remain in the incomplete task-systems may keep them at a greater degree of organization. The two factors which Zeigarnik sets against each other are not mutually independent; recall depends to a high degree, as Harrower has proved, upon the organization possessed by a trace, and the Zeigarnik tensions are a factor which contributes to the preservation of such organization.

PERSISTENCE OF THE TENSIONS. How long will these tensions persist? That must depend upon the persistence of the walls which separate the sub-system from the rest of the Ego. And this, in its turn, must be a function of the initial firmness of the walls and the forces which attack them. Since, however, at least during our waking life more and more tensions are created and relieved within our total Ego system, the constraining walls of any one sub-system will be constantly exposed to pressure from the outside so that we shall expect the tensions within to disappear unless the walls are strong enough to withstand such perpetual battering. It is not likely that the sub-systems created in Zeigarnik's experiments were of that nature and therefore we should expect the superiority of the incompleted tasks to disappear if the recall is made sufficiently long after the original performance. This prediction was proved to be true by special experiments. Eleven subjects, tested for recall 24 hours after the original work, had an average P of 1.14, and eight of these, who had six months previously taken part in a normal experiment with a P of 2.1, now had a P of 1.13.

That time qua time is not responsible for the difference, but only inasmuch as it contains other occurrences, is proved by new experiments with a much shorter interval between work and recall (10-30 minutes), which, however, was filled with highly emotional experiences; the subjects' systems were, as Zeigarnik puts it, thoroughly shaken up. Six such subjects had an average P of .64.

It would be interesting to see whether an interval of twelve hours would have a different effect on the conservation of the stressed systems if it was passed in waking or sleeping; experiments performed after the pattern of those by Jenkins and Dallenbach on retroactive inhibition should decide this issue. That tensions of not too high intensity in small sub-systems may disappear through mere "leakage" due to a loss of the wall-stability has thus been proved. But one should be cautious in generalizing from these cases to others where higher tensions and larger sub-systems are involved. One might indeed be tempted to explain the rather trivial saying that time heals all wounds by this principle. But where very strong needs belonging to the core of the Ego are concerned the dynamics of this leaking process may be of quite a different kind.

COMMUNICATION WITH MORE CENTRAL PARTS OF THE EGO. THE SELF. This leads us to a last point in connection with Zeigarnik's work. So far we have attributed the tensions exclusively to the subjects' acceptance of the tasks put before them, i.e., to their intention to solve these tasks. There are two other possibilities: (1) the incompleteness of the tasks as such, apart from the original intention to solve them, might produce a stress towards completion. This cause, which we shall discuss later when we treat of thinking, has probably been virtually negligible in Zeigarnik's experiments. (2) The tasks may not be as isolated as we assumed but may be in communication with other and deeper systems of the Ego. Zeigarnik found among her subjects nine persons who seemed particularly ambitious. The average P for these subjects was 2.75, as compared to 1.9 of the general average, with a variation from 6 to 1.5. What does that mean? For an ambitious person to miss the solution of a task means "failure," means that the achievement has fallen below his "personal standard," means therefore a definite affection of that part of the Ego system which we shall now call the "Self." The importance of this Self system, its dynamics in behaviour, and its relation to success and failure will be discussed much later. Here it must be emphasized that if the tasks of the experiment were in communication with the Self either through ambition or through other channels, then the tensions of the incompleted tasks became particularly strong, whereas such subjects as excluded their Selves completely from the experiment, who despised these childish occupations, had tensions far below the average, their P being 1.1 (six subjects).

Conclusion for Complex Structure of Ego. Thus these experiments have led us far beyond the original confines. Over and above the relatively temporary sub-systems which they investigated, they led us straight on to a permanent sub-system, the Self, whose tensions are much greater than those of the other sub-systems, representing real needs as opposed to the quasi-needs of our superficial intentions. And this gives us a new insight into the nature of the complexity of the Ego: the sub-systems do not simply exist side by side, they are organized in various ways. One principle of organization is that of surface-depth organization. The Ego has a core, the Self, and enveloping this core, in various communications with it and each other, are other sub-systems, comparable to different layers, until we come to the surface, which is most easily touched, and most easily discharged. Another principle of organization concerns the communication between the different systems, a third relative dominance.

THE EXECUTIVE

Action, we said before, results as a process of relieving existing stresses. This aim may be achieved in a great variety of ways for which we shall introduce the name "the executive."[11] The executive comprises, then, all the ways in which action can relieve stresses or contribute to such relief.

Not All Relief of Stresses Is Action. Not all relief of stresses, however, is action. Sensory organization, with its interplay of forces resulting in a minimum of remaining tension in the sensory field, is a relief of stress without action. Action occurs in such organized fields and frequently reduces the stresses within them. But it may even be that after a first sensory organization has been achieved the stresses within it are so strong as to change it without action, i.e., without interference of the executive, and we shall find similar events in processes of thought. We shall disregard these cases and turn instead to the workings of the executive. In most cases the executive will relieve stresses by producing movements of the body or some of its parts. Thus in vision the executive works through accommodation, fixation, and convergence; the stress which makes me write my letter is relieved by the actual writing of it, which includes actual bodily movements. And the same is true in so many other cases that the question arises whether it is not true in all cases, namely, that the executive is the power of the psychophysical field to initiate and regulate the movements of the body. But the an-

[11] Lewin uses the term "Motorik" which can only be translated as "motor system." I shall not adopt this term for two reasons. On the one hand the addition of the word "system" in English would introduce an ambiguity, since the executive does not constitute a system in the sense in which we have used the word. On the other hand, tensions can be relieved by other means than actual movements of the body or any of its parts. Therefore I prefer the wider term of the text.

swer to this question must be negative. I can think of at least two classes of stress relief where ordinary motor phenomena play either no rôle at all or not the decisive one. To the one class belong the attitudes, to the other thoughts. Let us begin with the latter. We have mentioned before that my wish to write a letter may be temporarily satisfied by my writing the letter merely "in my head," i.e., in thought. True enough, as a rule this will not definitely assuage my desire, but it certainly is a process which to a certain degree lessens the existing tensions. Now in this action no actual movement need occur, or where it occurs, as the incipient vocalizations of internal speech, these movements qua movements do not relieve the stress in the way in which accommodation does, or my taking off my overcoat when I feel too warm. It is the thought process itself that has the decisive function in our case, and those vocal movements are of significance only as far as they are necessary for thought. Another example: I am faced with a scientific problem which I want to solve. A stress exists, and again it is relieved by mere thinking. What kind of process this is we shall discuss in another chapter. But whatever it is, it may belong to the executive.

Let us now turn to attitudes. We are shown a puzzle picture like that of "my wife and my mother-in-law" published by Boring. We see one face and we are curious to find the other. What can we do to relieve this tension? Just remain directed towards the picture, changing perhaps the point on which our "attention" is centred, but keeping the pattern within the field of our interest, and waiting. The relief is accomplished when under this attitude the picture reorganizes itself so that we see the heretofore hidden face. Certainly our attitude may be more specific, we may try to see a certain line as a mouth, a certain area as a chin, and so forth, but all these attempts have only an indirect effect by facilitating the change of sensory organization. With these effects in my mind I defined the executive by stating that it either relieved pressure or contributed to such relief.

Direct and Indirect Effects of the Executive. This gives us one criterion by which we can discriminate various executive functions, direct and indirect, a distinction which cuts across our first division according to the kind of process involved. For motor performances also may have only an indirect effect; in our last example of the puzzle picture, e.g., a change of fixation may help to produce the change of organization, or switching on the lamp may relieve the stress of discomfort which we feel when we read at dusk. And the same point of view is, as we shall see later, applicable to thought.

Our two examples have made it evident that the indirect way of relief may have various forms, which in their turn might serve as a principle for classifying actions and their dynamics.

The Control of the Executive. Three Cases. But there is another equally important point of view for differentiating between different forms of the executive. We compare three examples: accommodation, the writing of the letter, and the flight from a danger. In the first the stress is entirely limited to the sensory field; it is relieved by a movement which is started and regulated by this field-stress, and has nothing to do with the Ego. In the second case the stress resides completely within the Ego system; the relief is started by this stress, the actual execution of the action which it entails may be regulated by the field, my pen, paper, support and so forth. In the last case the stress arises *between* the Ego and a field object, say a snake. This stress starts the movement, which again will be more or less directed by other field forces. The relation of the executive to the Ego is different in each of the three cases. In the first it has nothing to do with it, in the second the Ego is its main cause, while in the third the stress exists between the Ego and an object and disappears normally with the removal of the object.

Two Possible Interpretations of the Last Case. This last case, which we have not considered before, raises a difficult problem. In the first the executive was clearly under the control of the sensory field, in the second equally clearly under the control of the Ego. But how is it in the third? Two alternatives appear: the first being that the Ego-object stresses control the executive, the second that in this case also the actual control belongs to the Ego. The argument for this second possibility would run like this: the snake creates fear, i.e., a certain strong need for flight within the Ego, and it is this Ego need which initiates the actual movements. This interpretation could point to the fact that often the action persists long after the object which produced the stress has disappeared from the field. One might run for dear life for a long time after one was out of any danger, and the fright emotion might not subside even then. Furthermore, very strong reactions to particular field objects or events may leave tensions in the system which will break out again and again as neurotic symptoms. In short, there is sufficient evidence for the assumption that in such cases one or more of the Ego systems have been strongly affected and that it is their tension that is responsible for the behaviour, that the executive is entirely under Ego control.

LEWIN'S THEORY OF THE RECIPROCAL RELATION BETWEEN NEEDS AND DEMAND CHARACTERS. Lewin's theory of the reciprocal relation between a demand character and a need also seems to adopt this interpretation. Thus he says: "To a certain degree the two propositions: 'this or that need exists' and 'this or that range of objects possesses a demand character for these or those actions' are equivalent" (1926 a, p. 353).

This proposition is derived from a number of facts in which the demand character disappears with the satisfaction of the need, the relief of the particular tension. The most delicious food ceases to attract us after a copious meal, and the letter box, which just now interrupted my conversation and made me cross the street to post an important letter, leaves me completely cold when I pass it again on my way back. Furthermore "a person's world undergoes a fundamental change when his fundamental aims are changed" (Lewin, 1926 a, p. 353), because all demand characters change; things which were indifferent become attractive and important, repulsive ones may become indifferent, the attractive ones repulsive, and so on.

THE OTHER POSSIBILITY. However, neither of these arguments is absolutely conclusive. The first may mean no more than that in many such cases where the original stress derives from a field object the Ego becomes charged so that its own stresses participate in the control of the executive and may eventually have complete control over it, although originally the executive was under the influence of the object-Ego stresses. On the other hand Lewin acknowledges the type of action which he calls "field-action," "i.e., an action which takes place directly according to the field forces" (p. 378).

If we grant that the object-Ego stress can charge the Ego, we admit a direct effect exerted by the object on the Ego. It is, then, an equally plausible assumption that this same stress may affect the executive. As a matter of fact it seems quite likely that this effect is quicker than the other, that it takes more time to charge an Ego system with tensions which will in their turn control the executive than it does to influence the latter directly. The fact that frequently a quick action provoked by the situation precedes the emotion seems to support this interpretation. But we shall have to go into the nature of the demand characters before we can with greater conviction decide for this alternative.

What, then, does Lewin mean by demand characters? Let us approach this question from a very general point of view.

THE DEMAND CHARACTERS. Our description of the total field has so far been incomplete. We have emphasized the articulation of the field into a number of separate objects, those which form the behavioural environment and that which composes our Ego, but we have failed to emphasize explicitly that the product of organization is a unity, though in this unity the various parts have a greater or smaller degree of independence. As far as the behavioural environment goes this independence is often very great. The removal of the telephone from the right-hand corner of my desk does not change the aspect of the books right in front of me, and innumerable other examples prove the same point. On the other hand to put a pile of cigarette boxes next to an Egyptian statuette spoils to some extent the effect of the latter, also we do not hang side by side a picture by Renoir and one by Dürer, or set a Chinese vase on a modern steel table. This indicates that the segregation of the behavioural objects is not complete, that each object has around it a "field" which it determines, so that conversely it will be affected if this field is distorted by another object or its field. As a matter of fact we have already discussed a striking illustration of this, the Jastrow illusion (Chapter II, pp. 32 f.), and have seen that this influence exerted by one field object on another is not restricted to human fields but has been proved also for chickens. In one respect, certainly, the Jastrow illusion is different from our other examples. In the illusion the effect is "silent," to use again Köhler's term; we see two ring sectors of different size without any direct knowledge that this difference is due to their interaction. In the other instances, on the contrary, the actual effect of change is much less striking than in the case of the illusion—it is, for instance, much more difficult to describe in what respect the Dürer picture has changed by the introduction of the Renoir picture—but the mutual influence appears in experience itself as that feeling of incompatibility which prevents us from hanging our pictures in such combinations.

One must not object to this argument that there would be many people who would neither detect a change in the Dürer picture when the Renoir is hung by its side nor feel the slightest incongruity in such an arrangement. The influence we speak of is an influence existing between the pictures not as geographical but as behavioural objects, and the behavioural objects depend also upon the organism whose behavioural objects they are. The old maxim: *Si duo faciunt idem, non est idem,* has its counterpart in the maxim: *Si duo vident idem, non est idem.* A Renoir can affect a

Dürer only if both are seen "properly," and not just as two pictures, or as two *objets d'art* worth so and so many thousand dollars.

An Excursion into Aesthetics. The question what their "proper" appearances are belongs rightly to aesthetics. But we may devote a few words to it, particularly since this discussion will help us later in the solution of the problem which at the moment holds our main interest.

The "Proper Quality" of a Work of Art. Is there, so many psychologists and relativists in general will ask, a "proper" way in which a picture should be seen, a piece of music heard, a poem or a drama understood? Can science do more than describe as fully as possible all the various ways in which these products of art, in the widest sense of the word, are apprehended? How can science discriminate between persons and attribute greater weight to one man's apprehension than to that of another? How can science introduce value, objective standards, according to which one could say to any one person: You *should* see this picture in this particular way and not in that?

This relativistic argument sounds very plausible; it gains added weight from the fact that aestheticians and critics who stood up for and stuck to absolute standards have so often been mistaken when they rejected as fraudulent impositions on a gullible public works which afterwards were recognized as some of the great masterpieces of all times. Does not this failure of the critics, which has occurred with almost every new movement in any of the arts, prove conclusively that the scientist can do no more than register the different reactions without any evaluation of their intrinsic worth? Were the critics who refused to take van Gogh seriously and kept him from selling a single picture during his lifetime so much more stupid than our critics who now appreciate him?

We can easily reject so simple an explanation without accepting the consequence which the relativists would derive from such a rejection. The relativist's argument neglects in the first place the distinction between the picture as a geographical and a behavioural object. But the mere fact that critics disagree with regard to a behavioural object does nct even indicate that they find different things beautiful or ugly, if we now mean by things behavioural ones, which are the only ones that can directly affect their aesthetic judgments. For it may happen, nay, it must happen, that the geographical object produces two radically different behavioural ones in our two critics. If our two critics are called A and B, the geographical picture, or other work of art, P, and the two behavioural art-objects P_a and P_b, then A, who likes P, does so on the ground of P_a, and B, who dislikes it, is guided by P_b. It is still possible that A would dislike P_b as much as B, and B like P_a as much as A, if either of them could realize these behavioural objects. Now, although it is impossible to make any P_a absolutely like a P_b, it is possible to make it so in fundamental respects, fundamental enough at any rate to make B change from condemnation to admiration, or A from praise to contempt. A great deal, if not the most important part, of our education in art appreciation attempts just this, and, as I believe, with a fair amount of success. The aesthetician should therefore ask his question of the existence of general standards first with regard to the P_a, P_b, and then turn to the relation between these, $P_{a,b}$ and P, a question which he cannot avoid since the artist creates a P and can produce the $P_{a,b} \ldots$ only through the medium of P. We can only take up the second question as to the relation between the painting on the canvas and the experience of the picture, because it is a more general formulation of our former problem whether there is a "proper" way of seeing a picture, hearing a piece of music. Whether such a proper P_a, if it exists, is good or bad will depend upon the circumstances; why it is good or bad is a question which we must leave unanswered, since the theory of art is not our topic.

We return to the fact that the $P_{a,b} \ldots$ are not simple functions of P, but also of the A, B . . . We may express this by the formula $P_n = f\ (P, N)$, which is only a brief form of applying our general theorem that every behavioural object depends upon the external and internal conditions to the case of art-apprehension. In order to understand the variability of the P_n with a constant P we must, then, examine the variability of the N. If we confine the range of our N to normal individuals, we exclude such variations as colour-blindness, lack of power of articulation, and similar ones. But there remain others of greater importance for our particular problem. For each N is an organism with its history. Each critic, to return to the concrete case, has seen many pictures and has formed his taste by them. What does that mean? We have, in order to answer this question, to introduce a new concept, a concept akin to our framework category. To do so we must again envisage each individual person in his full reality, which includes time, and we shall thereby add another new characteristic to the behavioural world itself. When we described it as composed at any moment of a number of well segregated objects we gave a true picture. But when we go beyond the moment, another statement must be added: temporally considered, most objects which appear in our behavioural world are not completely isolated; a new object appears, it is large, yellow with purple trimmings, ornamented with silver clasps and what not; in short it is different from everything we have seen before, and yet it is a *book*. We walk through the streets of New York, and we see men and women although they are perfect strangers. Generalized, the behavioural world, temporally considered, consists of a great number of class-objects which is very much smaller than the number of all individual objects. Such a class is a very real psychological reality, because it determines the actually appearing individual object. To us a Chinese or a Papuan in his native dress looks strange, and similarly we look outlandish to Chinese or Papuans who come in contact with white people for the first time. In these cases there exists a conflict of forces: on the one hand, the person of the other race still appears with the claim to be a human being; on the other he does not fit the class schema of human beings as it has been built up. The results of this conflict may take various forms, only two of which will be mentioned. Provided that the conflict does not remain a more or less isolated occurrence but becomes fairly regular, the class schema itself will be affected: a human being will now be something that may have any colour of skin and whose main characteristics will appear equally well in different forms. But although this is the most stable resolution of the conflict, it is not, unfortunately, very easily achieved. As a rule the class schema remains unaffected and determines the characteristic of the individuals who, although they raise the claim to belong to it, deviate from it in certain striking aspects. The class schema, then, forms a sort of framework, or standard, and what does not fit into the framework, or does not conform to the standard, appears as inferior. The stranger is the barbarian; he is inferior in every respect, simply because he is different from the type; he is less intelligent, less honest, less sensitive, and so forth.[12] The application to our art critics is simple. When we see a picture, we do not only see this particular object, different from all other objects, but we see a picture, i.e., a member of a class. And therefore its quality will depend to a large extent upon the degree to which it fits into our picture schema. In Mohammedan countries, where pictures have been newly introduced and where there are consequently no standards, this innovation is greeted with acclaim, and every picture is desirable. Thus in Samarkand one sees

[12] Another reason for the aversion to strangers will be discussed in a later chapter.

the streets lined with photographers who have the most atrocious backgrounds, canvasses painted in the most vulgar manner and representing ugly objects, against which the patrons stand to have their photographs taken. And that in a city which harbours a great number of superb Islamic buildings with glorious façades. The reason is simple. The Islamic religion forbids the taking of pictures. Therefore the people there grew up without pictures; with the old political order the religious order collapsed also, pictures were introduced and as a part of the new order were in themselves something good. The result may, of course, all too easily be that the picture schema which these people build up will be a very bad one indeed. That one cannot explain this delight in horrid pictures by the innate lack of taste of these peoples is clearly proved by the fact that they do not accept jazz music. They had their own music, and to that they faithfully stick.

Our critics, however, have a picture schema. And if their schemas are as rigid as most of our schemas are, they will necessarily perceive as inferior a new work of art which does not fit into them. But schemas, historically considered, are not immutable. The more works of the new kind are produced, the more will they contribute to the picture schema, particularly since the different schemas are not unrelated to each other. The same needs that make one or more painters paint new pictures will make architects erect new buildings, musicians compose new music, poets write new poems, and even the dressmakers invent new fashions. Consequently the same forces appearing in different fields, moulding different class schemas, will support each other mutually. Moreover, there will always be men whose schemas are not so rigid as to remain unaltered by the appearance of a new object. Thus, if our critics delight in van Gogh it is not because they are of themselves better critics, but because they have had a chance to develop other schemas than those who held his pictures up to ridicule when he painted them.

Summary: The Class as a Temporal Characteristic of Our Whole Behavioural Environment. Let us pause for a moment to consider what we have so far achieved. We have added a category to the description and explanation of our behavioural environment which, quite apart from its value in aesthetics, is of paramount importance in introducing time into the structure of our world. Style, fashion, manners, frequently enough even morals, are all manifestations of the same fundamental principle, the development of class schemas with their particular "levels." These class levels play a part perfectly comparable to the spatial framework, inasmuch as they also "put things in their places."

By introducing the class level and demonstrating its effect upon the appearance of things we have at least opened the door for the introduction of absolute standards in aesthetics. For if a work of art is condemned because it does not fit the schema, it is not condemned on its own merits. Expressed in our old terminology: the work P is rejected because it appears as $P_{non\text{-}s}$, as a P determined by its deviation from the schema s, and not as it would appear without any schema or without the particular schema of the critic.

Class Schema and Absolute Value. The relativist may grant all this and interpret it as an argument in support of his own position. He will say: Each P_n has to be taken for what it is, an experience occurring under special conditions. We can even go further and find that historically certain P_n are apt to appear first and gradually to disappear in favour of others. By studying the causes of these changes we may even be able to explain the history of aesthetic appreciation, but nowhere shall we get beyond the mere facts into a realm of value, at no point of this whole investigation will the question as to the "proper" P_n emerge. But this argument forgets the artist, the man who created P, and who in doing so wanted to create something definite, who in his work was guided by an idea of his picture which we shall call P_a. We are not concerned here with the question whether any particular P_a is good or bad, nor whether such a distinction is valid; neither do we consider the question whether the P which he has created is an adequate expression of P_a, i.e., an object which will in the proper persons produce a P_n which is fundamentally like P_a. Our point here is only that the existence of the P_a introduces a criterion by which we can discriminate between the P_n. For those will be the most proper among them which come closest to the P_a. This would be a perfectly valid criterion if we knew what the P_a is. But as a rule the artist leaves us the P and nothing more. Still, the mere existence of the P_a justifies our distinction of proper and improper apprehensions of works of art, even if we cannot in a given case decide which is the proper one. This may seem a small gain which for all practical purposes would leave the relativist's position unshaken. But we can go a step further, although I can do no more here than indicate the direction this step will have to take.

We go to a concert and hear a pianist play a piece of music. The critics will then say whether he has played it well or not. What does that mean? One criterion would be that he has played the score correctly, i.e., all notes of the score as they stand, with the proper tempo and rhythm. But this is neither sufficient nor even necessary for the judgment that the pianist gave a good performance. One man may play with perfect technique and literally correctly, and yet the critics and the audience will be disappointed, his reproduction will appear empty and shallow. Another man may play with great freedom, not sticking always to the score, but he will produce an effect which will stir the audience and make the critics say that despite his inaccuracies he has rendered the spirit of the work more faithfully than the correct player. And I have no doubt that the composer would agree with this judgment of the critics. Often enough a famous virtuoso or conductor will present a piece better than the composer could, as the composer will gladly admit. That seems to indicate that in a great work of art the P demands a certain P_n rather than another, and that the performance of the artist, which mediates between the P, the score, and the P_n, is judged according to its capacity of producing the proper P_n.

This is nothing entirely new. When we discussed the laws of perception we saw that for the majority of stimulus distributions there is one most stable organization. When we look for the first time at the picture of Fig. 50 (p. 173) we are puzzled; something in the pattern is not right. We may discard it as a silly jumble of lines, but when we see it again and again we shall be dissatisfied with its chaotic nature. There seems to be something within it which demands a better order. As soon as the face appears everything is all right. The strain has disappeared and we shall find it very difficult to see the original chaos again when we are presented with the same pattern. Now it seems clear that in this example the face is the proper P_n, the chaos of lines an improper one. And then we see how on purely psychological grounds we must acknowledge that there are proper and improper ways of apprehending a work of art.

Return to Non-Silent Forces in the Behavioural Environment. Let us now return to our main problem, the non-silent influence exerted by one object in the behavioural environment on another, the incongruity of an Egyptian statuette and a pile of cigarette boxes. We say that persons who feel such incongruities and arrange their rooms in such a way that such incongruities do not appear have good taste. By this we mean that they are capable of seeing things in their proper way and of seeing greater parts of the behavioural world in unity. It may be necessary to do the first without the second as in an auction room where all sorts of objects are put into view. Here the proper attitude of the expert who wants to buy is to isolate each object as much as possible. But the rooms in which we live will look the better, the more we are able to perceive them as unities in which the "fields" of the different objects do not clash with each other. The less a person perceives a room as a unit, the less will he experience such clashes, and the less taste are his rooms likely to reveal. But the fact that for some persons any combination of objects is possible does not prove that for those others who are grossly offended by incongruities of style or quality these characters of ugliness and bad taste do not exist. These "incompatibilities," then, are true properties within the behavioural world of those who experience them. Thus we see that even within the behavioural environment organization is not entirely silent.

Dynamic Relations Between Objects and Ego. Objects Determining Our Behaviour. From the fields of forces which surround the objects in our behavioural environment and affect other objects therein, we now turn to the dynamic relations which exist between the objects and the Ego. A description of the objects within our behavioural environment would be incomplete and inadequate if we omitted that some of these objects were attractive, others repulsive, and others indifferent, the terms attractive and repulsive to be taken in the broadest sense. Now for an object to be attractive means that there are forces within the field starting from the object which tend to shorten the distance between it and myself; the opposite is true of repulsive objects, whereas the indifferent objects exert no such pressure upon me. Within the two groups of attractive and repulsive objects there exists again a variety of special characteristics. A handle wants to be turned, a step invites a two-year-old infant to climb it and jump down from it (Lewin), chocolate wants to be eaten, a mountain to be climbed, and so forth. There is less differentiation in the repulsive group, naturally, since a negative behaviour will depend much less in its detailed execution upon the particular object by which it is started. Nevertheless we can distinguish the group of escape and avoidance reactions, ranging from a mere turning of the eyes to panicky flight, and the destruction reactions, which may be regarded as lying between the limits of tearing up a piece of paper and the drum fire of modern warfare.

The Origin of These Forces. At any rate the things in our environment tell us what to do with them; they may do so more or less urgently and with any degree of specificity. But their doing so indicates a field of force between these objects and our Egos, a field force which in many cases leads to action, and which is in most cases of the non-silent kind. What is the origin of these forces?

Examples: (1) Letter Box. In order to answer this question we have to discuss several examples. We begin with the letter box which attracts us when we are carrying a letter in our pocket but is an indifferent object once the letter is disposed of. In this case no property of the letter box as a visual object is responsible for our action. The red pillar in England will have the same effect as the green receptacle in the U. S. or the blue boxes in Germany. I must have learned that these objects are letter boxes, in other words these objects must have acquired a definite relation to my behaviour. In the second place, however, these objects, once they have acquired the character of being letter boxes, will influence my behaviour directly only under special conditions, viz., when I want to post a letter. Their dynamic function then is to effect the actual execution of a deferred action; they affect the Ego in such a way that a system—intention to post a letter—which up to that moment was under tension and did not control the executive, gains that control. The action itself, however, derives ultimately from the intention, i.e., from the tension within the particular Ego system. This case is typical of a great many. It exemplifies Lewin's theory of the reciprocity of a need and a demand character, for the very aspect of the red or green or blue object which makes me approach it and drop a letter into it is called by Lewin its demand character. Indeed, without the need to post a letter this object, although it appears in my field not as a coloured object but as a letter box, does not have this particular demand character. The dynamic situation, then, is this: I have a need which for the moment cannot be satisfied; then an object appears in my field which may serve to relieve that tension, and then this object becomes endowed with a demand character—the emergence of the particular object and its endowment with a demand character may actually be two different moments, but it may also be that the object emerges simultaneously with the demand character, in which case the need would have been effective in the very first organization of the object; since we have as yet no exact knowledge of the condition under which either of these two cases is realized, we neglect this difference.

The next step is that our behaviour changes, the unrelieved stress gets command of the executive; but the action is regulated by the object with the demand character; in other words, the executive must be also under the influence of the force which, as demand character, issues from the latter. Thus, dynamically speaking, this case is very complex, because of the rôle which the Ego plays in it. At first, through a tension within one of its sub-systems, it determines the field organization, and then its actions are codetermined by the object which it has endowed with the attractive (or repulsive) force. Even in this case we cannot describe the situation, however, without granting to the forces between the Ego and the object some influence on the executive, although the Ego tension which pre-existed before the object appeared, is the prime mover, the chief commander of the executive.

(2) Food. Let us turn from momentary quasi-needs, intentions, resolves, etc., to more fundamental motives. The hungry animal will be attracted by food, the animal after a good meal will leave the same food unheeded—again a close correlation between need and demand character. How delicious a beefsteak looks when we return from a long walk, and how cold we feel towards it after a sumptuous repast. It no longer looks the same, having lost its demand character. There remains, however, one question: Why does the beefsteak and not the napkin or a candlestick look delicious to the hungry man? It seems a silly question to ask, for we can eat the former, but not the latter, as we know by experience. But I did not want my question to be taken quite so literally. Why does a young hungry animal, like a chick, peck at certain objects and not at others? How can the chick know that the things it pecks at are eatable? It is easy to quash this question by the counter-question: How do I know that the animal knows?

Instinct vs. Reflex-theory. This antithesis of point of view is the quintessence of a good deal of the discussion of instinct. Those psychologists who try to keep that orderliness and purposiveness in their theories which they observed in the behaviour of animals would speak of instinctive activities in such cases as we are discussing now, while those who try to exclude orderliness from their premises would speak of mere reflexes, i.e., stimulus-response connections. The difference between these two interpretations, as far as it affects us here, comes to this: whereas the reflex theory connects behaviour directly with the stimulus, the instinct theory connects it, in our terminology, with the behavioural environment of the animal, or with its psychophysical field, and that in such a way that it ascribes to the particular field-part such qualities as make it arouse the specific reaction. Thus MacDougall says: "Reflex action is response to a stimulus; instinctive action is in many cases a response to an object," and the capacity for perception "is given in the innate constitution of the animal and is as essential a part of the total instinctive disposition (or instinct) as the capacity to execute the train of bodily movements which catch our eye"; and lastly: "We may therefore define 'an instinct' as an innate disposition which determines the organism to perceive . . . any object of a certain class, and to experience in its presence a certain emotional excitement and an impulse to action . . ." (1923, pp. 75, 99, 110). In our terminology this would mean that because of its instinctive endowment an animal will see certain objects as things to be eaten, others as things to be killed, others again as things to run away or hide from. In other words the adherents of a true instinct theory would claim that because of their instinctive endowment animals see certain objects with certain demand characters. We can easily avoid the disputable term instinct and yet retain the gist of this theory, for we have all along declined to explain action in terms of stimulus-response connections and have instead established the dependency of action upon properties of the psychophysical field or the behavioural environment of the animal. Thus our question as to the reasons for the animal's selection in its search for food is a perfectly legitimate question. The animal, under the stress of a hunger need, approaches certain objects which it eventually swallows. This means that there must be something in the object that makes it attractive, even if it possesses this demand character only when the animal is hungry. Since from the very first there is some selection, since not all objects are endowed with demand characters, and certainly not all with the same ease, there must be something in these objects to account for this selection. In formulating our conclusion thus, we put the reason in the (behavioural) object and not in a mystical knowledge of the animal's, a point worthy to be mentioned in consideration of many attacks levelled against instinct theories. But if it is so, then the demand characters cannot all be entirely dependent upon the needs and preacquired knowledge of the animal. Rather must we assume that certain objects have, qua behavioural objects, certain demand characters. We recall the fact established by Götz (see Chapter III, p. 88) that chicks prefer the larger to the smaller grains. It is more than unlikely that this can be explained by experience; for quite apart from the intrinsic difficulties inherent in such an explanation, the same preference is shown by rats to sunflower seeds, where the difference of size resides only in the uneatable husk and not in the real seed (Yoshioka).[13] Since it takes more time and effort to unhusk the seeds from the larger than from the smaller husks, experience, if it had anything to do

[13] See also Tolman, pp. 30-31.

with the matter, should favour the smaller rather than the larger pieces. Therefore we may safely assume that the preference for the larger morsel of food is not acquired. Then it can only mean that the larger has the stronger demand character. Again, moving objects have much stronger demand characters than stationary ones. In short, our assumption that certain behavioural objects possess by themselves demand characters seems to be confirmed by the facts. The relation between demand character and need is still there, but we see that it is not sufficient to explain the arousal of a demand character.

Silent vs. Manifest Organization in These Two Examples. Let us consider the demand characters and their corresponding needs and quasi-needs (intentions) from another point of view. We saw at the end of our discussion of the latter how complex the dynamical situation is. How much of this complexity is silent, how much "manifest"? The intention, or need, is manifest, or will be at least in a great many cases; similarly the demand character will be manifest; i.e., we see the letter box as the proper object we needed to carry out our intention; the piece of steak looks most appetizing; and lastly the relation of our actions with regard to both need and demand character is again, in most cases, manifest. When we cross the street in order to get to the letter box, we know why we are doing it, and when we lift the piece of meat to our mouth we are also well aware of the meaning of this action. The functional relation between demand character and need, however, is silent. When we are hungry we do not know, except perhaps indirectly on account of rather sophisticated experience, that those delicious dishes spread on the table will have lost all their glamour after we have eaten; and we are not aware that the letter box owes its force of attraction to our intention to post a letter. Finally the inherent demand character, which we found it necessary to assume, belongs to the object in the same way as its shape and colour, i.e., because of silent organization. If we can accept our feeling of forces which make us do things as true indications of actual field forces, if, in other words, our concept of the manifest organization is correct, then indeed our executive must be subject directly to forces existing between the Ego and the field.

(3) The Telephone Bell. Signals. Let us turn to a third example: we hear the telephone bell ring and we rush to the instrument, or, when we have just settled down to a nice afternoon nap, we still experience the claim and grow angry at the disturbance, even if we do not actually obey the summons. That the specific demand char-

acter of the bell is a product of experience is obvious; also that it appeals to certain of our needs. But again this does not seem to be the whole story. With this "signal," as with many others, we have to raise the question why it has been selected. And in our attempt at answering this question we shall find that we choose our signals often enough because they are particularly suitable to be signals, because they possess certain demand characters by themselves which make them fit to assume a specific meaning. The suddenness, intensity, and recurrence of the bell are such characteristics.

Attention. All these three characteristics have been listed as "conditions of attention," together with several others of which we shall only mention quality: certain qualities, like a bitter taste, the smell of musk, and the colour yellow having a particularly strong effect on attention. The discussion of the conditions of attention which twenty-five years ago was carried on with great vigour and played a leading rôle in the psychological drama has ceased to interest psychologists. The reason for this change seems to me to lie not so much in the facts which supplied the matter for this discussion as in the concept or concepts of attention which set their mark upon it. It would serve no useful purpose to review these old conceptions. Instead we shall define attention in conformity with our general system, thereby achieving a definition which is in perfect accord with the meaning of the word as used in ordinary language. When we encountered attention before (Chapter V, p. 206) we said it was a force starting within the Ego and being directed towards an object. This is, of course, what we ordinarily mean by it when we say: "Please pay attention to what I am saying," or "Please concentrate on your problem." To treat of attention (as Titchener did, 1910) as a mere property, attribute, or dimension of field objects, called clearness, robs it of its main character, its Ego-object relationship. And if we define attention as an Ego-object force we can do justice both to so-called voluntary and to involuntary attention. In the former the force starts from the Ego; in the latter, primarily from the object. This way of looking at attention is, naturally, not absolutely new. It was kept from gaining its due weight by the psychologists' wish to keep the Ego, and with the Ego all psychological dynamics, out of their science. But when we read Stout's definition: "Attention is the direction of thought to this or that special object in preference to others" (1909, I, p. 203), we recognize the same general idea. True, we must substitute the Ego for Stout's "thought."

Intensity, suddenness, recurrence, as conditions of attention assume a very definite meaning under our definition. Attention as a force within the total field cannot be aroused by stimuli directly, but by field objects which in their turn owe their existence to stimuli. Consequently we must say that such objects as are produced by strong, sudden, recurring stimuli, and by stimuli of particular qualities, possess characters by virtue of which they affect the Ego. If these old statements about the conditions of attention are true, they indicate again that demand characters may belong to field objects apart from Ego needs which produce them.

(4) Physiognomic Characters. A last group of examples will raise this conclusion which has been forced upon us again and again to a state of certainty. We go to an interview upon which our whole future may depend. We are determined to be as nice and amiable as we can, and then we come into the presence of a man whose face makes it quite impossible to carry out our resolutions. True enough, we force a smile and use polite language, but inwardly we shrink with aversion and have to make the greatest effort not to betray our real feelings. It is unnecessary to multiply examples of this kind—and it would be just as easy to find instances where the demand characters of the face were as positive as they were negative in our case. But I will remind the reader of an experiment which Köhler performed with his chimpanzees. He had prepared a painted cardboard copy of a Singhalese demon mask, a ghastly-looking face. When he entered the animals' playground, the apes, as usual, approached to greet him, when suddenly he held the mask in front of his face, with the result that with one exception all the animals disappeared into a box, where they were joined by the last animal after Köhler had approached a few more steps.

We conclude that objects in the field may possess characters which can be expressed in terms neither of shape and colour nor of practical use, and which are apt to exert a powerful influence on our behaviour. These characters are for us most pronounced in human forms, but may belong to almost any object. Our preoccupation with practical use and scientifically classifiable properties has robbed our world of a good many of them. A corpse has to the ordinary person a very strong character of gruesome awe, but no longer to the medical student who has dissected corpses by the score. On the other hand, if we can abandon our practical or scientific attitude, we become aware of more and more such characteristics. Among us the poets and artists are those who are most free from the craving for efficiency. And truly, for them the world is richer in such characters than it is for us. I have already referred to Wordsworth's daffodils (p. 326), and I could add any number of examples from poetry and prose, Rilke's novel "Malte Laúrids Brigge" being particularly full of them. How even a humble piece of furniture may possess such characters is revealed by a painting by van Gogh in the Tate Gallery in London, where we see a simple chair which seems to carry the pathos of the world.

It does not seem adequate to me to call these characters demand characters. I choose a term which gains greater and greater significance in modern psychology, viz., *physiognomic character*. Several psychologists have been led to the belief, which I consider well founded, that at more primitive stages of human development, for children and primitive peoples, these physiognomic characters play a much greater rôle than in our behavioural world (Scheler, Werner). The primitive behavioural world is, as Werner puts it, a physiognomic world, which means that the organization of the field is such as to enhance the physiognomic characters at the expense of those properties which we find as the outstanding features. Food, then, if it is selected without prior experiences, must possess physiognomic characters, which may reside in its looks, or as much or even more so in its smell. Thus our discussion of the demand characters which correspond to the real needs and of those which belong to signals has anticipated the introduction of the physiognomic aspect of our behavioural environment. If a girl has "sex appeal," she has a definite physiognomic character.

A Conclusion About the Classical Theory of Sensation. If we look at the classical theory of sensation from this point of view, it gains a very different aspect. Sensations and their attributes appear as products of a particular kind of organization achieved by human beings in highly developed civilizations, but no longer as the raw material out of which all consciousness is built. "We must assume that features like 'threatening' or 'tempting' are more primitive and more elementary contents of perception than those we learn of as 'elements' in the textbooks of psychology" (Koffka, 1928, p. 150). Or a quotation from Wertheimer: "Does a child or a primitive man experience a certain tint of red in the scientific sense of a quality of sensation? Surely his actual experience is much closer to 'exciting,' 'gay,' 'strong,' . . ." (1925, p. 15). Without such a view it would be hard to understand the magic-mystical world of primitive peoples or the behaviour of small infants.

Origin of Physiognomic Characters. Although, then, the existence of the physiognomic characters in our behavioural environment is safely established, we have to enter the field of mere hypothesis when we try to raise the question as to their origin. For a number of cases, those to which the term physiognomic is most pertinent, viz., the understanding of the other person's emotions, Köhler has given a satisfactory theory which we shall discuss in our fourteenth chapter. Here we shall try to approach our problem in an even more general way, advancing for critical consideration and possible experimentation an hypothesis which must necessarily be in keeping with our system. Our hypothesis must, in other words, be an hypothesis about the nature of the organization of the field. We take our clue from the consideration of the most pronounced physiognomic characters, the horrible, the majestic, the enchanting. Words like these describe objects with reference to ourselves. May we then venture the assumption that these characters arise in organizations which include the Ego? This does not mean that they belong to the Ego; we leave them where we find them, in certain objects, but we claim that these objects possess them only in an organization which also includes an Ego, and an Ego of a special kind. Such an hypothesis would well accord with the fact previously mentioned that on more primitive levels the physiognomic characters are far more pronounced than at our own level of civilization. For the separation between the Ego and its environment increases with the progress of civilization. The more unitary the total field composed of Ego and environment, the more should the latter be endowed with physiognomic characters. Lack of separation means ample dynamical interplay. Therefore the presence of an Ego in an organization should affect the environmental parts the more, the less the degree of separation of the Ego. This is again in full harmony with Wertheimer, who conceives of the original Ego-environment relation not as of a purely cognitive one, in which the Ego merely takes cognizance of objects, but as of a conative one, in which the Ego adapts its behaviour to the environment (1925, p. 15). Again we are tempted to refer to instinctive behaviour; the common man applies the term instinctive to this kind of situation: a person doing the right thing without knowing why and yet feeling that he had to. When we say: Women rely more on instinct than men, we mean just this, that in a woman's behaviour the Ego is less separated from the environment than in a man's, and that therefore the mutual interplay of forces which determines the behaviour on the one hand and the physiognomic characters on the other is stronger. How many men accept their wives' judgment about the character of new acquaintances and even their old friends, and how many women accept their husbands'? This popular usage of the word instinctive seems, therefore, to be well founded, to be perfectly compatible with the theory of behaviour. And in this meaning it is also well applicable to the instinctive activity of animals, which has led to so many controversies. Truly, the Ego will be much less separated in an animal than in man, and therefore we ought to expect a much more direct dependence of the animal's behaviour on its behavioural environment, less and less cognition, more and more direct response —but of course not in the sense of the stimulus-response or the reflex concept.

We return to the physiognomic characters. According to our hypothesis they arise in objects when these objects are in dynamic relation with the Ego, when, otherwise expressed, a state of tension exists between them and the Ego. It is important to keep in mind that the kind of tension will vary for the different physiognomic characters. Not only will it be different in sign—positive or negative —and in degree, but also in quality. The kind of tension will determine our responses: attack, flight, approach, succour, disregard, compassion, and so forth.

Gaps in Our Hypothesis. This reveals a first gap in our hypothesis, for as yet we can translate only a few physiognomic characters into kinds of tensions, and probably for a long time to come we shall have to be satisfied with a behavioural description of the physiognomic characters and their relation to action, without being able to assign to them very definite distributions of forces. But our hypothesis contains another and more serious gap: we do not know in ever so many cases why a certain object possesses its physiognomic character. We can link up the insistency of objects produced by intense and sudden stimuli with the sharp gradient by which they emerge from the field, which entails a large potential difference or tension; we may equally connect the physiognomic character of colours, particularly the impressiveness of red and yellow, with their hardness, which again means a better segregation and thereby a greater tension, but for most other cases we have frankly to admit our ignorance, hoping only that the explanations which we find possible in the more simple cases may serve as clues for the more complex ones.

We may even doubt the general validity of our hypothesis. Is it true that all physiognomic characters require an Ego-object organization; may not physiognomic characters also arise within the organization of the external field without participation of the Ego? I do not mean the case where organization has not reached the Ego-level. Tensions in such organizations will have to be described in behavioural terms as neither Ego-emotions nor physiognomic characters, but something from which either of these two kinds of experiences will later emerge. The total field, not yet differentiated into Ego and object, will as a whole be satisfactory or unsatisfactory, a state which we may approach in our transitions from waking life to sleep. I mean the opposite extreme, organization with a strong Ego separation. That under these conditions physiognomic characters deteriorate, we have already emphasized. At the same time the articulation of the field gains in many other respects. Should we then attribute the remaining physiognomic characters to the remaining Ego-object relation, or should we also envisage the possibility that they may be due to the interplay of forces in the environment? I shall be satisfied with raising the question without an attempt at giving an answer, which at the present time would be no more than guess-work.

Return to Problem of Executive Control. We are now prepared to return to our problem whether the executive can be controlled directly by the forces between the Ego and the surrounding field. For we have found that objects possess not only demand characters with which they are endowed by pre-existing Ego-tensions, but also physiognomic characters which do not depend upon any such specific stress, although in many, and possibly in all, cases they presuppose an Ego for their appearance. Perhaps this distinction might become a true terminological distinction; it grows ambiguous only in those cases where, as in the appetizing character of food, both factors seem to be combined. The attractiveness of an eatable object would have to be called a demand character, inasmuch as it disappears in states of satiety, and a physiognomic character inasmuch as it depends upon the properties of the food object itself. We leave the terminological question open, content with having pointed out the interplay of different forces. What then is our answer to the question whether the executive can be directly controlled by the object-Ego forces?

Complexity of the Dynamic Situation. The answer seems simplest in cases of direct reactions to physiognomic characters. Here, at least in the beginning, the executive seems indeed to be under the control of these forces. The Ego-field relation is unstable, and the executive changes the situation in the direction of greater stability of this relation. In actual fact clear-cut cases of this simple nature will be very rare. If the Ego-field relation is unstable, the Ego itself will become unbalanced also, i.e., the object-Ego stress will produce intra-Ego stresses, which in their turn will begin to control the executive so as to re-balance the Ego. Nevertheless it seems plausible in these cases to attribute the primary impetus to action or the original control of the executive to the Ego-object stresses.

That the situation is much more complex with typical *demand characters* follows directly from our previous discussion of the dynamic situation in these cases. In consideration of this complexity I am loth to attribute the entire control in these cases to the Ego. At least one would have to distinguish between a direct and an indirect influence of the Ego. The first follows directly from the need, the second by way of the demand character, which though it has been, at least partly, created by the need, is an Ego-object force.

TOLMAN'S THEORY OF PHYSIOGNOMIC CHARACTERS AND THE ACTIONS CORRESPONDING TO THEM. Is it possible to simplify our interpretation and at the same time make it more adequate? Tolman proposes a theory which, in our terminology, would exclude the object-Ego stresses from the control of the executive, reserving this to the Ego itself. I quote:

"Similarly, the state of agitation to be called fright . . . does not arise merely, or primarily, as a result of danger-threatening 'disturbing stimuli,' but rather as a result of an initiating internal physiological state which, for want of a better name, we may call *timidity,* and which must be present in order to make the animal sensitive to such 'disturbing stimuli' " (pp. 273-4).

Tolman's main reason for such an interpretation seems to be that the same real object may arouse different emotions with their corresponding reactions, e.g., fright and pugnacity. I quote a few more passages:

"Both fright and pugnacity are gettings-away from their respectively evoking disturbing stimulus-situations. But the manner of getting away is characteristically different in the two cases." "This difference in the characters of fright and pugnacity is particularly obvious and pronounced when it is one and the same environmental object . . . which happens in the one individual to arouse fright, and in another pugnacity. . . . Given equal or similar past trainings, . . . if he (the animal) have a large dose of the initiating physiological state which we have designated timidity, then his fright impulse will be aroused. . . . If, on the other hand, . . . he have a large dose of the initiating state of pugnaciousness, his pugnacity impulse will be aroused" (pp. 280-281).

I shall try to discuss this view in our terminology and within our system, disregarding the fact that "large doses of initiating states of timidity or pugnacity" can hardly be accepted as final explanations.

We must, to appraise Tolman's argument, distinguish two cases; in the first the same *real* object appears to two different people with two different physiognomic characters, in the second the physiognomic characters are the same, yet the reactions are different.

For our first case we choose the following example: two persons have an encounter with the same ruffian. One of our two persons is a writer who never takes any physical exercise, the other a first-rate prize-fighter. To the first the ruffian will look formidable, to the second he will appear as a weak boaster. Why? Because the first possesses a great dose of timidity, is, to put it bluntly, a coward, and because the second has an equal dose of pugnaciousness, is, again, in blunt words, a rowdy? I do not admit for a moment that this explanation, though it is possible, is necessary. Our writer may be extremely pugnacious and our prize-fighter, like Cashel Byron after his marriage, a perfectly peaceful man, and yet the ruffian may appear formidable to the first and despicable to the second. Our hypothesis of the physiognomic characters allows for an explanation of this possibility. We derived the physiognomic character from the particular object-Ego organization achieved at the moment. This organization will, as all organizations, depend upon the relative properties of the objects organized. Now in the writer's field there is this bulky and heavy fellow, i.e., a physically large person, and his Ego, which is physically small and weak: a good reason for the ruffian to look formidable. Conversely, for the prize-fighter the physical Ego may be considerably larger than that of his opponent, with the result that the ruffian's physiognomic character is that of a sham power. Thus we agree with Tolman inasmuch as we also accord to the Ego an influence on the physiognomic character of the other person, but we disagree with him in our interpretation of this influence.

But we shall follow our example a little further. What will the two men do in their encounter with the ruffian? Should not, in Tolman's theory, the writer try to make his escape, and the prize-fighter "sock the ruffian in the jaw"? Again a real possibility. But it may just as easily happen that the writer gives fight and is badly beaten up, while the fighter turns away with a contemptuous shrug of the shoulder. These types of behaviour are particularly interesting, because they reveal a new complexity of behaviour which we have not yet discussed. We are, however, well aware of the fact that all action affects the existing organization and tends to maintain the organism intact. We have also applied the same conception to the Ego-part of the total field. What would happen to the Ego of our writer if he ran away? Most probably he would avoid physical injury, but certainly he would feel humiliated, an effect which everybody understands and which we shall treat systematically later. It is enough here to say that flight would set up new stresses within the Ego system, more specifically within the Self, and that if these stresses are strong enough, our writer will not turn to escape but will face the danger. Unnecessary to apply the same trend of thought to the prize-fighter. Our discussion has shown us that Tolman's basis of discussion is too narrow, that the complexity of behaviour is dynamically far greater than his system allows.

And let us now turn to the second case. An object looks threatening. There are then, as the discussion of the first case has shown, two or more ways of action. Which of these will actually be taken depends upon a host of circumstances. The effect of the action upon the Ego is one of them, but others may be equally effective; thus the fact that our reaction would produce relief in the quickest and simplest way may determine the actual selection. The case in which a condition of dynamic stress has only one way of relief, the problem only one solution, is extremely rare in mental and organic life. We found this same situation even in perception when we studied ambiguous patterns. In short, it seems not an adequate explanation to derive flight in all cases from a pre-existing state of timidity, fight from one of pugnaciousness. The dynamical situation is much more complex, and in this dynamical situation Ego-object forces may play an important part in controlling the executive.

The Actual Control of the Executive. Complex as the dynamic situation appears when we consider all the factors which control the executive, it is in reality still more complicated. For at any one moment there are numerous other factors which, although they are not in control, might be so. The Ego, being the complex structure we have shown it to be, contains a great number of sub-systems under pressure, all of which could be relieved by some action or other. Naturally most of these stresses must, for the time being, remain unrelieved. So the question arises which of all the possible factors—and we must include among them the pure field forces and the object-Ego forces as well as the pure Ego-forces—will at a given instant of time gain control. It is impossible to give an answer to this question at the present state of our knowledge. But such an answer, when it is available for a number of concrete cases, will have to take into account not only the individual factors by themselves, but their interplay, the structure and interconnection of the Ego systems, the results which any one action will have not only with regard to special forces but also with regard to the whole Ego and its relation to its environment.

GENERAL PRINCIPLE OF ACTION

All action is a process by which stresses existing in the total field are decreased or removed. Because of the multiplicity of such tensions and their mutual interdependence the possibilities of action are practically infinite. And small actions .may have enormous effects. An action may relieve a stress in an Ego system which at the moment was isolated from the rest of the Ego and in full command of the executive. The result of this action may revolutionize the whole life of the agent.

CHAPTER IX

ACTION

Adjusted Behaviour, Attitudes, Emotions, and the Will

The Task of This Chapter. The Problem of Adjusted Behaviour. How the Behavioural Environment Directs Behaviour. The Circular Process. The "Adequacy" of the Behavioural World. Cognitive Value of Manifest Organization. Manifest Organization in Phenomenal Behaviour. Its Cognitive Value. Insight. Silent Ego-organization. The Special Problems of Localization with Moving Eyes. Directed Action. The Force Diagrams. Variability of the Dynamic Characters. The Functional Characters of Behavioural Objects. Attitudes and Their Effects on the Behavioural Environment. Emotions. Silent and Manifest Organization. The Dynamic Theory of Emotion. Experimental Evidence. The Will. McDougall's Hormic Theory. Lewin's Concepts. Conclusion and Outlook

THE TASK OF THIS CHAPTER

In the last chapter we have taken up points (3) and (4) of our programme formulated in the second chapter (p. 67). We have studied the Ego and we have demonstrated the forces which connect the Ego with its environmental field. Both studies have to be continued. With regard to point (3) we must discuss the place of emotion and sentiment in the Ego, which so far has been mentioned rather incidentally, and with regard to point (4) we have to discuss the Ego-field relationships in greater detail, particularly the steady transformation which the field undergoes under the influence of the Ego, its needs and quasi-needs, its desires, wishes, resolves and attitudes. Lastly, we must add a discussion of our fifth and last point, the relation of behaviour to the geographical environment, the cognitive or adjustive aspect of behaviour.

THE PROBLEM OF ADJUSTED BEHAVIOUR

We shall begin our discussion with this last problem. In our theory behaviour was determined by the properties of the total psychophysical field, i.e., by the dynamic structure of the Ego and that of its psychophysical environment. Why is it, at the same time, *adapted* behaviour? Why does behaviour, leading to ever new stabilizations within the psychophysical field of the organism, also fulfil the task of preserving the real organism in its geographical environment? The answer must, necessarily, lie in the relations between the geographical and the behavioural or psychophysical environment and in the changes which, owing to this relationship, the latter undergoes in any behaviour act.

I see an object flying through the air in my direction. I either step aside or hold out my hand so as to catch it. In the first case the object, say a ball, will fly past me in my behavioural environment and in my geographical one; in the second case, on the contrary, it will, provided I am skilful enough, be caught in my hand, again both behaviourally and geographically. Under normal conditions, then, certain results in the behavioural field can come about only through corresponding results in the geographical environment. Only when the real ball is in real contact with my real hand will the behavioural ball appear in my behavioural hand. Therefore behaviour, directed by and adapted to the behavioural world, must in cases like these also be adapted to the geographical world.

How the Behavioural Environment Directs Behaviour. The question may be raised here, how the behavioural world manages to direct behaviour or, in our terminology, how it controls the executive. If an object comes hurtling towards us, no doubt we move so as to avoid it. But what is the actual occurrence in our nervous system? How does the perception of this moving object innervate our musculature?

STIMULUS-RESPONSE THEORY REJECTED. We discussed a similar problem in our theory of reflex action. There we found the traditional pathway or connection hypothesis according to which such innervation was explained as the simple transmission of the nervous excitation from the centripetal to the centrifugal part of the pre-established reflex arc. A similar hypothesis would be advanced to explain our last example; possibly some psychologists would even be inclined to take over the reflex arc concept without any modification; they would explain our stepping out of the path of an approaching missile as due to an original connection between the stimulus and the response. But such a simple transfer of the reflex arc theory is possible only by the surreptitious introduction of the words stimulus-response. The reflex arc hypothesis is an anatomical hypothesis, the reflex arc is a nervous structure with its real centripetal and centrifugal parts which are joined at a definite place in the nervous system. An excitation started on a certain point of the sense surface is conducted to a definite place in the centre and there switched over to a special centrifugal neuron. But if we react to a flying stone, the initiatory part of the reflex is not the stimulation of a point or a pattern of points on our retinae, but a *process* of motion produced within the central nervous system (see Chapter VII) by a real motion. Therefore the terminal point at which the excitation is to be switched over from the centripetal to the centrifugal branch of the arc is missing. Otherwise expressed, the reflex is not produced by a stimulus, the efferent impulse is not started at a particular *place* in the centre, but arises out of a process which in its turn has been caused by a spatio-temporal stimulus pattern. In short, the traditional reflex-arc or stimulus-response conception has to be modified to fit this case. It is, truly, impossible to reduce it to the simpler instances from which the reflex concept was originally derived. Such a reduction could only take the form of connecting the *point* of excitation with the response. Just as the old theory postulated a separate connection between each retinal point and the oculomotor system to explain fixation (see Chapter VIII, p. 312), so the *position* of the moving object at the moment our avoidance reaction was started should, through the retinal point on which it was at that moment projected, determine the path of the efferent impulse. A theory which claimed this would at least be self-consistent. But it would be equally absurd. At the risk of being criticized for defeating a bogus opponent, I will give my argument *in extenso,* because it may help the reader to be cautious in the application of the stimulus-response concept in cases which are less simple. In the first place, the position of the stone at the critical moment by no means determines the stimulated point of the retinae. This depends also upon the position of the eyes at the moment. And yet, the response may be quite independent of this position of my eyes; I will step aside, whether I had previously looked straight at the stone or at an object to its left or right, above or below, in front or behind it. Practically every point of the retina will, in this manner of speaking, be connected with the same reaction. In the second place, the same retinal point will lead to different reactions, including no reaction at all, according to the whole path and the velocity of the flying stone. If, in the accompanying figure, E stands for the person, P for the point at which the stone sets up the excitation in the afferent part of the reflex arc, and the three lines 1, 2, and 3 three different trajectories, then the

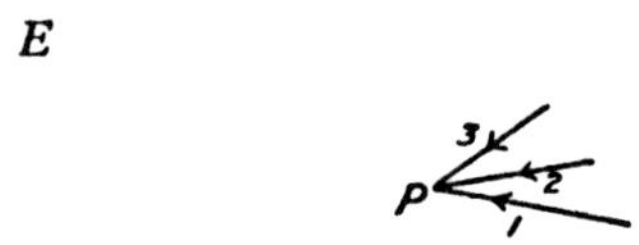

Fig. 91

same stimulus—the same because P is projected on the same retinal point in all three cases—will produce three different responses in the three cases: in 1 the person may step either to the left or the right, in 2 he will step to the left, and in 3 he will not move at all. And this leaves differences of velocity out of account, whereas such differences are of the greatest importance for cases 1 and 2 and quite irrelevant for case 3.

Thus the strict application of the simple reflex arc theory is impossible. Any modification would have to accept motion as a stimulus, that is to say not motion of the external object, not even motion of the retinal image, but motion as a process within the brain. But this modification is tantamount to a complete abandonment of the original reflex-arc hypothesis, since it has replaced the excitation in the afferent branch by a process in the brain, and has thereby destroyed the whole concept of connectionism.

I shall not strain my imagination to invent hypotheses which would preserve enough of the old conceptions to be still called reflex theories. Instead I shall now try to give the kind of answer which solves the problem without any new hypothesis.

THE DYNAMIC THEORY. The flying stone, if it comes in the proper direction, will set up a strong force in the field chiefly directed towards the Ego. If, on the other hand, its direction is different, no such force will arise. Consequently, in the second case, no movement will be made, since there is no force to initiate it.

ORIGIN OF THE FORCES. Before we proceed in the discussion of the case in which the force is set up, we must raise the question why these forces arise. Probably the reader will be inclined to seek the cause in experience. The person or animal has learned that an object possessing certain characteristics will eventually hurt him if he does not react to it. That such cases exist is not to be denied, but equally strongly it will be maintained that no proof whatever has been given that they are typical of all cases. On the contrary, Wertheimer has proved in his classical experiments (1912) that a motion within a field exerts a force on other field objects near to the path of the motion. In one of his ϕ-experiments (see p. 179) he exposed the following pattern of successive stimulation (see Fig. 92), *a* representing the object presented in the first, *b* that in the second exposure, and *c* an object which was shown either only together with *a* or *b*, or in conjunction with both. If then the conditions were such that one line was seen turning from the vertical to the horizontal, it frequently happened that *c* made a centrifugal

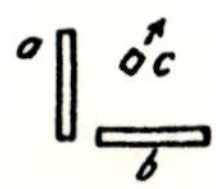

Fig. 92

movement as indicated by the small arrow. Since we have proved that in many respects, and particularly with regard to motion, the Ego must be treated as a field object, we have no reason to exclude the possibility that the moving object directly, without any experience, exerts a force upon it, a force which must depend upon the direction and velocity of the motion. Moreover, since we had good reason to believe that the total field was the more unified the more primitive the organization, we should have to conclude that such direct influence would be stronger at primitive than at highly developed levels. Experiments in child- and animal-psychology must eventually decide whether our deduction is correct or not.

DIRECTION OF FORCE AND RESPONSE. INFLUENCE OF EXPERIENCE. A force is a vectorial magnitude, i.e., it has a direction. It is hard to understand how in the case of an object moving straight towards one this direction could be any other than the direction of the motion itself. But that raises a difficulty: Why do we not run away from a hurtling stone but sidestep it instead? I am inclined to explain this response by experience, believing that the first reaction would indeed be that of direct flight. Again experiment will have to give the final decision. But casual observations seem to confirm this view: every motorist's patience has been severely tried by chickens and other animals on the road who tried to escape the approaching car by running away from it along the road. I remember a precious half hour lost in this way out West on account of a small herd of untamed horses. How such behaviour, the result of the direct field forces, gives way to the more rational behaviour of turning to the side cannot be treated here. It will be taken up in a discussion of learning.[1] For by regarding this modified form of behaviour as a product of experience we do not, at this point, consider it to be really explained. No recourse to experience is an explanation before a theory of experience or learning has been developed, and such a theory will be very different indeed from the traditional associationistic one.

THE DYNAMIC THEORY CONTINUED: DYNAMIC CONNECTION BETWEEN SENSORY AND MOTOR FIELD. We now return to the discussion of our hurtling stone when, because of the direction of the motion, a force between the moving object and the Ego is set up. How will such a force determine the behaviour of the organism; how will it control the executive? For the behaviour of the organism under the stress of such a force is dynamically very different from the behaviour of the small field object close to a motion field in Wert-

[1] See Chapter XIII, p. 645.

heimer's experiment recently described (pp. 371 f.). The latter occurs in the behavioural but not in the geographical field, and it is a *direct* effect, by which the object as a whole yields to a stress in the field. On both counts the behaviour of the *organism* is different. The change in the object-Ego relation within the behavioural field is here brought about by a change in the object-organism relation in the geographical field, and this change is not direct; the organism is not pushed or pulled as a whole, as by a gust of wind, but has to effect the change by the innervation of certain parts of its musculature, which leads to limb movements. But in this respect our case is no different from the case of eye-movements which we discussed at the beginning of the eighth chapter. Therefore the same kind of explanation that fitted that case will also fit our new one. In the case of eye-movements a stress in the environmental field was relieved by eye-movements. All we had to assume in order to explain this was a connection between the visual field and the oculomotor system. In our present case the stress exists between the Ego and the object, and is relieved by a movement of the organism's body. Therefore all we have to assume is that such stress may be in communication with the motor centres in the brain or a lower part of the central nervous system. In that case the motor system would be thrown into action, and the form which the ensuing behaviour takes is thereby determined. For such movement as would not be "adapted" would either leave the stress unaltered or increase it, whereas the "adapted" movement will decrease and eventually relieve the strain. Thus the adapted movements must be made for purely dynamic reasons. They alone are changes in the direction of equilibrium, whereas the unadapted ones are not. They can only happen when other forces, stronger than those which we are considering, are operative at the same time. Thus, without any specific knowledge of the actual anatomical and physiological conditions, we can derive the adaptedness of behaviour.

THE CIRCULAR PROCESS. Köhler (1925 b) has, for the case of eye-movements, described the "circular process" involved in such behaviour. We shall apply his conception to our case of field-behaviour. We distinguish the distant stimulus S_d, the proximal stimulus S_p, the field aroused by the latter, F, and the movements executed by the animal M, and we shall designate by indices 0, 1, 2 . . . the different moments of time. At first then we have the constellation S_d S_{0} F_0. Now movement is started. It results in a new relation between the distant stimulus object and the organism, therefore we have now M_1 S_{p1} F_1. M_1 was the effect of F_0. it has changed F_0 by changing S_p and can have done so only by making F_0 lose some of its power of causing M; i.e., the force between F_1 and the Ego must be smaller than that between F_0 and the Ego. F_1 will in its turn produce M_2 which will lead to S_{p2} and thereby to F_2 according to the same principle, and so forth, until a relation between the organism and S_d is reached in which the S_{pn} produces an F_n which is free of that strain which caused the movement. Of course in reality the process is continuous; the different moments of time with their respective characteristics are no real entities, but fictitious abstractions made for the purpose of elucidating the principle. The main point in this argument is that the direction of the change from F_{n-1} to F_n is determined by the dynamics of the situation. F_n must be in a condition of lower tension than F_{n-1}. To assume the opposite would be equivalent to the assumption that water would, by itself, run up the hill. Truly, we can pump the water up, but that fact does not prove that by itself the water will not run down; on the contrary, the forces which pump the water up must be stronger than the forces which pull it down. Exactly the same is true of behaviour. New forces may be introduced, and if these are stronger than the original field forces, then the F_n will be under greater stress than the F_{n-1}. The prize-fighter who leaves his corner to meet his opponent is in this very position, or the soldier who has to "go over the top." The will to fight, the discipline of the soldier, are the new forces which are responsible for these effects. But no new principle is required to explain them, just as little as we need a new kind of physics to explain the pumping of water. In our last examples also the movement actually made is such as to decrease the *total* stress, much as partial stresses may be increased by it. However, cases like our last ones introduce a new possibility of behaviour. The partial stresses which are increased by behaviour may become so strong as to equal the other stresses. Then movement will stop, or rather the behaviour will change, for then the total stress to which the organism is exposed will be enormous, and discharge may take any course that is opened by the complexity of the total field. The Ego itself may give way and be severely injured as in cases of shell shock, again comparable to our hydrodynamic example, where the walls of the pipes may burst.

MOLAR, BUT NOT MOLECULAR, BEHAVIOUR PREDICTABLE. Our dynamic interpretation of behaviour, as opposed to the traditional machine interpretation,[2] allows still another inference well supported by facts

[2] For this antithesis see Köhler, "Gestalt Psychology," Chapter IV.

Wherever we are able to predict animal or human behaviour, we are able to predict the behaviour as a molar phenomenon (see Chapter II, p. 25 f.), but very rarely shall we be able to predict the molecular aspect of behaviour, the actual limb movements or muscle contractions. We are, e.g., able to predict that an animal will move towards a lure, or build a nest, that a person will write a letter or fly into a rage, but we cannot predict what actual limb-movements they will perform and even less what muscle innervations they will effect. The latter depend upon a host of secondary conditions, entirely beyond our ken, which in most cases will not affect the final result or the general direction of the action.

ENERGY RELATIONS. STEERING. We have to add a last word about the actual dynamic situation. In our theory the forces in the total field direct the bodily movements of the organism. This cannot, of course, mean that the energies consumed in these movements derive from the total field, for energy consumed in our muscles is of a different order of magnitude from the energies in the brain field. The dynamic relation must therefore, as Köhler has pointed out, be that of release and *steering*. The release conception is perfectly familiar to traditional psychology, but the conception of *steering* is not, whereas it is just this function which explains the actual relation between field and action. How large energies can be steered by small ones is exemplified by numberless technical steering processes, e.g., by the driving of a motor car.[3]

RELATION OF FUNCTION AND STRUCTURE IN OUR THEORY. We can express the meaning of our dynamic theory of behaviour briefly by saying: the anatomical structure does not determine which muscles are to be innervated, what action is to take place, but the action required by the momentary field conditions determines the anatomical substratum in which the last part of the total process will take place. To show that such an interpretation was at least foreshadowed in the theorizings of other psychologists, even of extreme behaviouristic leanings, I shall quote a passage from an article by J. R. Kantor: "Does the neural apparatus control the muscles any more than the muscles and glands control the neural apparatus? Is it not a fact that the specific pathways involved in any reaction are involved because certain muscles or glands need to function?" (P. 28.)

The "Adequacy" of the Behavioural World. We can now return to our initial problem, why behaviour directed by the organization of the psychophysical field is adapted also to the geographical en-

[3] See also our earlier discussion in Chapter III, p. 99.

vironment. We have already seen that its solution depends upon the nature of the directing forces and upon the relation between the geographical and behavioural environment. After having discussed the former we must now, once more, turn to the latter and regard it from the point of view of "adequacy," after having studied the laws which regulate this relation in Chapters III-VII. The organization of the behavioural world was there found to depend upon the distribution of the proximal stimuli. "Adequacy" of the behavioural world, an organization which makes adapted behaviour possible, must therefore depend upon the properties of the distant stimuli which through the corresponding proximal stimuli produce the organization. Since the problem involved has been solved in Köhler's lucid presentation (1929, pp. 172 f.), a few words will suffice here. Real objects are separated from their environment by differences of material and structure which in all normal cases will appear as differences in surface structure and therefore in inhomogeneities of proximal stimulation along boundary lines which will produce segregated objects in the behavioural field. What is true of external articulations is equally true of internal ones. Thus under normal conditions the geographical objects will produce organizations of the psychophysical field suitable to arouse action which is adapted to the geographical one.

CORRESPONDENCE VERY INCOMPLETE. But we must be careful lest we overestimate the correspondence between the two fields. The conditions under which organization occurs in the two fields are very different indeed, and therefore in many respects the behavioural organization may not at all repeat the geographical one. We have given enough examples in our previous discussion (Chapters III-VII). Therefore we add here only one point of view: whereas the shape of a geographical object at a given moment may not be at all due to the forces expressed in the law of good continuation—a rocky ridge, for instance, owes its present state to the effects of erosion which attacks, roughly speaking, each part by itself—the behavioural objects are always due to such forces; thus the rocky ridge as we see it is, as an organization within the psychophysical field, a dynamical shape and as such subject to the law of good continuation. Camouflage, which we have previously discussed, is an artificial device to produce such discrepancies and thereby lead to non-adapted behaviour.

Thus the problem of adapted behaviour has led us to the problem of cognition in perception. And although we could sketch only very briefly the solution of this problem, our sketch should have shown how such a solution can be worked out on a larger scale. It is clear, however, that perceptual cognition can only be very incomplete. Even though the perceptual objects repeat to some extent some of the properties of the real objects, they are far from being perfect replicas. On the one hand they will possess characteristics which the corresponding real objects do not have, on the other hand they will lack all those properties of the real objects which find no expression in such macroscopic surface qualities as can affect our sense organs.

TEMPORAL PROPERTIES. MOTION. But we must not forget that in this formulation we have neglected time, and yet the temporal characteristics of the distant and thereby the proximal stimuli are equally important for organization as the spatial ones. Thus motion of a real object will in most cases produce motion of a behavioural object. Again cognition arises through the occurrence of a psychophysical process similar to the real process. And yet the two events in the geographical and the behavioural field, even though they correspond, have different causes, as becomes clear when we remember the theory of perceived motion. The case of the rotating wheel is particularly illuminating (Rubin, 1927). Each point of the wheel passes through a trajectory which is a cycloid. And yet we do not see this cycloid path, but instead a combination of a translatory motion of the hub and a circular motion of the rim. (See discussion in Chapter VII.) This is from the point of cognition very often the truer picture. If a carriage is pulled or pushed by horses or a locomotive engine, then the force applied is a rectilinear one and under this rectilinear force applied to the carriage the wheels begin to turn around their axles; or when the car is propelled by its own power, the forces applied to the wheels make them revolve in circles round their axles and a translatory movement ensues. The light which is transmitted from the rolling wheels contains, of course, no information of these processes. If the eye of the observer is kept steady, then, apart from perspective distortion, each part of the wheel describes a cycloid on the retina, the curve which results from the combination of the circular and translatory movement. But whereas we see a cycloid when a wheel with one luminous point on its periphery rolls in complete darkness, normally we see *two* movements, a circular and translatory one. Of course the fact that we see this is not directly caused by the objective motion, but is due to the internal forces of organization. The correspondence between the events in the behavioural and the geographical world is therefore no direct picturing of the one by the other, but due to the fact that different causes may produce corresponding results. Since, however, different causes will as a rule not produce similar results we have to be very careful in accepting the data of our behavioural world as true information about the geographical, even when for purposes of behaviour the former may be adequate.

FORCE, CAUSALITY. We now consider two bodies colliding in such a way that they influence each other's relative motions. The simplest case is that of one billiard ball hitting another which formerly was at rest and imparting its motion to it. In the real world we have an actual exchange of motion, which we usually express by saying that the moving ball in the collision causes the motion of the resting one. What happens in the behavioural world? The naïve person will say that he saw that process of causation, that he perceived how one ball *pushed* the other, how its force was transmitted to it.

THE POSITIVISTIC ARGUMENT AND ITS REFUTATION. But since Hume we have been taught that the naïve person is mistaken; that he could not possibly *see* such transference of motion or force, because in the stimulating conditions, in the light waves, there is nothing that could produce such a perception. Forces do not emit or reflect light waves, only bodies do, and therefore all we could possibly see was one ball moving till it struck the other one and then lying at rest while the other began to move. Moreover, having been told that we can see nothing else we thereupon *may* see just this and no more. This argument has had a profound influence on the development of the philosophy and the philosophic atmosphere of the last, let us say, hundred years. It is one of the cornerstones of the positivistic attitude towards science which we had so many occasions to attack. But its strength and unassailability are only apparent. To be consistent we should have to say: We cannot see motion, for motion is nothing that reflects light. Indeed, behavioural motion is the result of field processes, i.e., processes occurring within the brain, which need not at all be produced by really moving bodies. Therefore, as far as the argument goes we ought to deny that motion can be seen, a position which some psychologists have indeed taken (Driesch, Lindworsky). But such a view is in too strong a contrast with our everyday experience, our knowledge of animal behaviour, and our experimentation. What highly artificial and complicated hypotheses should we have to make, to mention only one point, in order to explain the results of Brown, whose subjects had to match the velocities of moving objects, if we did not admit that motion with its velocity can be seen, that it is a part of our behavioural environment?

Therefore we can accept the general view that motion is seen, although it is devoid of any special stimulus. But if that is admitted, the positivist argument is invalidated. Our behavioural world is indeed possessed of an inexhaustible number of properties for which no special local stimulation exists. A circle is "round," the edge of this page "straight," an arrow "pointed," a decorative pattern "symmetrical," to name but a few such properties.[4] The positivist might just as well claim that there is no such thing as roundness, or symmetry, because neither roundness nor symmetry reflects light. And if one looks at the history of psychology one has not to turn very far back to find a period where these characters, like shape in general, were treated as non-existent entities. In our fourth chapter we took great pains to prove the reality of shape, and we had to do it, because under the positivistic bias shape had tended to vanish from the sight of the psychologist.

But then, if we refrain from expelling shape and motion from the domain of our science, what reason have we to exclude the experience of force or causation from it? Must we not say instead that as some spatial stimulus distributions produce various shapes, and some spatio-temporal ones the experience of motion, so will others arouse the perception of force and causation? When in the beginning of our third chapter we gave a survey of our behavioural environment we enumerated "forces" among its constituents. We have now seen how these forces have to be treated by the psychologist, although this field is in sore need of experimental investigation, owing, naturally, to the prejudice against causality reared by positivism. Child psychologists have begun to study the field, thanks largely to the pioneering work of Piaget. In Huang's careful investigation which was based on Piaget's work, some rather concrete and definite experiments have been performed which begin to throw a light on the dynamical processes actually occurring (pp. 168 f.).

THE DOUBLE ASPECT OF THE COGNITIVE PROBLEM INVOLVED IN CAUSALITY. With the acknowledgment of causality as a trait of our behavioural environment we have, however, not yet solved the cognitive problem involved. Indeed, this problem has two sides, with regard to the geographical and the behavioural, or rather the psychophysical environment. About the former only a few words are

[4] For a fuller discussion see Köhler, 1929, Chapter VI.

in place. Since in many cases behavioural motion is a true index of geographical motion, there is no *a priori* reason why behavioural causality should not under certain conditions be also veridical with regard to geographical causality. This may mean either of two things: even if we were forced to abandon the idea that causality was an adequate category for the description of the real world, having to be replaced by mere regular sequence, behavioural causality might be an indication that we were in the presence of a case of such regular sequence. But there remains also the other and more important possibility, the possibility, namely, that behavioural causality gives us a true clue as to the constitution of the real world. That would mean that positivism has been too sceptical in its selections of behavioural data from which to build up a theory of the real world. We all accept motion as a true characteristic of the real world, and in doing so think of motion more or less in terms of the motions which we know in our behavioural world, and not merely as a distance-time function; and similarly our concept of velocity is still deeply rooted in our experience of behavioural velocities and not confined to the abstract expression $\frac{ds}{dt}$. Again, there is no *a priori* reason why behavioural force should not give us some direct hint of what real force is, even though we can define it as $m\,\frac{d^2s}{dt^2}$. This line of thought cannot be pursued further, since we are not dealing with epistemology. Our remarks, however, will suffice to revive the question as to what kind of material we can legitimately use for the construction of our world picture. And we are not alone in claiming that possibly we have overshot the mark in our critical attitude. I need only mention Whitehead, philosopher and mathematician, as supporting such a view.

The other side of the cognitive problem of causality, however, concerns the behavioural world, or rather the psychophysical field, itself. We must raise this question: If in our behavioural world an object A exerts a force on B, by setting it into motion or affecting it in some other way, are we justified in assuming that A as a process in the psychophysical field actually affects the psychophysical process B? When we think of our billiard ball example it may appear that such an assumption is unnecessary. For the second behavioural billiard ball will stay at rest, however strong the force with which the first behavioural ball hits it, unless the second *real* ball actually moves. The motion of the real ball is therefore a necessary condition for the motion of the behavioural ball, and it seems unnecessary to add to this patent cause another purely hypothetical one. On the other hand we know from Wertheimer's experiment reported on page 371 that behavioural motion may produce another behavioural motion without a corresponding real motion (or its equivalent, kinematographic shift of phase). Our assumption of a direct effect of the moving behavioural ball upon the stationary one is, therefore, not quite so hypothetical, not entirely unsupported by fact. If our assumption is right, the motion of the second ball should, in its initial stage, be somewhat different whether it is experienced as due to the impact of another or not; and it should not be impossible to test this conclusion by experiments.

Before the experiment has spoken there remain then three possibilities: the experience of a causal connection between A and B may be (a) a sign that there is an actual causal dynamic relation between the two psychophysical process organizations A′ and B′, or (b) a sign of some other interrelationship between them, or (c) no such relation between A′ and B′ exists, and the experience of causality derives from secondary causes. The second member of this disjunction seems, at the moment, so improbable by itself that we will exclude it from further consideration. Should we, then, choose between (a) and (c), or leave the question completely open? (c) is the traditional view, closely connected with associationism, which we shall later on reject for good reasons. (a) is perfectly consistent with our whole theory of field organization, and at the same time a clear-cut example of isomorphism. Moreover, we shall presently discuss cases where indeed the experienced connection and the actual ones coincide. Therefore, fully aware that the experiment will have to give the final verdict, we accept (a). As a matter of fact we have done so already in our last chapter when we introduced the *manifest* organization within the behavioural environment. We feel, to recall one of the examples discussed there, the disturbing influence exerted by a Renoir picture on a Dürer, and no doubt this feeling is well founded, for the disturbance disappears when we separate the two pictures sufficiently.

Cognitive Value of Manifest Organization. Manifest organization has then a cognitive value that goes beyond that of silent organization; for it gives us some *direct* information about events in a part of the geographical world, viz., that part which we call our brain; whereas silent organization gives us only indirect information about the same part of the world.

This direct information is never complete. It tells us very little of the actual dynamical interplay, and as often as not it will give only a part of the effective forces; the organization is, in other words, as a rule partly manifest and partly silent. Therefore it can be as easily overrated as underestimated. But the knowledge that this source of information may be misused must not prevent us from using it correctly.

Manifest Organization in Phenomenal Behaviour. Its Cognitive Value. Insight. We can now turn to the manifest forces between the field and the Ego which we have already amply discussed in the last chapter. This discussion ought to have made it plain that here a correspondence[1] exists between the behavioural and the psychophysical force, whether the former appears in the form of a need, a signal, a demand-, or a physiognomic character. Manifest organization has a particularly important cognitive value, for it presents us with a picture of the dynamics of our behaviour. We do not only act, but we know why we act. "Wherever this is the case we apply the term 'insight,'" said Köhler in a very similar connection (1929, p. 371). Thus, in this terminology, the existence of manifest Ego-field organization is tantamount to insightful behaviour. Again, however, one has to examine the cognitive value of such insight. How far is it an indication of the forces that underlie real behaviour? The reader who remembers the early part of this book will recall that we did not accept it there as a sufficient indicator. In the second chapter (pp. 50 f.), we discussed types of action in which the manifest forces were at best a small part of the real forces, where insight, taken at its face value, was deceptive. We have, unfortunately, no guarantee that all effective forces become manifest. But again the fact that insight may be wrongly employed must not prevent us from employing it correctly and attributing to it that importance which it possesses. Through insight, phenomenal behaviour (defined on p. 40) becomes meaningful, just as real behaviour becomes meaningful through the conservative tendency of the organism as formulated in Humphrey's principle (p. 308). On neither side, the real or the phenomenal, do we meet a mere haphazard sequence of events, on either side we find the events definitely directed. Does this not lend support to isomorphism?

consciousness without insight. Have I succeeded in impressing the reader with the importance that manifest organization possesses for our phenomenal behaviour? Let him picture a person endowed with consciousness, but without any kind of manifest organization, and compare such consciousness with his own. This person would be surrounded by objects and would feel himself approaching one, avoiding another, having pleasure in one set of conditions and being angry in another. But that would be all. He would, let us say, feel thirsty and drink a glass of water, and then feel his thirst quenched, but he would not know that he drank the water *because* he was thirsty, nor that his thirst vanished *because* of the drink. He would see a beautiful woman, would approach her, hear himself make the most clever and alluring speeches, find himself in flower shops ordering bunches of long-stemmed red roses addressed to that lady, he might even hear himself propose, be accepted, become married, but in the words of the baron in Gorki's "Lower Depths," "Why? No notion." Of course he could not really say these words because he would not know what "why?" means, a why presupposing manifest organization. Provided such a person could become a scientist and a philosopher—although I do not see how he could—what would his philosophy be? Without a doubt an extreme positivism of the Humean kind. But why should we, whose experiences are so different from and so much richer than the experience of this imaginary person, develop a similar philosophy?

The picture of this kind of consciousness shows us clearly that the possession of consciousness *per se* is nothing valuable. This person would be just as well off without it, if not better. Thus we have returned to a point which we raised at the end of the second chapter, where we discussed the alleged materialistic bias of isomorphism (pp. 64 f.).

INSIGHT APPLIED TO BEHAVIOURAL ENVIRONMENT. In the world of our imaginary person there would be no forces. One billiard ball would run, come in contact with another, stop, and the other would begin to roll. A pure sequence of events. Two trains would collide, leave the tracks, the cars turn turtle and become wrecked; another mere sequence. We need not continue. The behavioural world of this person would be poorer than ours in the same proportion in which his phenomenal behaviour would be. For we experience manifest organization also in our behavioural environment, there also "not only the result is experienced, but also very much of its 'why' and 'how' is felt. . . ." In short Köhler's definition of insight fits this aspect of the behavioural environment as well as phenomenal behaviour. Our behavioural world is ever so much more full of insight than that of the fictitious person, ever so much more meaningful.

SILENT EGO-ORGANIZATION

The problem of cognition will be resumed when we treat of memory and thought. We continue the discussion of this chapter by taking up another aspect of the problem of silent and manifest organization. We have seen that at least most manifest organizations include the Ego. But it would be wrong to infer from this fact that all organizations in which the Ego takes part are manifest. As a matter of fact we have previously, in Chapter VI (pp. 216 f. and 219 f.), discussed the Ego localization in its spatial framework, which is truly a case of silent organization.

Ego and Framework in Behaviour. We shall discuss this Ego-framework localization now with regard to action. Already we have seen that the framework is as constant as the conditions allow. When we act we change the position of our real body and thereby the retinal distribution. To this change of the *conditions* of our behavioural world a change in the total behavioural world must correspond, but it does not follow which part of this world will change. As we have pointed out in Chapter V, the change is the invariant, a definite amount of movement or change in the behavioural world must result from a given change in the effective conditions, but not necessarily a change in the behavioural *environment*. As a matter of fact, in normal cases of body-movements the framework will remain constant, and the Ego will be the carrier of the motion. We walk through our rooms, our retinal images change constantly, but the behavioural room remains at rest, the behavioural Ego is experienced as in motion. Duncker's work on induced motion has shown why this must be so. If real relative motion occurs between two objects, S and E, it is, *ceteris paribus,* E, the enclosed one, and not S, the surrounding one, which will appear as moved. We can express this also by saying: Our actions change our relation to the geographical environment and thereby the proximal stimulation which we receive from it; but the behavioural world arising out of this changing stimulation is such that the framework remains constant, while the Ego and possibly some of the objects are in motion.

The Special Problems of Localization with Moving Eyes. Duncker has also applied his theory to an old problem of space perception. The classical theory of localization had to distinguish localization with steady gaze and with moving eyes, of which the second one is at the same time the normal case and that which offered greater difficulties to the theory. Why is it, this was the main question, that the behavioural objects stay in their places when owing to our eye-movements the retinal images on account of which we see them move across the retina? Hering's theory, ingenious though it was, shows the additive character of the theorizing of his time (1879, pp. 531 f.). With normal position of the eyes each retinal point has, in this theory, as we have previously seen, a definite space value. The fovea F, e.g., has the space value 0, and L, a point to the left of it, say, the value + x, i.e., it appears to the right of the "straight ahead" (see Fig. 93). When we now turn our eyes to the right through an angle which corresponds to the distance FL, the object which was formerly projected on L is now projected on F, and that originally projected on F is now projected on a point R, FR = FL, with a space value (approximately) = —x. If the retinal points preserved their space values during the eye-movements, our two objects ought to have undergone a displacement to the left. In reality they appear at rest. Consequently Hering assumes that during the eye-movement all space values are changed in such a way that they are displaced by the exact amount of the motion. This is an adequate description of the facts in terms of this theory as will be clear from the following table, in which we list the space values of the three retinal points, F, L, and R, before and after the eye-movements.

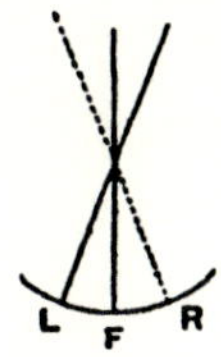

Fig. 93

TABLE 11

Retinal point	Before the eye-movement, object A on F, B on L	After the eye-movement, object A on R, B on F
F	0	+x
L	+x	+2x
R	—x	0

The eye, turning to the right, has added to each retinal point a "right" value corresponding to the amount of the eye-movement. The result is that the objects remain in their places, the shift of retinal points on which the objects are projected being exactly compensated by a shift in the respective space values of the retinal points. The object A was originally projected on F with the space value 0 and appeared in a certain place characterized as straight ahead. After the movement it falls on R, which originally had the space value —x; i.e., an object falling on this point before the movement was made would appear to the left of the straight ahead. But through the movement all space values have been changed by +x; therefore R, the point on which A is now being projected, has the resultant space value $-x + x = 0$, i.e., the object appears where it appeared before.

As a pure description this scheme fits the facts. But it wanted to be more than a mere description, it claimed to contain the explanation of the phenomenon. Therefore it had to assign a cause to this change of space value which the retinal points undergo. This cause lies, according to Hering, in *attention*. When we move our eyes voluntarily our attention accompanies or rather precedes our eye-movements and causes this change of the space values. Hillebrand has even attempted to show why a change of attention should produce this change of space values, but his theory is too complex to be reported here. Neither shall I criticize the details of this theory except by pointing out that it omits one essential part of the data: after we have moved our eyes we see indeed the objects in the same places in which we saw them before, but at the same time we are aware that *we* are no longer looking straight ahead! This last fact has been entirely neglected by the Hering-Hillebrand theory. And yet it is directly derivable from Duncker's theory in the same way in which we derived the constancy of the framework during actual body movements from it. The ocular system is a part of the Ego. The motion which results in the behavioural world on account of a displacement of retinal patterns may as well be carried by this *part* of the Ego as by the whole Ego, if the conditions are such as to keep the rest of the Ego constant.

There is, however, one fact that lent particularly strong support to the Hering theory and which therefore must now be harmonized with Duncker's. In cases of recent paresis of the eye muscles the patients see the objects in their field of vision in motion when they move their eyes. The connection with Hering's theory is very simple. Let us assume the right external muscle to be the paretic one. Then the eye will not completely obey the innervation of a movement, the actually executed movement will be smaller than the "intended" movement. This must, according to the Hering theory, lead to a displacement of the objects. Let us glance back at our table (on p. 385). The change of space values will, in the case of the patient, be the same as that indicated in our table, because it depends upon the *intended* movement, that is, the change of attention which is characteristic of our intention. But the shift of the objects over the retina will be different. Thus object A instead of being transported to R will be brought only to R′ with the space value $-y$, $y < x$. On the other hand, owing to the shift of attention all retinal points will have shifted their space values by $+x$. Consequently the place at which A. will appear after the eye-movement will be $-y + x$ which is > 0, i.e., the object is moved in the direction of the eye-movement, it has run away, so to speak, from the eye. This fact, as also that we see the objects moving when we move our eyes by pressing our fingers against the bulbs, proves that the theory cannot be quite so simple as we presented it. The difference between the normal and the last two cases is this: in the last one the eyes are moved without the participation of the oculomotor system, in the preceding they are moved by a partly disabled motor apparatus, while in the first the movement and the resulting shift of the retinal image takes place through the normal functioning of nerves and muscles. That looks as though under these conditions the eye-system of the Ego becomes the motion carrier only to the degree that the oculomotor system is involved, independently of the effect that is eventually achieved. Therefore, when the oculomotor system does not participate at all, as in displacements of the bulbs by pressure, the eyes will not be experienced as moving, and the full amount of the stimulus shift will appear in motion of the objects. On the other hand, in the case of the paretic muscle the eye-system will carry a movement greater than is warranted by the actual shift of the retinal image, i.e., the relative motion between object and eyes would be too great if the object appeared at rest, since the amount of experienced displacement was to be the invariant, determined by the amount of actual displacement. Therefore the objects must also appear to move in the same direction as the eyes. The reader may find it hard to understand this deduction. Therefore I shall give my argument in another way. In reality, and on the retina, the two objeqts A and B are in relative motion with regard to each other; the relative displacement, after time T, having the magnitude S. Then, according to our invariance theorems, a motion of the extent s should be *perceived,* distributed among the behavioural objects a and b according to the special conditions. Let a and b move along the line ab, during the time T. Then the path traversed by a will be s_1, and that traversed by b, s_2. And therefore the change of distance between a and b, at the end of the motion, $= s_1 - s_2$. This is, according to our invariance theorem,

$= s$; $s_1 - s_2 = s$. Naturally, if $s_1 = 0, -s_2 = s$, and if $s_2 = 0, s_1 = s$, representing the cases where one object is seen at rest and the other as the sole carrier of the motion. It is evident that in these cases the motions of either of these objects must be in opposite directions, s_1 being positive, s_2 negative. If $s_1 < s$, then $-s_2 > 0$, and therefore $s_2 < 0$; again the objects move in different directions. But if $s_1 > s$, then s_2 must be > 0, i.e., both objects must move in the same direction. We can apply this directly to the case of eye-movements, s_1 being the experienced movements of the eyes, s_2 that of the objects, and s, determined by the retinal displacement S, the total relative shift between the behavioural eye-system and the objects. In the normal case $s_1 = s$ and therefore $s_2 = 0$. In the case of the paretic muscle $s_1 > s$, therefore $s_2 > 0$, the objects must move in the same direction as the eyes. In the case of the eye moving through pressure of the finger $s_1 = 0$, therefore $s_2 = -s$, the objects are the sole motion carriers and move in a direction opposite to that of the eye. Finally we may consider the case of complete paralysis of the eye muscle. Here $S = 0$ and therefore $s = 0$, no displacement between objects and eye-system can be experienced. But $s_1 > 0 = x$, then s_2 also $= x$, the patient feels his eyes and the objects moving in the same direction and with the same angular displacement. This case is instructive because it shows that our presentation was oversimplified, for here we have $S = 0$ and yet a perception of motion, indicating that a third system, the body-system, must be taken into account. $S = 0$ would be perfectly compatible with no movement being experienced, either of the objects or of the eyes. In reality the latter is experienced and therefore also the former. The cause of the process, therefore, cannot be the shift of the retinal image alone, for if it were we could not understand why in this case any experience of motion occurs. Instead we must assume that intra-Ego forces become operative and determine directly the extent of the s_1. Then, because of the invariance theorem, the s_2 is also determined.[5]

In favour of our explanation we can add two facts. The first, mentioned in the third chapter, when we discussed the zenith-horizon illusion, is that perceptual properties, like size, depend upon the condition of the oculomotor system (pp. 94 f.). Therefore we are not raising an entirely new claim when we now attribute to the oculomotor system a decisive influence upon the localization and motion of objects. The second is the fact that paretic patients know of their disability only through the disturbing behaviour of the

[5] See also Köhler, 1933.

objects around them and not through any feeling of being hampered in moving their eyes. Even a person with complete paralysis of the rectus externus will have the impression that his eyes, actually immobile, move to the right.

There are still other cases where the eyes seem to move although in reality they do not. In Duncker's experiment it happened frequently that the fixated one of two objects was seen in motion, even when in reality the non-fixated one was the motion carrier. The primary effect here is the induced motion of the fixated object; from this, motion of the eyes must follow according to the invariance theorem, in the same way as in our previous cases. Since there is *no* displacement, no relative motion between eyes and objects can be experienced. Since, then, the objects appear in motion, the eyes must appear in motion also; the subject believes that he follows the moving object with his eyes when in reality he fixates steadily a non-moving object. This case fits our interpretation perfectly well, for in this case the oculomotor system is in direct connection with the perceptive one, since, as we have seen, without such a connection fixation would be inexplicable.

EFFECTS ON THE EGO OF AN UNSTABLE FRAMEWORK. All these effects were effects of silent organization including the Ego or one of its sub-systems. They were governed by the rule of the stability of the framework. In an unstable framework all action is severely hampered, because posture and balance are seriously affected. It is astonishing how little attention psychologists have paid to this point. And yet the simplest kind of experiment demonstrates the importance of a stable spatial framework for the maintenance of our bodily balance. It is quite easy for any normal person to stand on one leg as long as he keeps his eyes open. But try it with closed eyes, and you will be surprised how difficult it is, how soon you will have to use the other leg to keep yourself from toppling over. It is no exaggeration to say that we stand on our eyes as we stand on our feet, or perhaps better, that we balance with our eyes, and lean with our eyes against the surroundings as we do with our hands. This reminds us of one of Hartgenbusch's examples, the failure of the heavy athletes to break the existing records because of the lack of articulation of the walls at which they had to look (see Chapter II, p. 45). The most impressive demonstration of the support which our balance gains from sight is obtained when we try to stand upright on a narrow peak with a drop of hundreds or thousands of feet on either side. I quote from Thouless (1928), who has published a delightful paper on this and similar problems: "If the novice is urged to stand upright on the top of Napes Needle, the balancing difficulty appears to him to be insuperable. Indeed he need not go so high as that. If he mounts an isolated flat-topped rock eight feet from the ground, he will find great difficulty in standing upright on it" (p. 162). In the first case there is no visual frame to lend support to the mountain-climber, in the second, the framework is distorted by the fact that an articulated field exists "behind" the person standing on the rock, but not in front. Therefore the person will be in danger of falling forward over the edge. Thouless's explanation, slightly different in detail, also deduces a dislocation of the visual vertical.

Since we depend so much for our very balance on a fixed framework, any instability or change of it will have profound effects on our behaviour. Watson lists loss of support as one of the two primary stimuli to produce fear reaction. This fact becomes intelligible from our point of view. Loss of support means an instability of the framework, for as we have also pointed out previously, our space is by no means entirely visual (see Chapter IV, p. 121). This refers particularly to the spatial framework, which depends to a considerable extent upon the factors indicated in the passage just referred to previously. Loss of support will affect primarily the vestibular and the deep sensibility factors, which in an infant with a very poorly articulated visual space are the main foundations of the framework. Therefore loss of physical support means for the infant a loss of behavioural support through instability of the framework, with the very violent effects described by Watson. We can duplicate this experience by purely visual means. The revolving room used to be a popular attraction at county fairs. Here the visitor intent on being thrilled was led into a perfectly normal-looking room whose walls suddenly began to rotate at great speed with the result that the visitor became thoroughly dizzy, as much as if he had been rotated himself.[6] The effect of the shift of the framework is clear. I derive another example from rock climbing. When one climbs a fairly steep ridge—an experience whose relation to our problem has been well discussed by Thouless—and then comes to a horizontal resting place where one can stand upright quite easily, one feels at the first moment rather uncomfortable: the world has, for a second or so, lost its stability, it begins to rock and one is tempted to rock with it. The explanation is again

[6] Recent investigations have shown that this effect is strongest with a certain range of velocities, viz., one revolution in three to five seconds under the special conditions of the experiment, where a drum with alternating black and white stripes of 1.5 cm. width was the rotating object. (Vogel.)

a shift of the framework. While one is climbing, the ridge is phenomenally vertical or nearly so; it forms the main part of one's spatial framework. When now one stands up, the framework has to shift and the shift is not well defined, since on either side the ridge is surrounded by air and the nearest objects are far away.

Summary: Framework and Posture. Thus we see how important the framework is for action. For although all specific activity is directed towards objects and not towards the framework, yet posture and balance, without which action is impossible, depend to a very large extent on the framework. Posture is, of course, also action, maintained by a constant interplay of innervations. The maintenance of posture is, in other words, also a task of the executive, and in this task the executive seems primarily controlled by the framework-Ego forces.

DIRECTED ACTION. THE FORCE DIAGRAMS

If now we turn from postural to directed action we find the objects in the field of paramount importance. For each individual situation one has to try to discover the forces at work and the constraints in the field which limit the freedom of action. With great consistency Lewin and his school have applied this method, presenting various fields by special diagrams from which the resulting actions can be deduced. A relatively simple example is that of a child confronted either with an attractive but forbidden object, or with an unpleasant task for which he will be rewarded. The reader will find the respective diagrams in Lewin's article of 1931.

The objects within such a field have various characteristics with regard to the behaviour of the Ego; there are goal objects, paths leading to the goal, tools, signs and signals, barriers, detours and so forth, a number of which have been aptly discussed by Tolman, although in my opinion this author oversimplifies the picture by his concept of the *sign-gestalt,* by which he attributes primary importance to signs, whereas they seem to me but one among many different kinds of dynamic objects. Our description of field behaviour in Chapter II (pp. 43 f.) should be reread from the point of view of our last discussion.

Variability of the Dynamic Characters. In thinking of our fields in this dynamic manner we must avoid the error of overestimating the constancy of the dynamic characters of objects. We have already seen how the demand characters will change with needs. But this is only one of the possible changes that may and will take place. A detour may become the direct route, a barrier a stepping stone, a toy a tool, an attractive object a repulsive one during the progress of one action, depending upon the momentary conditions. These changes will occupy us in our discussion of learning, for they may be more or less permanent. We have to stress here only one point, because it is significant for action.

The Functional Characters of Behavioural Objects. When we recall the discussion of the behavioural environment presented in our Chapters IV and V, we may feel that something of great importance was left out there. We treated behavioural environment largely as though it consisted of squares, circles, ellipses and other shapes in various colours and at different places, also of cubes, spheres and other solids. But the laws of organization there derived did not explain why we see chairs and tables, houses and bridges, or post-offices, letter boxes, motor cars, etc. They could not give such an explanation because they treated only of forces within the external or environmental part of the psychophysical field, and these forces cannot possibly produce by themselves the objects of our daily use. For the characteristic of all the objects that we mentioned as neglected by our previous theory is that they bear a relation to our own activities. To a stranger the red pillars in the streets of London are just curious red pillars; it is their use that makes them letter boxes, and a Bushman suddenly transported into New York harbour would think that he was approaching a wild mountainous country. Conversely, for an artist a house may become a cube, a mountain a cone, and that not only for a cubist. Thus, like most of the physiognomic characters, these "functional" characters are products of an object-Ego organization, different from the former by the fact that they are not primary results of such organizations but can emerge only when the particular object has functioned in a behaviour act. Therefore these characters depend on pre-existing needs like the demand characters, but again in a different way. The demand characters will, as a rule, come and go with the need. The functional characters will, as a rule, be permanent and disappear only as a result of special forces, like the particular attitude of the artist. I believe it to be a true proposition that all demand characters presuppose either physiognomic or functional characters. Thus the *green* box over there will not make me deviate from my course in order to get rid of my letter, but the *letter* box; I will not use this T-shaped object for driving a nail into my wall, but this hammer; and so forth. Nevertheless, there must have been a time when such a T-shaped object was just a T-shaped object, and when, because of its possible use as a tool, it became a hammer. But let us return to the relation between functional characters and needs. As long as no need arises for using a hammer, there will not be any hammers, however many suitable T-shaped objects there may be around. But to us a hammer is a hammer even when we do not need it, although then it will not determine our actions through its hammer properties; if it enters into our behaviour it may do so in many ways, as a mere obstacle to be removed, as a paper weight, and so on. Its "demand" character has varied all the time, whereas its functional character has remained constant. This must mean that through its use the object has undergone a permanent change of organization, by virtue of which it is no longer an Ego-independent thing, like the squares and crosses which we used in our former demonstrations, but a thing with a permanent relation to the Ego. And it means secondly that such a reorganization may become permanent. The general meaning of this statement we shall discuss in our chapter on memory (Chapter XI); at this place the remark must suffice that the behavioural environment of a living being at any one moment of his life depends also upon the behavioural environments at earlier moments of his life. This in itself is a trite statement. There is no psychologist who has not taught that perception depends upon experience and memory; as we know from our discussion in the third chapter (see p. 85) traditional psychology *defined* perception by the participation of memory and distinguished it thereby from sensation. But this theory is radically different from the one we are advancing here. On the one hand it sticks to the constancy hypothesis (see p. 86) for its explanation of sensations; on the other it explains perception by the *addition* of new elements, images, to these sensations, in the assimilation hypothesis (see p. 103). We have in our third chapter rejected all these traditional hypotheses, and now we have put in their place a new one which, vague though it has to be at the moment—and even our later discussion will not be able to make it much more definite—escapes all the objections raised against the old theories and is perfectly consistent with our fundamental hypotheses. In this new theory experience has its place. Had it not, our theory would indeed be foolish. But in our theory the effect of experience is not that of adding new elements to old ones, but of changing a prior organization.

We possess as yet very little experimental evidence for supporting our theory of the functional characters. From human experiment we might adduce work done on the "quality of pliancy" ("Gefügigkeitsqualität") by Ach (1930) in which he established functional characters of nonsense syllables by the manner in which the subjects had to react to them. As far as I can see from Ach's short report, his results, as far as they go, are in good agreement with our theory. But the conditions of this experiment were too artificial, the relation between the material and its functional characters too arbitrary, for making these experiments the basis of generalizations. Animal experimentation since Köhler's classical work with chimpanzees has been more relevant. In animal psychology the *new* use of familiar objects by animals has been enforced, and therefore, if we are allowed to go by analogy, new functional characters in their behavioural environment have been produced. Unfortunately this inference by analogy can never be verified directly, although some ingenious experimenter may invent new methods of corroborating it indirectly. Meanwhile it would not add weight to our argument if we enumerated details of these experiments, which, besides, are familiar to most psychologists. We shall have to wait for good experiments on human subjects; they are, for our purposes, to be preferred to animals not only because they can speak and therefore report the changes which the behavioural objects undergo, but also because they have so many more needs, and are capable of creating ever new ones, so that functional characters corresponding to an enormous variety of such needs could be created.

ATTITUDES AND THEIR EFFECTS ON THE BEHAVIOURAL ENVIRONMENT

Although, then, we have no direct experimental knowledge of the arousal of functional characters by Ego-object forces, we are in a much better position with regard to the more general problem whether the Ego can influence the behavioural field. Not only everyday experience, but well controlled experimental evidence compels us to answer this question in the affirmative. In Chapter IV we have already referred to the fact that the visibility of a point depends upon the attitude of the onlooker (pp. 148 f.); during the first period of experimental psychology the problem arose whether attention could change the intensity of a sensation, and the result of experiments designed to solve it showed the existence of such an effect.[7] The fact that clangs can be analyzed, their overtones heard, under a special direction of the attention, belongs to the oldest store of knowledge our science possesses, although the actual explanation of this effect was not achieved till some years after the war (Eberhardt, 1922). For the problem of organization was unknown to

[7] See, for instançe, the discussion by Stumpf, pp. 71 f.

the older psychology, at least in the form in which it has followed us through this whole book. And changes in the behavioural environment, whether they be due to attention, attitude, or what not, are primarily changes of organization. As such a factor of organization, attitudes have been most thoroughly investigated by Gottschaldt (1926 and 1929), and Köhler has discussed under this aspect many examples taken from everyday life.

Attitude and Attention Defined. Before we present Gottschaldt's experiments, it will be fitting to define what we mean by attitude and attention. From our previous discussions of both these concepts it is clear that we mean by them actual *forces* that participate in the total dynamic situation (see pp. 149 and 206), actual forces that exist between the field and the Ego. It seems to conform to good usage if we attribute the more general meaning to the term attitude, the more special to the term attention. Attention would then be a special attitude, namely that of simple unspecific directedness towards an object, whereas other attitudes would be more specific, like expectation of something more or less definite, putting the centre of gravity in one place rather than another, being suspicious, curious, etc. In discussing attention we distinguished the cases where the origin of the force was in the Ego, voluntary, and, where it lay in the object, involuntary attention. Whether this same distinction is applicable to the other attitudes will not be decided here; surely, in many cases these attitudes originate in the Ego, its needs or quasi-needs. The degree to which these attitudes reveal themselves in consciousness is variable. In Gottschaldt's experiments the existence and efficacy of attitudes was proved by their effect and not by reports of the subjects, whose attitude varied between an active searching and mere passive conviction that a certain pattern would be shown to them.

Gottschaldt's Experiments. From the great number of different experiments performed by Gottschaldt I shall only report a few. We will begin with those which followed immediately upon his experiments already reported in Chapter IV (pp. 156 f.). On the day after the subjects had for the first time been shown the *b* figures (the reader will have to turn back to Chapter IV for an explanation of the method and terminology), the first group, who had previously seen the *a* figures 3 times, were shown them another 2 times, while the second group, who had seen the *a* figures 520 times, were presented with them another 20 times. Both groups were then shown the *b* figures for two seconds each with the instruction to search for one of the previously seen *a* figures. We present the results in the same way as before (see Table 6, p. 157), adding the figures of our old table in columns I and III. The results are very significant. A comparison of II with I and IV with III shows the effect of the new instruction, a comparison of II and IV, just as formerly the comparison of I and III, shows the ineffectiveness of the accumulation of repetitions, the figures in column II and IV show by themselves the amount of success of the new instruction. Clearly the search attitude has some influence, whereas mere repetition has none whatever, but equally clearly in the majority of

TABLE 12

	Group I		Group II	
	neutral 3 repet. 92 cases	searching 5 repet. 93 cases	neutral 520 repet. 242 cases	searching 540 repet. 248 cases
a has some influence	6.6	31.2	5.0	28.3
a has no influence	93.4	68.8	95.0	71.7
	I	II	III	IV

cases the forces corresponding to this search attitude are not sufficient to overcome the internal forces of organization within the figures. However, attitude may have an effect upon organization, an effect which is not reducible to experience.

In another paper Gottschaldt published new experiments devised to bring out the influence of attitude. Among other methods he used the device described on page 143 by which figures were exposed with a gradually increasing degree of distinctness. The subjects had to stop the experimenter as soon as they saw anything new and had to draw on paper what they had been seeing. Thus the gradual development of figures could be studied, and it could be determined whether, provided an *a* and a *b* figure had different histories of development, the history of the *b* figure could be influenced by frequent experience of the *a* figure contained within it. The results were again entirely negative as long as special attitudes were excluded but changed radically when such attitudes were aroused, not by special instructions, but by the temporal course of the experimental series. Two main *a b* combinations were used, as represented in Figs. 94 and 95.

Let us call the first the cross-square, and the second the arrow-circle pattern. The *b* figure of the former developed normally in such a way that first the square was seen to which the vertical dash was added considerably later. Similarly in the second *b* figure the circle preceded the arrow-part. Then a long series of exposures was arranged in which the two *a* figures alternated 12 times. If we give a number to each exposure the first 24 exposures would then be simple alternations of the *a* figures, the cross appearing in the odd, the arrow in the even places. There was only one slight interruption of this sequence, inasmuch as after three alternations, i.e., at exposures 7 and 8, not the *a* but the corresponding *b* figures were

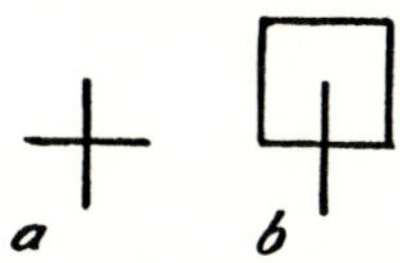

Fig. 94

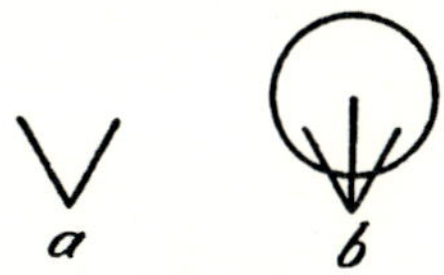

Fig. 95

shown. All six subjects saw, in contradiction to the normal history of these figures, first the cross and the arrow respectively, and the experiment was stopped before they had seen the complete figures, so that the sequence of alternations was not really interrupted as far as the subjects were concerned. But after the 24th exposure another change was introduced: either No. 25 was a *b* figure, but this time the circle instead of the cross, the latter following as No. 26, or No. 25 was still regular, the simple cross *a* figure, but was followed by the *b* figure of the *same* pattern (cross-square), No. 26, and the series concluded by 27, the *b* circle figure. Now five out of the six subjects saw these figures arise normally, the square and the circle preceding, quite uninfluenced by the practice of the corresponding *a* figures of which there had now been much more than at the beginning, when the *a* figures had determined the appearance of the *b* ones. Moreover, in the second alternative, the *b* square figure, No. 26, followed immediately upon the *a* square figure, No. 25, and yet in all three cases the square appeared first and not the cross. This experiment proves that mere repetition qua repetition has no effect on the perceptual organization under the conditions of this experiment, where the internal forces of organization are fairly strong, but that the attitude of the observer at the moment of the exposure has a very direct influence. For what is the difference between the first and the second exposures of the *b* figures? In the first they occurred in the place of their corresponding *a* figures; these latter were expected, and thereby the organization of the *b* figures was changed. In the second experiment the *b* figures appeared where not the corresponding *a* figure but another *a* was expected. Here no influence of the *a* figure appeared, since the expectation did not fit with any possible organization producible by the stimulus. Two other such series of exposures are represented in Fig. 96 a and b. In the first the temporal structure of the series is such that after the first exposure of the cross (No. 11) another cross was expected, with the result that the square *b* figure began to develop with the cross, despite the fact that a simple square had been presented five times immediately preceding the first cross exposure. Conversely, in the second series the *b* cross-square figure appeared directly after the cross *a* figure, which during that series had already been shown eight times, but in such a way that the subject expected a new figure. The result was that this *b* figure developed normally, the square and not the cross taking the lead.

Conclusion. Thus Gottschaldt's truly elegant experiments prove that forces originating in the Ego can exert an influence on the behavioural environment of the Ego by influencing its organization. At the same time Gottschaldt proved that there are very definite limits to such an influence. The *b* figures used in the three series described last were all such that the *a* figures were either real parts of them, arrow-circle pattern, or were in no great conflict with the *b* organization. In other words the production of *a* figures under these conditions had to contend against relatively weak forces only. As Gottschaldt has shown in special experiments—as also in those with search instruction reported on page 396—the attitudes will not be able to overcome strong internal forces of organization, i.e., they will not produce an *a* organization when the *a* figure is by structural principles completely lost in the *b* patterns.

Application to Clang Analysis. Since we have mentioned the case of clang analysis as a classical example of the effect of attitude upon the behavioural environment, we may add that this effect is also a case of change of organization, as Dr. Eberhardt has experimentally proved. To "analyze" an overtone is not to make a pre-existing tone-sensation "noticed," but to change the result of the stimulation by replacing a unified and rich clang by a duality of tone experiences.

The Influence of Attitudes in Non-experimental Situations. Attitudes, then, have a definite influence on the field organization which may overcome contrary forces of internal organization. Naturally, the weaker these counterforces are, the more will the field be de-

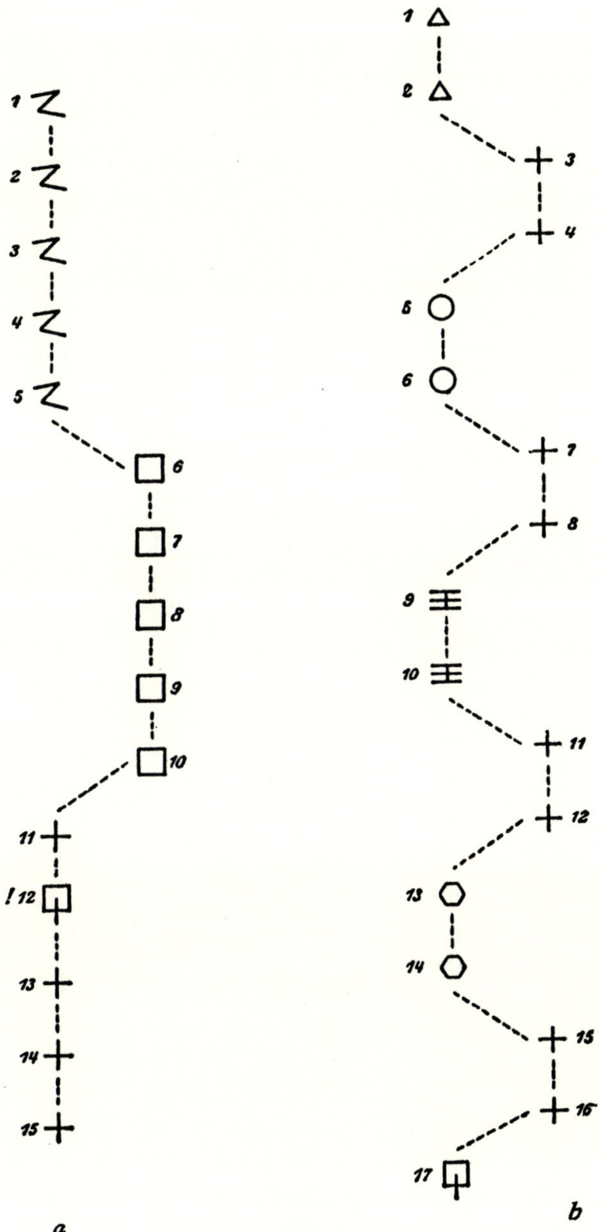

Fig. 96

terminable by attitudes. As a matter of fact the cases which Gottschaldt investigated and in which the internal forces of organization were still relatively strong are very rare in the field of perception, though they may play a greater rôle in the field of thought. Outside the laboratory we have little occasion to change one figure into another. Nevertheless, our previous discussion (pp. 148 f.) of the effect of attitudes on the perception of points proves that such reorganization of the field through attitudes plays some part outside the laboratory, and the reader will be able to augment this example by many others. But as a rule our attitudes influence field organizations where counterforces either do not exist or are very weak. The case, taken from Köhler, where I group the couples sitting around a table either by perceiving the two opposite or the two next to each other as partners, gives a good demonstration. If I consider them as bridge players, N and Miss S, E and Miss W, will form a subgroup, if as a merry party, N will be grouped with Miss W and E with Miss S. There is nothing, or at best very little, in the actual configuration which would favour either organization at the cost of the other and therefore organization follows attitudes very easily. Now this case is perpetually realized, since we always look around us with definite attitudes. Since attitudes themselves may vary enormously the possibility of changes produced in the field by attitudes is practically unlimited.

EMOTIONS

On page 395 we have enumerated a few such different attitudes, and these attitudes, like suspicion, curiosity, and even expectation, definitely imply an emotional tone. In other words we have already approached the field of emotions and sentiments, for just as an attitude of mere attention may influence the field, an attitude of hatred or extreme distrust may produce reorganizations, not only different from but also greater in degree than the changes brought about by mere attention. Hatred and mistrust are called sentiments in their lasting and latent stages, and violent emotions at moments when they break through and dominate the executive. We must, therefore, turn now to a discussion of emotions and sentiments, concentrating our efforts on the former, since our knowledge of the actual dynamic situations is not great enough to allow for their differential treatment.

Traditional Treatment of Emotions. The psychological theory of emotions is highly unsatisfactory. The reader will find two excellent presentations of the experimental and theoretical work done in the field of emotion in the two modern text-books by Wheeler and Woodworth, two presentations which will confirm my judgment. On the one hand, psychologists were bent on describing, analyzing, and classifying the emotions; on the other hand, they studied their physiological symptoms. The first attempt led to the distinction of simple and complex, and of primary and derived, emotions; the second brought to light a number of facts about different bodily functions like respiration, heart-beat, internal secretion, but no co-ordination between the findings of the two kinds could be established. Of course, for a long time the work in this field was profoundly influenced by the famous James-Lange theory, which despite certain merits was a typical product of nineteenth century psychology. I see the merits of this theory in its opposition to an abstract "structuralism," an interpretation of the emotions as special mental elements, or special compounds of special mental elements. What I regard as the only real achievement of the theory is its insistence upon the fact that emotions are more than just contents of consciousness, that they are processes pervading and often enough swamping the whole organism. But the theory went wrong in sticking too close to the view it tried to combat, in explaining emotions as the sensory knowledge of such organic processes. Much as James must have enjoyed the paradox that to be sad was to sense the activity of the tear glands, it is an absurd proposition, the great authority of James notwithstanding.

The theory of emotion has suffered from what I would call the static attitude of the psychologists. An emotion was considered as a sort of *thing,* the psychologists "indulging our natural tendency to reify whatever we name" (McDougall, 1923, p. 314), a tendency which we discussed in the beginning of the third chapter. But, of course, emotions cannot be treated adequately with the thing category. We cannot take them and cut them to pieces to see what they consist of. Again we are in full agreement with McDougall. who emphasizes "the obvious fact that there are no such things as 'emotions'" and prefers the adjectival to the substantival form of the term, just as Wheeler's chapter headings are not "The Emotions" but "Emotive Behaviour." That means: to certain psychophysical processes we apply the term "emotional" or "emotive," these terms therefore being *dynamic* characteristics, in the same sense as "accelerated," "crescendo," "oscillating," are dynamic characteristics of processes.

Emotions to Be Studied from the Point of View of Dynamics of Organization. Psychophysical processes are processes in organization. The study of organization must proceed, as we have seen all along, by searching for the underlying dynamical principles and the special conditions which determine the particular process organization to which in each concrete case the general principles give rise. Classification has played a minimal part in our investigation, and therefore classification shall be our least concern in the field of emotion also. It may be useful for a provisional mapping of the field of research, but it can give us no ultimate knowledge about its objects before research has reached a stage of completion and perfection; then classification may give a systematic survey of the accomplished theory, but naturally our knowledge of emotions is far from such a state. Instead we shall have to study the organizations in their dynamic properties, i.e., we shall have to analyze emotional situations so as to discover the actual forces at work.

Silent and Manifest Organization. This task will be facilitated if we apply our distinction of silent and manifest organization. If we do we must see at once that, at least to some extent, the emotional aspect of behaviour is a manifest aspect of organization. That we do not overrate the importance of this manifest character we have emphasized frequently enough (see pp. 50 and 382). With this reminder we can now proceed to explain what we mean by the manifest character of emotions. When we feel excited, or otherwise expressed, under a high state of tension, our psychophysical field is also in such a state of tension as is evidenced by the readiness to explosive behaviour under this condition. Again our feeling of irritability has its counterpart in a state of great instability of our Ego system, whereas a feeling of happy satisfaction corresponds to a psychophysical field at a lower level of tension and of greater stability. Subjective feeling and objective observation of behaviour or of physiological symptoms are in the best possible agreement. This is fundamental for our theory of the emotions. If there were no such agreement, if we could feel excited beyond all possible control, when our psychophysical field were as calm as a mountain lake at noon under a cloudless sky, our theory of the emotions, nay, our whole psychology, would have to be entirely different from what it is. Then it certainly could not be isomorphic, whereas the real facts support our isomorphistic methodolgy.

We can, however, go a step further: when we are afraid, we are as a rule not simply afraid, i.e., our consciousness is filled with some specific emotional quality, but we are afraid of something, and as our overt, or at least our implicit, behaviour reveals, this something actually influences our action. From facts such as these, indeed,

Köhler has derived his concept of non-silent organization. Thus the manifest aspect of emotion may not only reveal the degree and kind of tension that exists in the psychophysical field, but also its direction.

McDougall's Theory. This fact has been clearly recognized by McDougall, who made it the cornerstone of his theory of emotions. "The emotional qualities have, then, a cognitive function; they signify to us primarily not the nature of things, but rather the nature of our impulsive reactions to things" (p. 326). Or: "When we are afraid, we feel the impulse to retreat or escape from the object that frightens us; when we are angry, we feel the impulse to attack the object that angers us; when we are curious, we feel the impulse to draw nearer and examine the object that excites our curiosity" (p. 321). Although the terminology is slightly different from ours, these quotations reveal a fundamental agreement with the position we have so far taken. This agreement, I should like to say, does not result from the fact that McDougall's general principles are the same as ours. McDougall published the fundamentals of his theory in his "Introduction to Social Psychology" (1908) long before gestalt psychology existed, and gestalt psychology, on the other hand, is in its systematic aspect different, and in many respects even fundamentally different, from McDougall's general theoretical position. The agreement on which I insisted with so much satisfaction is due, in my opinion, to unbiassed observation and the manner of using such unbiassed observation in theoretical thinking.

McDougall's name is, however, associated with a more specific theory of emotion than this, the theory, namely, "that the primary 'emotions' are essentially indicators of the working of instinctive impulses" (p. 325). What McDougall means by instinct we have previously quoted (p. 356), viz., an innate disposition of perceiving and acting. It is at this point that we cannot follow McDougall any longer; in fact he seems to me here to have fallen to some extent into the error which he has criticized with great discrimination in many other cases, the error namely of reification. For the instinct as a disposition is, after all, a lasting entity, something of the nature of a thing. Surely, McDougall's conception is not as crude as all that, but the definition of instinct as innate disposition runs at least the great risk of abandoning a truly dynamic interpretation of behaviour, i.e., an interpretation of the forces actually at work at a given moment, and substituting for it an entity which achieves certain goals. This, since it is not a machine in his theory, must be something "which is therefore radically different from the energies which physical science conceives as working always mechanistically" (p. 317). It is important to note the caution with which McDougall expresses himself. He avoids the claim that purposive behaviour is radically different from physical processes, he only distinguishes it from such processes mechanistically conceived, and in an earlier part of the book he admits the possibility that all processes in the world are of one kind, though he deems it unlikely that this can be mechanism (p. 203). I do not know whether McDougall would call our treatment of purely physical and of psychophysical, including purposive, processes non-mechanical. He has made no attempt to change what he considers the physicist's interpretation of physical processes, and therefore his concepts, introduced in order to preserve in psychology the non-mechanistic interpretation, appear irreconcilable not only with a mechanistic but with any kind of physics. His instinct concept proves, I believe, my contention. "Thus, when the instinct of escape is excited, the impulse vents itself, and attains its goal, primarily and chiefly by locomotion" (p. 322). Now I cannot regard this as in any way an explanation of what actually happens. What I want is a much more concrete description of the actual dynamics involved than the conception of the "excitation of an instinct." Moreover, only such a concrete dynamic description of actual fields will support McDougall's valuable contribution to the theory of emotions, his view of the manifest character of the organizations in which they occur. For as his theory stands, it is exposed to this objection, which has been frequently brought against it: it is not true that any instinctive action carries the emotion corresponding to its instinct. Rather will the emotion be the greater, the less the organism is capable of acting.

An Example to Prove the Necessity of Supplementing McDougall's Theory by a Dynamical One. I shall discuss an example which will elucidate this, and another point: an object A will excite the instinct of escape in the person P. P will therefore have the impulse of running away; if the impulse is "at work" he will run, and the indication of the impulse at work is the emotion fear. Now, so the objection runs, the fear will be the greater the less freedom of motion P has; there may be the extreme case of very swift flight without any fear. I do not think that this objection in itself is fatal to McDougall's theory, because he could say that through running the excitation of the escape impulse by A would be continually decreased, and thereby the emotion. Even so, he would have to make the relation between the object which excites the instinct and the instinct itself much more dynamic if the degree of excitation is to depend, let us say, on the distance between A and P. But "the instinct to escape" might be excited without any fear reaction at all, as when a fleet sprinter encounters a bulky and terrifying-looking enemy. Flight, i.e., functioning of the escape instinct, would result, but it would be accompanied by a kind of joy or elation, which McDougall would have to ascribe to the excitation of the assertive instinct. So two questions remain unanswered: (1) Why does the escape instinct have no accompanying fear emotion? and (2) What excites the assertive instinct?

It is my conviction that a theory of emotions can be developed which is free from such difficulties, and I shall try to show how it can be done. I shall discard instinct from the discussion for a while, and approach the problem as before suggested, by a consideration of the forces at work. Lewin's method of field-force diagrams, previously referred to (p. 391), is particularly applicable here, as is demonstrated by Dr. Dembo's work, which we shall discuss soon.

The Dynamic Theory of Emotion. The general attitude to be taken by this theory is this: the total field is permeated by forces which either hold it in equilibrium or produce change and action. This interplay of forces applies to the Ego as a sub-system of the total field. Emotional behaviour will, in our theory, be considered as the dynamics of these intra-Ego forces, conscious emotion as the manifest aspect of these dynamics. The dynamics of the intra-Ego forces will often transcend the limits of the Ego, the emotions being directed towards objects in the field, and of course we must include these object-Ego dynamics in our definition of the emotion. How such a view can be generalized so as to be compatible with our previous statement that emotions need not necessarily belong to the Ego but may also appear in other parts of the behavioural field, will be explained later. Such a view does not encounter the difficulties that obstructed McDougall's theory. Flight may be connected with fear or not, according to the general dynamic situation. In the case of our fleet sprinter the movements of escape would be quite unaccompanied by fear because, owing to the dynamic relations between his Ego and the dangerous object, no tensions would be aroused in the Ego.

Applied to McDougall's Classification of the Emotions. Generally speaking, the problem of emotions is not one of classification and introspective analysis, but one of dynamics and functional analysis. Therefore I do not see that, at least at the present moment, such distinctions as those between primary, secondary or blended, and derived emotions will be of much use to our progress in this field. McDougall's distinction between the two first is perfectly correct; thus he says: "Such a complex emotional experience [based upon anger and disgust] is not literally formed by the separate excitement, the coming together, and the subsequent blending of the two emotions, anger and disgust; rather it is the immediate response to the complex situation" (p. 331). This is perfectly true. The dynamics of the secondary emotions are different from those of the primary ones, and it is also true that by a change in the conditions they might be transformed into primary ones. The term "blended emotions" seems to me, for this and for McDougall's own reason, inappropriate, and even the term "secondary" is dangerous as long as one has not succeeded in establishing a valid criterion for simple and more complex sets of conditions. If this can be done, then there would be no objection to calling the emotions arising from the simplest set of conditions primary, those from more complex ones secondary, but at the moment I prefer to disregard this distinction. McDougall has to introduce his third class, the derived emotions, of which joy, sorrow, surprise, disappointment, are a few examples, because there are emotions for which no corresponding constant instinctive impulse can be found (p. 338). Since we refused to accept McDougall's theory of the instinct-emotion connection, we need not pursue the discussion of this new group of emotions, were it not that our author had used other characteristics to distinguish it from the two first ones, one of which seems to me significant and important. "The primary emotion may be spoken of (somewhat loosely but without serious error) as a force, since it is constantly accompanied by an impulse toward some specific goal. . . . The derived emotions, on the other hand, cannot properly be regarded as forces. They are merely incidents in the working of the instinctive impulses, which are the only true forces that prompt and sustain thought and action" (p. 346). If we disregard again the use of the term instinct, and if we leave open the question, until we possess further knowledge, of how true the application of this distinction is for the emotions actually discussed, then we are offered a valuable hint as to the dynamic nature of different emotions. We might perhaps rephrase this in our terminology by saying that emotions, at least as experienced emotions, may belong to different parts or aspects of the total dynamical situation. There may be emotions arising with creation of tensions, with their working, and with their relief. Thus expressed, the term "derived emotions" would indeed be inadequate, but this is altogether a minor matter.

Emotions That Are not Experienced in the Ego. Before we report the experimental material available for the support of our theory we must briefly deal with the apparent contradiction between our definition and a previous contention which we just mentioned. What about the emotions in the field? It will be admitted that emotions that are not Ego emotions are experienced most frequently and most intensely in other human beings and next to that in higher animals. This fact is, probably, largely responsible for the theory of empathy which we have rejected (Chapter VIII, p. 326) and for the theory of analogical inference which we shall reject later (see pp. 655 f.). The similarity between these objects and our Ego, which must have greatly influenced the two theories named, has, however, another aspect which will lead to another more direct and tenable explanation. For other human beings, and next to them the higher animals, are the most complex objects within our behavioural environment. At the same time, and probably at least partly owing to their great complexity, they are more than any other objects centres of force, and surrounded by fields of force. In these objects qua behavioural objects, there may then arise an intra-object and an object-object or even an object-Ego dynamics, comparable to the intra-Ego and the Ego-object dynamics which we have treated as the real basis of emotions. In this way our theory can be easily generalized so as to account for non-Ego emotional experience. How men and animals can, as behavioural objects, possess the dynamics we ascribe to them will be treated in a later chapter, when we discuss our knowledge of the other person's emotions. Our generalization must, however, be broad enough to include emotions in non-living behavioural objects, the sad landscape, for example. Our whole problem has a great deal to do with the problem of the physiognomic characters, and when we resume our discussion we shall go into this relationship.

Experimental Evidence. This theory of the emotions, though more or less expressed in my language, is largely the accomplishment of those theories which Lewin and his school have consistently developed during the last fifteen years. It is from two contributions made by this school that we shall gain our main support, the contributions of Karsten (1928) and Dembo (1931).

dembo's investigation. Dr. Dembo's problem was an investigation of the dynamic situation in anger. She has reported her results in a long paper (144 pages), of which only a few outstanding points can be mentioned here but which should be read by all who want to get a real knowledge of Lewin's method of fields of force.

Dembo's experimental method consisted in confronting her subjects with an impossible task (two different ones were chosen) and demanding a completion from them. Her experiment lasted between one and two hours and was usually continued on the following day. The experimenter and a special reporter were in the same room with the subject, the former sometimes interfering with the actions of the subject. In all cases very genuine emotions of anger were aroused, manifesting themselves in swearing, threats, wishes and acts of destruction, and even in one case in the subject's rushing out of the room and being found in tears in another.

Dynamics of Anger. The actual symptoms or expressions of this emotion varied from case to case, but some fundamental aspects of the dynamical situation were common to all. I quote from Dr. Dembo: "Heterogeneous as all these processes are, dynamically they can be derived from a few fundamental factors in a relatively unitary manner. On the ground of the topology and the field forces of the situation there arises a *conflict,* an opposition of field forces in very diverse directions. The increasing *hopelessness of the situation* produces strong *tensions* which at the same time bring about a *loosening and destruction of the boundaries of the total field"* (p. 117).[8]

Dembo's paper deals in great detail with all phases of the arousal of these tensions and their consequences. Let us single out a few points. What is the cause of these tensions? Dembo's answer is: the existence of barriers which constrain action. Of these there exist two: first, the internal barrier, which prevents the subject from solving the task. This may be, or be concentrated in, an actual physical barrier, it may simply be the insuperable difficulty of the task. This barrier soon becomes endowed with a negative demand character, so that the subject is in a conflicting field of force: he is drawn towards the barrier by the vector of the task and the positive demand character that the goal has assumed by his wish to fulfil it, and he is repelled by the barrier because of its negative demand character. The relative strength of these two vectors not being constant, the subject should be alternately attracted and repelled, i.e., he should move towards the barrier and again away from it. This vacillation was indeed "one of the most striking and absolutely regular phenomena in our experiments" (p. 63). However, if the negative vector of the barrier is stronger than the posi-

[8] Theories of emotions based on conflict are old and numerous, as R. P. Angier has pointed out (1927, pp. 390 f.). But they are all much less concrete than Dembo's theory.

tive one, why does the subject not go away for good? This is prevented by the second, the external barrier, which may again be either physical or, as in most cases, mental. In these experiments the external barrier was provided by the general social and professional situation, the fact that the subjects undertake to co-operate in the experiment. In ordinary life customs, manners, and morals will often constitute such external barriers. The external barrier limits the subject's freedom of movement, he cannot yield to the negative force of the internal barrier, but must stay within the field, i.e., stay subject to the field forces. So he begins again to run against the internal barrier, is again repulsed, and so on, with an ever-increasing tension. This tension determines the behaviour of the subject to an ever-increasing degree; it appears not only in his overt actions but also in his thoughts. The only way out of the increasingly painful situation appears to lead across the internal barrier, although heretofore it has defied all such attempts. Nevertheless hope persists for a very long time, and the greater the tension, the less foundation is required for such a hope (p. 63).

Expressions of anger as results of this tension occur at practically all stages of the process, often differing more in functional meaning than in appearance. The expression of the anger and the anger itself must not be identified. At first, expressions occur fairly easily. Such outbreaks are discharges of tensions in directions which bring no real relief and therefore tend to increase the tension by involving new Ego systems. The result is that the subject inhibits such outbreaks by shutting his Ego off more and more from the rest of the field. Thus a change of the Ego-field organization takes place which, by preventing discharge, helps to increase the internal tensions. Thereby the separating walls between Ego and field and between the different Ego systems are put under high pressure, to which they eventually yield. The aversion towards the barrier, part of which in these experiments was formed by the experimenter, spreads, the whole environment appears as an undifferentiated hostile field, the total field becomes more or less chaotic. At the same time the intra-Ego walls yield, the central nucleus, the Self, becomes more and more involved, the systems lose their isolation and discharge their tensions, irrespective of the other field forces: the subject will begin to confide to the experimenter her intimate personal secrets, although at the same time she hates her. When finally the tension becomes too strong, an explosion occurs which is the stronger the more the Ego has been cut off from communication with the field. Not every explosion brings real relief, which is all too intelligible since these explosions cannot really change the conditions which keep the tension up. Instead they will produce new tension; the subject will become ashamed of her action and suffer from the new tension due to this shame. How different would it be if the experimenter told the subject: Your task is impossible, you have done all I expected you to, you may go. This would relieve all the original tensions, although the tensions created by the anger actions might remain and become more strongly directed against the experimenter, who was the cause of all the trouble. We have, in this short survey, omitted all references to the social relation between subject and experimenter, since we shall return to that in a later chapter. But it should be mentioned that later experiments of Dr. Dembo's have proved that a purely "objective" anger, an anger without direction towards a person, can arise. In these experiments the subject was alone in the room and received her instructions from slips of paper, the experimenter being concealed in another room from which she could observe the subject.

KARSTEN'S INVESTIGATION. Karsten's earlier investigation is in good agreement with Dembo's result. Her problem was not the investigation of emotion itself but that of saturation, i.e., the fact that the increasing repetition of one and the same task will under certain conditions set up strong forces which obstruct and eventually block the continuation of the work. The subjects were given several tasks and told to work at them as long as they cared to. When they showed inclination to cease, they were, however, encouraged to continue. The main tasks among a great number of others were making strokes on sheets of paper, either without further specification, or in prescribed groups like 3 and 5 or 4 and 4, and the reading of a poem. The dynamic situation is in several respects similar to that in Dembo's experiments. The tasks, for reasons to be discussed presently, became endowed with a strong negative vector which would "drive the subject away." But again he cannot leave the field because of an external barrier constituted as in Dembo's experiments by the total situation. The result, as with Dembo, is strong tensions which frequently lead to emotional outbreaks.

The Dynamics of Saturation. The specific contribution of Karsten's work is, of course, the investigation into the origin of saturation, i.e., the attempt to explain why the continued execution of a task will set up forces against its continuation. The negative character of the internal barrier in Dembo's experiments was easy to understand: the internal barrier stood between subject and goal. Here nothing interferes with the execution of the task, and yet something akin to an internal barrier is produced, some factor prevents the execution of the task from relieving the tensions corresponding to the resolve, the quasi-need set up by the instruction, and thereby brings about a steady increase of tension. We can express this fact by saying that under certain conditions the execution, instead of relieving the tension, increases it. What are the conditions of this effect, and what is the reason for it? In order to answer this question it is well to compare these situations with those in which no saturation occurred. One subject refused after one hour and twenty minutes to continue the task of filling sheets with dashes. Long before that she had shown signs of impatience, her work had deteriorated and she had needed encouragement in order to stick to it. A few days later the same subject worked for two and a half hours without any saturation, the quality of her work being as good at the end of this period as at the beginning, and the interruption came through the experimenter, the subject being willing and able to continue longer. The paradoxical aspect of this result disappears as soon as we learn that the second time the subject had been interested to find out whether she would be able to continue the work *ad libitum,* whereas in the preceding test she had concentrated on the task as it was given. Dynamically the two tasks actually performed by the subject were thus quite different. In the second case, although the filling of a line, a page, a dozen pages, was not a real solution, yet each new page filled with dashes, each minute through which she persevered, brought her nearer to the completion of the task, i.e., to work *ad libitum,* until stopped. And when this happened, she had "won the game," the real task was fulfilled, and the tension completely relieved. Here there is no reason why the execution should increase tension. Conversely in the first sitting, which is typical of the experiments performed with students as subjects, the execution does not bring the subject nearer to her goal. After having filled one or two or even twenty pages, if she could fill so many, she is just as far from the goal as before, simply because there is no real goal in this occupation. Energy is being expended all the time, but the energy, not being able to change the situation which necessitates the expenditure of energy, remains within the system and thereby sets up forces which block the process. It becomes more and more difficult to pump air into a tire. If the pressure in the tire could become so great that it equalled the force of the person at the pump, the process would come to an end. Just so in our case. The tensions become so great that continuation of the work is impossible; instead explosions may occur, the pressure finds relief through other channels, just as in Dembo's experiments.

This explanation is confirmed by the fact that several unemployed, who were hired for this work, behaved like the subject at the second sitting. Some of them worked for four full hours, liked the work, and showed an evenness of performance which is in the strongest possible contrast to the untidiness of the normal subjects in much shorter periods of time. For these unemployed the task involved a real goal to which they approached by each new dash made. Energy flowed freely, no counterforces were set up, no saturation occurred.

This explanation is further confirmed by a comparison of the different tasks with each other. It would be plausible to expect that tasks which the subjects dislike would lead most quickly to saturation, whereas such as appealed to the subject would show the slowest saturation rate, the indifferent tasks having an intermediate position. But this expectation is not fulfilled. Nine different tasks were used, the number of cases for each task varying between 8 and 16, and with great regularity the indifferent tasks were those last saturated, the pleasant ones second and the unpleasant ones first. But both the very pleasant and very unpleasant ones were saturated more quickly than the pleasant and the unpleasant ones, and the very pleasant ones even more quickly than the unpleasant ones. This shows conclusively that the relation of the task to the Ego is the decisive factor. In the indifferent task the Ego is not "engaged," with the result that Ego tensions are less easily produced.

Another confirmation of the explanation derives from the fact, observed with all subjects who showed saturation, that very soon, as early as the second line in the dash experiments, the subjects began to introduce variations. The intervals between the lines are made different, the size of the dashes is increased or decreased, the direction of progress changes from left to right to right to left, etc. These variations which appear at first spontaneously and are afterwards anticipated in thought continue through the whole series, indicating that the process of saturation begins very soon, that the process of execution creates forces which block its continuation.

Saturation and Fatigue. We had anticipated these forces at the end of our third chapter when we discussed the conditions upon which psychophysical processes depend (see p. 102). We must now add a word to distinguish them from fatigue. Superficially saturation looks very much like fatigue, the subject complaining of cramps in her hand, inability to hold the pencil any longer, hoarseness after reading poetry, and several other similar symptoms. But a deeper analysis makes it impossible to interpret saturation simply as fatigue. The same muscles can make practically the same movements if these movements belong to a different task. We need only recall the lack of saturation in the unemployed and the student who wanted to test her own ability, to see the truth of this statement. We can, however, add more evidence: after one hour and ten minutes a subject who had had the task of making dashes alternately in groups of 3 and 5 was fully saturated. Earlier she had started to make the lines very light in order to spare her "overtired hand"; still she often slipped and made her lines very irregular. After her refusal to continue she was told to try a new pattern, namely groups of 4 dashes without alternation. "The same dashes, drawn with the same muscles, which before by their crooked and slipshod execution had presented the picture of a complete gestalt-disintegration are now produced in a perfectly tidy and correct manner" (p. 160). This example is typical of many. New confirmation comes from the period after complete saturation when the subjects refused to undertake any tasks connected with drawing because they could no longer hold pen or pencil. The experimenter, acquiescing, requested them to report their experience during the whole course of the experiment, when they would grasp the pen with alacrity and draw dashes with the greatest ease in order to demonstrate their previous behaviour. Saturation, then, cannot be fatigue, although it is highly probable that fatigue contains in most if not in all cases a saturation component. In pure saturation the act as a mere movement can still be done, it is blocked only qua *action* of a particular kind, which proves that there must be forces at work which shut the executive off from the particular task.

Saturation and Perceptual Blocking. We have met before (Chapter V, pp. 183 f.) with forces which are produced by a process and block its continuation. I mean the causes of the oscillation of ambiguous figures. Both Karsten (p. 244) and Köhler (1929) consider it probable that these forces and those that produce saturation are of the same kind.

Saturation Range. Saturation is not strictly limited to the particular task but very soon spreads over a wider range, so that the problem of saturation leads at once to the problem of the saturation range which has been specially investigated in Karsten's study. We can only mention this here, emphasizing that we shall meet with a similar phenomenon, the spreading of an effect beyond its original range, when we discuss learning and that particular aspect of learning traditionally called transfer.

Saturation and Success. Saturation is emotional behaviour. Its analysis revealed an interplay of forces leading to increasing tension within the Ego system, a tension which became manifest in less and less co-ordinate, more and more chaotic behaviour and in the emotional resistance experienced by the subject. It would be the next step to inquire more specifically into the conditions which rob an action of its relief function and thereby make it productive of greater and greater tensions. This would lead us to the problem of success. For this much is clear after our discussion of saturation: no matter whether success, as mere accomplishment, in the sense defined on page 37, has any psychological significance or not, success as behavioural, as *experienced* success, must play a determining rôle. This distinction has often been obscured in the literature on success, but it has been handled with great skill by Hoppe, another of Lewin's students. Since, however, the treatment of this problem involves social behaviour in its broadest sense, we shall defer the discussion of this investigation to our fourteenth chapter.

THE PHYSIOLOGICAL CHANGES IN EMOTIONAL BEHAVIOUR. We cannot close our discussion of emotional behaviour without adding a brief word about the physiological changes which occur during emotions.[9] It will be relatively easy to assign to them their place in our theory. In discussing the James-Lange theory (p. 401) we have clearly pointed out that emotional behaviour involves the whole organism. The reason is easy to see. Tensions in any part will have reverberations over the whole system. Functionally these reverberations may be of either of two kinds. On the one hand the tensions themselves will involve directly a greater and greater part of the system. This becomes apparent in the field of limb movements in the activity which Lewin has called "restless activity" which occurs whenever directed action is prevented by a barrier and the tension is strong enough. Thus, in Lewin's beautiful film an infant will circle round a circular pen in whose centre the lure is situated, or will vacillate back and forth when it is inside and the lure outside. But the direct action of these tensions is not confined to the skeletal musculature. Fear and anger interfere with digestion by inhibiting the secretion of gastric juice, and during excitement and pain

[9] For a much more detailed account I refer the reader, for instance, to Wheeler's very apt discussion in his Chapter VIII, pp. 207 ff.

adrenalin is discharged into the blood in excessive amounts, with the ensuing effects of diverting the blood to the external muscles and increasing the blood pressure. On the other hand the system will counteract the tensions which begin to penetrate the whole organism so as to maintain the old balance as much as possible. The opposite action of the sympathetic and the parasympathetic parts of the autonomic nervous system indicates this second possibility.

Thus these physiological changes lose nothing of their importance in our theory, and yet they are not constitutive of emotions—in good harmony with Sherrington's and Cannon's results. Lastly, even in our theory the possibility remains that such physiological changes might induce emotions. For if the tensions in some other part of the system are heightened, they might affect the Ego, just as the Ego tensions, in our theory, spread to outlying systems. To test this hypothesis Marañon gave human subjects injections of adrenalin and found that only in a few cases, which he explained by suggestion and predisposition, real emotions ensued, while other subjects showed no emotion at all, or only "cold emotion," a feeling "as if afraid," for instance. This work was repeated by Cantril and Hunt, who could confirm Marañon's results except for the fact that they could not explain the few cases of real emotion by Marañon's assumptions and therefore interpret them as a direct result of the adrenalin or its physiological effects. I shall quote an example for each "cold" and "real" emotion from these authors: "Feel as though I had had a big scare, not fright, but like a reaction after tremendous fright. Don't feel unpleasant. If there is any affective state it is somewhat pleasant. Certain bodily restlessness but no worries, cares, or mental anxieties" (p. 303). In contrast to this the following real emotion: "Extreme fear was present, but no content for it at the time. Probably an unconscious reason, but at the time nothing but fear. The strongest reaction yet. I found myself shaking, chest trembling, building up rapidly in intensity, whereupon I abruptly recognized that I was intensely afraid" (p. 305).

These experiments seem to answer our question in the affirmative. The tensions produced by adrenalin injection may spread and involve Ego systems and then produce real emotions. They may remain entirely outside the sphere of the Ego, no emotion ensuing; the third possibility, the cold emotion, lies somewhere between these two extremes; the Ego seems definitely affected without being strongly charged. Whatever the exact interpretation of this last effect may be, these experiments seem to me to confirm our interpretation of emotional behaviour and the rôle played in it by the physiological changes.[10]

THE WILL

We cannot close our discussion of action without introducing the concept of the *will,* or the distinction between voluntary and involuntary actions. We have deferred the introduction of these terms, because by their great ambiguity they would have made our argument much more difficult. The discussion which is to follow will again be based very largely on the work of Lewin, whose lucid and acute analysis of the problem[1] has probably been the strongest force in re-establishing problems of volition as primary problems of psychology.

McDougall's Hormic Theory. It would be unfair if we omitted McDougall's hormic psychology (1930) in this connection. McDougall has insisted again and again that behaviour cannot be understood without the drive behind it. Yet I feel that McDougall's claim, despite all the power and enthusiasm of its presentation, exerted little influence on the actual progress of psychology. The will, in McDougall's theory, or rather the primeval urge, the hormic *x,* is at least at the present moment too far removed from concrete scientific concepts to be widely adopted or even fairly criticized. It suffers, in my opinion, from the reification of the instincts which I mentioned and criticized before. McDougall's theory is much more than a special psychological theory, it is philosophical, metaphysical, it expresses a *Weltanschauung,* throwing down the gauntlet to intellectualism, and preaching a Dionysian as opposed to the Apollinian conception of the universe. Just because I am in full sympathy with McDougall's ultimate goals, because I believe, as he does, that fundamental psychological theories are, or ought to be, much more than special hypotheses built to explain a limited number of facts and restricted to the system of a special science, because the super-intellectualist attitude of modern psychology even in some of its latest publications shocks me to the quick, because, lastly, I admire the courage with which he has championed an unpopular cause, I feel reluctant to criticize his position. I must do so because as it appears now it seems to me too unstable to serve as a real basis for psychological research.

[10] The authors draw a different conclusion, regarding a primary autonomic reaction as the only *sine qua non* of an emotion, a conclusion not warranted by their results and in contradiction to the results of Sherrington and Cannon.

Criticism: Mechanism—Vitalism, Intellectualism—Anti-intellectualism. The reason for my judgment is that he has not solved the old mechanistic-vitalistic conflict. We have seen in our very first chapter how the acceptance of mechanism as the principle of all inorganic behaviour makes vitalism a necessity. McDougall does not necessarily accept this assumption, he considers it quite possible that inorganic processes are also hormic. But in one respect his theory is nevertheless a vitalism: its main concept is the very concept which one must form if one starts out with a mechanistic philosophy, discovers its inadequacy, and tries to remedy it by supplementation. McDougall's *horme* is, so it seems to me at least, such a supplementary concept, even though it be prepared to assume full possession. The same point of view emerges when we consider his attitude towards intellectualism. Intellectualism is the result of a special field organization achieved in our Western civilization, in which certain sub-systems of the Ego gain dominance and thereby influence the rest of the field and with it our philosophy. It presupposes a differentiation and isolation of sub-systems, and in a way thereby creates its opposite, just as mechanism creates vitalism. Therefore, again, the adoption of the opposite point of view seems to me no ultimate solution either, because it accepts the differentiation and gives undue prominence to the hitherto neglected part. Certain political tendencies of the present day confirm me in my judgment. As a matter of fact I believe that a complete renunciation of the intellect will lead to consequences much more dangerous and destructive than its glorification. The radical solution must in my opinion be developed by going behind that differentiation, by unifying what has become severed. Then the Apollinian intellect may well turn out to have Dionysian characteristics and the Dionysian urge be capable of assuming Apollinian clarity. And we should learn to understand why at certain periods, in certain persons, the Apollinian, in others the Dionysian, trend became dominant.

Lewin's Concepts. Our comments on McDougall's theory have raised questions which go far beyond our present discussion. Let us therefore try to treat the problem of will by the methods introduced by Lewin. We use the term voluntary action in at least two different contexts: on the one hand we contrast it with impulsive and instinctive action, on the other with automatic action (Lewin, 1926 a). Thus we do not speak of voluntary action when a dog to whom we show a morsel of meat snaps at it, nor when a man jumps aside to avoid the wheels of a motor car. In other cases we may be in doubt whether to call an action voluntary or not: thus with regard to our periodic putting on and off of our clothes, our sitting down to dinner, walking or driving to our offices, answering polite questions politely, etc. On the other hand the carrying out of intentions will generally be called voluntary action, but also the spontaneous, not foreseen and therefore not intended interference in a quarrel, or the giving of a polite answer to an impolite question. Examples like these serve a two-fold purpose. On the negative side they teach us to be wary in our scientific use of a popular term. Popular terms are as a rule full of meaning and relevance, but at the same time quite unfit to serve as a basis for a scientific classification. Thus we have seen that a clear-cut classification of all actions into voluntary and non-voluntary ones will prove impossible, i.e., the principle of classification must be wrong. Positively our examples give us indications of the complexity of our problem and acquaint us with some specific characteristics of those actions which we call voluntary.

Palpably it would be absurd to try to discover the essence of voluntary action by throwing all our examples together and abstracting from them the particular experience which is common to them all. More particularly would it be wrong to define as voluntary actions such as are preceded by an experience of "I will" or "fiat," and to measure or at least estimate the strength of will by the intensity of this experience. As Lewin has pointed out, the very intense resolve "I *will* do this or that" is more often than not an indication that I really do not want it, with the result that actually I shall not do it. This does not mean that under other conditions the decision to do this rather than that, the experience: "I will this," may not be a true indicator of strong and decisive forces.

Field Action and Controlled Action. But our procedure cannot start from these will-experiences. We must remember our examples which show that we call many an action voluntary which is not accompanied by any such experience. Instead we shall have to proceed by a functional analysis of the dynamics in the different situations. Such an analysis led Lewin to the distinction of "field-actions" and "controlled actions." This distinction refers to the forces which have control of the executive, but it is not the simple distinction of the cases in which action is controlled entirely by environmental or environment-Ego forces (i.e., field action) and actions controlled by Ego-forces (i.e., controlled action). For pure impulsive or instinctive action, like that of a hungry animal, is chiefly controlled by the Ego forces, whereas a truly controlled action, like the rescue of a person from a burning house, is under strong control of the environment. The action of a person who would rush into his burning house and come out with an old battered hat and without an irreplaceable MS. would not be a controlled action. On the other hand we shall hardly call an action voluntary in which the Ego is not dynamically concerned. But the difference is not that between actions with and without forces emanating from the Ego. It is a difference of organization of Ego and non-Ego forces which accounts for Lewin's distinction. In discussing the uncontrolled execution of an intention Lewin says: "In this case the process occurs as though to the pre-existing forces of the situation (the psychic field) the intention had been added as a new force, and as though the action itself ran its course in a perfectly impulsive, uncontrolled manner in accordance with this new distribution of forces" (p. 377).

INTENTION. The execution of an intention need not, as appears from our last quotation, be controlled action in this sense. If we call it voluntary action we do so because the act of making the resolve was "controlled." In this case the creation of the need was the controlled action, whereas its relief may still be either controlled or uncontrolled.

CONFLICT OF FORCES. If Ego and field forces have the same direction it becomes doubtful whether we should still speak of controlled action, for then it will make no difference which of these forces is stronger. I have resolved to be very friendly to A, whom I expect to be a conceited and overbearing person. A comes and is as jolly, simple, and pleasant as can be. My own friendly response is no longer controlled. Things are different when A lives up to my expectation. Here the field forces by themselves would provoke me to teach him a lesson, but my resolve pulls me in a different direction; my action, as long as I stick to my resolve, will be controlled. Controlled action thus implies conflicting forces, a view well in accord with those theories of will which derive it from conflict (e.g., Claparède, 1925).

VARIETY OF VOLUNTARY ACTIONS AS A RESULT OF THE UNDERLYING DYNAMICS. How such conflicts will be resolved depends upon the organization of the forces, which in its turn depends upon the Ego-field organization. With strong field-Ego unity there will be little or no conflict, field action will be the rule. If the Ego is strongly separated all depends upon the relative strength of the operative forces, and these again depend upon the nature of the particular Ego. In his "Outline" (pp. 443 f.) McDougall has most suggestively discussed a number of different personality types with regard to their volitional behaviour. There is the moral athlete who despises indulgence and acts against the environment so as to increase his feeling of superiority, and there is the beachcomber at the other extreme who lets himself drift because his Ego has lost all self-respect. There are innumerable other possibilities between the two, just as there are countless degrees of isolation between field and Ego. That is the reason why in many cases we cannot decide whether to call an action voluntary or involuntary. In the preceding pages we have criticized an exaggerated intellectualism which is typical of Western civilization. It is tempting to criticize a hypertrophied voluntarism, which has sprung from the same soil. To value a person who does a kindly act against his inclination higher than one who does it joyfully is the absurd result of this tendency of over-isolating the Ego and giving it too great a dominance in the total field. And we may learn from the Chinese student at a mission school who criticized the parable of the vineyard severely because for him the son who refused to go and eventually did was really much worse than his brother, since he offended his father by his refusal. The Ego-environment dynamics characterize not only individual situations, but also individual persons, and smaller and larger groups. They may throw light on the differences of national characters, and those of the great historical civilizations, ancient and modern, of the West and the East.

Special Problems: Forgetting, Habit. But our discussion of volition should also lead us to humbler tasks, tasks even more urgent, because they are necessary for a proper elaboration of our sketch. Psychological research work of a true experimental nature can be done on the basis of this theory. These ideas were indeed the foundation on which the work of the Lewin school was done, which we have referred to so frequently and which we shall encounter again. In this place I shall only mention, without going into the detail, G. Birenbaum's investigation of the forgetting of intentions. This problem is indeed a problem not of memory, but of volitional activity. The term forgetting has two radically different meanings in our idiom. On the one hand it signifies our *inability* to remember, on the other our failure at a given moment to do so despite an unimpaired ability. You may have forgotten Kepler's laws, no effort will make you recall them—an example of the first meaning. On the way to class you may have forgotten to post a letter, and now you remember that it is still in the pocket of your coat—an example of the second type. It is with this second meaning that Birenbaum's investigation is concerned. It produces a situation in which a resolve is carried out once, with the resulting relief of the tension, but must be carried out again and again. It shows under what conditions the need will be re-created, under what conditions not; in the first case the intended action will be carried out, in the second it will be forgotten.

Another problem which has been attacked experimentally is that of will vs. habit. We shall postpone it until we have discussed habit, i.e., until Chapter XII, and we shall discuss the general problem of forgetting in Chapter XI.

CONCLUSION AND OUTLOOK

Let us review in conclusion what our discussion of action has achieved. It has carried out our programme of describing behaviour in terms of the field forces. In order to do this we had to introduce the Ego and we had to augment our knowledge of the environmental field as it had been developed in the preceding chapters. The problem of behaviour resolved itself into the problem of the changes of the great Ego-field gestalt, the changes which the relation between its sub-systems undergo. Through our discussion of manifest organization and the dynamic characters of environmental objects we could at least indicate the true status and meaning of behaviour. We saw how even the boundaries between Ego and environment develop, how greater differentiation takes the place of a prior greater unitedness. And we understand how the Ego-object relation is falsified if it is considered primarily as a cognitive one (see p. 361, Chapter VIII). Even for the problem of cognition we could derive some important conclusions. Behaviour became intelligible in all its richness and variety, defying any such simple formula as that of the stimulus and response, but occurring always in conformity with the general laws of dynamics. And yet, our account of behaviour is still incomplete. We have occasionally met with three different gaps: in the first place we saw again and again that present performances depend upon earlier ones. Although we have attacked traditional empiricism incessantly we have insisted ourselves on the all-pervasive influence of experience. We have even introduced a new hypothesis of memory which was inextricably bound up with our main theory. But it remains to show how, according to our present limited knowledge, memory works, how experience is acquired, and how the past influences the present. Otherwise expressed, we must deal with the problem of learning in its widest aspect. The treatment of this problem will not, however, necessitate the introduction of any essentially new principle. Learning will follow from the laws of organization which we have so far established if more conditions are included in our consideration. It was the method of this book throughout to start from simple conditions and introduce more and more complexities. From this point of view learning has to be discussed at a later stage because of the great complexity of conditions which are operative in it.

The second gap which we have encountered is indicated by the word thinking. The environment in which we behave is not only the actually and palpably present behavioural environment, but also the environment which we "merely" imagine or think of. This environment is responsible for the greatest achievements of mankind. Without it neither the sciences nor the arts would be possible. Closely connected with this environment is our language and the similar symbolic functions which we have developed. And an ultimate explanation of the problems of thought and imagination will not be possible without a theory of language and the other symbolic functions. But we shall exclude the study of language from our treatise. This restriction is necessary, because it would be impossible to give more than an utterly superficial treatment to this problem, so rich in psychological interest.

The last gap concerns the social aspect of behaviour. The behavioural environment contains, among other things, our fellow creatures, be we men, or wolves, or bees. And these fellow creatures of ours determine our behaviour far more than any other environmental objects. Neither the behavioural environment, nor the Ego, nor behaviour can be really understood without a study of the social aspect. Only as a member of a group, as a part of society, has man produced through his behaviour civilization with all it entails. And since we set out to treat behaviour in such a way as to make these results intelligible, we shall have to sketch in as our last contribution a discussion of some problems of social psychology.

CHAPTER X

MEMORY

Foundation of a Trace Theory. Theoretical Section

The Rôle of Memory. Memory Not to Be Considered as a Special Faculty. Memory and Time. Can Memory Be Completely Reduced to Traces? Temporal Units. Stout's Theory of Primary Retentiveness. The Self-determination of Temporal Organizations. Good Continuation. Spatial and Temporal Organizations Compared. Objections to Our Trace Hypothesis. In Defence of Speculative Hypotheses

THE RÔLE OF MEMORY

No fact has challenged the psychologist as much as the fact that we have a memory. Through memory we are at every moment connected with the past and the future; without memory we could not learn but would face each situation as we faced it the first time; without memory we could not act according to plans and resolves. No wonder, then, that in the development of psychology memory assumed the rôle it has played to the present day. In the eyes of the psychologists and the psychologizing scientists memory became the chief cause of adjusted behaviour, memory seemed to be the specific factor which distinguished life and mind from machine-like nature. A horse driven a few times over the same road will know the way, and the coachman may, on his homeward journey, go to sleep, assured that the mare will take him back to the stable. But the driver of a motor car is in no such fortunate position. He cannot close his eyes trusting that his car will find the way. The horse has memory, the car not, and therefore, so psychologists concluded, the adjusted behaviour of the former was altogether due to memory, the unadjusted behaviour of the latter due to its lack of memory. Psychologists have even gone so far as to use the possession of memory by an animal as a criterion of its possessing consciousness, and some of the arguments in favour of vitalism have been based on memory. Thus the two radically opposed philosophies of vitalism and empiricism both originate in an acknowledgment of the unique properties and achievements of memory.

MEMORY NOT TO BE CONSIDERED AS A SPECIAL FACULTY

And yet, to the cold critic memory is but a word which labels a great number of different achievements without explaining them. And nothing is more dangerous to scientific progress than such a single word which tends to become reified, to be taken for an entity which produces all the different effects. Hughlings Jackson criticized the faculty concept of memory as early as 1866,[1] and implicitly the wish to escape from such a purely verbal explanation must have influenced all the various theories of memory that have arisen in the past. At the present time this determination has become conscious. Wheeler's attempt at eliminating the concept of the memory trace seems to me born from this desire; but it is most clearly expressed by Humphrey, who writes of the acquisition of the skill of typewriting: "Sometimes, indeed, it is said that he can type better today because of his 'Memory' of his lessons; or it is a 'mnemic accumulation' or an 'engram' that enables him to type better. Such special terms of course only push the mystery a little farther back. They are as harmful as was the mediaeval explanation that the water rose in a pump because nature abhors a vacuum" (p. 103).

MEMORY AND TIME

Instead Humphrey sees the final solution of the problem of memory in a view which takes into account equally space and time. "With certain reservations it is characteristic of higher forms of life that their behaviour is integrated over longer periods of time; and this possibility of relating events in the life history of an organism over longer time intervals corresponds objectively to one factor in what is meant by the possession of a 'better memory'" (p. 157). Memory, if this view were right, would not be a new and specific factor but a temporal aspect of behaviour itself. Let us follow up the clue.

The Difficulties in the Concept of Time. Zeno's Paradox. It was Henri Bergson who called our attention to the fact that intellectually we are much better equipped to deal with spatial than with temporal relations. The "real" is thought of as timeless, viz., as the spatial constellation at a moment of time, i.e., at a time without extent, which is neither real nor time. And yet we are apt to say: only the present is real, for what preceded it is now past, and therefore no longer real, and what will follow upon it belongs to the future and is therefore not yet real. Plausible as such a proposition is, it involves an absurdity. For "the present" is undefinable.

[1] See H. Head, 1926, I, p. 40.

We can think of an interval of time becoming shorter and shorter, but however short we make it it still remains an *interval,* it still has duration. Let us begin with a time interval corresponding to one vibration of a tuning fork of 100 vibrations per second. We decrease it so that it corresponds progressively to ½, 1/10, 1/100, . . . of such a cycle. Theoretically we can go on indefinitely, and we never reach the value 0. If we did we should have lost both the interval and time with it. And yet the human mind wants to make that transition. In human experience time seems to be separable from space and therefore the human mind committed again and again the fallacy of separating these inseparables. Everybody knows Zeno's famous arguments against the reality of motion, which are based on just this wrong separation. Let us recall his paradox that Achilles could never pass a tortoise once he had given it a start, however fast he might run. At the beginning Achilles would start from scratch and the tortoise from a line 10 m. ahead of him. If now Achilles ran ten times as fast as the tortoise, what would happen? By the time he came to the starting point of the tortoise, the animal would be one metre further, i.e., when Achilles is 10 m. from his start the tortoise is 1 m. from its. When Achilles reaches this point, after traversing 1 m., the tortoise will still be ahead of him, having raced through 1/10 m. during this time. And this goes on. Whenever Achilles reaches the place where the tortoise was before, the latter is just ahead, and although the difference between their positions becomes increasingly smaller, it can never become zero. The table given on the following page clearly represents this case. Δs indicates the distance between the two rivals, and Δt the time passed between two consecutive moments of time considered, taking the time which Achilles needs to race 10 m. as the unit. This last column shows that Zeno's argument proves the irreality not only of motion but also of time, for the total time passed between the start and any of the positions increases in the same way as the distance between the runners decreases, 1.0–1.1–1.11–1.111 . . . , and one sees that this argument covers only a very small fraction of time, certainly less than 1.11111111–2 units and having as its upper limit 1 1/9 units. Since the unit of time again can be made as small as one likes—one need only give a smaller advantage to the tortoise and a greater difference of speed to the two competitors, without changing the power of the argument—the time during which Achilles cannot overtake the tortoise can be made as small as one likes, and since the argument proves that he can *never* overtake it, time itself vanishes. And it is clear that in a world without time there can be no motion. This reveals the fallacy of Zeno. His argument involves a vicious circle, since implicitly it denies the reality of time and thereby of motion, which he then concludes from it. But its power is due to our inclination to separate space from time and accord reality only to the former. In other words, his treatment of the race presupposes what it sets out to prove, viz., that motion does not exist, for it lists the *positions* at which the runners *are* at various stages of their race. But a moving body never *is* at any

TABLE 13

Time	Achilles	Tortoise	Δs	Δt
0	0	10	10	1
1	10	11	1	.1
2	11	11.1	.1	.01
3	11.1	11.11	.01	.001
4	11.11	11.111	.001	.0001
5	11.111	11.1111	.0001	.
.	.	.	.	.
.	.	.	.	.
.	.	.	.	

one point, instead it *passes* through a point. To describe reality, then, we must have concepts which contain both spatial and temporal components. The simplest of these is the concept of velocity which because of the speedometer in our motor cars is perfectly familiar today to persons who know nothing of mechanics. If the speedometer points, let us say, to 50, it means that our car travels at this "moment" with a velocity of "50 miles per hour." How can we test the accuracy of our measuring instrument? We could mark on a straight road a distance of 50 miles, start our car so that the speedometer pointed at 50 when we passed the first mark, drive with constant speed and measure the time between our passing of the first and second mark. If it were exactly one hour, then our speedometer would be right. But that is not what we would actually do. In reality we should choose a much shorter distance, say a mile, and with our speedometer at 50 we should measure the time it took us to pass over that mile. If we measured $\frac{1}{50}$ hour = 1 minute and 12 seconds, our speedometer would be correct, our speed 50 miles per hour. Furthermore it would not make any difference where within our original 50-mile track our standard mile was, because as long as we go at the same speed the result of measurement must always be the same. We might reduce our interval and make it smaller and smaller, 1 foot, 1 inch, as small as our measuring instrument will allow us, that makes no difference to the final result; to each decrease of measured space there corresponds a proportional decrease of time consumed in traversing it, so that the ratio of distance over time $\frac{s}{t}$ remains the same. The result of our measurement is independent of our measurement, as it ought to be if the measurement is to represent something real. But one thing we cannot do, we cannot continue the diminution of our distance until it becomes 0. If *no* distance were traversed no time would be needed to traverse it; our quotient $\frac{s}{t}$ would become $\frac{0}{0}$, which has no meaning. To say, then, that our car has a definite velocity *at a certain point* of our track means only that we are free to choose the distance over which we measure the time of its passing, as long as the car does not change its speed, as it travels with uniform velocity. But taken literally, the statement is meaningless, because velocity and a mathematical point are mutually exclusive, a velocity always implying a definite distance, however small.

This becomes even more impressive when our car does not travel at uniform velocity but accelerates or decelerates. For here our former method of measuring breaks down, the result is no longer independent of our method of measurement. Not only must we start our measurement at a definite time, since if we did not our result would be different; our measured velocity will also vary with the distance over which we take our measurement. Here a true *point* velocity seems to be demanded by the problem, and yet a point velocity is as absurd here as in the case of uniform velocity. The solution of this problem led to the introduction of differential calculus, and to the reader who knows the calculus no further word is necessary. It would be easy to sketch the first steps for the other readers, but I forbear to do so, only insisting again that the concept of velocity, changing as well as uniform, refers to definite space distances and time intervals, not to non-existing time points. In the case of varying velocity these intervals have to be small, and this is symbolized by defining the velocity by the equation $v = \frac{ds}{dt}$.

If the velocity is uniform, this becomes equivalent with the equation $v = \frac{s}{t}$ from which we started.

Every Event Depends upon Preceding Events. Let us now return to memory. If we tried to define memory as the dependence of the later parts of an event upon the earlier ones, we should have robbed the term of all specific meaning unless we defined the term "event." For without such a specific definition the word memory would apply to *all* events. If you travel from London to Edinburgh the motion of the train from York to Newcastle presupposes its motion from London to York. It would change our definition of memory if we distinguished between such events as depend only upon the *immediately* preceding events from those which depend also upon events that have occurred in a more distant past. The latter we should call events with, the former events without, memory.

Memory in Physics. If we apply this definition we find purely physical events which deserve the name of memory.[2] We clamp a wire at one of its ends and twist it clockwise through a certain angle, holding it in this position for a couple of minutes. We then release it and observe it turning back into its initial untwisted position, whereupon we give it a counterclockwise torsion of the same angle, and after a short time we release it again. The wire will slowly unwind, but it will not come to rest in its untwisted state but will go beyond it, and that the more, the longer we held it originally in its clockwise torsion. The event after the release is evidently here determined not only by the tension at the moment of release but by a previous tension which had ceased to exist. No less a physicist than Boltzmann has applied the name of memory to this, and it has been possible to treat such events mathematically with the help of a "memory function." Nevertheless, the physicist is not satisfied, he does not want to introduce effects between events which are separated by time, and therefore he turns to the molecular structure of the wire for a more satisfactory explanation. When we have given our wire a certain counterclockwise torsion, its tension is the same whether we have previously given it a clockwise torsion or not. But tension is a "macroscopic" magnitude, and therefore the same value of this magnitude may correspond to a great number of microscopic or molecular distributions, just as the same temperature of a volume of gas is compatible with a great number of distributions of the molecular velocities within it. The macroscopic magnitude is the average of all the molecular magnitudes involved, and the same average can correspond to a great

[2] The following after Kármán.

number of different distributions of the terms which are being averaged. Thus the three groups: 5-5-5, 2-6-7, 2-3-10 have all the same average 5, and would be indistinguishable if their averages only were known. The physicist will therefore try to establish the molecular distributions as different in the two cases, thereby reducing the event to a non-memory event, one that is entirely determined by the *immediately* preceding events.

Application to Psychology; the Trace. This last argument has a very direct bearing on our problem. Our wire is in good analogy with Humphrey's typist. Her present performance depends upon much earlier performances, and is therefore called an achievement of memory. And yet, if we follow the method of the physicist, we must interpret this macroscopic fact by microscopic ones, and then memory should disappear from the typist's case as it did from the wire, unless we give it an entirely new definition. Of course most psychologists have more or less followed the physicist's example. The concept of the memory trace is an attempt at explaining the influence of the past by the condition of the present. Just as our wire has been changed in its molecular structure by being held in torsion, so the brain of our typist has been changed by her practice of typing. And just as the wire, when released, does what it would not do without the change of its molecular structure, so the typist when given copy will do what she could not do before her brain had been changed by her exercises. But then it is hard to derive a definition of memory from the case of the typist, of memory as a "special faculty of organized matter" as Hering called it in his famous address (1870).

In this explanation of memory events an event in time influences another event, which succeeds it after a finite interval, not directly but only through some effect which it has left behind and which, for brevity's sake, we will call a trace, without implying by that term anything about the special nature of this after-effect. In the case of our wire we should then say that its behaviour after the second torsion was due to the trace produced by the first, and we would ascribe the finished performance of the trained typist to the traces produced by her continued exercises.

Physical and Psychological Memory Compared Further. We can analyze our two cases still further: the wire with the trace will show in several respects a behaviour different from the wire without the trace, but by no means in all. Its conductivity, its permeability and many other of its properties which determine specific responses will not have been changed, so that in many ways the wire with the trace will respond in the same way as the wire without. Similarly the typist after her training will react in a number of situations differently from what she did before, whereas in a number of other situations she will not. She will, for instance, perform well with any kind of copy, although she had been trained only with a limited number of different copies, but the change in her response will be more or less limited to typing and will not even carry over to another finger activity like longhand writing.

However, this analogy may not be so close as it appears at first sight. Conductivity and permeability are macroscopic magnitudes which are compatible with many different molecular processes. The same conductivity and permeability of the traceless and trace-endowed wire does not, therefore, prove that processes of electric and magnetic conduction occur in them in identically the same way. It is therefore possible that the trace has changed the wire in all its responses. But the same cannot be said about the typist. Her household duties, her amusements, and her longhand writing will occur as though her training in typing had not taken place. Of course one might retort that this comparison was not fair, since the typist's performances which we find unaffected by the trace are all macroscopic phenomena, while the wire responses which we found to depend upon the trace were microscopic; indeed certain macroscopic phenomena of the wire were found also to be independent of the trace. We ought to compare either macroscopic or microscopic phenomena on either side, but not, unfairly, microscopic phenomena on the one side with macroscopic phenomena on the other. Logically valid as this objection would be, it would not do justice to the apparent difference between our two cases. For in the case of the typist we have no reason whatsoever to assume that her training influences even the microscopic aspect of her other activities while the case of the wire is different in this respect. Whereas in the first case we have no reason to assume that the different functions are in any way related, we know that the same molecules that are responsible for the memory phenomenon of the wire are also the carriers of electric and magnetic currents.

First Definition of the Transfer Problem. This difference between our two cases does not, however, destroy the analogy completely. It points only to the much greater complexity of organic as compared to inorganic memory. For the former there arise the questions: *Which* functions will be affected by the trace, and what makes the trace gain an influence in a specific case? The first problem is the general formulation of the transfer problem, the second has an application in a field different from the one we are discussing at present, as we shall see later.

The fact itself, that the trace influences only a part of all functions, must be connected with the facts of field organization. As we have seen, this organization produces a number of relatively independent sub-systems, the Ego on the one hand, the environmental field on the other, either of which is structured again according to the same principle. The trace must therefore be confined to one or several of such sub-systems and will consequently affect behaviour only to the extent to which these sub-systems take part in it.

Memory as a Problem of Traces. This discussion which has demonstrated our reasons for assuming "traces" in our explanations of certain achievements of memory has taken us a long way off the course of our first reflections. A trace, if it is rigid or unchangeable, may be said to be spatialized time, not in the sense that it is timeless, of course, but that it is independent of time, that it does not change with time. Thus the grooves on a gramophone record form a purely spatial pattern which does not change with time, but they were produced by a process in time, and can give rise to a reproduction of the process which produced them. As far as memory is reducible to traces, the problems of memory would be how such traces are produced and how they influence future behaviour, but the specific time aspect which we discussed in the beginning would have been eliminated.

CAN MEMORY BE COMPLETELY REDUCED TO TRACES?

TEMPORAL UNITS

But can memory be completely reduced to traces? Let us turn to another case in which a present event depends upon previous events which do not necessarily precede it immediately. We choose a rhythm tapped on a drum, a melody sung or played on an instrument. In rhythm each beat as an event in our behavioural environment depends upon the preceding beat. Thus the loud taps in the anapaestic rhythm ⏑ ⏑ – ⏑ ⏑ – ⏑ ⏑ – . . . gain their character as "accents" from the preceding soft ones, and the soft ones similarly their character from the preceding loud ones, or the whole preceding group. This is easily proved. For if we replace this rhythm by a new one – – ■ – – ■ – – ■ – – in which the single bars symbolize intensities equal to the intensity of the accented beat in our first rhythm, and the heavy bars correspondingly greater intensities, then the beats of the old intensity no longer carry the accent, which has now been taken over by the louder beats. And conversely if we produce a rhythm in which our original soft beat is the loudest, preceded regularly by two still softer ones, then this soft beat will carry the accent. Similarly, one and the same tone will have a different musical "meaning" according to the tones which precede it. For example, in one melody c may be the tonic, in another the dominant, in a third the "leading tone," and so on; moreover, different tones may have identical meanings—be practically indistinguishable from each other if they occur at the same place in a melody. Thus what g is in a tune played in c major, c is in the "same" tune if played in f major, and f sharp if it is played in b. We can easily call these effects memory effects if we mean by memory merely the fact that an event depends upon not immediately preceding events. In all our cases we have perceptual experiences produced by auditory stimuli, and in each of them the effect of stimulation at one moment depends upon the effects of preceding stimulations. If these prior effects had disappeared completely with the cessation of the stimuli, we could hear neither rhythm nor melodies, to say nothing of speech.

Stout's Theory of Primary Retentiveness. It is for this reason that Stout considers all these events as effects of primary memory, or, as he calls it, *primary retentiveness,* reserving the term memory to reproductive ideal revival. And in doing so Stout develops a theory of primary retentiveness which is akin to a trace theory of memory. I quote: "The effect of rhythmic repetition of the same stimulus is peculiarly instructive, because the external occasion of each successive impression is throughout the same, so that modification of consciousness arising in the course of the process must be due to the working of *retentiveness,* to the *cumulative disposition*[8] left behind by previous impressions. The sequence of physical stimuli is *a, a, a, . . .* , the sequence of mental states is a_1, a_2, a_3 . . . The mere fact that a_2 comes before consciousness as a *repetition,* as *another* of the same kind, constitutes an important difference between it and a_1" (p. 179). Or: "The last note of a melody may be the only note of which we are aware at the moment it strikes the ear. Yet in it the entire melody is in a sense present. It comes before consciousness as part of a quite specific whole and derives a specific character from its place in that whole. *The cumulative disposition*[8] generated by the ordered sequence of previous notes co-operates with the new stimulus to the organ of hearing, and the ensuing state of consciousness is the joint product of both factors mutually modifying each other" (p. 181). Again: "In reading a sentence or a paragraph when we come to the final word, the meaning of the sentence or paragraph as a whole is present to our consciousness. But it is only

[8] Italics are mine.

as a cumulative effect of previous process. *What is directly given as a special datum is the last word itself and its meaning*"[4] (p. 181).

Criticism of Stout's Theory. Much in these quotations, particularly in the second, sounds like gestalt psychology. And truly, Stout recognized many gestalt problems. To show why his system as a whole is essentially different from gestalt theory would disrupt the continuity of our argument. We shall merely take up his explanations by primary retentiveness of rhythm, melody, and a sentence. The particular words in his text which I have italicized betray its outstanding features: the concept of the cumulative disposition which co-operates with the stimulus in producing the conscious datum, and the reference to the datum as a thing of the present moment. Only the last note of the melody, the last word of the sentence, are actually present in consciousness, although because of the cumulative disposition they carry with them the whole tune and the whole phrase.

THE "ACTUALLY PRESENT." This, however, leads us at once into the difficulties implicit in the concept of the timeless present which we have discussed above. Let us choose a familiar example, the beginning of the anthem played in strict legato. When the third

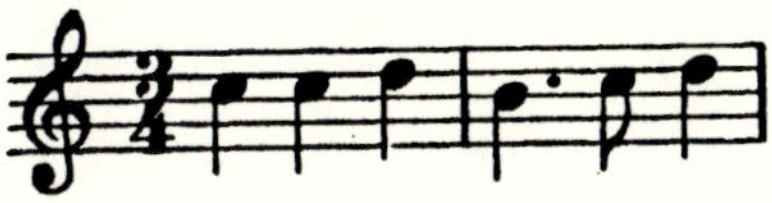

note is struck, it is "the only one of which we are aware." But awareness is a real event and therefore takes time. How much time? Probably we ought to answer, as much as the note is held by the player. But this is different for different notes, our fourth note being longer, our fifth shorter than the rest. That means our "present" depends upon stimulus characteristics; a shorter note has the shorter, a longer the longer presence. Moreover, the "meaning" of the note depends to a great extent upon its length, so that the meaning of the "present" datum depends upon the kind of presence which it has.

NEED OF THE CONCEPT OF ORGANIZATION FOR ITS EXPLANATION. But this is not the whole story. Time is continuous. If we break it up into small time intervals, there must be a principle operative by which these intervals are determined. Why, so we may legitimately ask, do the successive presences correspond to the successive notes?

[4] Italics are mine.

A priori it would be just as possible that one present moment began, let us say, in the middle of the second note and lasted till the middle of the third, to be followed by a new present moment which included the second half of the third and the first of the fourth tone. The problem is the same as the problem of unit formation in spatial organization. Inasmuch as each note is held to be "present," it is considered as a segregated unit, and this segregation is not contained in the stimulus! In the stimulus there is change, and to this stimulus change there corresponds perceptual segregation, just as in spatial organization segregation was produced by inhomogeneity of stimulation. In spatial organization homogeneously stimulated parts segregated themselves from the rest of the field and became units. Similarly, the note, as a stimulation homogeneous during a certain interval of time, is segregated from the other notes and unified within itself, by its homogeneity and its difference from the other notes. In other words, temporal wholes, like rhythms, melodies, sentences, cannot be theoretically discussed without the concept of organization. One other example is to demonstrate the likeness of spatial and temporal organization. This phrase will be heard as

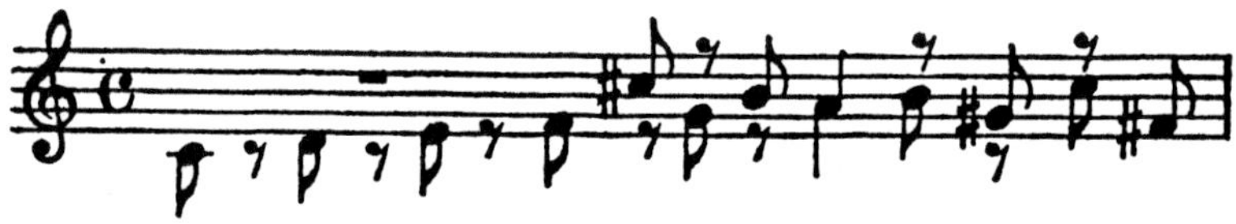

two staccato movements, one ascending from c to c′, the other descending from c♯ to f♯, the notes of the second falling between those of the first. The two movements meet in the note *a*. And this note a will *not* be heard as one long note, but as two notes of normal length, one belonging to the ascending, the other to the descending scale. Here the factor of uniformity or homogeneity has been overcome by the factor of good continuation. This last example, besides demonstrating the law of good continuation in temporal organization, should have brought out the difficulty of the "present" even more than the first. For here we meet with one case where the present does not coincide with one note, where instead one note gives rise to two presents.

A melody, like any temporal organization, cannot be described by successive states, as little as the race between Achilles and the tortoise could be described by considering the different places in which they *were*. As we said before, a moving body never *is* at one place, it always *passes through* places. Just so, a melody, until it is finished and comes, so to speak, to a stop, never *is* at one note but passes through it.

STOUT'S PRINCIPLES APPLIED TO THE THEORY OF PERCEIVED MOTION. The analogy of motion and melody can be followed up still further. For Stout's principle of cumulative dispositions might as well be applied to the perception of motion as to that of a melody. If an object moves through our field of vision so that it stimulates successively the retinal elements *a, b, c, d* . . . and is seen as an object in motion we might explain this according to Stout's principle by saying that each element if stimulated alone would give us the experience of a point at a certain place. But because of the serial stimulation each point stimulus after the first one would co-operate with the dispositions left over from the preceding ones. At any moment, so we might argue in conformity with Stout's principles, the experience of the last position should be the only one of which we are directly aware, but it comes before consciousness as part of a specific whole, the path of the motion, and thereby endowed with a specific property, its velocity. It is significant that Stout himself does not present such a view, because it would be incompatible with many facts on which he bases his own brief theory of motion, in which it is treated as a sensation (p. 220). Although our own theory was different from and much more concrete than this theory of Stout's, it is equally different from the theory we have sketched in conformity with Stout's principle of cumulative dispositions. We explained the perception of motion as due to a specific dynamic process in the psychophysical field, i.e., an event which never *was* at any place but passed through a range of places. In motion, then, we have a definite time-dependent experience which cannot possibly be explained by reference to individual "present moments." But if the existence of such processes is established, why should we then not look for similar dynamic processes in our explanations of other time-consuming events like melodies? In other words, in our explanation of such events we shall have to go beyond "primary retentiveness"—beyond memory in the sense of traces.

STOUT'S THEORY OF CUMULATIVE DISPOSITIONS. And this leads us to Stout's other fundamental concept, the concept of disposition. "We may regard mental dispositions as constituting a sort of mental structure which is constantly being formed and modified by conscious process and is in its turn constantly contributing to determine and modify subsequent conscious process" (p. 22). "We know of their existence through their effects, through their indispensable function as factors conditioning the flow of conscious life. In like manner mass and energy are known to the physicist only as being indispensable factors conditioning the motion of bodies in space. To the question, What are they? it is sufficient to reply that their nature is defined for us by their function and their origin . . ." (p. 24). However, we learn this much: "By far the greater part of our mental acquisitions are owned by us as mental *traces*[5] or dispositions and are not present in the form of actual consciousness" (p. 21). Stout, lastly, treats the dispositions as mental, although he admits the possibility that "that which is a physiological disposition is also a mental disposition" (p. 26). We see that, apart from the mind-body dualism of this system, Stout's dispositions are traces in the sense in which we defined the term. Peculiar to Stout is the use which he makes of these dispositions. By it he reduces a temporal process to a sequence of momentary processes, the later of which are influenced by the traces remaining from the earlier ones. "If we denote the sequences of specific items of sense experience . . . by *a, b, c, d,* then *a, b, c, d* by no means adequately symbolizes the process as a whole. For when *b* occurs, the resulting state of consciousness is the joint product of *b* and the persistent disposition or after-effect left behind by *a*. Similarly, when *d* occurs, the resulting state of consciousness is due to *d* in co-operation with the persistent disposition left behind by *a, b,* and *c*. We may denote the after-effect of *a* by m_1, the after-effect of *a* and *b* by m_2, and so on. The whole series may then be presented by *a*, bm_1, cm_2, dm_3" (p. 183). m_2 and m_3 are "cumulative dispositions." This is surely the best description that can be given of a melody if one breaks it up into elements and present moments.

Its Lack of a Principle of Selection According to Which These Dispositions Become Effective. But apart from the impossibility of this procedure which we have just demonstrated, it suffers from another incurable defect, for it does not contain any criterion to distinguish between dispositions which become effective and such as do not. Such a criterion, however, would be necessary; for item *d,* in Stout's example, although it will depend upon the preceding *a, b, c,* will not depend, or not depend in the same way, upon other items which also preceded it. Before the fourth tone of the melody is played the horn of a motor car may become audible, and yet the sound of this horn leaves *d* quite uninfluenced; it still appears, in Stout's terminology, as dm_3, dependent only upon *a, b, c,* and not upon the sound of the hooter, which was as good an experience as

[5] Italics are mine.

they and as liable to leave a trace. Or turn back to our second musical example. If for convenience we number the notes after the second voice enters, then we see that an odd note will depend primarily on the preceding *odd* notes, being their continuation in the scale, and *not* upon the preceding even ones, although one of these precedes it immediately, which no odd note does. The even notes may also have an effect upon the odd ones, and *vice versa,* but it is of a different *kind* from that of the odd ones. We see the same problem bobbing up again: Which items will go together to form units, from which others will they be segregated?—a problem which can be solved only in terms of organization.

The Self-determination of Temporal Organizations. Good Continuation. A melody is a whole, organized in time. That its later members depend upon its earlier ones is the exact counterpart of the fact that the right upper quadrant of a seen circle depends upon the left lower one. The difference between the two cases is only this, that in the latter we are dealing with a stationary distribution, in the former with a process which changes in time. The earlier notes of the melody have an effect upon the later ones, because they have started a process which demands a definite continuation. A melody, a rhythm, a spoken sentence, are not analogous to beads on a string, even if we assume, as Stout does, that the later beads depend upon the earlier ones, but they are continuous processes, and the dependence of the later parts of these processes upon the earlier ones cannot be treated in Stout's ultimately summative manner. A difficulty which besets the treatment of psychophysical time organizations derives from the fact that perceptual events, like heard melodies or rhythms, depend upon the appearance of ever new conditions created from the outside, viz., upon the "stimuli." But we have already seen that very soon these events have their own shape, which demands a proper continuation. How the law of good continuation finds its concrete application to psychophysical events like heard melodies will be elaborated later.

SOME EXPERIMENTAL PROOFS OF TEMPORAL ORGANIZATION. To this argument we add two more proofs. The first is taken from my dissertation. In this investigation I experimented with rhythmical experiences produced by light stimuli. In my third series, only very incompletely reported, I showed to my subjects a small number of light flashes, all of equal quality and intensity and appearing in the same place, but with different intervals between them, and asked the subjects to apprehend them as *one* rhythmical group which they were to continue first in their own minds and later on by tapping.

This is more than a test of accuracy of memory, for on the stimulus side the task is not fully determined. If three lights *a, b, c,* were presented with the interval p_1 between *a* and *b,* and p_2 between *b* and *c,* and if the subject had to continue this rhythm, he had to "create" an interval between the last perceived light *c* and the first reproduced light or beat *a,* and such an interval would recur after every group of 3. This interval p_3 had to be "created" because there was nothing in the stimuli to determine it. But five of the seven subjects were entirely unaware of this fact. To them the interval p_3 was as much a datum of the original presentation as the intervals p_1 and p_2. How the hypothesis of cumulative dispositions could explain this, I do not know; for this hypothesis explains the conscious effect at any moment by the co-operation of a cumulative disposition and a stimulus (see p. 432). But what stimulus exists in my experiments to co-operate with a cumulative disposition? If, on the other hand, we assume that the presentation of the lights started a process with its own "shape," then the result is a necessary consequence. My other proof that temporal events are organized events can be taken directly from Head. "One of the commonest defects produced by a cortical injury is this want of temporal definitions; a stimulus rhythmically repeated 'seems to be there all the time' " (1920, II, p. 754). This effect is perfectly analogous to the case of strongly reduced visual acuity. In the case of the latter a patient will see a line composed of a number of dots as a continuous line, just as Head's patients hear a continuous sound instead of a series of separate beats. We have shown in Chapter V (pp. 205 f.) that visual acuity is a matter of organization, and therefore we can use the example taken from Head as a new proof that a rhythmical series is a product of organization which gives place to another and simpler organization if the nervous system is injured in a special way. In this connection we might add that Goldstein and Gelb have found a patient who lacked the perception of motion; thus the connection which we established above between motion and melody or rhythm (p. 435) is well confirmed.

Spatial and Temporal Organizations Compared. The gist of our arguments, then, is that the explanation of temporally extended wholes cannot lie fully in the accumulation of traces, that these wholes are more than mere manifestations of "primary retentiveness." They cannot be treated without the concept of organization. Similar as their organization appeared in many respects to the purely spatial organizations which we treated in Chapters IV and V, they differ from these in one specific regard, inasmuch as they are temporal organizations. Therefore we have to examine this particular aspect. We shall discuss two simple examples, each time comparing a case of spatial and of temporal organization. (1) A white spot on a black surface—a constant tone sounding for a definite period of time in absolute stillness. We have seen before that the unity both of the spot and of the tone is a product of organization. We also know that the spot is held together, segregated from the background, by the fact that it is uniform within itself and different from its surroundings. We inferred that equal processes in contiguity exert forces of attraction upon each other, and that discontinuities between processes create forces which keep them apart. We can apply the same explanation, as also previously mentioned, to our tone; but a difference between the two cases remains, the very difference which we are now investigating, i.e., that between a spatial and a temporal unit. How does this difference appear in the process of organization? Where, in this process, does the difference between spatial and temporal homogeneity become manifest?

THE PROBLEM OF THE TEMPORAL UNIT OF ONE CONTINUOUS TONE RAISED. In order to answer this question we have to remember a fact which we have so far disregarded, the fact namely that all organization is a process in time. Concerned with the results of spatial organization, with stable forms, we could neglect this fact, because stable organizations are time-independent inasmuch as they no longer change with time. And yet, all these stable spatial organizations are held together by an interplay of forces, and the propagation of these forces, from every point to every other within the unit, takes time, short as this time may be. The introduction of this fact, however, will help us to clarify the difference between spatial and temporal organizations. With regard to time any two points within the spatial unit are equivalent; the force starting at *a* takes the same time to reach *b* as the force starting at *b* needs to reach *a*. And since the forces start simultaneously at *a* and *b*, *b* and *a* are also simultaneously affected by them. Therefore the whole process lacks *direction*.[6]

THE PROBLEM OF THE TEMPORAL UNIT OF A PAIR. One sees at once that it is quite impossible to apply the same description to our tones. Apparently there are no different points which interact with each

[6] One can use the term direction in two different meanings. It is perfectly legitimate to say that the avenues in New York City, have, approximately, the direction from south to north; but it is equally right to say that their direction is from north to south. On the other hand a bus on one of the avenues is either directed northwards or southwards, it is not both at the same time. In the text we use the term direction in the latter sense.

other, no forces propagated through space responsible for the organization of this unit. Before we try to explain this process we shall turn to our second example: two white lines in proximity on a black background and two taps in fairly close succession, both lines and taps being perceived as pairs. Little need be added about the two lines. They are held together, so as to form a pair, by forces produced by their equality (see p. 166), and these forces act exactly like those which we discussed in our first example. Let us then turn to the two taps. If we hear them as a pair they also must be held together by forces. But this case is different from the spatial one for two reasons: on the one hand the taps appear in the same place and on the other the first tap has ceased to exist when the second appears. Clearly no force can exist between something that is and something that is not. The mere conclusion that forces are required to produce the unit of our pair of taps compels us to assume that, although the first tap has ceased to exist, something must have remained which serves as one of the points at which the forces apply. In other words the conclusion that our pair of taps is a product of organization leads directly to the assumption of a *trace* left by the first of them.

PROCESS AND TRACE HAVE DIFFERENT LOCALIZATION IN THE BRAIN. But our conclusion leads us even a step further. We have to assume that the process of the second tap occurs at a place in the brain which is different, however little, from the place of the trace. If it did not, the case of the two taps would be specifically different from the case of the two lines. If the process of the second tap occurred in the same spot in which the trace of the first had been left, then we could not understand the formation of the pair. True, the second tap might, by occurring in a place filled by a trace, be different from the first tap, which occurred in a traceless area; this assumption would therefore fit Stout's theory. But pairedness is not one tap plus another tap with a new character. Moreover, if we continue our series of taps, the third tap can easily be heard as the first of a pair, the fourth as the second, and so forth. Furthermore, the temporal aspect of the perceived series will differ from the temporal aspect of the real series, the intervals between two members of one pair appearing smaller than the intervals between the second member of one pair and the first of the next.[7] If in Fig. 97 the upper dots represent the objective temporal sequence of taps, the lower ones will repre-

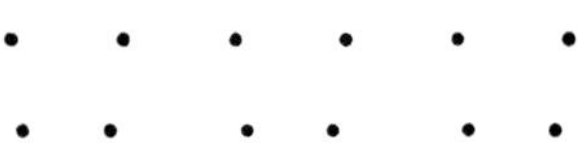

Fig. 97

[7] See, for instance, Koffka, 1908, p. 43.

sent the sequence as it is heard when subjective rhythmization in groups of two occurs. Such facts seem quite unintelligible under the assumption that the place of the trace is the same as that of the process, because if it were, the trace of the first excitation would be so completely changed by the second excitation that it would lose its identity. Our arguments against Stout's use of the traces lead to the same conclusion (see p. 446), most particularly that of the two intertwined ascending and descending scales. This fundamental conclusion, that the place of a process is different from the place of the traces, recently emphasized by Lauenstein, who derived it from considerations slightly different from our own, is different from most current theories of learning. "The theories to which allusion has briefly been made are all based on the assumption that when the organism performs a learned action on successive occasions the same cerebral cells must participate . . ." (Humphrey, p. 210).

ORGANIZATION DUE TO DYNAMICAL INTERCOURSE BETWEEN CHEMICAL DEPOSITS. The organization of two taps into a pair depends, according to our argument, upon the dynamic intercourse between an excited area and the trace of a former excitation. This makes it necessary to find characteristics of the two areas which make their dynamic communication possible. Lauenstein, developing Köhler's theory of psychophysical organization, has advanced an hypothesis which solves this problem and leads to rather far-reaching conclusions. The interaction may be due to a leap of electrical potential between the two areas, when they are in contact, or between each of them and the field between them, if they are not adjoining. If stimulation is different in two adjoining areas, then, according to this assumption, the chemical processes in the two corresponding psychophysical areas will lead to different concentrations of the reacting molecules and ions, which, owing to the different velocities of positive and negative ions, must produce a difference of potential.[8] If the two areas are separated by an area of different stimulation, then the whole field, comprising all three areas, will be a unitary dynamic field, depending for its properties upon the relative concentrations in the three areas. Lauenstein discusses the case of two grey spots (of different brightness) on a homogeneous ground (see Fig. 97*a*). In this case, if the two patches are in functional relation, some-

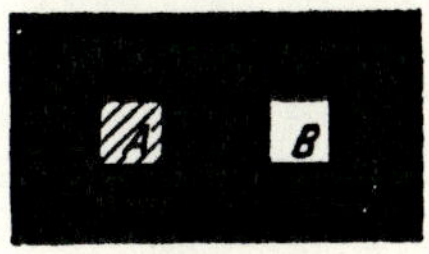

Fig. 97*a*

[8] The details must be gathered from Köhler's "Physische Gestalten" and from Lauenstein, 1933.

thing must happen in the field which depends directly upon the difference between the two patches and can therefore mediate the experience of their difference. He adduces several examples to indicate what *general kind* of event must be assumed in the intervening field. I shall reproduce the simplest example, although the concrete process in the brain must be very different: "Two containers with a large horizontal cross section, are filled with water up to different levels and communicate through a narrow pipe. Then the streaming velocity (or the pressure gradient) in each cross section of the connecting pipe can serve as a measure of the difference of level in the two containers" (p. 145). One sees that the theory also includes the case in which the two separate patches are equal; to it the velocity zero would correspond in the hydrodynamic example.

These hypotheses must be applied to our two taps, which correspond to the two separate patches rather than to the case of contiguous areas. At the moment of the second tap a certain concentration is produced in a brain area. The trace of the first tap, i.e., the sediment remaining from the first excitation, lies, as we have deduced, in a slightly different area; on the other hand it has its own concentration, more or less like the concentration produced by the first process,[9] and in between lies the trace of the interval with its concentration. In this respect, then, the case of the two successive taps has been reduced to the case of the two simultaneous patches: the two taps are a behavioural unit, because there exists a field process between the deposit produced by the second tap and the trace left by the first across the trace left by the interval.

So far our hypothesis explains the pair-character of the two taps: for at the time of the second tap we assume not only an excitation corresponding to it, but also a field excitation which connects this excitation with the trace of the preceding one. It ought to be well remembered that we correlate experiences with excitation, but not with traces. Therefore, the first tap is "in consciousness" only by virtue of the field excitation which is directed towards its trace, but not as an image, i.e., a separate experience.

Our theory contains an implication about the causes of this field process. Since we derived it from the difference (or equality) of concentration in the excited and the trace area, it is only indirectly connected with the process of excitation itself, viz., only through the concentration to which this process gives rise. Here the theory is

[9] We shall presently deal with the changes which this concentration undergoes after the cessation of the first excitation.

clearly incomplete. After the second excitation is past, its trace remains and therefore also the difference of concentration between the two areas. If, then, the field event depended only upon this difference, it should go on indefinitely; we should no longer hear any tap, but still be aware of the pair-character. We have previously contended that such experiences are possible,[10] but certainly they do not occur all the time, as they should if our theory were complete.

Before we continue this side of our theory we must correct another fault which was inherent in our presentation. We have treated the second excitation as a primarily independent event which secondarily came into communication with the trace of the first process. This was an illegitimate simplification, introduced only in order to make it easier for the reader to follow this difficult argument. In reality the excitation of the second tap will arise in the field determined by the trace of the first. This point will prove of great importance in our later discussion.

THE RÔLE OF EXCITATION IN TEMPORAL ORGANIZATIONS. In order to develop our theory further we will now distinguish four different cases: (1) The experience of the two grey patches, as in Fig. 97*a*. (2) That of the two successive taps. (3) The trace of the former and (4) the trace of the latter. Since we have not discussed (3) before, it will be well to consider this case now as a representative of the trace of a spatial unit. Spatial units were explained as corresponding to areas held together and segregated from the rest by the nature of the processes occurring within them. Since the traces depend directly on the processes, they will, so to speak, "map" those processes, and as such "maps" they will be segregated from traces of surrounding processes and be integrated within themselves. In other words, just as we had to deduce that a field process would continue between the traces of our two taps after the second tap was over, so we must assume that field processes occur within traces of spatial units. If they did not, these trace units would cease to be units.

In Chapter III we learned that unit formation involves *shape*. Therefore the shape of the original process distribution must also be preserved in a dynamical shape of the trace. Traces of spatial units, then, are systems under stress, a statement from which further conclusions follow, as we shall see later.

When now we compare cases (3) and (4) we find them in many respects essentially alike. In both cases the trace is a unitary system

[10] See page 180, the grin without the cat.

composed of three parts, corresponding to the two patches and taps, and the interval between them, which in the trace is in both cases a spatial interval. True enough, this spatial interval is due in the first case to the fact that in the original process, corresponding to the experience, the total event with its three parts was spatially extended, while in the second case it owes its existence to a time sequence, the excitations occurring at different places from those of the traces. But experimental evidence, which we shall discuss later, indicates that this difference of origin has no influence at least upon a number of effects which take place in this unitary trace system. Therefore we shall treat these two cases together.

As long as the trace is just a trace without a new excitation nothing in our behavioural field corresponds to it. But it is a condition for a number of future processes which are accompanied by experience, e.g., recognition, discrimination, and recall. On the other hand we were led to the conclusion that these unified trace systems are under stress. Let us symbolize the part in these systems which corresponds to the first member by *a,* that corresponding to the second by *b,* and that corresponding to the interval by *i.* Then, if *a, b,* and *i* are areas of different concentration, there will be a pattern of leaps of potential between them, which might produce processes of equalization, or other occurrences within the *a i b* system. On the other hand, there is nothing in experience to suggest the existence of such processes. Apparently our argument has led to a contradiction. This contradiction cannot, however, be abolished by eliminating our assumption of a dynamic state in the trace system from our hypothesis. As we shall soon see, a number of experimental facts as well as our deductions make this assumption necessary: such trace systems change with time, as can be proved by their after-effects. Consequently we must explain why these processes are not represented in our behavioural field, why, differently expressed, they are unaccompanied by consciousness.

We shall gain a clue for this explanation by including the first two cases in our discussion. In case (1) we experience a pair both of whose members are simultaneously present, whereas in (2) the pair is experienced while one of its members is already past. To this difference in experience there corresponds a difference in the dynamics of the process: in case (1) there are two excitations (or rather three, since we must include the interval between the two patches) and the dynamic field which connects them.[11] In case (2)

[11] This description with its distinction of excitations *and* the field is chosen only to emphasize a particular point; it is not a good description of the real occurrences in which the excitations and the field are not "and-connected."

there is only *one* excitation and a field process which connects this excitation with the traces of the two preceding excitations. From this confrontation of our two cases we must infer that the presence of one or more excitations in a field determines the temporal or spatial character of the field. If area *b* is, through the mediation of area *i*, in communication with area *a*, and if area *b* alone is the seat of an actual excitation, then this communication, besides accounting for the organization of *a i b*, lends to *b* the character of being *"later than a,"* or of being *"the second."*

Temporal Direction and Excitation. Thus we may say that the *"direction"* of the process depends upon the fact whether it contains one or more excitations, but this term direction must be handled with care, for there are process directions which are independent of the excitations. Thus if area *a* has a higher concentration than *b* the process will be directed from *a* to *b*, whereas it must have the opposite direction when *b* is the area of greater concentration, no matter whether *a* is an excitation or merely a trace. Indeed we can see *a* lighter or darker than *b* in our first example (according to the arrangement of the patches) and we can hear *b* stronger or weaker than *a* in our second (according to the relative intensities of the two taps). The direction which, in our hypothesis, must depend upon the number of excitations is the temporal direction itself.

Our hypothesis contains a difference between the cases, patches (1) and taps (2), even if it ascribes the field event to the difference in concentration between *a* and *b;* for if as in case (2) *a* is a mere trace, then its concentration is what it is, because it has been left over, because nothing new happens to it,[12] whereas the concentration at *b* is created and maintained by the excitation during the period of time through which the whole process lasts. In case (1) on the other hand, the concentrations at *a* and *b* are dynamically equal, both being created and maintained by excitations. This difference in the occurrences at *a* and *b*—in (2) a static condition at the one and a dynamic process at the other, in (1) two dynamic processes—must account for other differences which will directly explain the time direction of the process. To explain the difference between cases (1) and (2) on the one hand and cases (3) and (4) on the other we might assume that the process that occurs between two traces in the absence of any excitation is of different intensity, i.e., rate, or of a different kind from the one that takes place when at least one of the areas is in a state of excitation.

[12] We disregard again the changes which it may undergo through its communication with *b* and other parts of the field.

This would imply the assumption that a process has to be of a certain intensity, to occur with a certain velocity, in order to be represented in the behavioural field, or, in other words, to be accompanied by consciousness, an assumption which seems by no means impossible. It is, however, possible, if not probable, that the difference in rate is due to a difference in kind; one might, for instance, think that processes of pure diffusion—among others—would take place between "dead" traces, processes which would be far too slow to be considered as counterparts of experience.[18] In that case the property of a physiological process which made it the carrier of an experience would not necessarily be its velocity, or its velocity alone, but also its kind.

SIMILARITY OF SPATIAL AND TEMPORAL MEMORY. Before we close this discussion we must draw one more inference from the similarity of cases (3) and (4), viz., the traces remaining from two simultaneous grey patches and those from two successive taps. If our assumptions and the arguments based upon them were right, our memory of temporal sequences should be similar to that of spatial patterns, since in the traces time becomes spatialized. This inference seems to be largely confirmed by facts. In recalling events in my own past which followed upon each other, like the events of a day spent at the seaside, I recall them as spread out in different places, but although I *know* that they followed upon each other in time, this knowledge is an experience of a different kind from the spatial pattern which the events possess in my recollection. Whereas they are, in my act of remembering, spread out in a definite spatial schema, they lack the *immediate character* of being temporal sequences which distinguishes, for instance, the two taps which we have so fully discussed. The *knowledge* of their temporal relations seems much more to be a dynamic relationship which connects them with my Ego than one which holds them together among themselves. This statement, which as far as it goes adds weight to our inference, does not, however, exclude that memory of *true* temporal sequences may occur.

THE PROBLEM OF THE TEMPORAL UNITY OF A CONTINUOUS TONE SOLVED. Let us now return to our first example, which we abandoned for the discussion of the second, I mean the constant tone heard for a definite period of time. What gives it its unity? If our explanation of the pair formation is right, there can be only one answer to our question: just as the unity between the two taps is due to the processes occurring between the chemical deposits at the

[18] See Köhler, 1920, p. 16.

two areas corresponding to the two taps (and the area corresponding to the interval between them), so the unity of the one tone must be caused by the deposits produced in continually different places by the continuous vibrations. The organization is again spatial and derives its temporal character, like the other one, from the fact that the whole deposit unit consists of dead traces except for its "tip" where it is just being *made* by an excitation. Continually such excitations occur, therefore continually the column of deposits is increased. Normally the excitation will not be uniform for any length of time, one sound, e.g., will be followed by another. To such changing stimulations there must then, if our hypothesis is right, correspond pieces of the column, corresponding to the periods of uniform excitation, held together by this uniformity according to the law of equality which we discovered in our discussion of spatial organization (see p. 166). Change of excitation, on the other hand, accompanied by change of deposits, will segregate these pieces from each other, in perfect analogy to space organization. It would be a welcome confirmation of this hypothesis if the equivalent of Mach rings could be discovered in the temporal field. In acoustics one might look for such an equivalent both in pitch and intensity. One would have to produce a glissando, either of frequency or of intensity, and introduce a sudden change in the rate of this glissando. Our Fig. 48, page 170, will exemplify such cases, if the abscissa now means *time* instead of distance and the ordinate either frequency or intensity. If, then, a phenomenon similar to the Mach rings occurred, we should hear the stimulation of figures *b* and *c* as upward glissandos with discontinuities at the moments *p*, this discontinuity having, in figure *b*, the character of a sudden rise or fall (either in pitch or intensity) and in figure *c* of a sudden fall and rise. The experiment, however, is not crucial. Although it would lend great weight to our hypothesis, if its result were positive, a negative outcome would not invalidate our assumption, since the spatial organization in the deposit column need not be in *all* respects equal to that in a simultaneous spatial field.

Our hypothesis leads to another inference. If the stimulation is short enough, then, owing to the inertia of the system, there will be no time for "dead" deposits to remain while the excitation builds up new deposits. All that happens will be an excitation with its own concentration, followed by another excitation. This case resembles closely that of the "point" in space; such short sound, a telephone click, or a short note in music, has no duration, just as the point has no extension—phenomenologically, of course, not physically.

We must now return to the other member of our first example, the light patch on the homogeneous background. In the beginning we discussed it only from the point of view of spatial organization. But we must now remember that such a patch persists also through time; it therefore contains the same problem as the tone, and this problem must find the same solution. We have now to apply our hypothesis of the trace column to the spatially organized (shaped) deposit which corresponds to the patch, and the same is of course true of all permanent objects in our behavioural world.

Our Theory Compared to Stout's. In order to see how much we have achieved by our hypothesis it will be expedient to turn back to the criticisms which we raised against Stout and to see how our own theory escapes them. On page 433 we discovered that in Stout's theory the "immediate present" must be a function of the stimulus duration. Our hypothesis contains the reason why it must be so, why, as a rule, a temporal unit in experience will correspond to a continuous uniform stimulation. Moreover, as will be seen presently, our hypothesis is such as to imply a function different from mere geometrical correspondence between the duration of the stimulus and that of the experienced unit. The next point which we raised against Stout was that his theory lacked a principle of integration for immediate presents. And this principle has again been supplied by our theory. But how can we deal with the example of the two scales, one temporally inserted in the other? We used it in criticism of Stout's concept of the immediate present, his analysis of the melody tones plus after-effects (which he also calls their "meaning"), and of his failure to discriminate between effective and ineffective dispositions (p. 436 f.). All these aspects will now be considered together, they all pointed to the effectiveness of the law of good continuation.

Beginning with the first, one has to ask: Why, in our example, is the one long note heard as two short notes? Why, in terms of our theory, is the unity of this temporal experience broken despite the uniformity of stimulation which should produce a homogeneous and therefore coherent trace column? The answer is to be found in a previous statement (p. 443): our hypothesis would not be able to cope with the facts if it assumed that a stimulus-produced excitation and hence its deposit were independent of the preceding stimulations.[14] Therefore, as we emphasized before, each excitation has to be envisaged in a field of traces, at the "tip" of which it occurs.

What does this mean within the framework of our hypothesis?

[14] This would be a temporal constancy hypothesis.

We consider a sequence of stimuli that gives rise to a temporal unit. What happens at the moment when the *n*th stimulus takes effect? Immediately preceding this moment there exists a trace column produced by the first $n-1$ stimulations. This trace column forms a coherent and organized field, i.e., it is permeated by forces which hold it together, segregate it from the rest, and determine its own articulation. Now we know from the discussion of spatial organizations that the forces which bound and shape a segregated unit also permeate into the field outside. If the unit is "open" or "incomplete" then that part of the field which corresponds to the gap will be a seat of very particular forces, forces which will make the arousal of processes of closure easier than the arousal of any others. The closure will, of course, be that closure which is demanded by the rest of the figure, a closure of good continuation. And even where closure in a proper sense is not possible a structure will so influence its field that in its neighbourhood, notably at its ends, certain processes have a better chance to occur than others. If, for instance, the points *a–n* of Fig. 98 are exposed, then it will be easier to add point p_1 than p_2. Wertheimer has demonstrated this in unpublished threshold experiments. Our trace column, before the sequence has come to its natural end, is just such an open or incomplete spatial organization, and therefore it will facilitate such excitations as continue it properly and eventually lead towards closure. The organization being one of deposits in a trace column, it can be continued and completed only by new deposits. Therefore the excitation which the stimulus produces will be determined by the field forces in such a way as to produce *that* deposit which is a proper continuation of the existing trace column. In other words, excitation *n* will, in consequence of the field forces, tend to be such as to produce a deposit *n* which fits into the trace column created by the preceding $n-1$ excitations. Whether the *n*th excitation will actually be of that kind depends of course upon the nature of the stimulus. The latter is an external force of organization, while the field supplies internal forces. Even when the stimulus prevents the occurrence of the "proper" excitation, the field forces will prove effective. If, e.g., the stimuli are the notes of a melody and the *n*th note is too flat or too sharp, it will be heard as out of *tune;* and if it is entirely different from the fitting stimulus, then it will be heard as "a surprise."

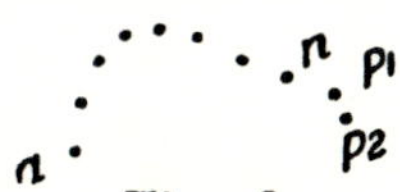

Fig. 98

The application to our example of the two scales is now simple. The long tone will be heard as two short ones because the two interlaced trace columns each favour the arousal of one short tone. In this case, as in all similar ones, the forces due to embracing field systems, following the laws of good continuation and closure, are stronger than the forces which are active in the isolated piece, forces due to mere homogeneity of process and acting according to the law of equality. In a sense our discussion has confirmed an aspect of Stout's theory: also in ours there *is* "co-operation" between traces and stimuli. But there is at the same time a principle which explains the *selectiveness* of this co-operation, which was lacking in Stout's exposition; this will soon be discussed more fully.

THE DYNAMIC CHARACTER OF TEMPORAL UNITS. A NEW RÔLE OF EXCITATIONS. If each member of a temporal unit depends upon the field produced by the preceding members as well as upon its own stimulus, then we can also understand why the direction of the unit becomes more and more determined the further the sequence proceeds. With each new member the field grows in extent and thereby in power.[15] The forces of the field increase continually in strength so that their share will become stronger and stronger in the compound effect the longer the unit lasts. Of course there is a limit to this effect. Just as spatial units have their limits, depending upon the particular conditions, so have temporal ones. In neither field can the units be made as large as we like. But the last agreement with Stout's theory does not mean that we accept his description of a melody as composed of tones with meanings. Such a description robs a melody of its dynamic character.

We must now explain why in our musical example on page 434 we hear two interlaced scales. The first four notes have established a trace field and a process which are both most properly continued by g, the sixth note, but not by c sharp, the fifth. When g is sounded it will, therefore, "come from" the direction determined by the first four notes and will extend this trace system, remaining relatively independent of the trace of the preceding c sharp. The next note, b, will conversely be closely connected with the trace of this, and so on. One might doubt how a process can continue through the presence of another process, i.e., how the motion of each of the two scales can survive the interpolated tones of the other scale. Again an analogy from vision, the so-called tunnel motion, will show that this is not a serious difficulty. It is easy to demonstrate an object

[15] Not only does the field become gradually organized, it may also become *re*-organized; thus the third tone may become the tonic, thereby forcing the first from this position, which it originally held.

moving through the field over an uninterrupted track although a part of the track is filled by a different object. The moving object is then seen to pass "behind" the obstruction as if it went through a tunnel. In a way this is another case of "double representation."

A New Rôle of Traces. Our introduction of the continuous process has still left the burden of the explanation on the trace system, just as Stout put it on his cumulative dispositions. We have avoided the criticism to which Stout's theory could be subjected, by treating the trace system as a system in organization, subject to the same laws of organization which we have studied in an entirely different field, and by deriving not only unit formation but also the specific dynamic character of temporal units from the trace field. The main feature of the theory is still that it ascribes the forces of organization to the trace field. The good continuation, according to our assumption, is not due to the movement qua movement, but to the field which favours certain motions rather than others. This seems necessary not only because of Newton's first law of motion, but also owing to the extreme degree of friction in the nervous systems, in which no motion can take place without forces, all inert velocities being destroyed.[16]

The assumption of a special process of motion is not necessary to explain *every* kind of temporal unit. We saw before that it is possible to explain the pair character of two taps entirely by processes between deposits (see p. 442). For a single pair the assumed motion would be the dynamical manner in which the second member appears, "rising" or "falling" from the first. Thus Lauenstein found it necessary to distinguish two types of processes of successive comparison (p. 149 f.); in one a pure dynamical relation between the two deposits produces the unification, in the other there occurs over and above this field condition a process of "motion," a "jump" or "drop" of the second member.

It is easy to see how the two hypotheses are to be applied in different cases. Wherever a musical phrase consists of a quick sequence of tones which produce the impression of an upward, downward, or undulating motion, the hypothesis of a unitary motion will be necessary: no tone lasts sufficiently long to "be" something by itself; it is merely a stage, a phase, in a larger motion. When on the other hand a tone is held for a relatively long time, as, let us say, the fourth note of Beethoven's fifth symphony, then the excitation hypothesis is not sufficient. True enough, the coming of this tone requires this hypothesis, the drop from e flat to

16 See Köhler, 1927 a.

c; but while c lasts, it retains its character of being at the bottom, and this requires for an explanation the deposit-gradient hypothesis. The pure gradient hypothesis, lastly, will suffice to explain cases of successive comparison with relatively long intervals between the two experiences to be compared.

Objections to Our Trace Hypothesis. Although our construction is not quite finished yet, it seems advisable to test the plausibility of our hypothesis by subjecting it to objections which can be raised against it.

(1) Spatialization of Time Would Require a Non-existent Fourth Dimension of Space. It was one of the features of our hypothesis that it spatialized time in the brain. This raises at once the following difficulty: our brain is tri-dimensional and we have assumed that to perceived tri-dimensional objects there correspond tri-dimensional process distributions in the brain. Where, then, is a place for the time dimension? If the temporal unity of any behavioural object depends upon a spatial unity of the traces which its psychophysical process builds up, how is it to be explained that a point can be remembered as a point, a line as a line, a surface as a surface, and not instead the first as a line, the second as a surface, the third as a solid; and how can we ever remember the duration of a solid? For, so we must argue, the traces of the point must be spatially different, so that each point, which has lasted in our behavioural world through an appreciable period of time must have left a trace which should be similar to the trace of a line seen for the shortest possible time, if the direction of the line corresponded with the direction in which the traces superimpose themselves on each other. Similarly a straight line should, by the accumulation of traces, become an oblong, a circle a cylinder, and since no fourth dimension is at our disposal, we cannot see what is to become of a solid, not even how we should in our hypothesis be able to experience the duration of a tri-dimensional object.

Powerful as this argument is, I do not believe that it is fatal to our hypothesis. As a matter of fact the difficulty concerns only the memory effect proper and not the perceived duration. For the continued perception of a point and the momentary perception of a line are in our hypothesis different psychophysical events. In the former the *excitation,* though it always occurs at the tip of a trace *line,* is at every moment but a *point* excitation, whereas in the latter the excitation itself is linear. Thus in perception our two cases must, according to our hypothesis, appear as different, and the same is true for the other examples. To add only a discussion of the solid:

Even though the "time direction," i.e., the direction in which the traces accumulate, must coincide with some direction of the solid, the trace column cannot distort the continued perception of the solid because the excitation itself remains unaltered.

But a more serious difficulty arises when we turn to the lasting memory effects. If the excitation of a point perception which has lasted for a definite period of time ceases, then the traces remain, and they form, as we have just now stated, a linear pattern. Similarly the trace of a momentarily exposed line has a linear pattern. Where then can the difference between these two trace patterns lie? For difference there must be, since we do not confuse in our remembrances a point looked at for 15 seconds and a line seen for a brief moment. This difference can only lie in one place, and that is the internal organization of these two linear trace patterns, i.e., in the manner in which they form units. The line trace was produced by a spatially extended process, we shall therefore assume that its trace is a spatially coherent trace, a trace in which no point is segregated from another. Contrariwise, the time pattern of the point traces was produced by an excitation of the smallest spatial extent.[17] We must therefore conclude that the temporal trace pattern of the point retains its punctiform character through its entire extent. Whereas the line trace is one, the temporally extended point trace can be considered as a great number of individual point traces, which in their pattern do not lose their point character. We know from Lauenstein's and von Restorff's investigations, to be discussed later, that equal or similar traces if close together influence each other, this influence taking the form of assimilation. We must expect an even stronger effect when the traces are continuous, but we cannot expect that the interaction of such traces, which undoubtedly occurs, changes their spatial or figural aspects by integrating them into new traces of a higher dimension. Interaction within a temporal trace pattern was a necessary assumption to explain temporal unity; it has been proved experimentally in different ways. But this interaction cannot be such as to destroy fundamentally the *spatial* boundaries of each part trace within the whole pattern. The change that takes place within a temporal trace pattern moves towards simplicity of the minimum kind; for when the trace system is left alone, it has in many cases no access to any outside energies. The building up, on the other hand, of structures of more dimensions from those of fewer would be a change towards simplicity of the

[17] We neglect for simplicity's sake that in reality both line and point are seen on their backgrounds, so that the whole trace is in either case spatially extended.

maximum kind. The actually observed changes (Lauenstein, von Restorff) are in full accord with this conclusion. In compound trace systems consisting not of equal but of similar members, these members are apt to lose their identity, to fuse into unitary systems.[18] Furthermore (another aspect of the same change) much of the temporal aspect of our experience is lost in memory, as previously mentioned (p. 446). We remember, e.g., that some time ago we saw a point here, a line there, a house in that landscape, and so forth, but as a rule we do not remember *how long* we have seen point, line, house.[19] So much for our first objection.

(2) The Relation of Lashley's Results to a Trace Theory. We now turn to an objection which may be raised against the assumption of traces based on Lashley's famous results (1929, pp. 100, 107, 109). Lashley found that maze habits acquired by normal rats are interfered with by cortical lesions in such a way that the degree of deterioration of the habit is a direct function of the *amount* of cerebral tissue destroyed but is virtually independent of the locus of such destruction. This fact may also be expressed by saying that this habit "seems to be non-localized" (Lashley, p. 87). It seems plausible to go one step further and say with Wheeler and Perkins (p. 387) that "the brain, therefore, is not a mass of structures each having its own particular and independent function. In face of these facts the trace theory is inconceivable." The first part of this quotation is indeed quite acceptable, if one emphasizes its concluding clause: no trace has an independent function, nor even an independent existence. But the final sentence of the quotation is by no means proven by Lashley's results nor does Lashley himself believe it. For what he found true for the maze habit he did not find true for three other habits, viz., brightness discrimination, inclined plane box,[20] and double platform box. In speaking of the latter Lashley says: "This habit thus resembles that of brightness discrimination in having a definite localization of the engram . . ." (p. 87). For these three habits are lost when after their acquisition *certain* parts of the cortex (occipital for the first, frontal for the two others) are destroyed, while injuries in any other region do not affect

[18] Concrete demonstrations will follow in Chapter XI.

[19] Language and conceptual thinking complicate this mattter. The statement in the text refers to recall as little influenced by these factors as possible. They give us *knowledge* of durations without recalling such durations.

[20] In the inclined plane box the rat has to run up an inclined plane on top of a box containing food in order to open its door; the double platform box "is a problem box provided with a door which is opened by successively pressing down in predetermined order two platforms attached to opposite sides of the box." (Lashley, p. 27.)

them (p. 121). These achievements, then, if once learned, have left definite parts of the brain altered, i.e., they have left traces which account for the retention of these habits, and these habits are, as Lashley points out (pp. 133 f.), simpler in nature than the maze habits. When Lashley says that maze habits are not localized he does not mean that learning leaves no after-effect, i.e., no traces whatsoever. It is perfectly compatible with his results that for maze habits these traces are distributed over the entire cortex. In the particular experiment which is relevant to our issue rats were trained in a maze until 10 consecutive errorless trials were obtained. Ten days later they were retrained and then immediately subjected to operations in which different amounts of the cortex were removed (with or without injury to subcortial regions). Ten days later they were again retrained. The average learning times obtained were in seconds:

for original training	*for pre-operative retraining*	*for post-operative retraining*
1,911	64.8	2,221

with an average destruction of 17.7%.

From these figures alone we might argue that these results gave no proof whatever that the operation had produced a deterioration of the habit through destruction of traces. The mere fact, also discovered by Lashley, that animals with brain injuries learn more slowly than normal ones and that their retardation is a direct function of the extent of the injury, might account for the result. The very fact that the third average is higher than the first seems to support this argument, which would claim that they did not measure a learning and a relearning achievement, but two acts of learning performed under different neurological conditions. But the argument would be conclusive only if this average coincided with the average of animals who *acquired* the habit after an operation of the same average extent, and if no, or only few, cases occurred in which the third average was lower than the first, though still significantly higher than the second. In reality nine cases of the last kind are to be found in Lashley's table[21] with the three averages: 3,386, 94, and 1,115. Here, then, the animals learned better after the operation than they did when they were first trained, and yet very much worse than in their first, pre-operative, retraining. Both facts can be explained only by the assumption that some effect

[21] His animals No. 70, 72, 74, 78, 90, 91, 99, 110, 112.

or trace had been carried over, but that a great deal of it had been destroyed by the operation.

I have also averaged the time of post-operative retraining for animals 88-114, with an average percentage of destruction of 22.6, ranging between 15.8 and 31.1, for which a control group can be obtained from Lashley's Table I, animals 10-25, with an average destruction of 24.5%, ranging between 16.1 and 32.0. These animals *learned* the same maze, after operation, that the other animals relearned. The figures are: relearning after operation: 3,630 sec., *learning* after operation 4,521 sec. The number of cases is probably not large enough to draw binding conclusions, but they give sufficient indication to refute the anti-trace argument from this side also; since the animals which had learned the maze before the operation relearned it more quickly after the operation than operated animals which had had no previous training learned it, the original training must have left effects which explain this difference, even though the time consumed in relearning was considerably longer than the average time of training of the whole group.

Thus Lashley's experiments, far from being incompatible with the assumption of traces, demand such an hypothesis. The difference between "localized" traces and such as are deposited over practically the whole cortex is easily explained as due to the processes which originally produced the traces. For the maze habit—as Lashley points out himself (pp. 132 ff.)—these processes must involve more or less the whole brain, while the significant aspect of brightness discrimination is a much more isolated affair. No wonder then that the traces of the former should be more widely scattered than those of the latter.

In concluding this argument we must point out two salient aspects of Lashley's experiments and results. In the first place they investigate the effect not of such simple trace patterns as we have so far mostly discussed, but of whole trace systems built up at different times, each new trial adding something to the traces of the preceding trials. Thus the problem of the accumulation of such trace systems arises. Quite evidently a repetition of a run, even if it occurs a considerable time after the last, does not leave a trace independent of the preceding ones. Learning, rather, depends to a great extent upon the manner in which new deposits combine with old traces. In the second place we must not overlook the fact that Lashley's method supplies him primarily with data of accomplishment and not of behaviour, these terms taken in the sense defined above (on p. 37), even though he supplements them with behavioural data.

Hence we do not know whether an identity of accomplishment corresponds to an identity of behaviour. All our knowledge of the effects of brain lesions seems to indicate that similar accomplishments are brought about by different behaviours of normal persons and persons with brain lesions. This has to be kept in mind for an ultimate evaluation of Lashley's results.

(3) WHEELER'S OPPOSITION TO A TRACE THEORY AND HIS ATTEMPT TO EXPLAIN MEMORY WITHOUT TRACES. We shall continue by casting a glance at Wheeler's position with regard to the assumption of traces. As already indicated, he rejects the trace hypothesis entirely. It seems important to discuss his arguments because he is the foremost American champion of gestalt theory and bases his position with regard to traces on these principles. His arguments are of very unequal value. The one taken from Lashley's experiments we have already refuted; on the other hand we gladly accept those directed against an atomistic or a synapse theory of traces. There remains only one important argument, which, though we have really dealt with it before (p. 440 f.), deserves a special discussion. "The brain is constantly being stimulated so that the 'traces' would be constantly changing toward finer and finer differentiations of pattern until, shortly, there would be a homogeneous condition in the brain and therefore no 'traces'" (Wheeler and Perkins, p. 391). We have forestalled this criticism by our assumption that the excitations do not occur in the place of previously deposited traces (see above). To prove their point, Wheeler and Perkins give an example from physics which I will partly reproduce in order to show the origin of their faulty conclusions.

"Suppose that a horizontal metal plate of some sort is fastened, on one edge, to an upright bar. The surface of this plate is covered evenly with a layer of sand. If, now, this plate is made to vibrate at a constant rate the vibrations will keep the sand equally distributed over the plate. But suppose that while the plate is still vibrating it is suddenly bowed with a violin bow on one of the free sides. . . . The bowing momentarily induces added vibrations which must adjust themselves to the other vibrations already going on. *The sand will now arrange itself into four equal areas, with two streaks which contain no sand bisecting the square plate into four equal parts.*[22] The original force applied to the plate continues to keep it vibrating at the steady rate set up before the bowing, so that when the bowing stops the sand will gradually approach the equally distributed condition existing at the outset.

[22] Italics in the original.

"This illustration helps us to understand the condition which exists in the brain under Köhler's theory of disequilibration. The original, equally distributed condition of the sand represents the original equilibrium of forces within the nervous system. The constant vibration represents the dynamic character of the condition. The bowing corresponds to the impinging of some external stimulus pattern upon the system. In the case of the plate the bowing sets up stress-patterns of four equal areas as indicated by the distribution of sand. There has been a mutual adjustment of two stresses, one set up by the first vibrating force, and the other by the bowing. *The consequence was a 'non-process condition' set up in the sand.*[23] This was the pattern formed into the four square areas. When the bowing stopped, however, the four sections began to disappear. The sand began at once to approach the condition of equilibrium again, and this was the equal distribution conditioned by the original vibrations" (pp. 389, 390).

Unfortunately this analogy with the Chladni figures of physics is totally false. The sand pattern, though an indication of the process of vibration, is never a condition of it; the plate vibrates as it does because of the two forces which in superposition result in that form of motion. The sand has nothing to do with it; remove it, and the plate vibrates as before. Therefore the sand is *not* comparable to a trace. Furthermore, the causal relation between sand and vibration being unilateral, the sand returns to its old pattern when the vibration resumes its old form. No physicist would call the Chladni figures examples of memory. One cannot use as analogies of memory illustrations from physics where a present event occurs without reference to past events, and that is what Wheeler does again and again.[24] Physics knows, as we have seen (p. 428), real analogies to memory effects, but in order to explain them, changes within the reacting system, traces of some sort, have to be assumed.

The rest of Wheeler's argument, based on the Chladni figures, may be omitted, because it adds nothing new, repeating the confusion of a mere effect of a process with an effect which at once becomes a codeterminant of the process.

If the Chladni plate were covered with a viscous substance much heavier than sand, then the analogy would be better. It would take some time before the substance had arranged itself in a stable pattern; at the same time, because of its weight and because it does not follow quickly the forces produced by the vibrating body, it will co-determine this vi-

[23] Italics mine. A non-process condition (a term introduced by me in an article on the structure of the unconscious (1927) is a trace.

[24] See the example of the air currents produced by candles in Wheeler and Perkins (W. P.), p. 388.

bration, it will be a real condition, and when it has reached a stable distribution with one sort of vibration it will co-determine the vibration of the plate under a new excitation, and thereby its own redistribution.

How, then, can Wheeler explain memory effects without the assumption of traces? His theory, as far as I understand it, overlooks again the main point.

"The story is often told of a horse that was being driven along a country road. At a certain place a newspaper blew across the road and the horse shied. About three weeks later it was being driven along the same road and when it came to this place it shied, but there was no newspaper" (W. P., p. 397). "Why should the horse . . . shy the second time if the original experience had left no impression? *The reason why he shied the second time was exactly the same as the reason why he shied the first time!* A newspaper was blowing across the road and the horse was responding to the *total situation*.[25] The total stimulus-pattern induced the response, which was configurational in character. The same stimulus-pattern, or one similar to it, is going to produce the response again for the same reason that it produced a response the first time. . . . If a trace were necessary to account for the second response, one would also be required for the first!" (W. P., pp. 398, 399.)

This quotation derives its apparent plausibility from the use of the term "total situation." It thus demonstrates how justified we were when we criticized this concept (see Chapter IV, pp. 158 f.). The fallacy becomes obvious when one asks the question why the horse did not shy at any other part of his route. Here the "total situation" was such that it pursued its trot undisturbed, and it certainly would have done the same also at the critical spot, had the newspaper not happened to blow across it. It is therefore not true that the horse shied at the place for the second time for the same reason it did so for the first. To make this point still clearer, we shall assume three trips, A, B, and C, instead of two. During A and C nothing happens at the critical point X, while during B the wind tosses the paper across the road. In A the horse proceeds undisturbed through X, in B and C it shies. This proves that the "total situation" of X, as it was both in A and C, is not responsible for the shying, for it did not provoke it in A. The only difference between A and C is that B has preceded C, but not A, and therefore I find it logically necessary to conclude that the difference in behaviour in A and C is due to the effect of B, i.e., to traces which have remained from the experience in B.

[25] Italics in original.

I am not certain whether I have represented the whole of Wheeler's theory of memory. In his first book (p. 273) there is a passage from which one might gather that he attributed the learning process either to growth or to the building up of chemical compounds. The first assumption has to be ruled out, at least for most memory effects, because growth is far too slow a process, while the second would be equivalent to a trace theory of the kind we propose, although Wheeler refuses to accept the name. However, such an intrepretation of Wheeler would probably either be wrong or no longer represent his present opinion, for in the second book he writes (W. P., p. 387), *"A given experience is not represented by a brain-pattern except when the stimulus-situation is keeping the pattern set up. The instant the stimulus is removed the brain-pattern disappears."* [26] In our theory this is true of the excitation pattern, but not of the trace pattern, while Wheeler seems in these lines to deny any persistence whatever to what he calls the brain-pattern.

(4) VON KRIES'S ARGUMENT. The most severe criticism of traditional trace theories dates back more than thirty years. It was first presented by von Kries, who did not use it against *any* trace theory, but only against those prevalent at his time and ever after; some years later it was elaborated by Becher, to whom it appeared an ultimate refutation of all trace theories and thereby a proof of a vitalistic interpretation of memory.

The decisive argument can be presented in this way: memory effects are as a rule not traceable to the individual original excitation, but to their form or pattern. I recognize a melody, which I have heard played in G major by an orchestra, when it is hummed in F or B or C major. All the sounds are different, and yet the memory effect is clear. The same is true of reproduction: if I try to sing or whistle a familiar melody, the key of my reproduction will but rarely coincide with the key of the original. Or a person who has some facility in reading will be more or less independent of the type or the handwriting he encounters, and he will be able to write, though clumsily, with a pen held between his teeth, as anyone can try for himself, although he never performed that particular activity before. Can a trace theory of memory account for these facts, which, far from being exceptional cases, are typical of memory effects?

THE RE-FUNCTIONING OF TRACES. The hypothesis which we have developed is better prepared to meet this difficulty than the old trace

[26] Italics in the original.

hypothesis against which von Kries levelled his argument. For in our hypothesis traces form *organized systems,* i.e., dynamical wholes whose *pattern* is as much of a reality as their material. To see how far this property of the trace system will lead us to solve our problem we have to consider what will happen when such a trace system is "reactivated," when it co-operates in a new excitation. To be consistent we shall have to assume that such a new excitation occurs at a place different from that of the trace system itself, but strongly determined by it. This assumption is necessary also because, in most cases, we shall be able to remember this individual process of recall or recognition, at least after a short period of time, without losing our capacity of recalling or recognizing the first occasion, a proof that this process has left a new trace without destroying the old. At the same time the new excitation must be strongly dependent upon the trace system in question. It is clear that this dependence must be able to assume a great number of different forms, according to the different functions of memory. It will be different in recognition and recall, different when the trace system supplies data for the solution of a new problem, different again in the case of an acquired skill. We shall for the present confine ourselves to the first two, recognition and recall.

SELECTION OF TRACES BY NEW EXCITATIONS. Since we have already emphasized that each new excitation occurs in a new place, the function of the trace system can in neither case be that of "re-excitation." In this respect our theory seems to be different from most or all previous trace theories, and superior to them, since it seems very difficult to understand how an excitation process could be started in a mere trace system. But the new excitation, occurring now, must be in communication with a trace system, both in recognition and recall. The question then arises as to the cause of this communication, and this problem contains as a part problem the question how the present excitation selects among the enormous variety of traces the "proper" one. It is this aspect in the functions of recognition and recall which interests us now when we are dealing with von Kries's arguments against a traditional trace theory. We shall pursue this discussion only as far as it is relevant to our present context and shall continue it in the twelfth chapter (pp. 597 ff.), when we have learned more about the function of traces.

There are two ways in which we might look for such principles of selection; on the one hand we might collect facts and try to derive our principles from them; on the other we might attempt to apply such principles of selection to our present problem as we have discovered before as operative in other fields. The second method, if it were successful, would have the advantage that it would from the outset envisage memory functions in a wider context. The principles which would be discovered by this method would not be just laws of memory, but laws which would be applicable to memory as well as to other events. Memory would lose the character of being something unique, something added to the non-memorial functions of the organism, and it is this very result which in the introduction of this chapter we proposed to achieve.

Therefore we shall use this method and look for familiar principles of selection. To find them will be an easy task. For the principles of spatial organization which we discussed in Chapter IV can be regarded as such. These principles gave us the solution of the following problem: if through a pattern of retinal stimulation a variety of excitations is produced, which of these excitations will become integrated? One sees the similarity to our present problem: there one process became integrated with certain other processes but remained separated from the rest, here a new process interacts with certain trace systems, but not with others. To both cases we can therefore apply the concept of selection. Formerly we discovered the laws of equality and proximity, and the laws of closure and good continuation. Are these same laws applicable to our new problem? Our answer to this question is facilitated when we remember still another set of facts, reported at the end of Chapter V, from Ternus' experiments, because in these experiments the kind of selection is more similar to the one that occupies us now than in the purely spatial organizations. In the Ternus experiments two stimulus patterns followed upon each other so as to produce apparent movement of a behavioural pattern. If the first pattern consisted of points a_1, b_1, c_1, d_1, and the second of points b_2, f_2, c_2, g_2, where the indices refer to the temporal order, whereas in other respects equal letters correspond to equal points, then under certain conditions excitation b_2 would not be integrated with b_1 nor c_2 with c_1, but, e.g., b_2 with a_1, f_2 with b_1, and so forth. These conditions were conditions which referred to the whole-processes produced by the stimulus patterns. If excitation f_2 possessed the same significance in the second pattern that b_1 had in the first, then these two would interact, and not the "absolutely" equal b_2 and b_1. The interaction of successive processes, then, was proved to depend upon the whole character of these processes, and "equality" had to be interpreted as equality of function within a whole.

If, then, we apply the law of equality to our problem of the selection of traces by excitations we shall expect this equality to be primarily equality of whole character. A process should, *ceteris paribus,* communicate with a trace system which possessed the same whole character. This must be a trace system which had been produced by a process of the same whole character, because we assumed that the trace retained the dynamic character of the process in the form of tensions or stresses. In our Fig. 43 (p. 165) we have demonstrated that similarity of whole character has such an integrating effect in spatial organization.[27] That the same effect takes place under much less simple conditions is evidenced by Fig. 99, where the similar

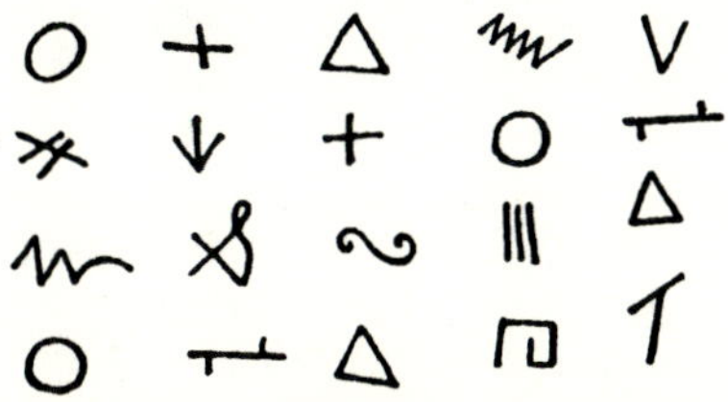

Fig. 99

shapes tend to fall together.[28] Therefore, if some integration can take place between an excitation and a trace pattern we should be justified in assuming that similarity of dynamic pattern would be one of the deciding influences. This would explain those facts of recognition which von Kries adduced as arguments against the traditional trace theory. For the pattern is, within wide limits, independent of size, colour and location, just as our recognition is. How much more we can say about the concrete process of recognition this is not the place to discuss (see pp. 591 ff.). We must also defer the discussion of recall and reproduction, but the present argument will serve to overcome the difficulties inherent in the older form of trace theories for the explanation of these effects. Only one more word need be added here: our theory of memory traces is in one radical respect different from the older forms. We have previously seen that psychologists wanted to reduce unit formation and shape to experience, i.e., ultimately to traces.[29] For two reasons such an attempt is impossible in our hypothesis. In the first place we had to assume the traces as organized systems, and that presupposes that the processes which produced the traces are organized themselves; their organi-

27 A similar pattern in Köhler's article in "Psychologies of 1925," p. 169.

28 Compare also the figure in von Restorff, p. 315, reproduced in Chapter XI.

29 See, for instance, our discussion of the assimilation hypothesis at the end of Chapter III.

zation can therefore not be a consequence of traces. In the second place we see that the selection of traces by processes, the laws according to which an excitation communicates with an existing trace system, depend upon the similarity of pattern between excitation and trace, and that implies again that an excitation must be patterned before it communicates with the trace system, for otherwise it would not be capable of selecting the proper one among the many traces which are constantly being left in the organism.

We have so far considered only the factor of equality, disregarding the factors of proximity, closure and good continuation. But all of them play their parts in the relation between excitations and traces. *Ceteris paribus,* old impressions are less well recognized and recalled than new ones, a fact which, though it probably depends also on other factors, demonstrates the laws of proximity. Good continuation and closure are clearly powerful factors of recall.

THE WIDE SCOPE OF THE LAWS OF ORGANIZATION. Our discussion of von Kries's arguments against a trace theory has done much more than to safeguard the assumption of traces, it has introduced the laws of spatial organization into the field of memory. The application of these laws has, however, a still wider scope than we have so far discussed. Not only the relation between excitations and traces is regulated by them, but also the fate of traces themselves, the changes which single trace systems undergo on account of their inherent stresses, and those which occur by virtue of the piling up of ever new traces. Experiments which will shortly be discussed will shed light on these events.

IN DEFENCE OF SPECULATIVE HYPOTHESES. To a critic who would object to all my hypotheses, who would say, Why so much speculation on so slender a basis of fact? I should reply: if I want to carry out my programme and give as systematic an account of the facts of psychology as is possible at the present time, I have to introduce the concept of traces in a concrete manner; this concept must be sufficiently well defined to admit of a concrete interpretation. It must face all the difficulties which are inherent in it and must try to overcome them in a way consistent with the whole system of thought developed and with the facts as far as we know them. I am convinced that in due course of time my hypotheses will have to be changed because they will conflict with newly discovered facts. But I am also convinced that without a system of hypotheses, as rigid and concrete as possible, even if they are speculative, no systematic research work will be possible. As I read the sign of the times, boldness, not caution, must be the catchword.

CHAPTER XI

MEMORY

Foundation of a Trace Theory: Experimental Section and Completion of the Theory

Experimental Evidence. Successive Comparison and the Time Errors. The Functional Effect of the Gradient. Von Restorff's Experiments: The Effect of Trace-Aggregation on Recall and Recognition. The Experiments by Wulf and His Successors: Changes Within Individual Traces. Theory of Traces Resumed: Insufficiency of Our Hypotheses. Acquisition of Skills. Reorganization in Perception. Learning a New Relation. Traces and the Ego. Forgetting. The Availability of Traces

EXPERIMENTAL EVIDENCE

Although the long theoretical discussion of the last chapter tried to keep in touch with facts all the time, it is now appropriate to supplement it by the experimental evidence. Experimental facts will serve two purposes: on the one hand they will supply a broader basis for our theoretical structure; on the other hand they will make it clear that these hypotheses, far from being speculative in the sense of being divorced from testable reality, have proved extremely fruitful for research. It has made a difference for experimental work that such hypotheses have been advanced, and I expect that the development of the next few years will add new proofs of their heuristic value.

Successive Comparison and the Time Errors. Since our trace hypothesis was largely based on the findings of Köhler and Lauenstein, it seems advisable to begin with their experimental work. It was started by a chance event. In the first volume of the "Psychologische Forschung" (1922) Borak published an article on the comparison of lifted weights in which he demonstrated and emphasized anew an effect which had been discovered long ago,[1] but whose real significance had fallen into oblivion. This effect had been called the *negative time-error;* it consists in the fact that if two stimuli are presented for successive comparison, the differential limen is

[1] References to the old literature on the subject are given in Köhler's article (1923), to the recent one in Lauenstein's.

found to be smaller when the stronger stimulus succeeds the weaker than when it precedes it. This means that if the two stimuli A and B, B > A, are sufficiently similar to each other to make their difference recognizable in less than 100% of all presentations, then the sequence A B will produce a greater number of right judgments than the sequence B A. It also means, as Köhler pointed out later, that even when the judgments are correct in both cases, the first sequence seems to involve a much greater difference than the second (l. c., p. 163).

Borak had tried to find a physiological explanation for his effect, but since his experimental test of his hypothesis proved it to be wrong he abandoned the attempt altogether in favour of a psychological theory. It is here that Köhler stepped in. He developed another physiological hypothesis, derived certain conclusions from it and confirmed them by new experiments. Finally Lauenstein, analyzing Köhler's hypothesis, distinguished two parts in it, one of which he accepted, while he found it necessary on the basis of his own experiments to reject the other one. His theory, grown out of Köhler's hypothesis, is more general. So much for the history. From now on we shall discuss the problem as it now exists, unconcerned with the historical sequence.

We have already come across Lauenstein's theory in our discussion of temporal units. Lauenstein developed it as an explanation of comparison, both simultaneous and successive. If we compare two items, these items must form some sort of unit, and the result of the comparison will depend upon the *kind* of these units. On page 441, we reproduced a figure from Lauenstein's paper, two grey spots on a homogeneous background in functional relation. Although at that stage of our discussion we did not go into the nature of this functional relationship, having in mind rather the "pair" character than the brighter-darker relation, Lauenstein developed his theory for this particular aspect. As Köhler (1918) was the first to point out, our two cases, pairedness and comparison, are in many respects so similar that their dynamic properties must be considered as of the same type.[2]

[2] We shall not go into the detail of this discrimination. A full discussion is to be found in Köhler's articles, 1923 and 1933. I will only mention that a comparison can also be accomplished in a manner different from the one treated in the text and by Köhler: the two items, instead of communicating with each other, come into functional relationship with a whole graded system, A with one part, B with another; and the comparison depends upon the relative position of these two points in that system. Thus, A may appear as a light grey, B as a dark grey, and therefore the person set on comparing A and B will say A is lighter than B although in the actual process A was not in direct functional relation with B.

Similarly I have introduced the concept of the step-wise phenomenon (1922) to describe and explain the process of comparison. When we compare the two grey patches of our figure, these patches form such a "step"; that is, a whole with two members between which there exists a gradient of potential. And when we compare two weights lifted successively or two tones, then this potential gradient exists between the concentration at the point of the new excitation and the trace of the preceding excitation. If this hypothesis is true, then it must make a difference whether the trace of the first excitation remains constant or undergoes changes during the interval between the application of the first and second stimulus. If, e.g., the two successive stimuli A1 and A2 are equal, then we should expect a majority of equality judgments if the trace of A1 remains unchanged until A2 appears. If, however, A1 were exposed to forces which change its constitution, then the concentrations a_1 and a_2 will no longer be equal, and correspondingly we should expect a majority of judgments A2 > A1, or A1 > A2, whether A1 has decreased or increased its concentration during the interval. The fact of the negative time error is identical with the alternative A2 > A1. If, as we have explained above, the sequence A B, where B > A, produces more right judgments than the sequence B A, then the judgment "the second greater than the first" is more easily elicited than the judgment "the second smaller than the first." Consequently, if the two stimuli are equal, the second one will still in a greater number of cases be judged as greater than as smaller. The negative time error would then be explained if we could assume that during the interval the trace of the first excitation decreased in concentration. We cannot test this assumption directly, but we can submit it to an indirect test: if the trace is exposed to forces, then the change in the trace will be the greater the longer these forces are allowed to work; in terms of the experiment, the negative time error should be a direct function of the interval. This prediction was amply confirmed in Köhler's experiments with telephone clicks, which showed that for small intervals (for some subjects up to three seconds) the time error was positive, while with longer intervals it became increasingly negative. The following table may serve as an example; it represents the percentage of "second louder" and "second softer" judgments of eight subjects for pairs of equal stimuli. The number of equality judgments has not been reproduced. It can easily be calculated as the difference between 100 and the sum of the two other kinds of judgment.

TABLE 14

(from Köhler, 1923, p. 152)

% of judgments with varying intervals between the two equal clicks A1, A2

Judgment	Interval in Seconds			
	1½	3	4½	6
Second Louder	4.2	29.2	54.2	62.5
Second Softer	62.5	50.	25.	8.3

The question then arises as to the cause of these changes. We shall for the moment disregard the changes which occur at first and give rise to the positive error, and concentrate on the other change which lasts much longer and caused in Köhler's experiments the negative time error. "We can either assume that all traces are gradually being destroyed by metabolic processes and that this causes the negative time error with longer intervals. Or we can assume that under the conditions of these experiments traces in proximity become assimilated to each other. In that case the negative time error would be explained by an assimilation of the trace of the first excitation to the trace of the state corresponding to lack of stimulation" (Lauenstein, p. 152).

Lauenstein seeks the decision between these alternative hypotheses in experiments in which the two critical stimuli arise from a homogeneous temporal ground which is produced by stimuli of the same quality as the two critical ones, but of a different intensity, being stronger in one set of experiments, weaker in another. He experimented both with sight and audition. In the visual experiments, he used Metzger's apparatus of the total homogeneous field described in Chapter IV (p. 114). The critical stimuli were given by pairing five different intensities of this field. In one set of experiments, these stimuli broke in upon a state of comparative darkness, the big screen being illuminated only by the diffuse light escaping from the projection lantern and the experimenter's reading lamp. In the other set of experiments the screen was illuminated by two strong lamps before, between, and after the exposure of the two critical stimuli. The following table illustrates the result. It indicates the average time errors of eight subjects for dark and light "ground" and various time intervals. The measure of the time error has been calculated in the following manner: The sum of all "second lighter" judgments has been subtracted from the sum of all "second darker" judgments; the difference has been multiplied by 100 and divided by the sum of *all judgments*. These figures measure therefore the relative preponderance of judgments of lighter or darker. When the former preponderate, the figures are negative; when the latter, positive—corresponding to the terminology of positive and negative time errors.

TABLE 15

(from Lauenstein, p. 157)

Figures represent relative preponderance of lighter (—) or darker (+) judgments

	Intervals in Seconds			
Ground	5	10	20	40
Dark	+3	—20	—24	—37
Light	+29	+27	+47	+62

In the acoustic experiments two tones of 80 cycles, sounded for two seconds, were the critical stimuli. In the two sets of experiments the ground consisted of the same tone that sounded before, between, and after the two critical ones. But in one set it was of a lower, in the other of a higher, intensity than the critical tones.

Table 16, on page 470, essentially like the preceding, summarizes the results of thirteen subjects.

The results are perfectly unequivocal. In both sensory fields there appears a positive time error with short intervals with both kinds of ground, and thereafter a time error—increasing with the length of the interval—which is negative only for the weaker ground and positive for the stronger grounds.

Thus two different kinds of changes in the traces have been demonstrated. (1) An initial change of short duration during which the intensity of the trace is increased; this effect, occurring as it does with both weak and strong ground, cannot be ascribed to an influence of the ground upon the trace. That is all we can at present say about this effect. (2) A progressive change, beginning after approximately one second, which assimilates the individual trace to the trace system of its background, thereby causing a progressive time error, either positive or negative, according to the nature of the ground. Thus with regard to this second change Lauenstein's alternative has been decided, and in the terms of his second hypothesis. As a matter of fact, this second alternative had already been anticipated and experimentally proved in 1899 by Bentley, as Lauenstein points out. Bentley's experiments with grey disks used only spatial grounds, so that by the inclusion of his results the empirical evidence for the assumed assimilation effect in the traces is more general.

TABLE 16

(from Lauenstein, p. 160)

Figures represent relative preponderance of louder (—) or softer (+) judgments

Ground	Intervals in Seconds			
	2	5	15	45
Soft	+15	—3	—19	—48
Loud	+12	+25	+29	+36

Köhler's results, negative time error with a background of silence, would, according to this interpretation, be explained by an assimilation of the sound-trace towards the stillness-trace. With this interpretation, Pratt takes issue on the ground of very interesting experiments. He argues thus: A stillness must be considered as the lowest degree of loudness. Consequently, if we compare a ground of complete stillness with a "soft" ground, the time error should be greater in the first case than in the second. In order to prove this, he evaluated two series of experiments. In the first, the two critical stimuli were noises produced by various heights of fall of a sound pendulum, the standard stimulus being set at 45°. The interval between the two critical stimuli was kept constant at four seconds.

Three sets of experiments were compared with each other: (1)

the normal, in which this interval remained empty; (2) loud, in which during the interval a strong noise was introduced, the pendulum falling through an angle of 70°; (3) soft, an intermediate stimulus of 20°. The following table contains a summary of the results, the figures representing the average Point of Subjective Equality of the second noise, calculated from Pratt's table.

TABLE 17

(from Pratt, p. 295)

Standard noise 45°. Point of Subjective Equality of Second Noise

Constellation	Normal	Loud intermediate noise	Soft intermediate noise
	44.1	48.8	42.2

In the second series of experiments, lifted weights were compared. This time only two different constellations were used, the normal and one with a light intermediate weight. The standard weight was 100 g., the interval between the two critical weights was four seconds. The next table summarizes the results. The figures this time are calculated as in the tables from Lauenstein, measuring direction and size of the time error in the same way. Again I have averaged the results of Pratt's three subjects.

TABLE 18

(from Pratt, p. 296)

Standard weight 100 g. Relative preponderance of heavier (—) and lighter (+) judgments

Constellation	Normal	Light
	— 16.7	— 38.9

The last two figures of the first table confirm Lauenstein's results for the new conditions of Pratt's experiments. Comparison of the first and third figures in the first table and of the two figures in the second contain, however, a new result. The negative time error is considerably smaller when the interval is empty than when it is partly filled by a stimulus equal in kind to the critical stimuli, but of lower intensity. From these results Pratt concludes that assimilation, such as Lauenstein has assumed in theory, occurs when the interval between the critical stimuli is filled by a stimulus either of higher or of lower intensity; "when, however, there is no intermediate stimulus nor appreciable background, the trace merely *sinks*"[8] (p. 297).

Interesting and suggestive as these experiments are, they have, in my opinion, done no more than to raise a problem; they have not proved Pratt's contentions. I will not stress the point that only one interval has been investigated in each series, and that an extension of the investigation to longer intervals might possibly alter the picture. Instead, I will emphasize that a third impression inserted between two others is not equivalent to a background which surrounds the two critical ones. It is very plausible to assume that, at least in the beginning, the influence of the former is stronger than that of the latter. When Pratt compares the empty constellation with that filled by a stimulus of weaker intensity, he compares in reality an influence exerted by a ground with one exerted by a new figure, and the difference in his results may well be due to this difference and thus may not support his own conclusions. Many more experiments must be forthcoming before the issue will be clearly decided, and I have no doubt that the near future will supply the information which is yet lacking. One of the experiments should take the following form. There should be, before and after the two critical stimuli, a background as used by Lauenstein, and between them emptiness. Then only would emptiness have the same function that it has in Pratt's experiments. We can symbolize Lauenstein's and Pratt's experiments graphically in this manner:

LAUENSTEIN PRATT

The experiment just proposed would then have the following representation:

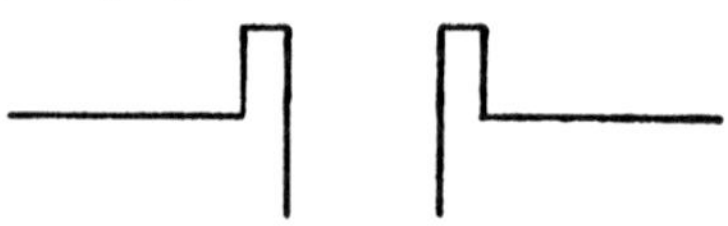

The Traces Dynamically Active. (1) Change of Time Error. Whatever the results of such experiments, Lauenstein has proved,

[8] Italics in original.

like Bentley before him, that the traces which remain after the excitations are over are not altogether dead, but are, at least under certain conditions, in functional relationship with other traces, by virtue of which they undergo changes. This same conclusion follows also from other effects apparent in both his and Köhler's experiments. Köhler found that if the experiments were continued over several days the negative time error became increasingly smaller. I reproduce in the following table some figures, calculated from one of Köhler's tables (on p. 159), which represent the relative preponderance of "second louder" (—) and "second softer" (+) judgments, determined as previously explained, which were obtained from five subjects on three different days. These figures summarize the results from three different time intervals, 3, 4½, and 6 seconds, while Köhler's shortest interval, 1½ seconds, has been omitted because for that interval the time error was already positive on the first day.

TABLE 19

(from Köhler, p. 159)

Preponderance of Louder or Softer Judgments

Date	2/12/21	5/12/21	6/12/21
Relative Preponderance	—38	—22	+17

The result is perfectly evident. It is accompanied by a marked change in the appearance of the clicks. On the first day, the series seemed to contain a vast majority of "ascending" steps, many of them quite large, while on the third day a great many "descending" steps appeared, and the ascending ones were without vigour. These facts reveal another functional property of traces over and above the one which was proved by Lauenstein: traces produced by "similar" excitations do not remain independent of each other but form larger trace systems which influence newly formed traces in definite ways. For a trace which on the first day would have changed towards lower concentration during the intra-pair interval, so as to produce a negative time error, will on the third day have increased its concentration during the same time, and therefore now produce a positive time error. This statement implies two different propositions: (1) the very obvious one about the interdependence of traces within a larger system. (2) The claim that the dynamic organization of traces does not solely follow their temporal arrangement but depends also upon intrinsic properties of the traces themselves, in the case under discussion upon their similarity. Which tones are similar will depend upon the total conditions, so that equality of stimulation is not a sufficient criterion for equality or similarity of excitations and processes. The circumstance, however, that trace organization is determined by intrinsic trace properties is of the utmost significance for the theory of memory. It shows the utter inadequacy of the old analogy of the wax tablet on which experience traces impressions. For whereas on the tablet each impression would remain independent of all the others, the traces, whose sequence may be perfectly contingent, organize themselves according to intrinsic properties; a purely temporal chance arrangement is replaced by well ordered systems. To avoid a possible misunderstanding, I will only add that the principle of equality is by no means the only one that governs the organization of trace systems.

(2) THE "CENTRAL TENDENCY." Lauenstein could detect in his results still another effect within the trace systems, an effect which has been known for a long time and which Hollingworth has called "the central tendency of judgment." Since I have described Hollingworth's experiments before (1922), I shall refer to them only briefly. He investigated the "indifference point," i.e., that stimulus within a graded series which is reproduced or recognized correctly, whereas smaller ones are over-, larger ones underestimated. In one form of experiment the arm of his subject was moved over a variable distance and the subjects had to reproduce this arm movement; in a second series, the subjects were presented with a square of variable size and after an interval of five seconds had to choose this square from memory from 30 simultaneously presented ones. In both sets of experiments certain small stimuli (movements and squares) were overestimated—i.e., the reproduced movement and the selected square were larger than the original, other large stimuli were underestimated, while one stimulus was at the indifference point. The positive contribution of Hollingworth's work was the proof that the position of the indifference point is not determined absolutely, but corresponds always to the centre of the range of stimuli employed. Therefore the same stimulus may either be over- or underestimated or be at the indifference point, according to the *series* of stimuli to which it belongs. This

proves, of course, an influence of the trace system on each newly created trace, and an averaging effect within the trace system.

Lauenstein demonstrated a similar effect in the following manner. In his second acoustic series he used clicks of five different intensities with soft and loud ground. He calculates the relative preponderance of "louder" and "softer" judgments for objectively equal stimuli and compares the value for the two lowest intensities (I and II) with those for the two highest. I reproduce in the following tables an extract from his results.

TABLE 20

(from Lauenstein, p. 172, Table 7)

Relative preponderance of "louder" and "softer" judgments for pairs of equal stimuli with different time intervals. I is the softest, V the loudest stimulus. Ground soft.

	Interval in Seconds					
Pairs Compared	1	2	3	5	10	20
I-I and II-II	+38	+23	+20	+23	+8	−10
IV-IV and V-V	+8	−35	−23	−70	−80	−100

TABLE 21

Everything as above, only ground loud

	Interval in Seconds					
Pairs Compared	1	2	3	5	10	20
I-I and II-II	+43	+60	+75	+75	+80	+78
IV-IV and V-V	−8	+13	−3	0	−8	+10

In both tables, for soft and loud ground, the louder pairs are more negative, or less positive, than the softer ones. Now in the experiments of the first table each individual trace was exposed to the assimilative influence of the softer ground, as we have previously shown, while in those of the second table they were assimilated to the louder ground. Therefore the first table should contain predominantly negative, and the second predominantly positive, time errors. In reality the first conclusion is true only for the loud pairs, the second only for the soft pairs. Consequently, there must have been other forces at work which affect soft and loud pairs in opposite direction. These forces must have their origin in the trace system not of the ground but of the preceding individual clicks. If, as we concluded from the "central tendency" experiments of Hollingworth, such trace systems undergo an averaging effect, then the trace of the first member of a soft pair should be "raised," that of the first member of a loud pair "lowered." Therefore the loud pairs with soft grounds should be preponderantly judged as "ascending" (negative time error), since the traces of the first members are lowered both by the ground- and the averaged click-traces; similarly the soft pairs with loud grounds should be judged as descending in the vast majority of cases, since the traces of their first members are subjected to two forces which raise them. In the two other cases, the two forces are in conflict, so that the total effect is less clear.

This averaging effect within a trace system is of high significance. It explains the so-called "absolute" judgments, according to which a weight seems "heavy" or "light" without being compared to a specific other one, a tone loud or soft, and so on. That the "absolute impression" had to be explained by a reference to larger trace systems had already been Köhler's conclusion. The absolute impression has a close relation to the "class" concepts which we encountered in Chapter VIII (p. 349). But in saying this I do not mean to imply that concepts are such averages, but merely that we possess within our store of traces many systems which, through a process of condensation and assimilation, form the basis for "class" perceptions, for the "normal" and the "unusual." To generalize from this that all our concepts are nothing but such averaged trace systems seems to me, however, erroneous.

The Functional Effect of the Gradient. The preceding arguments which proved a functional interdependence of different traces rested on the assumption that the comparison is based on a *gradient* of concentration (or some other property) between the two terminal members of the comparison. The more firmly this assumption is established, the greater also the conviction carried by our arguments. Therefore, before advancing new evidence for the functional character of traces, we shall report such experimental results as will strengthen our fundamental assumptions. The fact that we derive the dynamics of comparison from the gradient means, as M. H. Jacobs and Köhler (1933) have pointed out, more than the assumption of a mere difference of potential at the two respective places. The gradient is a function both of this difference and of the spatial distance between the two points or areas. Therefore, with a constant difference the comparison should still be a function of the distance between the excited areas.

More than five years ago I tried to establish such a difference directly. If A1 B1 and A2 B2 are two pairs of grey squares, such that A1 looks like A2, and B1 like B2, but spatially A1 is further away from B1 than A2 is from B2, then A1 and B1 should appear less different from each other than A2 and B2. We should find the paradoxical relation: $A1 = A2$, $B1 = B2$, but $A1 - B1 < A2 - B2$. The experiments, which were largely carried out by Dr. A. Mintz, failed to verify this prediction, because of the extremely complex relations within the field with its four figures, in which the spontaneous organization was in conflict with the organization to be enforced for the purpose of the necessary comparison.[4] Therefore these experiments were never published. But the experiments of M. H. Jacobs gave an indirect proof of our general assumption: the difference threshold, as measured by the number of uncertainty and equality judgments, increases directly with the spatial distance between the two objects to be compared, and this is exactly what we should expect if the experience of difference depended upon a *gradient* of potential.

The theory which we have developed demands, however, even more. As Lauenstein has pointed out, in successive comparison the difference threshold should also depend upon the time interval between the two stimuli, because in our theory a temporal distance is transformed into a spatial difference, since the traces form a "trace column" (see p. 447). Lauenstein mentions that his experiments bear out this conclusion. I have calculated from Lauenstein's tables the numbers of uncertainty judgments, and reproduce a summary in the three following tables. (See pages 478 and 479.)

The general tendency of the figures is well marked in all three

[4] Another result, however, was indicated: It seemed to make a difference for the apparent difference between A1 and B1 whether another difference A2 B2 was in the field or not, an effect which did not depend upon the mutual "contrast" influence of the individual members upon each other. One process seemed directly to influence another.

tables; the uncertainty judgments increase with the magnitude of the time interval. Thus far these results of Lauenstein's are a good confirmation of our conclusion, according to which temporal intervals should play the same rôle as spatial ones because the time interval is transformed into a spatial distance in the brain.

However, if in accordance with these results we correlate the impression of the greater and smaller with the gradient between two places, the explanation of the time errors becomes more complex than it appeared

TABLE 22

(from Lauenstein, p. 157, Table 2)

Number of uncertain judgments, optical experiments. Eight subjects

Ground	Interval in Seconds				
	5	10	20	40	Sum
Dark	0	0	1	3	4
Light	2	0	1	6	9
Sum	2	0	2	9	13

TABLE 23

(from Lauenstein, p. 160, Table 3)

Acoustic experiments, otherwise like preceding table. Thirteen subjects

Ground	Interval in Seconds				
	2	5	15	45	Sum
Soft	2	1	2	7	12
Loud	2	6	5	15	28
Sum	4	7	7	22	40

TABLE 24

(from Lauenstein, pp. 163-166, Tables 4*a, b* and 5*a, b* combined)

Acoustic experiments, as last table, 18 subjects

	Interval in Seconds									
Ground	0	.2	.5	1.0	2	3	5	10	20	Sum
Soft	3	1	0	3	8	5	4	9	12	45
Loud	6	9	11	14	11	9	24	41	48	173
Sum	9	10	11	17	19	14	28	50	60	218

in Köhler's and Lauenstein's treatment, because the time interval has two different effects which can be variously combined. In the one case the time interval acts as mere time during which the process of assimilation within the trace system progresses—this is the Köhler-Lauenstein explanation—in the other case the time interval produces a spatial distance between the places of the new excitation and the trace of the preceding one, thereby *flattening* the gradient. If the two stimuli are equal, the first factor is responsible for the time error, negative when the trace sinks, positive when the trace rises, and this effect must vary directly with the length of the interval. On the other hand, an increase in the time interval flattens the gradient so that it takes away from the full effect of the difference in concentration which results from the first effect. To understand the co-operation of the two factors in the case where the two stimuli are unequal, we have to distinguish the four possible cases: I, ground lower than the stimuli, stimuli descending (Ld); II, ground ditto, stimuli ascending (La); III, ground high, stimuli descending (Hd), and IV, ground ditto, stimuli ascending (Ha). In I, Ld, the trace of the first excitation sinks during the interval in the direction of the new excitation, so that the longer the interval, the smaller the difference between the two potentials, therefore the judgment "second smaller" has less and less chance. At the same time, quite independently of this effect, the gradient flattens out with an increasing interval by an increase of the spatial distance between the trace and the new excitation. Both factors work in the same direction to produce a negative time error. In II, La, the trace of the first excitation sinks away from the second, so that with increasing intervals the chances for the judgment "second greater" become increasingly favourable. At the same time, the flattening of the gradient must tend to reduce the effect of the increased difference in potential, the two factors work in opposite directions as regards the end effect. Similarly III, Hd, shows conflict, and IV, Ha, co-operation of the two effects in the resulting positive time errors; the general rule being that whenever through the effective forces the trace of the first becomes, in the lapse of time, increasingly similar to the second, the two effects reinforce each other—where the first trace changes during the interval so as to become more and more different from the second, the two factors are in conflict.

It may be possible to verify these conclusions from the raw data of Köhler's and Lauenstein's results, but the published figures allow no such verification.

Our last three tables contain, however, another significant result which has some bearing on the general assumption of our last deductions. Since the two stimuli were, as a rule, not applied in immediate succession, the gradient was mediated by a field with properties of its own (see pp. 441 f.). It is at the outset very unlikely that the properties of this intervening field should have no influence upon the gradient. As a matter of fact in all our tables the number of uncertainty judgments is considerably greater when the ground is "high" than when it is "low." (See, for instance, the last columns in our tables.) This opens up a new and interesting line of research.

A last point, however, must be mentioned. We used the experimental results of Jacobs and Lauenstein to prove our contention that spatial and temporal (spatialized) gradients were essentially similar. In doing so we have, so far, neglected one difference between the results of these two authors. Jacobs found that the sum of uncertainty judgments and equal judgments increases with spatial distance; Lauenstein, that the sum of uncertainty judgments alone increases with temporal distance. The circumstance, which Lauenstein emphasizes, that the majority of Jacobs' judgments were "uncertain" and not "equal" does not entirely remove the difference between their results, for in Lauenstein's the equal judgments decreased so much with increasing time interval that the sum of equal and uncertain judgments also shows a marked decrease with the length of the interval. Therefore, if we take this sum instead of the number of our equality judgments, Jacobs's and Lauenstein's results would contradict each other and thereby our theory. I should not have presented Lauenstein's results in the manner in which I did—which agrees with his own interpretation as far as it goes—did I not believe that this contradiction is merely an apparent one. For there is an explanation that accounts for the decrease of Lauenstein's equality judgments with increased interval. The unpublished work of Mintz, to which I referred previously with regard to my theory of comparison, had one positive result which supplements Jacobs's results for very small spatial distances which she did not investigate. The minimum of the difference threshold does not lie at the smallest spatial distance; instead, when one decreases the spatial distance continually, a minimum of the difference threshold is reached, such that with a further decrease of this distance the threshold begins again to rise. If the two objects to be compared are too near each other and sufficiently similar, then they will become assimilated to each other, proximity appearing again in its rôle as a unifying factor. Now the traces of events following upon each other with a short interval must be very close to each other indeed, so that a new factor must become operative under these conditions which will favour equality judgments. If this deduction is true, then the behaviour of the equality judgments in Lauenstein's results does not invalidate our conclusions, but it introduces a new complexity into the process of successive comparison.

Von Restorff's Experiments: The Effect of Trace-Aggregation on Recall and Recognition. We return to the study of the dynamic connectedness in trace systems. The experimental proofs so far advanced rested on results of successive comparison. But if traces form real systems, dynamically interconnected, then this characteristic of theirs should also become manifest in other memory effects like recall and recognition. In an investigation by Köhler and von Restorff, distinguished by a rare combination of ingenuity and utmost simplicity, such effects have become demonstrated as the causes of three well-known effects: (1) the great difficulty of learning series of nonsense syllables, (2) retroactive inhibition, (3) forward-acting inhibition.

In discussing the Köhler-Lauenstein experiments which used the results of successive comparison as their criterion for the fate of the traces, we discussed the theory of comparison on which the deductions were based. Similarly it might seem appropriate to discuss the theory of recognition and recall before we present these new experiments. This, however, we shall not do. We shall not break up our discussion of the trace systems by considering the processes which they make possible, but shall defer such discussion to the next chapter. Such a procedure is possible because the conclusions which we shall draw are independent of such a theory and presuppose merely that these functions depend in *some* way upon the traces, an assumption which we have defended before. It may appear as a drawback of our procedure that we shall have to introduce several facts about the processes of recognition and recall into our discussion of traces, but this drawback of mixing the treatment of one subject with that of another is unavoidable whatever procedure we follow. The traces can be studied only through the processes; the latter can be understood only through the former.

THE DIFFICULTY OF LEARNING "MONOTONOUS" SERIES. Therefore we turn to the question why it is so difficult and highly unpleasant to learn series of nonsense syllables. All previous attempts to answer this question have centred around the fact that the syllables are *nonsense,* i.e., that no natural bridge leads from one of them to another, whereas meaningful material is distinguished by these very bridges. No doubt, this factor plays a part. And yet, as Restorff has shown, it is not the only, and in the classical memory experiments not even the decisive, factor. In Chapter IV (p. 167) we have encountered a fact which in a way anticipates this conclusion: in discussing spatial organization we found the extraordinarily strong influence of mere spatial proximity upon organization (cf., for instance, Fig. 44). If, then, the same laws of organization hold for memory that govern perception, then mere contiguity should be a strong organizing factor even when natural bridges between the different terms in contiguity are missing. Therefore the extreme difficulty and unpleasantness of learning the standard nonsense series of experimental psychology cannot be regarded as satisfactorily explained. These standard series are not only nonsensical but also homogeneous, i.e., they consist of elements which are all of the same *kind*. Restorff has proved that this second aspect of theirs, their homogeneity, and not, as previously thought, their nonsense character, is chiefly responsible for their refractoriness, and that the effect of the homogeneity results from processes in the traces, the formation of larger trace systems in which the individual traces become absorbed and lose their independence and individuality.[5] Thus a problem of process or accomplishment has been transformed into a problem of trace action; the formation of trace systems has been proved by the experimental analysis of an old-established fact.

Nothing could be more complete than Restorff's proof that homogeneity of material is of itself a factor that interferes with memory functions. In a first set of experiments the subject had to learn, by reading them two or three times, series of the following type: There were eight pairs of terms in each series, four of which consisted of the same material, while the four others were of different material. The terms so associated were: nonsense syllables, geometrical figures, two-digit numbers, letters, and small oblongs of different colours. Thus in one series four pairs of nonsense syllables were

[5] It seems as though Woodworth had a similar, though much less concrete, theory, when he explains by "inhibition" the fact that we can retain eight digits after one reading, but need considerably more than one to retain twelve or sixteen digits (1929, p. 76).

combined with one pair of each of the other materials; in another series the figures occurred in four pairs, the rest in one, and so forth. Five different sets, each containing five series, corresponding to the five different kinds of material, were presented, each to four or five subjects, so that at the end twenty-two subjects had been tested. The result was the same for all five sets, which differed from each other in certain technical aspects. Therefore it will be sufficient to reproduce here a brief summary of all the results that were obtained by testing the subjects after various intervals by the method of paired associates.

The following table contains the number of "hits" for all subjects in all sets for each material according to whether this material was "isolated" (I) or "repeated" (R). Both absolute and relative figures are given, the latter being the percentage of the actual hits among all the hits possible.

TABLE 25

(from Restorff, p. 202)

The figures indicate absolute and relative numbers of hits. 22 subjects in all

	Syllables		Figures		Numbers		Letters		Colours		Total	
Material	R	I	R	I	R	I	R	I	R	I	R	I
Absolute	36	61	29	65	23	55	52	65	49	82	189	328
Per cent	41	69	33	74	26	63	59	74	56	93	43	75

Thus 41% correct answers were obtained from those syllables which occurred in the series in which the syllables were represented by four pairs, but 69% from those syllables which occurred in the series which contained only one such pair, etc. The results are absolutely consistent: whenever a material occurs in isolation it is recalled better as a paired associate than when it occurs in repetition. As a matter of fact these experiments proved an even greater superiority of the I over the R material. The I material was also better remembered than the R material of the same *series;* i.e., if the syllables were the R material, then the four test syllables gave fewer hits than the test figure, number, letter, and colour added together. This is particularly significant since it shows that the factor of repetition or isolation is stronger than any difference in the material which might make one kind be learned more easily than another.

If the difference between isolation and repetition is increased, the effect also increases. In a new set, with only three kinds of material, syllables, figures, and numbers, one kind always occurred in six pairs, each of the others in one pair. I reproduce in the next table the percentage of hits in this set, which was carried out with twelve subjects.

TABLE 26

(from Restorff, p. 305)

Relative number of hits

	Syllables		Figures		Numbers		Total	
Material	R	I	R	I	R	I	R	I
Per cent hits	27	85	18	90	31	85	25	87

Again the same superiority appears if we compare the R of one series with the I terms of the same series but of different material. The same result was confirmed in other experiments in which the testing was not carried out by the method of paired associates or hits but by the method of "retained members"; with this method the subject learns one or more series of unpaired terms and has, at a later time, to recall as many of the terms as he can without any prompting and without sticking to the original sequence.

The result of all these experiments is this: the difficulty of learning series of nonsense syllables arises largely from the fact that the sequence of homogeneous terms interferes with the learning effect by robbing the individual traces of their individuality. But this is only possible if the traces of the terms are not independent of each other but form interconnected systems in which each part is influenced by every other part. Learning of nonsense syllables is therefore anything but the normal case of learning: not only is this nonsense material devoid of "bridges" which facilitate the passage from one term to the next, but also by its homogeneity it sets up strong counter forces which affect its retention.

The interpretation of Restorff's results as due to the properties of the traces is corroborated by experiments in which retention was tested not by recall, but by recognition. In recognition experiments, the details of which I omit, the I material proved superior to the R material, although the differences were here considerably smaller than for recall.

The fact, however, that the I–R difference manifests itself also in recognition is of great theoretical significance. Had it been proved only for recall it might have been explained by the factors which are responsible for this function apart from the traces. But recognition is a different function, and yet the same effect, though in smaller degree, appears there also. Consequently such factors must be involved as play a part in both functions, and thus we are compelled to seek the explanation in the traces.

THE AGGREGATION OF TRACES. What kind of events in the traces we must assume and what forces responsible for these events, appears from considerations and experiments based upon the first results. The critical point lies in the definition of "isolation." When is an element isolated? Two answers seem possible: (1) When it is equally different from all other elements, no matter how different the other elements are from each other, or (2) when it is more different from each of the other elements than they are from each other. If A B C D . . . represent different materials, A1 A2 . . . B1 B2 . . . different specimens within each material, e.g., different syllables or figures, then the two kinds of isolation could be represented in the following way:

(1) A B C D E F G H
(2) A1 A2 C A3 A4 A5 A6 A7

What this difference means is obvious if we translate it into perceptual terms. Fig. 100 A and B, taken from von Restorff's paper, illustrate two perceptual arrangements analogous to our arrangements of learning material. In the first no term obtrudes itself more than any other, whereas in the second, the third figure emerges at the first glance, while the others form a fairly uniform aggregate in which no special member stands out by itself. The different degree of prominence of the third member in the two patterns is, therefore, evidently not due to its relations of similarity or dissimilarity to the other members, since the difference between the critical members and each of the others is not smaller in the first than in the second pattern, but to the fact that in the second the other figures form an aggregate, which they do not do in the first. Why they form such an aggregate in the one case and not in the other is clear from our law of similarity in spatial organization.

Whether this analogy from perception holds for memory must be tested in special experiments, in which series of the type (1) must be compared with series of the type (2). If in these experiments type (2) proves to be superior to type (1), as it is in the field of perception, then we have good reason to ascribe the superiority of the critical element over the other elements to the fact that these others have formed an aggregate in which they have lost some of

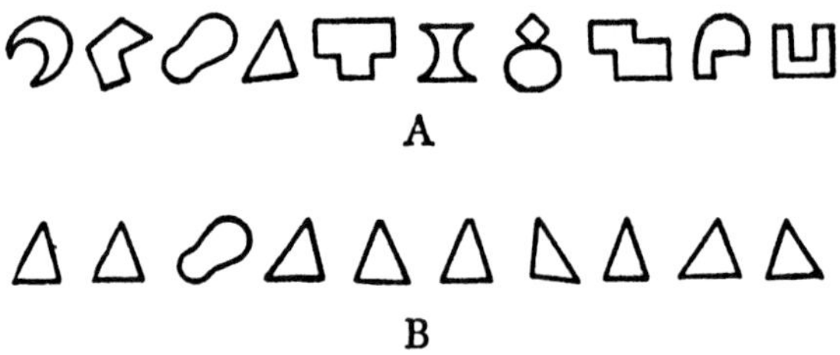

Fig. 100

their individuality, and against which the critical member stands out, whereas in type (1) no *such* aggregation could occur, and therefore no difference between the critical members and any of the others.

Several such experiments were carried out by von Restorff with positive results. Only one will be reported here:

On three different days, the fifteen subjects were shown once one of three series of ten elements. After the presentation of the series the subjects had to learn a meaningful text for ten minutes, whereupon they were asked to write down as many items of the series as they could remember (method of retained members), a time of thirty seconds being allowed for this performance.[6] On the first day they learned series (1), consisting of ten different elements, viz., a number, a syllable, a colour, a letter, a word, a small photograph, a symbol, a button, a punctuation mark, and a name of a chemical compound. On the two other days either of the two series (2) and (3) were presented, (2) consisting of one number and nine syllables, (3) of one syllable and nine numbers. Fifteen subjects took part

[6] Afterwards they were tested with regard to the text memorized, so that they could not suspect that this activity was not important for the experiment as such, but used only as a standardized filling of the interval between presentation and recall.

in this experiment. I reproduce von Restorff's table as a summary of the results. The figures represent the number of elements remembered. Since in series (2) and (3) the repeated elment occurred nine times as often as the isolated one, one must divide the number of R elements by nine to make it comparable to the number of I elements.

TABLE 27

(from Restorff, p. 320)
Figures indicate numbers of elements remembered

Series	(1)	(2) and (3)	
		R	I
Syllable	6	34 ÷ 9 = 3.8 (series (2))	12 (series (3))
Numbers	6	24 ÷ 9 = 2.7 (series (3))	9 (series (2))
Sum	12	58 ÷ 9 = 6.5	21
In %	40	22	70

This table contains a number of results to be read off by comparing the figures in the different columns with each other. The comparison of the second and third columns gives confirmation of the first result by the new method which we mentioned above: the superiority of the isolated members compared with the repeated ones. Comparing the first column with the third, we find that isolation of a single element in a group of similar elements is almost twice as effective as "isolation" of one element in a group with others which are as different from each other as they are from the critical one. It is, as a matter of fact, not adequate to speak of an isolated element at all in this constellation. Since each element is as different from the others as every other one, they ought all to be equal with regard to their recall value; this is borne out by these experiments: 40% of the "critical" elements of series (1) (i.e., syllables and numbers) were recalled, while the average of recall for all the other elements in the same series was 43%, an insignificant difference.

Finally, comparing columns one and two, we find that the elements of series (1) were better remembered than the repeated elements of series (2) and (3). The explanation of this difference is obvious: we have explained the inferiority of the R elements compared to the I ones by the assumption that the former became aggregated. The inferiority of all the elements of series (1) suggests the same interpretation: all the different members of this series form an aggregate without any outstanding members. That the terms of this series are superior to the R elements of series (2) and (3) must then be explained by the further assumption that the aggregate of the *different* members of series (1) possessed a lower degree of cohesion than that of the similar members in series (2) and (3). This assumption is not introduced as a sort of *ad hoc* hypothesis to explain this particular effect, but follows directly from the law of similarity: if aggregation is caused by similarity, then the degree of cohesion must be a direct function of the similarity.

This relation between memory effects and processes in perception raises the very important issue as to its nature. Is the memory effect *due* to a perceptual organization, the trace merely retaining a structure which characterized the excitation which produced it, or are the same factors that determine distribution of process in perception operative also in the formation of trace aggregates? The latter interpretation implies a more dynamic nature of the traces than the first, since according to it there will occur in trace systems events which give them an organization that the original excitations did not possess.

The procedure in von Restorff's experiments practically excluded the first interpretations and thereby compels us to accept the second. The different elements were shown successively, the series in which all elements were different from each other preceded those in which one element (or in another series two different ones) stood out from the remaining similar ones, and this outstanding element appeared in the second or third place of the series. Therefore the subject could not possibly know that it would be the isolated element, he could not even know that the series would contain such an element. There is therefore absolutely no reason why perceptually the critical element should be isolated. The fact, then, that its isolation proves to be an effective factor in recall seems to demand the interpretation that it became isolated in the trace system; and that in its turn means that processes of organization occur within trace systems following the same laws as the organization of perceptual excitations. This is the proof of the applicability of our laws of organization to traces which we promised some time ago (p. 464). True enough, our proof pertains only to the law of similarity; that proximity has an effect in memory as in perception follows from the close relation of these two factors which appeared in our first discussion (Chapter IV, pp. 165 f.); the discussion which is to follow will add experimental proof. The efficacy of the other laws in the transformation of traces will likewise be demonstrated in the presentation of new experimental material.

Two more aspects of the changes which occur in trace systems are emphasized by von Restorff. (1) It seems an inevitable assumption that the transformation which single traces undergo by being incorporated in a larger trace system may go much farther than perceptual transformations of relatively independent parts. (2) The nature of these transformations is a problem by itself. In Restorff's experiments the formation of aggregates had a nocuous influence on recall, but she points out that this case, occurring under very special conditions, must not be regarded as typical of all cases; formations of aggregates are possible which *increase* the recall value of the aggregated members, a point which we shall take up later.

The Effect of Trace Systems after Longer Time Intervals. Let us return to von Restorff's experiments. We have so far considered traces which belong to one and the same series. We found that in such a series similar traces form aggregates even when they are not next to each other, i.e., when the excitations which produced them were separated by intervals filled with other excitations. Thus in the first five sets of experiments which we reported, the four repeated pairs of each series did not follow one upon the other but were separated from each other by one or two other pairs. The question then arises: is the effect of aggregation limited to such relatively short intervals, or does it occur also after longer periods of time? The answer to this question can be attempted in two ways. In the first an I R series is learned, and soon afterwards a series in which the I elements of the first series are R elements. If aggregation between corresponding traces of the first and second series occurs, the I elements of the first should lose some of their superiority. The second way uses the converse method of presentation. The R elements of a first series appear as I elements in a second. Aggregation between the corresponding traces of the two series must have taken place, if the I element of the second series is inferior to I elements in series which have not been preceded by another in which these elements were the repeated ones. Actually both these effects occurred.

RETROACTIVE INHIBITION. I shall describe briefly one of the first kind: 28 subjects had to memorize a series, presented four times, which consisted of two pairs of syllables, two pairs of figures, and five pairs of numbers. Afterwards they were presented once with four other series, which were different for the two groups into which the subjects were divided: for 13 of them the series consisted of 6 syllables and 3 numbers, not arranged in pairs, for the remaining 15, of 6 figures and 3 numbers. Then, 8 minutes after the last presentation of the first series, the subjects were tested by the method of paired associates. If aggregation had taken place, then the first group of subjects should show a better recall for figures than for syllables, because the 4 following series had contained the latter, but not the former, and correspondingly the second group of subjects should show a superiority of syllables. The following table summarizes the results, the figures indicating percentage of hits.

TABLE 28

(from Restorff, p. 331)

Percentage of Hits

Group	I (Syllables in post-series)	II (Figures in post-series)
Syllables	54	90
Figures	69	43

Whether one reads the table horizontally (same material, different subjects and post-series) or vertically (same subjects but different materials), one finds the same result: elements which have been succeeded by series containing similar elements in repetition are at a disadvantage compared with elements succeeded by series with different kinds of elements. Thus these experiments indicate that aggregation occurs over greater time intervals than those previously employed. On the other hand the effect proved in these experiments is by no means new, but perfectly familiar as retroactive inhibition. But whereas the traditional method of testing this effect used the standard series of nonsense syllables, or similar material, which in itself creates unfavourable conditions for recall by primary aggregation within the original series, Restorff's method subjects material of a high recall value to this effect. At the same time it proves that retroactive inhibition is a function of the similarity between the materials learned, i.e., the nature of the interacting traces. That figures influence syllables and *vice versa,* to some extent, was shown by another set of experiments in which a third way of filling the time between the learning and the testing of the main series was added, namely, occupation with difficult thought problems. This activity had a much smaller effect on the recall of syllables or figures than the syllables had on the figures, the figures on the syllables.[7]

Thus the nature of retroactive inhibition has been clarified. It arises from the aggregation of similar traces, just like the difficulty of learning monotonous series. If, as Müller and Pilzecker originally believed, retroactive inhibition were entirely independent of the kind of processes occurring after the learning and depended only on their intensity, then the theory would be wrong. Conversely, the proof that the *kind* of material accumulated after the learning is of decisive importance makes it necessary to explain retroactive inhibition as an effect due to specific organization of traces. The further result that there are different degrees of similarity, and that, as far as this effect goes, relatively different material—figures and syllables, for example—must still be regarded as similar is important for a future study of the difference in processes.

According to von Restorff's theory an element should succumb the more to retroactive inhibition, the more isolated it had been originally; for if it already formed a part of a large aggregate the fact that this aggregate was increased should have less noticeable consequences than the fact that an element which was isolated becomes aggregated or that a member of a small aggregate becomes part of a much larger one. Restorff's own experiments were based on this conclusion. But the fact itself had been discovered before by Robinson and Darrow, who found that the longer a learned monotonous series was, the less its recall was affected by retroactive inhibition.

Another conclusion from the theory finds support in an experiment by Jenkins and Dallenbach. According to that theory retroactive inhibition should fail to appear if, under conditions otherwise identical with those that produce it, the old trace system could be prevented from aggregating with the new one. The two authors

[7] For the history of the problem of retroactive inhibition, cf. Hunter, 1929, pp. 599 ff. With regard to the factor of similarity, Hunter summarizes, "At present, experiments clearly indicate that one interpolated activity may differ markedly from another activity in its effect upon retention, but the reasons for the difference are as yet undetermined" (p. 603).

just mentioned conducted an experiment in which a subject was hypnotized during the learning and recall of a series of ten syllables, while during the intervening time he was in his normal state. After two, four, and eight hours he reproduced the series completely, while two other subjects of the same authors had reproduced, on an average, after the three intervals, 3.1, 2.3 and .9 syllables, under conditions identical except for hypnosis. Since events in the hypnotic state seem to be but little connected with those of normal life, the failure of retroactive inhibition to appear in these experiments confirms, as far as it goes, our conclusion.

There remains, however, one fact about retroactive inhibition which has puzzled psychologists for a long time. In 1914 Rose Heine discovered that if the learning were tested by recognition instead of by recall, no retroactive inhibition could be found. Restorff repeated such experiments under her conditions in which, owing to the absence of those factors which by themselves interfere with memory, a clearer retroactive effect should have appeared, and also failed to establish clearly the existence of this inhibition.

However, even this result is no longer as paradoxical as it appeared, for the effect of repetition itself proved in her experiments less detrimental for recognition than for recall. Therefore it seems plausible to assume that repetition after an interval (the condition for retroactive inhibition) will produce an effect on recognition too small to be discovered by our present methods.

This interpretation gains some support from the experiments of Jenkins and Dallenbach and of Dahl. The former authors tested the recall of learned series after varying intervals which were filled either with the normal occupations of waking life or by sleep. In the latter case recall was superior. These experiments were repeated by Dahl with the difference that he tested not recall but recognition. He also found a slight but consistent superiority of the sleep constellation, particularly for the longer intervals of four and eight hours. After Restorff's experiments it seems plausible to interpret Dahl's results as effects of retroactive inhibition, while the author himself, relying on the previous failure to find such inhibition for recognition, is inclined to doubt that the effect discovered by Jenkins and Dallenbach is due to that cause.

FORWARD-ACTING INHIBITION. The second time-effect of trace systems derived on page 489 was equally confirmed in von Restorff's experiments. An evaluation of the series of the first set of experiments showed unmistakably that I members were better recalled if they had not occurred as R members in previous series than if this had been the case. A new excitation, even if it is preceded and followed by different excitations, will leave a trace which is drawn into an aggregation of traces left by similar excitations which occurred at a considerably earlier period. This effect seems to decrease when the time between the new excitations and the older ones increases. That a positive effect of "forward-acting inhibition" occurs proves anew the existence of processes within trace systems, their organization according to similarity, while the influence of time on the effect demonstrates the factor of proximity.

THE EXPERIMENTS BY WULF AND HIS SUCCESSORS: CHANGES WITHIN INDIVIDUAL TRACES. True enough, we cannot observe the traces themselves; the evidence as to their nature which we have derived from the preceding discussion of various experiments is indirect. But indirect evidence gains in weight by accumulation. And it is the accumulation of indirect testimony that seems to me to lift the hypothesis that we developed out of the realm of pure guesses or vague surmises. This accumulation of evidence goes even further than we have so far reported. An entirely different line of experiments, originating in 1919, fits in with the results and theories of the recent ones. In that year F. Wulf started an investigation of the changes that traces undergo in time, and his paper, published in 1922 from the University of Giessen, gave rise to three similar studies, made in different places by J. J. Gibson, Gordon Allport, and F. T. Perkins. Wulf's problem was originally not what would happen to a trace by its connection with other traces, but what would happen to it quite apart from such influences, although his work and that of his followers, notably Gibson's, sheds light on this problem also. The connection with our present context appears from Wulf's conclusions: "Gestalt-laws govern memory also. Just as not any gestalt can be perceived, so not all those perceived can be preserved in memory. Therefore, what remains in memory, the physiological 'engram,' cannot be regarded as an immutable impression which can only become blurred with time, similar to a drawing carved on a brick. Rather this engram undergoes changes by virtue of gestalt laws. The originally perceived gestalten are transformed, and these transformations concern the gestalten as wholes" (p. 370).

METHODOLOGICAL ASSUMPTIONS; RELATION OF REPRODUCTION AND TRACE. Wulf's test of the state of the traces at consecutive periods of time was actual reproduction of designs which the subjects had been shown once. The deviations of these reproductions from the original were considered as indicative of the changes which the respective traces had undergone. The value of the results depends therefore upon the validity of the criterion. We have deferred the discussion of the actual process of reproduction to a later chapter, but we have already emphasized the point that each new reproduction is a *new* excitation occurring in a new place, different from the place of the traces, an excitation, however, which depends upon certain traces. From this formulation it follows that the reproductions obtained from Wulf's subjects were not necessarily influenced exclusively or even preponderantly by the trace of the one excitation corresponding to the exposure of the original. In his results, and even more so in Gibson's, we shall find other and older trace systems partially, or even preponderantly, influential. One fact, however, which appeared in Wulf's, Allport's, and Perkins' experiments, and in Gibson's wherever the conditions were favourable for it, makes it necessary to attribute to the original trace a very definite influence on the reproductions, and to ascribe changes in the latter to changes in the former—the fact, namely, of the *consistent direction* which the change takes, a later reproduction deviating from an earlier in the same direction as this deviated from its predecessor or the original.

In one respect, however, all four investigations are incomplete: They examine only one function of the trace, reproduction. We have previously pointed out how our conclusions from experimental results as to the nature of traces are strengthened when we find the same laws operative for different memory functions, e.g., recall and recognition. It will therefore be necessary to supplement the results obtained by the method of reproduction by the method of recognition. This necessity is the greater since long ago Claparède found a marked difference between recall, i.e., description of previously shown objects, and their recognition. In his experiments objects which were very badly described, i.e., recalled with many errors, were correctly recognized when shown again together with other similar objects. It is to be regretted that these pioneer experiments have been overlooked by Wulf and his successors, for they illustrate again how different processes of recognition and reproduction must be—a point which Claparède set out to prove. In themselves Claparède's results go no further, but they raise the serious problem as to the rôle of traces in reproduction and recognition. Indeed, if recognition were *always* right and specific where reproduction is faulty, we could not draw inferences from the errors of reproduction to changes in the traces. Fortunately, however, we know from Wulf's experiments that this is not true. For Wulf, although he concentrated on reproductions, introduced one modification which brought in recognition. A week after the first exposure of all but the first four figures the subjects were shown *parts* of these figures and asked to draw the full figures, using the shown parts if they thought them to be correct, but changing them if they considered that necessary. In fourteen cases the part patterns were changed by the subjects, in more cases they were not recognized at all. Figs. 101 and 102 give examples of the alterations, the original and the newly exposed part being drawn in full lines, the changes and completions in broken ones.

Since only parts of the original figures were re-exposed, these results are not entirely conclusive, but they indicate that recognition is not so entirely different from reproduction as one might have concluded from Claparède's experiments. I hope to produce new evidence in the near future to settle this point.

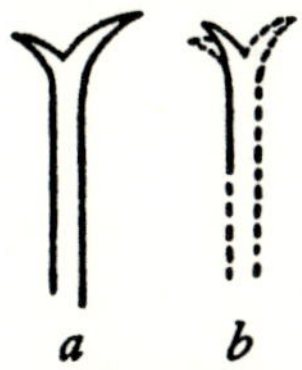

Fig. 101

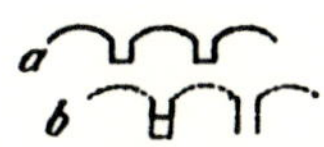

Fig. 102

PROCEDURE OF WULF, ALLPORT, AND PERKINS. Let us now turn to the experiments themselves and first describe in more detail the method employed. Since Wulf's method was more or less closely adhered to by Allport and Perkins—with the exception that neither of these investigators used representations of partial figures—we will describe it first, pointing out later the differences of the methods employed by Gibson.[8]

Twenty-six simple patterns, composed of straight and curved lines or of points (4 patterns), were drawn on white cards 8 × 10 cm. sq. The greatest extent of these patterns was 6–7 cm. They were shown to the subjects for a period of time varying between five and ten seconds, the first and simplest drawings receiving the shortest exposures. The six subjects[9] were told to look at these carefully, since they would be required to reproduce them later. During the first six meetings only two different drawings were shown; later four patterns were always presented at each sitting, but even this was done without strictly "serial" presentation, in which one pattern follows immediately upon the other. Repro-

[8] Allport, who published before Perkins, gives a very good comparative survey of his and his two predecessors' methods.

[9] The author of this book, four students without any psychological training who had never taken part in a psychological experiment, and the wife of the author of the paper.

ductions were asked for thirty seconds after the presentations, 24 hours later, again after a week—at that time for all but the first four figures parts were re-exposed as explained above—and again after a longer interval, ranging from two weeks to two months.

Allport used two patterns only (truncated pyramid and Greek Key), drawn on the same card side by side, with a total size of 7″ × 2½″ and exposed for ten seconds. His subjects, 350 children of an average age of 11 yr. and 4 mo., reproduced those designs immediately after exposure, after two weeks, and after four months.

Perkins used two sets of five drawings, one for each group of adult naïve subjects (98 in one group, 52 in the other). The figures, whose size is not reported, were drawn on large cards, 14 in. × 11 in., shown one directly after the other to groups of 20 subjects simultaneously. Reproduction was demanded 20 seconds after the exposure, and at 1, 6, 7, and 14–19 day intervals.

It may be added that both Wulf and Allport tried to induce their subjects to use as much visual imagery as possible for this reproduction, while Perkins instructed his only to reproduce as accurately as possible.

THE CHOICE OF THE PATTERNS AS A DETERMINING FACTOR. The general plan of experimentation, then, was the same for these three experimenters, although each of them used different patterns. The choice of patterns, however, is of the utmost significance if we remember the summary of Wulf's results as quoted (p. 493). If traces change according to gestalt laws, then it will be impossible to find a law according to which every pattern will change in exactly, i.e., *absolutely,* the same manner. If Wulf's conclusion is right the change which any pattern undergoes must be determined by the pattern itself, the pattern, i.e., in the behavioural, not of course in the geographical, environment. Thus according to the nature of the pattern lines may gradually become straighter or more curved, longer or shorter, etc. If any perceived form is a product of organization, ensuing upon a certain kind of stimulation, such a form is, as we know, sustained by real forces. According to the kind of stimulus distribution these forces of organization will be balanced in different degree; in cases of very irregular patterns the internal forces of organization will, as previously discussed (Chapter IV, p. 139), be in conflict with the external ones; the perceived forms will be under stress. Therefore, if the trace retains the dynamic pattern of the original excitation, it will be under stress too, and the changes which occur within it will be such as to reduce those internal stresses. Hence these changes depend upon the distribution of stresses within the trace, and eventually on the nature of the originally perceived forms. If, then, this whole theory is right, changes which appear in reproduction can be used as indications of the stresses in the traces and therefore in the perceived forms. And conversely, phenomenal characteristics of the latter which ought to be correlative to such stresses, like asymmetries, irregularities, patent gaps, etc., should determine the gradual transformation which occurs in reproduction.

Thus Wulf and Perkins both selected figures with definite asymmetries, Wulf's figures often being more asymmetrical than Perkins', and Gibson used several figures with gaps. Such a procedure is perfectly justified. True induction is not a collection of any random cases, but search for facts guided by explanatory principles. Many more different figure-characteristics should of course be investigated; for, as we shall see, Allport's results brought out a new factor.

REPRODUCTION AND RECOGNITION METHODS COMPARED TO THE METHOD OF SUCCESSIVE COMPARISON. From the point of view of method this procedure is in a way a continuation of the successive comparison method which also tested the changes in the trace system. So far the two procedures have been different in two respects: on the one hand the periods of time during which the change could occur were very considerably shorter in the comparison than in the reproduction method, on the other the former has so far been restricted to very few aspects of the compound items, heaviness of weights, intensities of tones and noises, whiteness of neutral colours, whereas the latter has been concerned with figural characteristics exclusively. As regards the first point, a method of recognition could be developed which would be similar to the reproduction method by being able to employ long time intervals, and similar to the successive comparison method by presenting to the observer a number of more or less different patterns, including the original, for selection. As regards the second point, the comparison method might easily be applied to figural properties. A first such step was taken in 1929 in my research laboratory for size of simple lines, but the results were entirely inconclusive, size of such lines as we used being, apparently, a very ambiguous determinant. Conversely the reproduction method or a modification of it could be used for the intensity and quality aspect so as to verify the result obtained about these characteristics by the comparison method. For such problems the recognition method would often be more adequate than the reproduction method. Actually Wulf carried out some experiments with colours of different saturation, but although his first results were significant enough, he did not have the time to develop them systematically so that they were never published. Katz, however

(1930, p. 255 f.), points out that if a subject is to select from a series of tints and colours the one that is equal to the blue of a friend's eyes, the black of his own hat, the red of his lips, he will as a rule select too saturated a colour.

THE DIRECTION OF THE CHANGES. Let us now turn to the actual results: corresponding to the similar nature of their original patterns (see p. 497) Wulf, Allport, and Perkins obtained similar results. "It became evident from detailed examination of the data that all changes were in the direction of some balanced or symmetrical patterns," thus Perkins (p. 475). "Perhaps the most striking of all the results is the tendency for the figure to retain, or to achieve, symmetry," this from Allport (p. 145). "With the exception of eight cases out of about 400, six of which yielded either no reproduction at all or an entirely unrecognizable one—the comparison of the reproductions with the original reveals *throughout a clear deviation of the former from the latter in the direction of either sharpening or levelling.*" This statement of Wulf's (p. 340) needs some amplification. Terminologically, he means by sharpening an increase or exaggeration, by levelling a weakening or toning down of a peculiarity of a pattern. Thus, in many cases, levelling coincided with a tendency towards symmetry, since the peculiarity was the particular asymmetry of the figure. Secondly, Wulf's statement coincides with those of his two successors only in one half of his alternative, the levelling; but he found an equal number of changes occurring in the opposite direction. This, however, must not surprise us, when we remember that Wulf's figures were constructed so as to contain greater asymmetries than those of the two other authors. Moreover, Allport also found in his material examples of sharpening.

THE NATURE OF THE CHANGES. If three different investigators working in three different countries, Germany, England, and America, two with a great number of subjects, obtain so similar results, the facts themselves are clearly established. How are they to be interpreted? To this question Wulf devotes the greatest part of his paper, distinguishing three different causal factors, which he names *normalizing, emphasizing* or *pointing,* and *autonomous* changes.[10]

[10] Wulf's terms are: *Normalisierung, Pointierung,* and *struktive Veränderung.* The English equivalent of the first, used in the text, is taken over from both Allport and Gibson; the two terms used in the text for the second are Gibson's and Allport's, respectively; while the third is my own translation, since Allport gives no translation, though a good description, and Gibson one that seems to me slightly ambiguous.

Autonomous Changes. Normalizing occurs when the reproductions approach successively a familiar form; pointing, when a particular feature of the pattern, which strikes the observer as such when he perceives it, becomes more and more exaggerated; autonomous changes, lastly, are such as derive from neither of the two other sources but are inherent in the trace pattern itself, a result of its own intrinsic stresses. The last class of changes is that described on page 496. Wulf regards it as proved by the fact that such autonomous changes occur against the forces of normalization and pointing. The tendency towards symmetry would then be such an autonomous change, a view held also by Allport and Perkins.

As an example of this change towards symmetry I reproduce one of Perkins' figures. As an example of sharpening I reproduce one

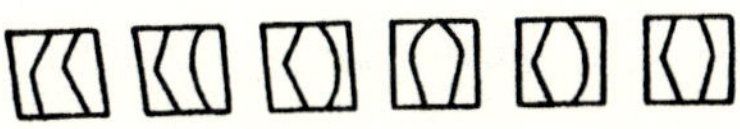

Fig. 103

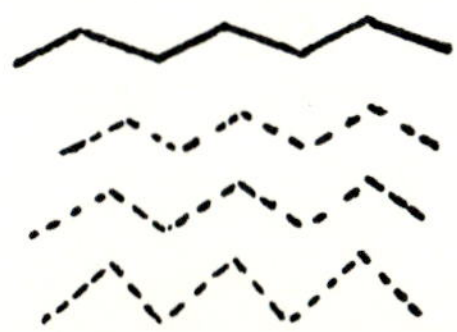

Fig. 104

of Wulf's figures. To understand this autonomous change one might think of a spiral spring which has been pulled apart and therefore possesses a stress towards contraction. Five of Wulf's subjects showed the same direction for this figure, a fact indicative of the strength of this tendency. One subject, however, reproduced this figure with a progressive flattening. The reason for this effect is clear from the reports. Whereas the other subjects perceived this pattern as a zigzag or something similar, this one subject saw it as a "broken line," i.e., as a modification of a straight line. Naturally it is the form as perceived, and not as a mere geometric drawing—which is no gestalt at all—that is under stress and therefore determines the successive changes.

Another autonomous change was found by Allport: "As many as 95% of the children displayed at least a 20% reduction in the size of their third drawing of the pyramid as compared with the original stimulus" (p. 144). We remember that Allport's figures were the largest used by any of the investigators. After excluding several other possibilities Allport says: "The phenomenon seems more readily to be explained by the hypothesis that shrinkage with time is one of the definitely 'dynamical' properties of traces" (l. c.). Since none of the other investigators found this change, it must be confined to certain definite ranges of size. One might, however, expect that very small figures would manifest the opposite tendency, i.e., to expand. Since Gibson's figures were relatively small his negative result might contradict this expectation, were it not for the special method of this author, which rather excluded such an effect; in his experiments the figures were exposed under the narrow slit of a Ranschburg memory apparatus, so that their size was definitely fixed by the size of the opening, which was a constant factor in all his experiments. This problem, therefore, is still waiting its experimental test.

Pointing. What is the cause of pointing or emphasizing? Why is it, in other words, that specially noticed peculiarities of figures are so frequently exaggerated in successive reproductions? The fact is established beyond a doubt. G. E. Müller (1913, p. 378) described it long before Wulf under the name "affective transformation" and explained it as an affair of attention, an explanation the insufficiency of which has been proved by Wulf.

A true explanation, even if it is not complete, can be found in our principle of autonomous change. Emphasis on a particular aspect of the perceived object means that this aspect possesses particular "weight" in the total pattern. The same pattern perceived either with or without such emphasis is therefore, qua dynamic pattern as well as qua behavioural datum, *not* the same; two different psychophysical patterns correspond in these cases to the same geometrical pattern, and therefore the autonomous changes of their traces must be different. Pointing, then, indicates that such changes do not necessarily take the direction of symmetry but may, when the original pattern exhibits pronounced dominance of parts or aspects, increase the weight of the dominant parts or aspects. Since, however, pointing does not always occur when the original perception contained especially noticed peculiarities, giving way to a levelling effect, we see that in explaining the changes we cannot look only at any one characteristic of the pattern, but must always consider the pattern as a whole. As long, however, as we possess no more detailed or quantitative knowledge about all the factors concerned, this last remark is no more than a methodological, it is not yet an explanatory principle.

In accordance with Katz's own interpretation, though in different terminology, we interpret his findings of the exaggeration of colours in memory, reported on page 498, as examples of pointing, which fall well under our explanatory principles.

The Effect of Verbalization. More Than One Trace System Effective in Reproduction. However, it would be an illegitimate simplification to claim that pointing is nothing but a special kind of autonomous change. The subject, on perceiving the pattern, gives it a verbal characteristic, e.g., "a very narrow triangle," "bracket, large below and small above," etc. And this verbal characterization exerts a direct influence upon the reproduction. This fact introduces a new point of view: it would be wrong to assume that a reproduction is based on *one* kind of traces only. Particularly when the subjects possess language, and so far no other subjects have been employed, the language factor will in all, or at least in many, cases become effective in reproduction. To deal with language qua language is outside the scope of this book, although we shall not be able to avoid meeting this factor again and again in our next chapters. Whatever language as a psychological function is, its efficacy in reproduction proves that the process underlying this accomplishment is based on a complex set of conditions, and does not depend merely upon a single individual trace.

Normalization. This point becomes still more manifest when we turn to the last mode of change, the normalizing. For to explain these changes we have to recur to traces different from the individual trace of the original pattern and not purely verbal. When Wulf's pattern 23 (Fig. 105) was apprehended as "bridge with two pillars" (by four subjects) and consistently changed in such a way that the indentures, as pillars, become deeper and deeper, then we must assume that the trace system of bridges has in some way or other influenced the reproduction. A fifth subject apprehended the same pattern as a battlement and her reproductions showed not deeper but wider indentures, proof that here a different trace system was operative.

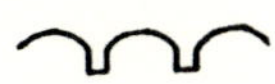

Fig. 105

The Influence of "Outside" Trace Systems. The influence of these "outside" trace systems on reproduction may be of different kinds. In the first place it may be indirect inasmuch as it does not affect the reproduction directly but the trace of the original percept. Such an influence would be of the same kind as that investigated by von Restorff and Lauenstein: the trace of the original pattern would come into communication with other trace systems and be changed by this communication. In the second place one might, as in the discussion of pointing, think of a direct influence, the trace of the original pattern being unaffected by the other trace system but co-operating with it in the act of reproduction. Lastly, of course, any combination of these two effects is possible, and this is, in my opinion, by far the most likely case. That a trace may undergo changes by communication with other traces has been proved by Lauenstein and von Restorff, and results of Allport's and Gibson's lead to the same conclusion. Allport presented his two designs simultaneously on the same card. "In a few cases the features of one of the designs appeared to be incorporated into the drawing of the other" (p. 137), and in Gibson's experiments, for reasons to be discussed presently, this kind of change was more frequent than any other.

It seems therefore a necessary assumption that communication of a new trace, with an old trace system, such as we have described above, *may* lead to changes in the trace. That such changes can assimilate the new to the old was again proved by Lauenstein and von Restorff. Normalization, therefore, if interpreted as an effect within the traces, is derivable from our general principles. These principles, moreover, permit communication to produce changes other than normalization. Communication between traces will affect either or all of the interacting traces; assimiliation is, of all possible effects of such interactions, a very special and easily realized case, but by no means the only possible one. If, e.g., I apprehend a certain design as a bottle, I may at the same time apprehend its peculiarities; it may not really be a bottle, but only something like it. This kind of communication between the trace of the design and the trace system of bottles, being of a particular kind, will have its particular effects. We do not know any details of the processes involved, but we know from Wulf's experiments that the reproduction of such a design may consistently become more and more symmetrical and at the same time less and less bottle-like. Generally speaking, the change produced in a trace by communication with an older class trace system will depend upon the relative properties of the new trace with regard to the old system. To give an example: if a class trace system has a definite property Sn, say a certain normal size, and a new object is experienced as belonging to this class and possessing the same property with the degree S, then the relation of S and Sn will determine how S will change in the new trace. Roughly speaking, when S is not very different from Sn, then, *ceteris paribus,* assimilation = normalization will occur. If, on the other hand, S is much greater or smaller than Sn, then this difference will become exaggerated: sharpening, contrast. Many exaggerations in the spreading of gossip and rumours may find at least a partial explanation in these intertrace dynamics. What properties must a "normal" system have? If we are right, it will be a normal system not because of its greatest frequency, but because of its greatest stability. Autonomous changes will modify traces and trace systems until their stresses have become as well balanced as possible—stresses, that is, within their interior and between them and their surrounding trace systems. The "normal" is dynamically unique. (Compare our discussion of normality in Chapter VI, pp. 221 f.)

Good examples of reproduction in which evidently old trace systems influenced the *act* of reproduction directly and not by way of the specific traces are contained in Gibson's article, particularly under his caption "Verbal Analysis." Fig. 106 is a good illustration: (a) the original was characterized by the subject as "pillars with

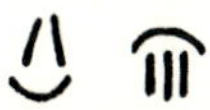

a *b*

Fig. 106

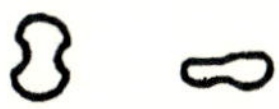

a *b*

Fig. 107

curve," and reproduced as (b). Reproduction and original are so dissimilar as geometrical patterns that it is safe to assume that (b) owes its existence not to a change in the original trace but to the fact that the older trace systems, "pillars with curve," exerted the main influence on the reproduction. The test would be whether the subject responsible for this drawing, if confronted with (a) and (b) and possibly a number of other similar designs, would choose (a) or (b) or another pattern as the one originally presented to him. It seems to me very unlikely that he would choose (b), an opinion which is strengthened by the results of Claparède's experiments previously mentioned. Another example from Gibson's "Object Assimilation" (Fig. 107): (a) is again the original, designated as "footprint on the sands of time," (b) the reproduction. In most similar cases, however, the reproductions do not seem to be so exclusively determined by the old trace system, the new trace of the pattern itself exerting a noticeable influence. Whether this trace itself had become changed through its communication with the older system is, of course, impossible to derive from the drawings.

The process occurring at the moment of reproduction depends, therefore, on a very complex set of conditions, which it is impossible to unravel in each particular case. Experimentation will have the task of establishing as simple conditions as possible so that "pure" cases may appear, i.e., cases in which one of the many conditions has a dominating influence. Such pure cases would reveal the actual factors at work. But it is wrong to say: "The issue is this: Is the change in a reproduction of a perceived form caused by the influence of past perceptions on the perception and memory of that form, or is the change caused by the nature of the form itself?" (Gibson, p. 35.) There is no such alternative in reality. We must study *all* the traces and trace systems on which an actual reproduction depends, and the changes which each of these has undergone either autonomously or by communication with other systems. Therefore the fact that *sometimes* we can prove an influence of an older trace either directly on reproduction or on a newer trace does not prove that autonomous changes never occur.

GIBSON'S METHOD AND RESULTS. We shall close the discussion of this section by an analysis of Gibson's results. His method differed from those of the other investigators in many decisive respects, some of which have already been mentioned. Apart from some subsidiary experiments he carried out two full series, each having two groups, A and B, of fourteen simple designs; the patterns of group A were made up of straight, those of group B of curved, or curved and straight, lines. Each of these series was presented to the subjects in the standardized fashion of a memory experiment: they were serially exposed on a Ranschburg apparatus, where each figure appeared for 1½ seconds, to be immediately followed by the next. The subjects' task was "to look carefully at each figure and at the end of each series to draw as many figures as he remembered in any order he wished" (p. 7). On the first day the two groups were presented two or three times, each presentation followed by as many reproductions as the subject could accomplish; presentations were then continued on later days until the subject reproduced all figures. Five weeks and a year later the subjects were once more asked to furnish reproductions. In the second series each group of figures was presented and reproduced only twice.

It is not surprising that his results differ in many decisive respects from those of the other investigators. The renewed presentations would necessarily interfere with the change processes in the traces, and therefore one could not expect the continuity of these changes found by the three other authors. This is borne out by the results, although such continuous changes also occurred (no figures given by Gibson; cf. p. 36). But a much more powerful factor was the mode of presentation itself, the arrangement of the material in long monotonous series. True enough, von Restorff's results were not known at the time of Gibson's experiments, but all of the other investigators avoided this mode of presentation, aware of the fact that a series is not a sum of elements, and that therefore changes in the trace of a series would be largely dependent upon the serial nature of the trace systems. To present all figures in the same opening of an apparatus must necessarily increase such an effect. For by being surrounded by the identical (behavioural) object, the top of the exposure instrument, the members of the series must become particularly strongly unified. With our present-day knowledge we must expect effects of aggregation such as von Restorff found, besides the natural influence of figures upon each other. Both expectations are fulfilled by Gibson's results: "It should be mentioned that, as a result of this method of presentation, retroactive inhibition occurred during the exposure of the series. The observers often complained that each figure as it appeared 'blotted out' the preceding figure" (p. 26). Learning of these figures was therefore very difficult and often led to a voluntary effort "to think of objects by means of which the figures could be 'understood'" (p. 14). "Figure assimilation . . . is the most frequent kind of change to be found in the reproductions" (p. 25), i.e., changes in the reproduction of one figure so as to make it more similar to another occurred more frequently than any other kind of change. Thus the influence of aggregation which we could predict is amply confirmed, and the fact that so frequently the reproductions were not so much due to the trace of the original design as to other older trace systems—connected with the design by "object assimilation" or "verbal analysis" (see our two examples on p. 503)—is another effect of aggregation; for in order to memorize the figures against the destructive forces of aggregation the subjects had to use these special devices.

To have established figure assimilation in so unequivocal a manner is one of the main merits of Gibson's experiments. He errs, however, when he believes that his results contradict Wulf's theory. As a matter of fact he himself found several changes which under the conditions of the other experiments would have to be regarded as at least largely autonomous, viz., changes towards symmetry (p. 30), rectilinearity (p. 30 f.), and completion of gaps (p. 261). The particular method of his experiments, however, makes it impossible to classify these changes as necessarily autonomous.

Summarizing our experimental evidence we see how a consistent dynamic trace theory is capable of explaining systematically a great number of facts, and how experiments based on such a theory have contributed to a more concrete and detailed elaboration of it. Last not least: experiment and theory in systematic connection have raised a number of problems ready to be attacked by the art of the experimentalist.

THEORY OF TRACES RESUMED: INSUFFICIENCY OF OUR HYPOTHESES

Acquisition of Skills. We have now to resume our theory of traces, for we have not developed it far enough to make it capable of explaining all functions of memory. The foundations of our hypotheses so far were threefold: temporal units, recall (reproduction), and recognition. But at the beginning of this chapter we have encountered other modes in which memory manifests itself, viz., the acquisition of skills, e.g., the learning to type. In such accomplishments the past plays a rôle different from that in our three aforementioned functions. In these the past is in some way present in the accomplishment of the moment: a tone of a melody, as a *later* tone, follows upon and stands in a definite dynamic relationship to preceding ones. I recall a former experience, I recognize a present object as having been encountered sometime in the past; in both these cases the past is also contained in the datum. Not so in the acquired skill. When I type a letter today, my typing as an experience has, as a rule, no such backward reference to former experiences of typing; and the greater ease and perfection of my typing today, though it is functionally connected with the clumsy performance in the past, is not experientally, or behaviourally, so connected. Moreover, the application of a skill to a new task has a much less *specific* relation to the past than the three functions so far discussed. Acquisition of the skill of typewriting does not mean the ability to write a specific text, but to type *any* text. Similarly, as Bartlett has insisted, a practised tennis player has not learned to make a small number of very specific movements, but to strike the ball in the proper way in the ever-changing situations of the game.

Reorganization in Perception. We find the same characteristics also, absence of a reference to the past and lack of specificity, in memory functions which do not concern motor skills. Of these I shall exemplify two. Turn back to page 173. You will see the figure on this page at once as a face, whereas when you saw it for the first time it appeared as a jumble of lines, and it took possibly quite a long time for the face to emerge. The effect of which this example is a simple illustration has not yet been studied by special experiments. And yet such a study is highly desirable if we want to elaborate our trace theory. We do not, at the present moment, know how specific this after-effect is. That it is not restricted to the individual pattern with which the original reorganization took place is certain. When in the summer of 1929 I was shown into my office at the University of California I saw on the blackboard, to my great surprise, a rough drawing of this "face" which I recognized at once as a face without any period of transition. And yet this drawing was by no means an exact replica of the pattern. Such an individual case is of course no more than an indication of what we may expect to find in systematic experiments. I should not be at all surprised if the range of patterns influenced by the reorganization of one pattern, though limited, were considerably wider even than one would conclude from this incident.

But even now, while we lack detailed knowledge about this effect, we know enough to recognize the serious difficulty it presents to our theory. A pattern of lines if presented for the first time gives rise to the impression of chaos, replaced, as a rule, by a well-organized and articulated pattern only after we make an effort to organize the chaos. The same pattern—and a similar one—if presented for a second time will appear in good organization at the start. What properties must the trace have to produce this result?

Greater Survival Value of Better Organization. This same case has another aspect which is more easily understood. If one has seen the face once or several times, it is impossible to see the pattern as a chaos, or to recall the chaos, although it has once been experienced and was at that time very persistent and difficult to destroy. True enough, this statement is based on ordinary observation and not on systematic experiments, but I feel convinced that such experiments, even if they bring to light new facts, will not seriously affect my proposition. If we accept it, we must conclude that traces of chaotic processes have a much lower "survival value" than traces of well-organized processes. And this conclusion is in good harmony with our general trace theory. For if traces are exposed to forces which connect them with other traces, then highly unstable trace structures will be destroyed. Choatic patterns have neither a well-defined boundary, to keep them unified and segregated, nor interior stability. Therefore they can have but little power of resisting outside forces. This principle seems fundamental. It sheds a new light on the results of von Restorff and of Wulf and his successors. If preservation of a trace is a function of its own stability, then traces will gradually change from less to more stable forms (Wulf and his followers), and badly articulated trace structures will simply deteriorate (von Restorff). A monotonous series of nonsense syllables or numbers is such a badly articulated semi-chaotic structure, whereas an isolated element within an otherwise monotonous series gains definition and stability by its character of isolation. The aggregation which von Restorff has investigated is aggregation into a state bordering on chaos. The less articulation the series possesses, the more chaotic will the aggregation become, and the series will therefore be the harder to learn. This conclusion is well supported by experimental facts: it has proved impossible to learn series of nonsense syllables without rhythm, i.e., without the least vestige of articulation (G. E. Müller, 1913, p. 43 f.).

Finally we recall one of Zeigarnik's results, discussed previously (Chapter VIII, pp. 339 f.), viz., the fact that a well-organized trace, the trace of a completed task, is more stable and therefore more effective than that of a less organized one; thus uncompleted tasks, which usually, owing to the stress towards completion, were more frequently recalled than completed ones, were, because of their less perfect organization, inferior to the better organized completed ones when that special stress was lacking. More evidence will be adduced in Chapter XIII, pages 621 f.

Complexity of Articulation and Survival Value. If we accept the survival value of a trace as a measure of its stability, then we cannot simply correlate degree of articulation with stability. For, unfortunately, we forget not only chaotic experiences but also the most highly articulated ones of which we are capable. It is a common experience that one is unable to repeat an argument which one has understood perfectly well when one listened to its presentation. I find this particularly amazing in the field of mathematics. One may understand a proof perfectly and yet be unable to reconstruct it, even if one remembers one or two of its steps.

Such observations are confirmed by experiments. Köhler found that when chimpanzees reach the limit of their ability they will no longer "learn," i.e., they will attack the problem in the same way whether they have solved it before or not. Such a problem was that of lifting a ring from a long nail. It could be solved "intelligently" when the ape had a good day, but the animal's performance did not improve with repetition.

Such facts, far from contradicting our theory, could have been derived from it. Articulations of a highly complex kind can be produced only under special conditions, when the organism, through its "attitude," supplies part of the effective forces and an ample store of energy. The traces of such processes, which lack these added Ego-forces, are therefore not stable; instead they will sooner or later disintegrate, part systems losing their connections with each other, so that the whole is destroyed. How complex an articulation can be without losing its stability depends necessarily upon the kind of system in which it is produced. What we call differences of intelligence may consist, among other things, in differences of stable articulation, although in this sense intelligence would be also a function of experience, since the stability of an organization will depend upon the trace structures already existing.

Learning a New Relation. We return to our main argument and discuss the second example of a non-motor memory function for which our present assumptions are insufficient. Dallenbach published in 1926 a short note on the learning of a relation which was followed in 1929 by a more formal investigation carried out by the same author in conjunction with Kreezer. Dallenbach asked his six-year-old boy whether he knew what "opposite" means. Refusing to accept the boy's negative answer, he asked him to name the opposite, first, of "good," then of "big," and obtained the answers "boy" and "man," both of which were called "wrong." Thereupon he told the boy the correct answers, and then proceeded to ask him the opposite of "black," "long," "fat," "little," and so on. The boy now produced immediately the correct answers. Again this case, whose significance was confirmed by the later investigation of Kreezer and Dallenbach, who worked with one hundred children, stands merely as an example of a whole class of cases. Furthermore, in this chapter we are not interested in what happens at the moment when the child "understands" the relation. Our point here is that the child can do something after this "understanding" which he could not do before. Therefore the child's brain must have been changed by this process of understanding, a trace must have remained from it, and the nature of the trace must account for his new behaviour. What must the trace be like to produce the new response? To this question accrues, just as in the case of the face pattern, the other question *how* this trace with its particular characteristic determines the new process. We shall take up this question in our next chapter when we discuss the functions of memory themselves rather than the traces. The first function, however, belongs to our present context, just as the same question arising from the discussion of the face pattern does (p. 506). It seems wisest to admit that at the moment we can give no satisfactory answer, that indeed the trace theory is here face to face with a difficult problem of immense importance. For without a solution of it we shall not be able to understand learning, an accomplishment which only in rare cases consists in the exact repetition of a previous process. I may add, however, that the case of learning a relation seems in some ways related to the case of transposition of a melody which we have already discussed (p. 460).

Trace Theory Developed to Fit These Cases. Trace Determines the Field. We may summarize the discussion of all three examples, of motor skill, perception, relational thought, by saying that the new performances take place in a field which is determined by previous experiences. More concretely we should have to say that the field of the present process comprises the traces of previous processes. If we interpret our cases in this way, we have at least some experimental evidence that sheds light on these processes. That a process is determined by the nature of the larger field in which it occurs has been proved before. I recall only a number of optical illusions which demonstrate this effect and will add another instance: the direction of perceived motion depends on the surrounding field, as proved by Annie Stern for movement through the blind spot. If the field is framed or articulated by straight lines, the motion is rectilinear; if frame or articulation is curved, the motion follows the shape and direction of the curves. A similar effect had already been discovered by myself (1922, 1931, p. 1185) for ordinary ϕ movement. In all these cases, however, the field which influences a perceptual process is itself a perceptual field. We possess, however, also some evidence that the effective field can be a trace field. I refer to one of Hartmann's experiments (pp. 375-6). Hartmann exposed in succession a special kind of triangle and a circle in such a way that if presented successively they would have appeared as the pattern of Fig. 108*a*. The times of exposure of the two figures were equal and stood in the relation of 8.5:20 to the time of the interval between them. When the latter was around 155σ the observers saw the following phenomenon: "At first the triangle appeared, then it was suddenly gone and there came a 'pear' or a 'shamrock leaf.'" (See Fig. 108 *a* and *b*.) The indentations of the distorted circle correspond to the places where the two corners of the triangle had been in the first exposure; thus the shape produced by the circular stimulus must be due to the field created by the fresh trace of the preceding triangle.

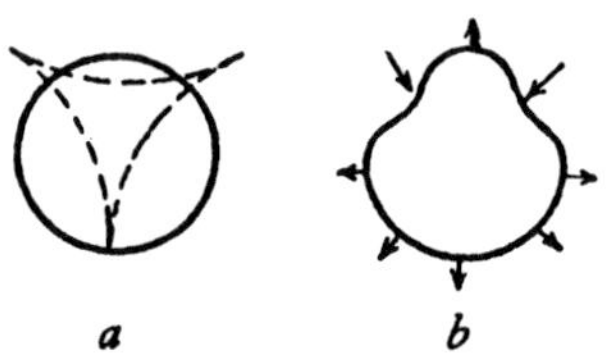

Fig. 108

Three of Wertheimer's experiments are still closer to the problem which concerns us now. The two first are very old indeed, being contained in Wertheimer's classical paper on the perception of motion (Wertheimer, 1912, also Koffka, 1919). In both cases an effect was produced in the perceptual field by a cumulative effect in the trace field. In the first a simple ϕ experiment (two lines, parallel or at an angle, successively exposed) is performed a number of times, whereupon, without the knowledge of the observer, the second exposure is suppressed. Under ordinary conditions the observer would then see an object at rest, but under these conditions the observer continues to see the object in motion though over a shorter distance; repeated exposure decreases this distance until the object eventually appears at rest. In the second experiment, illustrated by Fig. 109 *a* and *b,* the subject is first shown for a number of times the

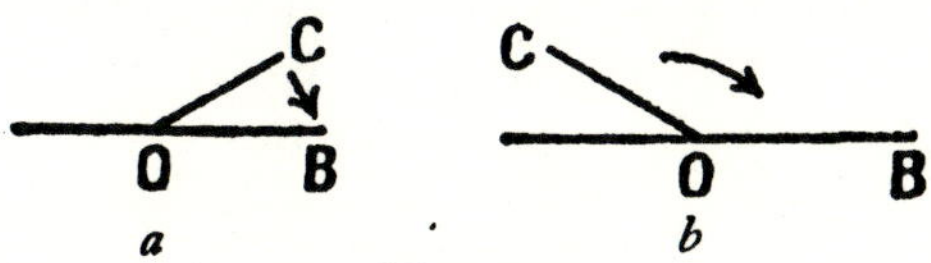

Fig. 109

successive exposures of the lines of Fig. 109*a*. He sees the short arm turning to the right. Then in succeeding exposures the angle between the short and the long arm is increased until the two lines reach the position of Fig. 109*b*. The arm continues to turn to the right, whereas without the previous exposures it would now turn to the left.

In both cases we have an influence of the trace system extending over a longer period of time than that demonstrated in the Hartmann experiment. In both cases this influence is best understood as one upon the field in which the new process takes place. This field must be so structured, through influence of the recent trace systems, that it forces a single excitation to move, or to favour one direction of movement rather than the opposite. Motion as a process has left a trace which influences the field in its neighbourhood in such a way that it produces processes of motion under conditions under which "normal" fields would not produce such processes. The term neighbourhood is here used for the neighbourhood of the "time axis" (see pp. 452 f.). That our proposition is also true if we use "neighbourhood" in the ordinary spatial sense is proved by other experiments of Wertheimer's; therefore it is a fact that a spatial field in which motion occurs in one place is a field more apt to produce (or allow) motion in other places than a field without any motion. This fact supports our trace theory in two ways. On the one hand it makes the field explanation of the after-effect no new *ad hoc* hypothesis; instead it links up anew "spatial" and "temporal" fields. On the other hand it tells us something about the nature of particular trace systems which is responsible for the after-effect. For if the original movement field itself has the property of being particularly favourable for the occurrence of motion, and if the trace retains, as we have supposed, the dynamic properties of the excitations, then the *trace* of the motion field will have the same property that distinguishes the motion field itself. Thus we have succeeded in transforming the problem of a trace property into a problem of a process field property. The difficulties inherent in the problem are thus no longer specifically those of a trace theory, but pertain to the theory of field organization in general.

Wertheimer's third experiment (1923, p. 319 f.) proves a similar influence for stationary organization. In this experiment one pre-

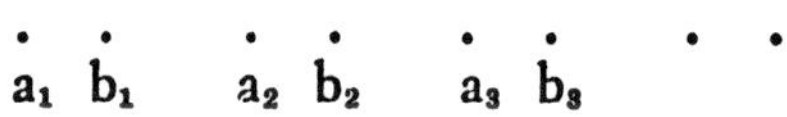

Fig. 110

pares a number of point patterns, modifications of Fig. 110. In this figure the distances between members with equal indices are considerably smaller than those between members with consecutive indices ($a_1 b_1 < b_1 a_2$, etc.). Starting from this pattern one produces a number of new ones by leaving the distance a_1 a_2 (generally a_k a_{k+1}) constant and changing the other distance (a_k b_k and b_k a_{k+1}). Doing this by small steps, one reaches a point where these latter distances are equal, i.e., where all points are equidistant from each other; then the distances between members of equal indices become longer than those between members of consecutive indices, until finally the relative distances are completely reversed, a_1 b_1 in the last pattern $=$ b_1 a_2 in the first. This series of patterns is presented to the observer one by one, starting with either the first or the last, the observer's task being to indicate the natural grouping. At some point in this series this grouping will change from a_1 b_1 to b_1 a_2 if the subject starts with the first series, and from b_1 a_2 to a_1 b_1 if he starts with the last series. The question is, at which point in the series will this change occur? The result is that as a rule the change in grouping takes place sometime after the neutral pattern (with equal point distances throughout) has been passed; i.e., such serial presentation has the effect that grouping will, for a time, occur against proximity but in accordance with previous grouping. Again we must assume that the dynamic character of the trace system of the preceding groupings affects the field in which the new grouping takes place, and it is the *character of the grouping* in the trace which determines the new field.

These experiments demonstrate an effect of traces on perceptual organization. They are therefore directly relevant to that case of perceptual memory, the face of the man, which was one of the starting points of our discussion. In principle this case is hardly different from that of Wertheimer's experiment described last, apart from the fact that the time interval between the successive presentations of patterns in this last experiment is relatively short, whereas in our case it can be very much longer, altogether of a different order of magnitude. However, this aspect does not affect our immediate problem as to the nature of the trace which produces the effect. It enters only when we try to envisage how an *old* trace can influence a new field. The nature of the trace must be such as to be able to produce a certain field condition in which some organizations are favoured over others, and this characteristic of the trace must derive directly from the dynamics of the original process.

This general conclusion as to the nature of the trace is applicable to our two other principal cases as well, the motor skill and the thought relation. In these cases, as in the first, the problem remains how the new field can be influenced by the old trace system; this problem involves the special problem how the new excitations select, so to speak, among the vast mass of traces the one that will influence its own field so as to give it the organization actually achieved. To this problem we shall turn in the next chapter.

Still our discussion has been fruitful. It has shown that our trace theory is, at least in principle, capable of dealing with effects which were not taken into account when we developed it. Moreover, our new development of the theory implies that the effect of traces may be very different from a mere reproduction of the original process. If the trace determines directly the field of an event, then it does not thereby determine the event itself *completely*. This train of thought also will be continued in the next chapter.

No doubt, the results which we reached are not entirely satisfactory. We are still far from knowing in detail what properties the traces must have to exert the observed influences, even though we could lay down a general principle. Psychology is still in a very unsatisfactory state, and it is a Socratic gain to become aware of such unsatisfactoriness by formulating questions which have to remain unanswered.

In a former publication (1925) I introduced "gestalt-disposition" as an explanatory term to account for such phenomena. A gestalt-disposition would be the after-effect of a gestalt process by virtue of which the organism would produce processes of a similar gestalt- or formal nature which it could not produce before, or would produce them now more easily. Thus the concept of the gestalt-disposition labels a very definite problem; but in the framework of a concrete trace theory it offers no satisfactory explanation before we see what gestalt-disposition means in terms of traces.

TRACES AND THE EGO

After having pointed out these gaps in our trace theory we shall now try to fill in another one by taking up a thread started in Chapter VIII (pp. 331 ff.). There we found it necessary to assume a permanent substratum of the Ego, a substratum moreover which as a segregated unit could exist only as part of a more extended substratum, that of the Ego's environment. Our trace theory has so far been developed without any regard to our previous conclusion. Nevertheless, viewed in its light it may be said to account for the environmental substratum. How, then, will the permanent Ego fit into our theory? On the earlier occasion we based the permanent Ego-substratum on our general principles of organization. We can now give it a new foundation by referring to facts observed and beautifully interpreted by Sir Henry Head (1920, II).

Head's Schemata. Three frequent results of brain injury supply the empirical evidence for our hypothesis: voluntary movement and postural tone may be impaired or destroyed, appreciation of posture and passive movement may be greatly reduced, and the localization of touch on the surface of the body, apart from the momentary position of the limb touched, may be lost. The first two symptoms are always concomitant and therefore point to an identical underlying cause. The difference between the second and the third may be illustrated by an example. In the second case the "patient may be able to name correctly, and indicate on a diagram or on another person's hand, the exact position of the spot touched or pricked, and yet be ignorant of the position in space of the limb upon which it lies" (II, p. 606). In the third case, "the patient complains that he has no idea where he has been touched. He knows that a contact has occurred, but he cannot tell where it has taken place on the surface of the affected part" (l. c.).

What functions have been damaged to produce these symptoms? We begin with the first two, which, as just mentioned, must have a common cause. Head argues that "it would be impossible to discover the position of any part of the body, unless the immediate postural sensations were related to something that had preceded them" (p. 604). He excludes the explanation that the new postural sensation gains its special meaning by reference to a visual or motor image (pp. 605-723), and therefore concludes as follows: "Before the apparent processes caused by movement of a joint can evoke a change in consciousness, they have already been integrated and brought into relation with the previous physiological dispositions, due to antecedent postural changes." "For this standard, against which all subsequent changes of postures are measured before they enter consciousness, we have proposed the word 'schema.' By means of perpetual alterations in position *we are always building up a model of ourselves*[11] which constantly changes" (pp. 723, 605).

The two symptoms under discussion, impairment of voluntary movement and knowledge of the spatial position of our limbs, are thus explained by injuries to this schema, this "model of ourselves." Head's theory seems to me in perfect harmony with the trace theory which we have previously developed. In particular, his schema shows obvious similarities to our explanation of time units, like heard melodies, a fact which is not surprising since voluntary movements are the motor counterpart of perceived tunes. Thus the term "movement melody" has been used to emphasize this similarity. We could not perceive a melody if each new tone came to consciousness as an entirely new event. And quite in harmony with Head's principles we explained the perception of the melody by the trace system to which it gives rise. The close agreement between Head's and our theory is further borne out by a remark he makes in his later book on aphasia, when he draws explicitly the distinction between what we have called process and trace: "It must not be forgotten that the theory of schemata involves two conceptions, the schema building and the schema built. The first is an activity corresponding to all those processes discussed in this work, the second is a state which results from the activity" (1926, I, p. 488, n. 2).

There is still another similarity between melodies and schemata. A person with no particular musical ability will forget a new melody rather quickly; not only will he be unable to reproduce it, in many cases he will not even recognize it when it is played the next time. Melody traces are therefore short-lived. Even if they do not disap-

[11] Italics are mine.

pear completely, so little of them remains as to be insufficient for any direct after-effect.[12] Similarly the schemata do not endure very long. My movement and postures of five minutes ago are no longer reproducible or recognizable, and that is true even of such movements as were in the centre of attention, expressing at the moment the main impulse of the person. At least I cannot recall my movements during my climb of the *Winkler Riss,* although other aspects of this extremely vivid experience still stand out fairly clearly in my memory. In some respect the *causes* of the transitoriness of schemata and melody traces are similar also. A schema has fulfilled its function when it has given rise to a new movement which leads to a new schema. This new schema has then taken over the task of directing posture and movement, the old is dead inasmuch as it can exert no more influence. A similar situation obtains in an extended piece of music where one theme is followed by another. For the composer and the highly trained and musical listener even a long piece may be such a perfect unity that each new theme is experienced with reference to all that preceded it. Not so for the less trained and less musical person who hears the piece for the first time. For him one theme ends at a certain point and another one begins. For the arousal of this new one the trace system of the old one is no longer material, it has no function. It is therefore plausible in both examples to correlate the forgetting with the loss of function. What this forgetting is, is of course another matter, to which we shall devote the last section of this chapter. Here we shall only relate the fate of these "forgotten" traces to von Restorff's results. Schemata as well as melodies in a long piece of music have the general character of "monotonous" series in Restorff's sense, albeit the monotony is of a lower degree than in a series of nonsense syllables. Therefore, if the analogy holds, aggregation between traces should take place, and forgetting should be not absolute obliteration but absorption into a large and little differentiated aggregation in which individual trace systems lose their individuality. This assumption seems necessary when we now turn to that aspect of Head's theory which we have emphasized by italicizing. In Head's theory schemata are *models of ourselves,* a phrase which he manifestly uses in full consciousness of its import, since he repeats it several times.[13] And by this term Head's theory stands out as a clear anticipation of our own

[12] The fact that a melody heard frequently will eventually be remembered indicates that, at least in many cases, the trace is not entirely lost since it can be strengthened by cumulative effects of the process.

[13] In the "Studies on Neurology," where the concept is introduced, as well as in his later work on aphasia.

which postulated a permanent Ego-substratum. Bartlett (1932), who, as we shall see, makes a wide and generalized use of Head's schemata in his own theory of memory, does not do full justice to it when he refers to the term "model of ourselves" as "picturesque phraseology" (p. 203). Schemata, then, are parts of that Ego-substratum which our theory demands, and they are at the same time organized trace systems (Head, 1920, p. 607). How seriously this view is taken by Head appears from another point in which he anticipates our theory. In Chapter VIII we remarked upon the variable boundaries of the Ego, and exemplified this *inter alia* by reference to clothes, which often belong to the Ego. Quite in accordance with this view Head writes: "Anything which participates in the conscious movements of our bodies is added to the model of ourselves and becomes part of these schemata; a woman's power of localization may extend to the feather in her hat" (p. 606).

We need only a few words to explain the third symptom, loss of localization of touch. From it Head concludes the existence of "another schema or model of the surface of our bodies which also can be destroyed by a cortical lesion" (p. 606). Although the movement and the surface schemata are not identical, they must normally be in close interconnection, both being closely related parts of the same Ego system. The surface model is much less transient than the postural one, it survives more or less intact even when a limb has been amputated; such patients possess for a long time "phantom limbs" which can be carriers of movement and pain. It is interesting that one of Head's patients who had lost his leg before his brain lesion, and had experienced movements in the phantom leg and foot, lost his phantom when, through a stroke, he lost all recognition of posture (p. 606). This seems to indicate a very close connection between the surface and the posture schemata, although we do not know whether the abolition of the posture schema would also have destroyed the localization of pain in the phantom leg.

Bartlett's Generalization. Before we proceed a few words are in place about the interpretation and amplification which Bartlett has given to Head's theory. Although I am not sure that I understand Bartlett correctly, I believe that two aspects can be distinguished in his attitude. On the one hand, because of his theory of remembering as an active process which we shall discuss in the next chapter, he is, to say the least, wary about the notion of traces; on the other hand he seems to employ the term schema in a sense which goes far beyond Head's intention, although it is not in contradiction with it.

Bartlett's Position with Regard to Traces. The Store-house Conception. As regards the first point, I am not certain whether Bartlett wants to eliminate the concept of traces completely. Though many of his passages may be read this way, I do not believe that this is his real purpose, while on the other hand I cannot find out what he considers to be the nature of such traces as must be kept in his system. Head had spoken of the sensory cortex as a "store-house of past impressions," and this notion of a store-house is severely criticized by Bartlett with arguments very similar to those which I employed against the same idea in a discussion of memory: "The unconsciousness has been likened to a store-house. But what a strange store-house we find it to be! Things do not simply fall into those places into which they are being thrown, they arrange themselves in coming and during their time of storage according to the many ways in which they belong together. And they do more; they influence each other, form groups of various sizes and kinds, always trying to meet the exigencies of the moment. A miraculous store-house indeed." (1927, p. 66.) This quotation from my old article is evidence of my perfect agreement with Bartlett as regards the store-house idea as such. But in arguing against this conception Bartlett goes so far as to give the impression that he argues not only against the store-house, but also against traces. "All that his [viz., Head's] experiments show is that certain processes cannot be carried out unless the brain is playing its normal part. But equally those very reactions could be cut out by injuries to peripheral nerves or to muscular functions. One might almost as well say that because nobody who is suffering from a raging toothache could calmly recite 'Oh, my love's like a red, red rose,' the teeth are a repository of lyric poetry" (p. 200). This attitude is reminiscent of Wheeler's, which we have previously criticized. It is hardly necessary to point out that a removal of the offending tooth, which would stop the toothache, would restore the ability to recite Burns' love song. The plausibility of Bartlett's argument rests on his phrase "unless the brain is playing its *normal* part." Here the word "normal" obscures the issue. What is the brain's normal part? Since it is different today from what it was yesterday by virtue of the experience of the intervening time, we have to assume traces as previously explained. But, as I said before, other passages in Bartlett's book indicate that he does not reject traces altogether. "It now becomes possible to see that, though we may still talk of traces, there is no reason in the world for regarding these as made complete at one moment, stored up somewhere, and then re-excited at some much later moment. The traces that our evidence allows us to speak of are interest-determined, interest-carried traces. They live with our interests and with them they change" (pp. 211-12). Again the reader will find the negative part of this quotation in perfect agreement with the theory here propounded. How near our theory comes also to the positive aspect, the influence of interest on traces, will become manifest soon. My only criticism is that Bartlett, if he is interpreted literally, seems to go too far. There are, as we have pointed out, autonomous changes in traces; also it seems quite unwarranted to assume that a trace is obliterated as soon as our particular interest which was active at the time of its formation has died.

SCHEMA AS ORGANIZATION. This leads us to our second point, Bartlett's generalized use of the word schema. Whereas Head definitely restricted this term to postural and surface models of ourselves, Bartlett gives a much wider meaning to the word: " 'Schema' refers to an active organization of past reactions, or of past experiences, which must always be supposed to be operating in any well-adapted organic response. That is, whenever there is any order or regularity of behaviour, a particular response is possible only because it is related to the similar responses which have been serially organized, yet which operate—not simply as individual members coming one after another, but as a unitary mass. . . . There is not the slightest reason, however, to suppose that each set of incoming impulses, each new group of experiences persists as an isolated member of some passive patchwork . . ." (p. 201). The term schema thus has acquired the meaning of past experience as *organized.* It covers our aggregations and all other forms of communication and unifications between trace systems and thereby reveals a great affinity between Bartlett's theory of memory and our own. Two critical remarks must, however, be added. In the first place the last quotation undoubtedly attributes too much to memory. Memory is made responsible for any "order or regularity of behaviour." But we have shown at length how order and regularity *must* occur without memory. Bartlett seems to allow too much to traditional empiricism when he makes this statement. He goes far beyond this traditional empiricism in his theory of *organized* memory, his schema. But it is hard to understand why organization should be the privilege of memory. Once organization is admitted into the system as a real factor, such a restriction is *a priori* quite arbitrary. *A posteriori,* it does not fit the facts, and it makes the concept of organized memory itself almost untenable, since, as we have shown, organized memory depends upon organized experience, even though memorized and perceptual organization need not always coincide.

INSUFFICIENCY OF BARTLETT'S EGO THEORY. In the second place, Bartlett's generalization of the term schema omits the differentiation into Ego- and environmental trace systems which Head's concept of schema so happily introduced. Thus Bartlett's position seems less concrete than Head's. "If this view is correct, however, memory is personal, not because of some intangible and hypothetical 'self,' which receives and maintains innumerable traces, restimulating them whenever it needs; but because the mechanism of adult human memory demands an organization of 'schemata' depending upon an interplay of appetites, instincts, interests and ideals peculiar to any given subject" (Bartlett, p. 213). In my opinion Bartlett's opposition of a permanent hypothetical self and his schemata depending upon appetites, instincts, etc., tend to obscure the issue. To whom do the appetites, instincts, interests belong? Probably Bartlett would answer: To the organism, for in his exposition it is the organism that remembers: "An organism has somehow to acquire the capacity to turn round upon its own 'schemata' and to construct them afresh" (pp. 206, 202). But the schemata are parts of the organism, as well as the perceptions and interests. One *part* of the organism, that which embraces the interests, is, in Bartlett's theory, responsible for remembering, and this part is the one we call the Self or the Ego. This Ego develops in the trace structure along with the environment; to say that it receives traces can mean only that certain traces contribute to its continuous development, while other traces are not received by the Ego at all but accrue to those trace systems which form the non-Ego parts of the total field. Bartlett's theory, if it is to be a truly concrete theory, demands such a separate Ego, just as ours does; only in such a separate system is there a place for those factors which in his theory rightly play a dominating rôle, viz., the appetites and interests. Such an Ego system, both in process and trace, was introduced in Head's schemata. True, Head's notion has to be amplified: the Ego system is much more than those body schemata, and it is enclosed in and segregated from "environmental schemata." The theory here defended can therefore be regarded as a form of Bartlett's generalizations which includes the difference of Ego and environment in the trace system.

Ego- and Environment-Trace Systems Dynamically Interdependent. This point must be elaborated. In our theory the total field of excitation is divided into two major sub-systems, each containing numerous sub-systems of its own: the Ego and the environment. And the trace field which is created by the excitation field contains the same dichotomous organization. But these two partial systems are not independent parts, but sub-systems in the larger system of the total field and as such in dynamic interconnection, both in the process and in the trace phase. Therefore events in one of the systems will have their reverberations in the other: changes in the Ego, his desires and interests, will produce changes in the environmental system, and *vice versa* modifications of the former will affect the latter: the Ego of a person who has never left his own village must for that very reason be different from the Ego of a person who is at home in every country of the world. Although the relation is mutual, it need not be symmetrical; the Ego system may, as a rule, very well be the dominant one. Furthermore, the growth of the two systems, the changes which they undergo during the period of the organism's life, must be very different from each other. The directedness of the Ego which was formerly mentioned (Chapter VIII, p. 332) contrasts with the more contingent character of the successive environments. Therefore the organization of these two sub-systems must follow different lines; nevertheless, even here the mutual influence exerted by the two sub-systems upon each other must not be neglected. Changes in the environmental trace system depend upon the conditions within the Ego system.

Aall's Experiments. This statement is substantiated by experiments of Aall's. He investigated the influence exerted on recall by the attitude of the learner. In one group of experiments the subjects were told that they would be tested the next day, in another that a test would be made at some indefinitely later time. In the first group the subjects, instead of being examined on the following day, were told that unfortunately the experiment could not be carried out; in both groups, however, a test was taken four or eight weeks later. The material to be remembered was in one set of experiments a story, in another a group of ten or six objects. The results show a strong tendency for that material to be better remembered which was learned with the attitude that it would be tested at an indefinitely later time. When, however, in new experiments the subjects of the first group, expecting to be tested on the following day, were told that the test would have to be postponed to a later period, the difference between the two groups decreased considerably. Aall's highly suggestive experiments and theoretical considerations, which in some respects foreshadow some of Lewin's concepts and methods, are a first attempt at connecting memory processes with conative ones. Naturally they leave many important issues unsettled—among them, the influence of the learned material, although incidentally Aall reports that the two different attitudes gave no very clear difference in the recall of meaningless material. Positively, they seem to establish the fact that the trace systems depend upon their relation to the Ego system, being influenced by stresses within it that correspond to the purposes of the learner. Thus they confirm and supplement the much later results of Zeigarnik which we have previously discussed (Chapter VIII, p. 337) and in which stresses within the trace systems themselves and between the trace and the Ego-system also exerted an influence on recall and consequently in all likelihood upon the trace systems.

OTHER CONSEQUENCES. This interrelatedness between the trace system of Ego and environment has many consequences of which we shall discuss but a few. If an object in our behavioural world stood in a definite relation to our Ego, this connection will persist in the trace system, so that when we encounter the same geographical object the corresponding behavioural one will be produced in a field determined by this trace and will therefore carry the old Ego-relation. This is the theory of the permanence of the functional characters which we have indicated in the ninth chapter (p. 393).

Furthermore, if an environmental trace is in close connection with the Ego system it will not only be in communication with the particular time structure of that system with which it communicated at the time of its formation; but because of the coherence of the whole temporal Ego system it will be in communication with later strata also. These relations, however, may be different in kind from those which connected the trace with the contemporaneous Ego, since the later strata are different from the earlier ones. It is tempting to use this conclusion in explanation of the well-known fact that we are apt to idealize our youth and all its surroundings. The home of our childhood days, which at the time was the "normal" and more or less "indifferent" environment, often acquires in later years a sort of halo. It seems at least plausible to interpret this as an effect of the communication between the old trace system of the home and recent strata of the Ego.

FORGETTING. THE AVAILABILITY OF TRACES

Of all the changes within trace systems none has received more attention by psychologists than that which manifests itself in what we call *forgetting*. And yet, the relation between forgetting and the changes in the traces is by no means simple. It will be the last problem of this chapter to clarify this relationship.

The term forgetting, like so many psychological terms taken over from common speech, refers to an accomplishment, even though it be a negative one, and not to a process. We speak of forgetting whenever a previous experience is not available on a present occasion, although its co-operation would help our present response. This lack of availability may have a number of different causes and therefore psychologically forgetting may entail a number of different processes. We have already (Chapter IX, p. 420) pointed out two different kinds of forgetting, cases where we fail to remember, although we might have remembered, and cases where we are really unable to remember. We must now follow up this clue and shall do so by investigating the causes responsible for inability to remember. In terms of our trace theory this means that the present process cannot come into communication with an older trace or trace system. This may be due to three causes: (1) The trace has disappeared, (2) the trace cannot exert an influence upon the present occasion, (3) the present occasion cannot communicate with the trace. Let us discuss these possibilities one by one.

(1) **Disappearance of a Trace.** Whether a trace can totally disappear or not, i.e., whether after a lapse of time the organism will be exactly the same as if the trace had never been formed, it is impossible to decide. A trace may, however, disappear in another way, viz., by being so transformed that it loses its individuality, and even its identity. Complete disappearance must therefore be considered as a limiting case of trace transformation. Two questions then arise, that of the causes of such transformation, and that of its nature. It has been an assumption, implicit if not explicit in traditional trace theories, that traces undergo gradual destruction by organic processes which attack each trace independently: the grooves in a scratched tablet are being gradually worn away by the "ravages of time." It is impossible in the present state of our knowledge either to prove or to refute this hypothesis. Thus it may well be that general metabolic processes which have no specific relation to traces will gradually exert a destructive influence upon them. But it seems safe to assume that by far the most powerful forces that transform our traces derive from the specific nature of these traces, their intrinsic structure, and their dynamic connection with other traces. Such influences may be destructive in various ways. We think in the first place of the low survival value of chaotic units discussed on page 507. If the coherence of such a figure is very weak, it may well disappear in the trace, which would then actually vanish as a trace of that particular chaotic figure. Since our be-

havioural field contains all the time a mass of more or less chaotic parts, a great deal of our experience will be forgotten by such a process of dissolution of traces. However, when we remember the example of the face (Fig. 50) from which we derived the low survival value of chaotic forms, still another possibility of destruction of traces obtrudes itself. We may raise the question: Does it make any difference to the trace of the original chaotic impression whether afterwards the figure has become well organized, the face discovered, or not? Unfortunately, as in so many cases, we possess as yet no experimental evidence to decide this question; but it remains possible, I should say even probable, that the reorganization of the pattern interferes directly with the recall of the old pattern, i.e., it exerts a direct influence upon the old trace. If this assumption were right, new processes could affect old traces, if for some reason or other they were in communication. This conclusion seems highly plausible. It would explain the fact that it is often very difficult, if not impossible, to recall the old condition of a building, a street, after it has been rebuilt. In this case the old trace has not disappeared completely. Enough of it must have remained to enable us to remember that there was an old building, different from the present one, which we entered a certain number of times—in many cases this kind of memory will not be entirely carried by the language system, although this can never be totally excluded—but the old trace must have been severely affected by our new recurring perceptions of the new building to justify the proposition that in a sense the old trace has given place to a different one.

To these two possible causes of destruction of traces, autonomous through lack of cohesion and heteronomous through communication with a new process, we can add a third: heteronomous through communication with other traces. This case is realized in the aggregations investigated by von Restorff. Here a trace disappears by losing its individuality in a larger, badly articulated aggregate. Such aggregates, again, must be formed continually, because our lives contain innumerable repetitions. The traces of such repeated occurrences must form aggregates, just like the repeated elements in von Restorff's series or the repeated impressions in a series of threshold experiments (Lauenstein). An everyday experience which many of my readers may be able to confirm: Every night before retiring I wind my watch. And every night before turning out my light, I check up whether I have actually wound it. A fe · minutes after the act the trace is still intact as the trace of having wound it *tonight;* but soon it disappears as such and melts into the aggregate of traces of having wound my watch without temporal locus. It has lost its individuality.

Many psychologists have pointed out the benefits which we derive from forgetting and which to some extent balance the disadvantages. Our discussion has revealed a number of causes why such forgetting is necessary owing to the properties of the traces themselves.

(2) **Unavailability of the Trace.** The second point: unavailability of the trace at the moment, though it is of enormous significance, has as yet hardly been investigated. Probably there are many different reasons which may prevent a trace from influencing a present field. Here we take up a few examples to discover some of the causes. How can we explain our search for a name, a process which has been frequently discussed in psychological literature (notably by G. E. Müller)? For some reason or other I happen to think of a person, a mountain, a town, but I cannot recall its name. Half an hour, four hours, a day later, the name will suddenly emerge, a proof that the failure to recall it originally cannot be due to a true loss of the trace. The fact that the name comes to consciousness later may also shed some light on the causes which shut off the old trace from the new process. The situation of failing to recall a name is a situation of an incompleted task, i.e., the psychophysical field contains a part system under stress which can only be relieved by the recall of the name. That eventually such recall takes place forces us to assume that this stress in the (Ego-) trace system must have had an effect on the name trace system. We might venture to assume that this stress in the Ego system has broken through a barrier which shut off the name trace from the present field. If this assumption is near the truth—and we have already shown why we have to assume an influence of the Ego system upon the trace systems—then we must conclude that the temporal stratification of traces is one of the factors which determine their availability. A trace within its stratum is connected with the Ego of the same stratum, but may be far removed from the Ego of a later stratum. Such an hypothesis would explain certain effects of frequency and recency upon recall. If a process occurs at frequent intervals, then through aggregation of the respective traces the developing trace system will be in communication with different strata of the Ego system, and will be more readily available for that reason. If the trace, on the other hand, is of recent origin, its stratum will not be very far removed from the present stratum, so that the barrier which might separate it will be less strong.

Mere temporal sequence, however, is but one factor in this complex dynamic connection. Availability of the trace, in cases considered at the moment, depends upon proper connection between the trace system and the Ego. Now this connection depends upon a host of factors, among which the so-called conative ones are probably of paramount importance. If a trace is derived from a process which was directly connected with a person's interests, then it will have its place in a field formed by processes of high intensity and will be in particularly close connection with the Ego system. Such traces then are favoured for many reasons. Belonging to a sphere of interest, these traces will find ready a trace system with which they will communicate, and ever new traces will be formed which communicate with the same system, enlarging and stabilizing it continually. For aggregation with its detrimental results is but one of many ways in which traces can communicate. Instead of mere aggregates, in which the individual members more or less lose their identity and individuality, articulated gestalt systems may be built up in which the individual members preserve their individuality qua significant parts, in which they may even gain new dynamic properties as the whole whose parts they are is enlarged. Moreover, if aggregation takes place not between different members of the same class, as in von Restorff's experiments, but between more or less identical experiences, then the mere aggregation will have a conservative effect on the trace, a conclusion which is borne out by the results of Perkins's experiments which we discussed above. The change towards symmetry was more rapid over a long time interval when during this period no reproductions were made than when during this time the figures were reproduced once or several times.

Furthermore, as long as the interest lasts, not only do these factors remain operative, but ever new Ego strata are being brought into relation with the trace system, and this again makes it possible for the trace system to communicate with more and more other, non-Ego, trace systems. When the interest dies, all this is changed. The large system which has been gradually built up may disintegrate because parts of it may become connected with other interests. The original trace will become more and more isolated and more and more separated from the stratum of the present. In this sense we can therefore subscribe to Bartlett's thesis that traces are "interest-determined, interest-carried" (see p. 519).

In our discussion of the executive we distinguished several cases according to the origin of the forces which started and controlled it (Chapter VIII, p. 344). There were forces within the Ego system, forces within the environmental field, and forces between these two parts of the total field. The same distinction has to be applied to our present problem: the availability of a trace may depend upon either of the three factors, whereas so far we have only discussed the third, the Ego-environmental forces. But what is true of these is equally true of the others. How the survival of a trace depends upon its connection with larger, environmental, trace systems, we have already discussed. Its availability will also depend upon this factor. A trace strongly organized within a larger trace system will, on many occasions, be less available, though it has a higher survival value, than a trace that has preserved a greater degree of independence. We shall revert to this in the next chapter when we discuss thinking.

The same principles apply to pure Ego traces. Parts of the Ego may gradually lose their connection with others, so that those traces which belong to the isolated parts become less available. To some extent this is a normal process, resulting from the development of the Ego. The effects are, however, particularly striking in abnormal cases, where the separation of some part of the Ego from the rest has acute emotional causes. The fact that in such cases recall of events, totally "forgotten" in normal life, is possible under hypnosis, fits well into our theory, if we assume that in the hypnotic state radical transformations of the Ego system occur.

(3) **Failure of the Process to Communicate with an Otherwise Available Trace.** Whereas the first two causes of the non-availability of traces for present processes lay in the traces themselves, the third resides in the processes which fail to communicate with a trace which other processes may easily connect with. Again there must be various causes which account for that failure. Their nature will become clear only after we have answered the converse question as to the factors which produce communication between a present process and a trace. The little that is known about this interaction will be discussed in the next chapter. This last point, however, is no longer, strictly speaking, a case of *inability* to remember, but one where we fail to do so. And whether the cases of our second point should be considered as the one or the other is a matter of taste, depending upon our definition of inability. As a matter of fact, our discussion of the causes of the non-availability of traces has shown the relation in which the two types of forgetting which we formerly distinguished stand to each other. We need hardly add that our

three points are not meant to be mutually exclusive. In each concrete case all factors play some part, either conflicting with or reinforcing each other.

With this discussion we have established our theory of traces. In the next chapter we shall investigate more specifically the rôle which the trace systems play in actual processes.

CHAPTER XII

LEARNING AND OTHER MEMORY FUNCTIONS I

Definition of Learning. Learning as Accomplishment and as Process. The Positions of Lashley and Humphrey. Learning as Process. When Does It Take Place? Learning and Traces. Learning and Repetition. Three Problems Involved in Learning. Learning Defined by Process. Consolidation of Traces. Availability of Traces. Formation of Traces. The *New* Process. The After-effect of Traces. Acquisition of Skills. Associative Learning. The Doctrine of Associationism. Theory of Rote Learning. Summary: Arbitrary Connections Replaced by Dynamic Organizations. Association as a Force. Lewin. Other Types of "Associative Learning." The General Field-Influence Exerted by a Trace upon a Process

DEFINITION OF LEARNING

In our last chapter we developed a theory of "memorial fields," i.e., we tried to establish certain principles which explain why the psychophysical field at any one moment is affected by events which occurred in the past. We shall now test our trace theory by examining what light it sheds on those processes which evidently depend upon previous experience. In common parlance the term *learning* is used to denote this problem. For a long time learned activities were sharply distinguished from original or inherited ones, and a number of theories were proposed to explain this difference and with it the nature of learning. Lashley distinguishes five major types of such theories, some of them including several special modifications, and finds none of them acceptable in view of the established facts (1929 a, pp. 556 f.). It will not be necessary to repeat the criticism of these theories after Lashley's trenchant and lucid discussion, which was preceded and followed by other attacks (e.g., Koffka, 1928, and Tolman). Instead we shall discuss the meaning of the term learning in order to have a safe basis for our own theory.

"Learning amounts to a change or modification of behaviour" (Woodworth, p. 163), or more fully: "In general, however, we may say that learning is taking place wherever behaviour shows a *progressive change* or *trend,* with a repetition of the same stimulating situation and where the change cannot be accounted for on the basis of fatigue or of receptor and effector changes" (Hunter, p. 564). Humphrey, to quote lastly from this author, claims that modification of behaviour, though a necessary criterion, is not a sufficient criterion of learning. "Where there is learning the later actions of the series ordinarily differ from the earlier ones in the direction of the organism's advantage." And: "In order then to exhibit learning, a series of organic actions must first of all be such that later terms presuppose earlier ones, which is the same thing as to say that modification has taken place; but in addition the series will generally show a general approximation to an optimal term, optimal, that is to say, from the point of view of systemic conservation" (p. 105).

LEARNING AS ACCOMPLISHMENT AND AS PROCESS. THE POSITIONS OF LASHLEY AND HUMPHREY

All three authors, and the last most clearly and consciously, define learning as an *accomplishment* and not as a process or performance. Thus by their definition they raise the problem as to the nature of the process or processes which account for this accomplishment, a problem which Lashley formulates in these terms: ". . . we are justified in raising the question whether the concept of learning or of memory embraces a unitary process which can be studied as a single problem, or whether it may not instead cover a great variety of phenomena having no common organic basis" (p. 525). Humphrey, on the other hand, intends to find such a common principle in all learning accomplishments. We have seen in Chapter X that he rejects any theory of learning which introduces a specific new factor different from those that explain other types of behaviour. His positive thesis is that learning can be explained as an *integrated* reaction, integrated not only in space but also in time. ". . . it may be repeated that starting from the conception of the organism as reacting or adjusting to a single stimulus or situation, learning must be considered as the process of making an adjustment or total reaction to a total series of such stimuli or situations. It is essentially similar to the process familiar as the act of responding to a situation by means of an integrative process. It involves no new principle, but merely the extension of one already known" (p. 104). "All integration is four dimensional, it is integration of organic processes, events, corresponding to external changes that are four dimensional also. . . . If, then, we regard the act of 'associative memory' not in itself but together with the preceding acts that go to form the total relevant series, we have a unified total Response to a four-dimensional Situation, requiring four-dimensional integration of neural impulses" (p. 117). "Köhler's chimpanzee connected into a unity two sticks and the banana which were simultaneously presented in space. The animal's reaction is to the total spatio-temporal situation including these three specific elements, which the creative, integrative activity of the animal has interrelated. In the same way the animal learning by repetition effects a similar creative integration involving the similar elements in the repeated situation" (pp. 119-20). "Learning has been defined as the act of adjustment to a complex repetitive situation" (p. 124). The difference between Lashley and Humphrey is more apparent than real. It hinges on the term "common organic basis." If this is to mean that special "mechanism" involved in different acts of learning, Humphrey would agree thoroughly with Lashley; but by his unitary theory of learning he means a community of principle or law, which under different conditions, i.e., for different performances and in different individuals and species, may lead to very different actual occurrences, but as such is nevertheless the same in all of them. And this, Lashley in his turn might easily accept.

Criticism of Humphrey. As previously stated I am in full accord with Humphrey in his attempt at explaining learning, or memory, without the introduction of a special faculty. But his solution, as presented in the preceding quotations, seems to me at least incomplete. I am not certain whether I understand Humphrey correctly; therefore the following critical remarks, although aimed at him, may not strike him; even so they would not be entirely lost inasmuch as they deal with a position which it is tempting to take.

Four-dimensional Organization. We have argued ourselves (in Chapter X) that reality cannot be treated in terms of space alone, that the time dimension must necessarily be included. From this insight it is easy to pass on to a theory in which the four-dimensional space-time continuum plays the same rôle which the three-dimensional space continuum plays in spatial organization, a rôle in which all four dimensions are absolutely equivalent. Such a theory, if it were tenable, would solve many of our problems much more directly and simply. We might, e.g., consider a one-dimensional structure in this four-dimensional continuum different from a point, like a melody. And then we could say that the melody was organized in the time dimension just as a curve is organized in space-dimensions. I resisted this temptation in the case of the melody, and other temporal units, because it seemed to me to be no more than a formal analogy devoid of a concrete dynamical meaning. Since I shall now criticize Humphrey's application of a similar conception to learning I shall omit a detailed discussion of my refusal to treat time units in this manner. Moreover, several of my reasons are implicitly contained in my earlier arguments. My criticism of Humphrey starts from his concept of the total four-dimensional situation to which there is a total and *unified* response. The quotation from page 105 given on page 530 continues: "Because the series consists of related terms it is a unity." I find both terms, "total situation" and "four-dimensionally integrated reaction," inadequate not because they are intrinsically bad, but because without further elaboration they are not concrete enough. How is the "total situation" to be defined? We saw the difficulty inherent in this concept when it is used in a purely spatial connotation (see Chapter IV, pp. 158 f.). How much more difficult does it become when the time dimension is included! Without modification the "total situation" is the whole spatio-temporal life history of the person. But no process is explained if it is referred to this practically infinite mass of events. Humphrey, very appropriately, speaks of repetitions of a stimulus situation which form a total situation in their entirety, i.e., he specifies "total situations" so as to mean something different for each special occasion. If I learn to type, the former occasions on which I practised, together with the present, form the total situation; if I try to learn to play tennis, all my efforts in this direction make the total situation, etc., etc. Therefore, the specific total situation cannot simply be taken for granted; instead we must explain why certain past events and not others join with the present occasion to form a total situation. The mere recourse to four-dimensional space-time avails us nothing in the solution of this problem. The same conclusion arises from a different starting point. Not all objects "learn," although they all occur and behave in the four-dimensional continuum. A billiard ball is "as good" when it is brand new as after it has been used for years, because it is so elastic that it regains its original shape after each deformation produced by cue or cannoning ball. For the billiard ball the past does not exist. Therefore, objects which have memory, be they pieces of wire or human organisms, must be different from billiard balls, in the sense that they *never* regain their old status completely, once they have been affected. We called the change which cannot be completely annihilated in objects with memory, a trace. By means of this concept, finally, we were able to overcome another difficulty inherent in Humphrey's four-dimensional total situation: the difficulty, namely, how the past can affect the present (see Chapter X, p. 429), a difficulty which seems to me not solved by the mere reference to space-time.

Let us now turn to the second term, the unity of the learning series, the four-dimensionally integrated reaction. While our attitude to the first, the four-dimensional total situation, was to consider it incomplete without the assumption of traces and a principle of selection, our attitude to the second must be somewhat different. The term applies very well to melodies and other temporal units. But does it apply in the *same way* to the progressive learning series? Humphrey, although he has not discussed the example of the melody, has seen this difficulty. He compares an ordinary purposive activity with learning activities and claims that they are essentially similar in nature. "The fact that learning ordinarily implies an intermittent series of actions, the animal being put into the maze three times a day, for example, while in the interval it is in its cage, does not constitute an essential difference between the purposive and the learned activity. For many 'purposes' are interrupted in the same way" (p. 127). Now one may well admit that interruptions qua interruptions do not constitute an essential difference between the two kinds of activities and yet may withhold assent to the statement that therefore the two activities are essentially similar. For a purposive activity or a melody completed after an interruption is still one and the same action or melody. The dynamic situation is such that the completion is demanded and that the interruption has the function of an obstacle. But the repetition of a purposive action or of a melody is not the same action or melody as the first; there need be nothing in the dynamic situation that demands repetition. The second occurrence, besides being numerically different, will also in many cases be qualitatively different—that is what we call learning, and that is what we want to explain. To call the first and the second event together a total reaction seems to me neither to be correct nor to supply that explanation. It is not correct in the sense in which *one* action or melody is a total reaction, for in these all parts demand and support each other in one continuous process, or if the purposive act is interrupted before completion, at least in one directed tension. Particularly in the melody the end requires the middle and the beginning and derives its meaning from them, while in the repetitions of one and the same event no such relation necessarily holds. If, for instance, a person could execute a perfect tennis stroke the first time he made it, all the training that is ordinarily necessary would be superfluous. A perfect stroke is a perfect stroke and no different whether it is executed after much or little practice. Furthermore, often enough the repetition occurs undemanded by the earlier occasions. That means: the later process, which derives some of its characteristics from the earlier ones, often requires the occurrence of some event in the geographical environment that is contingent or adventitious with regard to the previous events. These previous events are over and done with, they contain in themselves no factor that can produce an occasion for the renewed occurrence of a similar event. A very simple example: a person comes for the first time in his life to a place where there is heavy snow. He will find walking through the slippery streets a very difficult task. If the snow stays on the ground, he will gradually become more sure-footed, but his action of walking on it is over when he has reached his destination, and whether the snow stays or goes or whether a new blizzard presents him with new opportunities for "practising" has nothing to do with his accomplishment. This contingency of the occasions that are necessary for the repetition of the processes again makes it impossible for me to accept the sum of the subsequent repetitions as one total response.

Learning as Process. When Does It Take Place? This criticism of some of Humphrey's concepts does not, however, imply that we disagree with him in his general position that learning must be explained without the introduction of a new specific principle. To see this, and thereby how close our position is to Humphrey's, we shall analyze some learning activities raising the question *when* in these activities learning takes place. Since the greater part of learning occurs without the intention to learn, we shall choose cases of this kind. They include all animal learning, for an animal in its trials runs for food or to escape punishment, or to explore, or for some other reasons, but certainly not in order to learn. The same is true of many human activities, such as the one last discussed, the improvement of a person's ability to walk on slippery streets, and also of the acquisition of language by an infant, or the "learning of the lesson of experience" in the social situations of the adult; here the behaviour is directed towards good and tactful conduct, and again not towards learning.

But let us start from a simple example. How does the stranger from a more clement climate learn to walk safely over frozen ground? Let us, for simplicity's sake, assume that already on the second occasion he is more skilful. Is this second performance the learning? Certainly not; it is, as everyone will agree, a learned activity to the extent that it is dependent upon the first. Then the first performance must be the learning activity, and yet it had nothing to do with learning qua learning, but served only the purpose of going from one place to another. As such, then, it has no claim to be called a learning activity, whereas viewed retrospectively from the improved second performance it must be so called. What is true of the first holds equally for the second, for a third performance would show a new improvement, and so forth.

Learning and Traces. This case is typical, and it shows that *any* activity might be called a learning activity, provided it fulfilled some special conditions which we shall state later. This proposition might look like a purely verbal solution of a real problem, but this is not its intent. We can show in what respect, or why, an activity is a learning activity. Supposing that the organism, after a process had occurred in its psychophysical field, returned completely to its old state, like the billiard ball of our previous discussion. Then each process occurring on repeated occasions would be similar to the first process, differing from it only inasmuch as the external conditions, or the desires and interests of the organism, were different. But the former performances could not be responsible for improvement in the later ones: the same system exposed to the same forces for a number of times must react each time in exactly the same manner. As a response to the set of external and internal conditions the first response is thus *not* a learning response, for it might be the same as it is now if the organism were totally "elastic," i.e., if it re-instated its old condition completely after the performance is past. But we know that the organism is not of this kind; it cannot return to its old state because the process itself effects a permanent change in it, the trace. Such a changed organism, if exposed a second time to the same stimulus situation, must, qua different organism, behave differently the second time from what it did the first time. Therefore the first performance, inasmuch as it leaves a trace, is a learning process, provided we use modification of behaviour as synonymous with learning, a usage which Humphrey has criticized for good reasons, reserving the term learning for such modifications as show "improvement." Improvement looks like a purely pragmatic criterion. Although I agree with Humphrey that it is not, but points to a much more essential feature of the modification, I shall leave this point open for the moment. At present it is sufficient to point out that the process by leaving a trace must modify later processes in some respects, improvement being but one of the possibilities. But all possibilities of modification, whether we dub them learning or not, must be derivable from the same principle, the special kind of modification depending upon the particular nature of the case in a manner to be discussed presently.

Our Theory Consistent with Humphrey's Main Principle. But first it will be worth our while to consider how far we have lived up to Humphrey's principle that no new factor is to be introduced to explain learning. The result of such reflection must be that we have not violated this postulate. We included in our explanation nothing but the process itself with its effect on the organism, called a trace. This is no new assumption. It is not self-evident that a process should leave no trace, and therefore the assumption of such a trace is not the introduction of a new factor. The organism is in this respect similar to many inorganic systems. Therefore, if we use the term in the widest possible sense, it is perfectly correct to say that every process is in some respect a learning process.

Learning and Repetition. This wide use of the term has, however, its disadvantages. To quote again from Humphrey: "A burnt child that used its experience in order to acquire deftness in plunging its hands into the flames would be a candidate for an institution" (p. 105). To give a different example: repetition may lead to bad habits as well as to good ones; thus it is very difficult to learn to pronounce a word correctly once one has acquired the habit of pronouncing it incorrectly, a fact I know well from my own experience.[1] The same is true in acquiring a motor skill, be it the proper stroke at tennis, the position of the body in skiing, or anything else. One may easily start "wrong" and then acquire bad habits which will prevent one from really "learning" the desired activity. In such cases practice does not lead to an "optimum," regarded from the point of view of adjustment to the specific situation, even though the modifications produced by such bad practice may have a direction towards a final term. And so we can now resume the question which we held in abeyance as to the causes which determine the rôle of practice or repetition; whether it leads to real learning in Humphrey's sense, to bad habits, or has no effect at all. An example for this last case is taken from Köhler's anthropoid work. The reader may remember that one of the problems set to the apes required the stacking of boxes for the attainment of the goal. This activity became a real pastime for the animals, which practised it continually over a long period, with the striking result that they showed no improvement whatever. Their stacking was, at the end as at the beginning, a mere piling of one box on top of one or two others without any regard to the stability of the structure achieved. Only because of their great skill and uncanny bodily balance were they able to reach the suspended fruit before the shaky edifice on which

[1] This is in no contradiction to Dunlap's position that a bad habit is most easily broken by repetition. For in the cases considered by him the bad repetition takes place with the knowledge that it is bad, and that introduces of course an entirely new set of conditions.

they stood collapsed. Köhler's film and to some extent the pictures in his book show the nature of this performance which will raise the hair of the spectator. Why, however, was there no improvement? Why did the traces of the previous performances not influence the execution of the later ones so as to make them progressively better and better? Why, otherwise expressed, was the practice of the apes in box stacking so different in its effects from the practice of a human pupil in a typewriting school?

Repetition of Accomplishment and Repetition of Process. No explanation can be given as long as one thinks of these activities in terms of accomplishment. If one activity improves through practice while another one does not, the reason must be that the traces are different in the two kinds of practice in such a way that this difference accounts for the difference in the effect of practice. This does not mean that the traces of the two *accomplishments,* typing and box stacking, are thus different; for one could think of conditions under which practice with the typewriter causes no gain in typing ability—e.g., when a child plays with it before he can read or write—and conversely box stacking by human beings may very well be improved by practice. Therefore the processes which produce the traces must be different in two activities which show such different effects of practice, no matter whether these processes correspond to the same or to different accomplishments. In the case of the apes, box stacking was merely the action of getting one on top of the other; the aspect of doing this in a mechanically stable way, involving definite spatial relationships of the top of the lower and the bottom of the higher box, was totally absent from their behaviour, i.e., from the processes which actually occurred in their psychophysical field, and therefore also from the traces which these processes left behind. But the trace field as a remnant of a process distribution has nothing in it to influence a new process occurring under similar stimulus conditions that would make the process distribute itself in a direction different from the one to which it owes its existence. Rather, the ordinary facts of practice prove that repetition of activity A will create an aggregated trace system of such a kind that activity A will become more stable and regular and thereby exclude variation into a very different activity B. Applied to the box stacking this means that improvement of this performance can occur in the direction of greater stability of the structures created only when at one stage in the series of building activities the process itself has something to do with this stability so that the trace left by it can influence the following performance. Generally speaking, if an accomplishment X involves the aspects A, B, C . . . , then improvement can occur only in those aspects which were, in however low a degree, also represented in the *process* and were thereby left in the trace system. Since every accomplishment is of this type, repetition can lead to improvement only to the extent to which the partial aspects are present in performances. If, in accomplishing X, I have not *performed* A, although I have *accomplished* it, this performance will have no practice effect for the future accomplishment of A, however much practice effect it may have on other aspects of X which were part of my actual performance.

Repetition of Occasion. Its Two Functions. Consequently repetition of the same accomplishment may have very different effects if during this series an aspect A occurs for the first time. Before this occurrence repetition can have no effect for A; afterwards it can. Repetition of the *occasion,* therefore, has a double function for learning. On the one hand it gives a number of opportunities for the particular process to occur for the first time. Up to that point it has no influence on later performances of this process. On the other hand, once the particular process has occurred each repetition will add to the particular trace system or aggregate and thereby exert an influence on later performances. Since repetitions have thus a different function before and after a critical occasion the mere counting of repetitions *per se* does not seem to be valuable for a better understanding of the learning process unless the experimenter knows beforehand that the process in the development of which he is interested occurred at the first repetition. Therefore, much experimental work on memory possesses less significance than has been attributed to it.

REPETITION OF PROCESS AND TOLMAN'S POSITION: THE LAW OF FREQUENCY. According to our theory repetition affects learning directly only qua repetition of the process. This seems at first sight to be in contradiction to Tolman's position, although a closer inspection seems to me to reveal that the two positions are more or less identical. Tolman distinguishes between two meanings of the law of frequency, one of which he considers correct; the other, the one usually given to it, he shows to be contradicted by the facts. "The Law of Exercise . . . holds, we shall assert, when that which is meant by exercise is frequent and recent repetition of the whole stimulus situation, irrespective of whether in the given trial the animal chooses a correct or an incorrect path. Exercise in this sense means the frequency and recency with which the whole problem, as a problem, is met and responded to" (p. 346). "In the second meaning of the Law of Exercise . . . what is meant by frequent and recent exercise seems to be frequent and recent 'differential' exercise upon the correct path at the expense of the incorrect paths" (p. 347). These statements might be read so as to contain a theory the direct opposite of the one here presented. Tolman's *true* law seems to treat repetition as repetition of an accomplishment, the false as that of a performance and process, whereas in our theory the rôles were exactly reversed. But as already pointed out, this impression would be erroneous. From Tolman's apt and trenchant refutation of the false interpretation it appears that in this form of the theory repetition really means accomplishment, and from the later statement of his own law, that the first interpretation really refers to performance or process. It is hardly necessary to devote much space to the interpretation rejected by Tolman, since its main supporter, Thorndike, has repudiated it himself on account of his own extended experiments. I shall only demonstrate by one example why Tolman's criticism can be translated into the terms: accomplishment vs. process. If an animal learns to run through the correct path because all blind alleys are blocked, then his *process* of running through these correct paths leads to the same *accomplishment* as that of an animal which makes a perfect run after having learned the maze with the blinds unobstructed, but qua process it is totally different. To run through the only open path is different from running over a path which at various points forks in two or more directions so as to necessitate a *choice*. Only when choice can occur during the learning will the performance have the "choice" character, otherwise it will not, and therefore an animal which has been trained with entrances of culs-de-sac blocked has *not* learned "the maze"; i.e., it will commit errors as soon as the blocks are removed. Tolman reproduces a quotation from Carr, from whose work this example is taken. With the omission of the first sentence this quotation follows: ". . . a certain number of errors must be made and eliminated before the subject is ever able to run the maze correctly. Correct modes of response are established in part by learning what not to do."

LEARNING WHAT NOT TO DO. Carr's highly instructive results offer a convincing argument against a wrong interpretation of the rôle of repetition. But Carr's words as just quoted do not do full justice to this significance, because Carr speaks in terms of accomplishment and not of performance. It is perfectly true to say, as he does, that in order to learn what to do we must also learn what not to do, but this statement, referring as it does to accomplishments, must be translated into terms of performance or process. Let us try to do this for the maze experiments under discussion. When the animal comes to a fork in the maze for the first time and enters a blind alley, this part of its behaviour is no different from the rest. When it then runs against the barrier and has to retrace its steps, something new *may* happen: the cul-de-sac may become a different kind of path from the ones it has traversed so far; and even its behaviour in running to the barrier may thereby become changed from "a continuation of the original run" into a "deviation." Now this change cannot, of course, occur in the process of this run itself, but in its recent trace system. The assumption that a recent trace may be changed by later processes is by no means introduced to explain just this particular case. It is a very common experience in music. Let a piece begin with the notes: c e d g . . . and after the second or third tone c will have become established as the "tonic"; but in another piece, which begins with c f e d . . . , f will assume this rôle and c that of the dominant. Another example is a statement such as this: "A motorist comes to a big sign: 'Fine for Parking' and there he parks." The last word of this sentence changes the meaning of the word "fine." Although puns are particularly fit for demonstrating this transformation, it occurs continually as we listen to speech; words gain their full meaning only from others that precede or follow after them.

Therefore we may now return to our maze. The wall at the end of the blind alley may retroactively change its behavioural characteristic and thereby also the behavioural aspect of the running through the alley, i.e., its nature as a process or performance. Thereby the other end of the fork will also be affected; in contrast to a "deviation" it will, eventually, become "the true path." Thus taking this path is, qua process, different for this animal which had the chance of entering a blind from what it is for an animal that finds all blinds blocked. Thus we have translated the "learning what to do by learning what not to do" from accomplishment language into process language. At the same time we have prepared an explanation of the rôle of success in learning.

Let us return to Tolman's two interpretations of the Law of Exercise. We see now that the second, which he rejects, is a law of accomplishment and therefore at fault. His first interpretation, viz., repetition of the whole stimulus situation irrespective of the fact of the animal's behaving correctly or incorrectly in it, is acceptable because it leaves room for the two functions of repetition which we deduced above (p. 538). Repetition of the same stimulus situation gives a chance for the arousal of the correct process, and after it has been aroused its repetition will strengthen it, because what is now repeated is the *proper* process and not a process which leads to the same accomplishment only under the particular conditions. But so far the Law of Exercise is, strictly speaking, not a law. When Tolman eventually formulates his law of frequency, he does it in terms of process: frequency and recency of the particular process will favour its recurrence. Since he expresses it in his own elaborate terminology which I do not want to explain here, I refrain from quoting his text (on p. 365 of his book).

THREE PROBLEMS INVOLVED IN LEARNING

We can summarize the preceding discussion in this way: the accomplishment of learning as a modification of behaviour can be analyzed on its process side into three different constituents: (1) the arousal of a specific (the "correct") process; (2) the trace of this process; (3) the effect of this trace on later processes. In an earlier analysis (1925 a, 1928) I distinguished two problems of learning: the problem of *achievement* and the problem of *memory*. The problem of achievement refers to the first point of our analysis, the problem of memory to the two last. In our present treatment we have already dealt extensively with point (2) of our analysis, the formation and change of traces (in the last two chapters). In this and the next chapter we shall discuss the first and third point. That learning necessarily implies all three points is easy to demonstrate. If no new process ever occurred, there would by definition be no learning. If the new process left no trace, a recurrence of the conditions would not lead to an improved performance and the same would be true if the trace failed to influence the newly aroused process. The interconnection of the three problems is still closer. True enough, the arousal of a new process does not necessarily presuppose the existence of traces. At some time or other in the early history of each individual organism new processes must occur without pre-existing traces, and that such processes would possess their own intrinsic order has been shown in the discussion of Chapters IV and V. It is quite a fascinating task to speculate how much a fictitious organism without any memory could achieve. We mentioned before that a person who, the first time he tried, could strike a tennis ball as well as a champion player would need no practice, and that means also no memory for this skill, and we might go on pursuing this line of thought. However, we shall leave this highly suggestive speculation to the reader who will, if he makes the attempt, discover easily enough for himself whether God needs memory or for which of his functions he needs it.

The Circular Relation Between Process and Trace as the Cause of Mental Development. We shall stay on this earth, and there new processes occur in systems already endowed with traces; it is this fact alone that makes mental *development* intelligible. For by occurring in trace-endowed systems processes will be influenced by these traces, and the *novelty* of a process itself may in a large measure be due to the traces. Such a *new* process leaves a *new* trace in its wake, which in its turn may contribute to the arousal of another *new* process which without it could not have arisen. Thus by processes making traces, and traces processes, the system is bound to develop if for the moment we mean by development the production of ever new processes. It is obvious that development in this sense depends entirely on the effects that traces can exert on later processes, i.e., on the solution of our problem (3).

Associationism and the Problem of Achievement. Traditional empiricism, which in the preceding chapters I so frequently made the butt of my criticism, has been the failure I consider it to be because it never recognized the full import of this problem. And this lack of insight is closely related to its complete elimination of the first problem, our problem of achievement. Empiricism has been based on two basic concepts: sensation and association. The first of these two has been criticized in an earlier chapter (Chapter III, p. 103 f.); the second one requires a few words of comment. I shall forbear to go into the long history of associationism. Suffice it to say that in this history the concept, while becoming more and more sharply defined, was at the same time narrowed down to one and only one type of relation. Whereas originally several kinds of association had been distinguished, viz., association by contiguity, by similarity, and by contrast, only the first survived in the process of development, reaching its climax in the concept of the conditioned reflex. Association by contiguity established a purely *existential* and *external* relation between *any* two events that happen to occur in spatial or temporal neighbourhood. The associative bond between the two items A and B is, according to strict associationism, due exclusively to their occurring together and is quite independent of the intrinsic characteristics of A and B. Radical associationism will even explain the differences between A and B, apart from differences in sensory content—blue, red, loud, sweet, etc.—by association: since association obtains as a rule not between "simple sensations"—a concept which was a crux in every associationistic system—but between perceived objects, these objects were themselves explained as complexes of sensations held together by particularly strong associative bonds. Thus associationists were by the very extension of their fundamental assumption prevented from ascribing any importance to the intrinsic qualities of the associated items, all such items differing from each other merely in associative combination and the sense qualities of their elementary constituents. Associationism was therefore bound to react violently against gestalt theory, which, as we demonstrated in the preceding chapters, has a very definite and important place for *real* intrinsic differences between behavioural objects, intrinsic differences which are not reducible to association. The most detailed and impassioned associationistic attack against gestalt theory came from G. E. Müller, who published a special monograph against it (1923). Since Köhler (1925 a) replied extensively to this attack, showing the inconsistencies of Müller's arguments and the *ad hoc* hypotheses which again and again he had to attach to his old system in order to deal with facts discovered by gestalt theorists, I need not pursue this matter any further.

The one important point for us to note about associationism is that it knows only one kind of connection or interaction between elements, that of association. Wherever parts of a larger whole are found to hang together in some way or other, such communication is described and treated as association, a purely external and existential bond. Thus the members of a learned series of nonsense syllables are not only associated one with the other—in various degrees, according to proximity and other factors—but also with the place they occupy in the total series, which in persons with imaginal diagrams like number-forms means association with a spatial locus, just as a quotation, whose position on the page we remember, is in this view associated with the particular part of the page. Similarly, if we see a square and not four lines, it is because these four lines have become associated, and so forth.

Such a theory can know no real problem of achievement. The new process which is to be learned, i.e., strengthened by repetition, is always a process of association, and since its one cause was considered to be contiguity, no problem even arose as to what produced such a new association. As far as I know, associationism, which based its theory on experiments of the rote learning type, has never felt the need to tackle this problem. A new situation for associationism arose, however, when the experimental base was changed. We gain a new point of view for evaluating the achievement of Thorndike's first animal experiments when we compare them with the experiments invented, refined, and almost endlessly repeated in Germany. For in Thorndike's experiments an animal has truly to learn something new which is not presented to it readymade as the nonsense syllables are to the human subject. Therefore something like our problem of achievement arose; how does the animal arrive at the correct response for the first time? But Thorndike's associationism prevented him from seeing the real significance of this problem, because he never doubted that associationism, or "connectionism"—an even more rigid form of the same general way of thinking—was the only way of explaining it. And so he invented his principle of multiple response, in which all responses that the animal can make in any situation are lying ready within the animal as inherited reflex connections. I have discussed Thorndike's theories in another book (1928, pp. 130, 138, 180 f.), and therefore refrain from repeating my argument. Against its critical tendency I want here to emphasize the great potential gain which psychology derived from the change of method introduced by Thorndike, a change of method which has prepared the way for the recognition of the true problem and has tremendously broadened the discussion of the problem of learning by the introduction of the much debated law of success which we shall discuss later.

LEARNING DEFINED BY PROCESS

Let us briefly summarize what we have gained, by giving a new explanatory definition of learning. Learning, as the modification of an accomplishment in a certain direction, consists in *creating* trace systems of a *particular kind,* in *consolidating* them, and in making them more and more *available* both in repeated and in new situations. This describes learning because available traces modify new processes and thereby achieve modification of behaviour and accomplishment.

Consolidation of Traces. Little need be said about the consolidation of traces, for we have discussed in various parts of our last chapter a number of causes which counteract consolidation. We may summarize these discussions in our present context by saying that consolidation will be achieved by stable articulate organization. Inarticulate organization, mere aggregation, is detrimental to consolidation, as von Restorff has shown, and similarly traces of chaotic processes are unstable. Articulate organization has two aspects. In the first place the individual trace may be more or less articulate, in the second the trace may be a more or less articulate and significant part in one or several larger trace systems. Thus repetition may play a third rôle which we have not yet discussed. If the same process occurs repeatedly in different contexts it may gain stability by the place it assumes in the trace systems of each of these contexts.

The rules which we have laid down for consolidation are not mere empirical rules but follow directly from our laws of organization. We know that segregation and unification require inhomogeneity and vary directly with the degree of inhomogeneity. In "aggregates" each trace finds itself in a quasi-homogeneous environment and must for that reason lack stability. Conversely, an "isolated" trace is a region of inhomogeneity, and for that reason stable. But we saw that degree of inhomogeneity is by no means the only factor determining organization. We found besides such factors as good continuation and closure. If we apply these to traces we are led to our rule that articulate organization favours stability. For a trace which forms a "good" part of a larger system is maintained by the forces of the whole system, while one that does not conform to the pattern of the whole will be exposed to forces within this whole which tend to change it.

A New Double Rôle of Repetition: A Paradox. Yet this cannot be enough. Repetition is without a doubt, to a certain extent and under definite conditions, a very powerful factor in stabilizing traces. This fact introduces into our theory a sort of paradox which we shall have to solve. For we saw that repetition cannot mean the strengthening of *one* trace but the building up of a trace system composed of as many members as there are repetitions. Thus we obtain necessarily an aggregate of traces which should interfere with consolidation. This seems paradoxical in view of the beneficial rôle which repetition plays in all learning, but in reality it is not. For the effect which we have just derived from our theory, interference with the stability of a trace by repetition of a process, actually occurs. There is loss of consolidation of the *single individual* traces which we are apt to overlook because it is accompanied by a gain in the stability of the *trace system*. When we learn to type, the individual lessons will soon be forgotten, and the clumsy movements which we originally executed will at a later stage be impossible; i.e., the traces of the first lessons have become changed by the aggregate of traces which has been produced by the many repetitions and is responsible for the improvement of the skill. Similarly, when we stay in a room for any length of time, we get a great number of impressions of it by moving about or merely letting our eyes roam. But only a few of them can be recalled. It is needless to give more examples. It is quite generally confirmed that repetition interferes with the individual traces, just as von Restorff's theory demands. At the same time, however, the trace system becomes more and more fixed, it acquires a greater and greater influence on future processes. It is therefore at least a plausible hypothesis to assume that the extension of the trace system is one of the factors which determine its efficacy, an extension which is steadily increased with each new repetition. Perhaps this conclusion should be correlated with Lashley's discovery that the extent to which behaviour deteriorates through brain injury is a direct function of the amount of tissue destroyed. Be this as it may, our paradox has been solved; we understand now how repetition can be beneficial to learning despite its destructive influence on individual traces.

Availability of Traces. Our discussion of the aspect of learning which concerns the availability of traces can be equally short. At the end of the last chapter we have said all we can say about the causes of availability. The applications to the learning process are too obvious to require further elaboration. Only one point may be added. In introducing the present topic we distinguished availability for identical or very similar and for different and new situations.

THE TRANSFER PROBLEM GENERALIZED. The latter has a great deal to do with the transfer problem. The name transfer implies that psychologists considered it as the "normal" case that a trace should influence a similar process, and therefore gave the name of transfer to cases where performances of one kind exerted, through their traces, an influence on different performances not separately practised. But this mode of treating the general problem, practical as it is for a number of special problems, does not seem to be entirely adequate to the fundamental problem of learning, if by learning we mean *any* influence exerted by a trace on a later performance. Viewed in this broad frame, the effect of a trace or a trace system on processes similar to those which have produced them is but a special case, and to consider it as the normal may easily distort our view of the problems involved. For we do not really know of what kind this influence is. It has to be studied in the same way as any other influence. Methodologically it is most simple to investigate learning by repetition of process, and the greater bulk of the vast literature on learning has used this method. But it would be wrong to ascribe a special importance or unique significance to a special case merely because it is most amenable to scientific treatment. A rat, to give an example, can be trained to go to the food box of a maze by being put into the entrance box in a hungry condition and being fed each time it reaches the food compartment. But experiments on so-called "latent learning," emphasized by Tolman (pp. 343 f.), have proved that a rat also learns the maze to a considerable extent if before the "critical runs," when it is hungry and finds food in the food chambers, it has been allowed to roam about the maze freely and explore it thoroughly. Here roaming around, following all sorts of different paths, has the effect that the "true" path is taken with far fewer errors than it would have been had the other activity not preceded the "critical" one. Cases like this demonstrate the inadequacy of the term transfer. If we called the effect of the latent learning a transfer, then we ought to know, or assume, what the direct, non-transfer, effect of the exploring runs is. Does the animal in these experiments learn directly to follow a very special path, an acquisition which can be "transferred" to a new, the "true," path? Certainly not. The animals do not, in these experiments, become fixed to any particular pattern of alleys before the critical runs begin. What they acquire is an orientation within the maze, a sort of "plan" of the maze. This acquisition, which has a direct effect on the discovery of the true path, is in itself a case where traces of one kind of process, i.e., roaming about, gradually produce another process, i.e., knowing the layout of the maze.

Possible Conflict Between Two Kinds of Availability. Drill. How traces become more available for such new processes is a question we cannot yet even begin to answer. All we can say is that it must depend upon the nature of the trace and the new process. However, one conclusion seems fairly safe: conditions which make a trace more and more available for mere repetition of one process will often make it at the same time less available for other processes. Thus the educator should be very conscious of his aims when he decides whether to apply drill or not. Drill will no doubt make the traces more and more available for one kind of activity, but it may at the same time narrow down the *range* of availability.

Formation of Traces. The "New" Process. We are then left with the first of the three effects found necessary for learning (see p. 544), the creation of the proper trace. Since traces are created by processes, this leads us to a consideration of process itself with regard to learning. We said before that *any* process might be considered as a learning process inasmuch as its repetition would, qua repetition, be different from the first occurrence. Therefore, when in our present context we treat of the *first* arousals of processes, we must be as inclusive as possible. We are dealing here with the problem previously named the problem of achievement; but this name is apt to bias our attitude towards the problem; we think of processes not easily aroused, achieved the first time with more or less difficulty, and by their very occurrence raising the intellectual level of the organism. But important as such cases are, they are not the only ones that must be considered now; we must include in our survey *every* new process, unconcerned with the degree of difficulty with which it is aroused. When we see an ink blot of a new shape, this perception is a *new* process; when we walk through a picture gallery and see new pictures, other new processes occur; again when we hear for the first time a new simple tune, or a complex piece of music. If we contrast with these cases the understanding of a mathematical proof or, even better, the discovery or invention of such a proof, we see the enormous variety of processes, different in quality and in ease of arousal; at the same time we see that with regard to the second point the difference is a graded one. There are not only cases where the process is aroused at once by the forces of the proximal stimuli and others where a long and laborious effort is necessary to produce it; there are numberless intermediate cases, as exemplified by the complex piece of music which we understand better with each new repetition. All cases, however, have one aspect in common: at a definite moment in the life history of the organism a certain process must arise for the first time and leave a corresponding trace which remains as a condition for an unlimited number of later processes. That this condition itself is not immutable we have discussed in the two preceding chapters, notably in our theory of forgetting. But the fact remains that potentially every new process may affect later processes through its trace, so that each process alters the organism, i.e., is a process of learning. Therefore our scientific attitude with regard to this accomplishment must of necessity be unduly limited if we view learning only as either rote learning or the acquisition of a motor skill, or the gradually improved performances in mazes or puzzle boxes. It is clear how emphasis on rote learning has led to the theory of associations, and how this theory in its turn has influenced the explanation of the other accomplishments first enumerated. If we free ourselves from the limitations imposed upon older theories by too narrow and one-sided a selection of empirical material, we shall gain a much broader view of the processes occurring in progressive learning.

"Innate" and "Acquired." At the same time the time-honoured distinction between innate and acquired processes gains a new aspect. As I have pointed out elsewhere (1932) it is wrong to speak of innate *processes*. What is innate is structure, structure which will carry processes only when special forces arouse them. Even the first processes, which occur when the organism has as yet no traces, cannot be called innate: they are the reactions of the traceless organism to a definite set of stimuli.

To stress this point may seem pedantic. Nobody can have meant anything else when he spoke of innate processes. But pedantry, as the making explicit of what previously had been at best implicit, may be very valuable by formulating the assumptions contained in a theory, so that one knows what they are and what they are not. In our case the formulation that structure is innate but processes are not, adds very definitely to the understanding of the nature-nurture dichotomy. For it makes it explicit that each process depends upon a *set* of conditions, of which the innate structure is one, the factual stimuli are another, and the laws of organization a third. That the second factor was extraneous to the dilemma of inherited vs. acquired would have been admitted by everyone, although it would not have appeared as a particularly important point. But that the third factor also lies entirely beyond this distinction has been overlooked for the mere fact that organization itself played no rôle in traditional systems of psychology. The result was that when gestalt psychologists introduced the concept of organization, other psychologists, accustomed to think in terms of innate and acquired, interpreted organization and its laws as something innate, thereby ascribing to gestalt theory a sort of psychological Kantian *a priori*. But as we have emphasized, the laws of organization fall entirely outside the scope of our dichotomy. The laws of electric potential, of surface tension, of maximum or minimum energy, hold for *any* system and are quite independent of the particular system considered, much as the nature of those systems will determine the actual processes which follow from these universal laws. To call these laws innate is therefore nonsensical; for innate can only mean: dependent upon the particular nature of the system as it is on account of its biological origin.

SEVERAL KINDS OF PROCESSES. (a) DIRECTLY STIMULUS-CONDITIONED ONES. We return to the processes themselves. Are we justified in including in our account of learning those which arise directly upon stimulation without pre-existing traces? If the stimuli alone can produce a certain process, how can the trace become effective when the stimuli are repeated; in other words, how in such cases can learning take place? This is really a *quaestio facti:* Does learning take place under these conditions, will repetition of the same stimuli produce the same process or not? The answer to this question cannot be in doubt: Learning does take place; the second experience is not, as a rule, exactly like the first. On the one hand the second experience is "familiar," it is being recognized, and as such it is different from the first. But at the same time it will also change qualitatively in some aspect of organization. This will even be true of the simplest possible process, the perception of, say, a white circle on a black background. All our knowledge of early stages of mental development indicates that the first process aroused by such stimulation will be far less sharp and defined than later processes; a vague circular blur will appear at first, where later a sharply bounded circle will be seen. The normal environment of the newly born organism does not, of course, contain such simple stimuli. No such simple process, therefore, can be aroused, but again it is impossible to believe that the infant perceives the mother's face from the beginning in the same way as it does later. Generalizing, we must say that a trace left by a process must affect the process occurring with a repetition of the stimuli, even when the first process was directly and exclusively stimulus-determined.

(b) TRANSFORMATION OF ONE PROCESS INTO ANOTHER. The nature of this influence of traces upon later processes will be discussed presently. At the moment we turn to the arousal of such processes as do not stand in such a simple relation to the stimulus. It is typical of these cases that a reaction R_1 to a stimulus complex S changes into the reaction R_2, and the question arises: Why does this transformation take place? Now in a majority of occasions this change will occur through the introduction of new traces into the field of the process, so that the solution of our present problem will be dependent on our discussion of the influences exerted by traces on later processes, though over and above this problem it involves the other, of how the trace field becomes extended, and why in the particular way which brings about the new process R_2. There are, however, other cases. The whole material may be presented simultaneously or quasi-simultaneously, i.e., within the scope of a temporal unit, and yet the proper process may not take place. "I try to explain to my students a somewhat difficult demonstration of a mathematical theory, putting all my sentences together with the utmost care in the right sequence and with all possible clearness. I shall probably not have much success in my first performance. Something remains dull in the faces of my audience." Some students may, however, "understand" the argument, and others will understand it after one or more repetitions, which in this case serve chiefly to keep the "material" present to their minds. Here a change takes place from processes R_1, all characterized by lack of understanding, to process

R_2, the process by which the theory is understood. We shall discuss the reasons of this change in the next chapter, which will be devoted to the theory of thinking, and there we shall also discuss such accomplishments as those of Köhler's chimpanzees, which in some respects are similar to our last example, also taken from Köhler (1930, p. 57).

(c) TRANSFORMATION BY EFFECT. At the moment we must point out a third class of cases, those where the process is transformed during its own progress by its effect. The puzzle box experiments introduced by Thorndike may serve as our example. In these experiments an animal by continued repetition learns to eliminate useless movements and to perform the "proper" one, i.e., that which will lead it to the lure. The question then is, what are the causes that transform its behaviour. The famous laws of frequency, recency and effect were formulated to answer this question. All three laws in their application to this problem have of late years been discussed so often that I can omit the various arguments here, the more so since I have treated this matter fully in my earlier book (1928, Chapter IV). Here I shall confine myself to a positive theory. Why does a cat in a cage, which originally manifests an extremely varied behaviour, eventually limit its activity to the turning of a latch or the pressing of a button? The question can be answered only in terms of process, not in terms of accomplishment. The fact that R_1, R_2 . . . are dropped while process R_n, e.g., the pressing of a button, is preserved and perfected, must be explained as a transformation of process. We recall our discussion of maze-running (pp. 539 f.) and distinguish in conformity with it the *accomplishment* of pressing the button, A_n, and the *process* of doing so, P_n. A_n can be achieved by many P_n, for instance, by stepping on the button accidentally while moving to another place within the cage, P_{n1}. Since it played no part in the process, the button as such can contribute nothing to the proper P_n, the deliberate pressing of the button. But it is possible that P_{n1}, by virtue of leading to success, may become transformed into P_n, just as in the maze example discussed above the run through a blind alley may, by the fact that the animal finds itself blocked, be transformed into a detour. This hypothesis does not imply that such transformation occurs completely on one occasion. It is perfectly within the frame of the hypothesis that the change in the process, or rather in the trace of it (see p. 540), be no more than a slight shift in the direction of the true process; any degree of such a shift, from the merest beginning to a complete reorganization, is perfectly compatible with our theory.

Thus in one fundamental aspect these cases are like those discussed last—mathematical argument and the intelligent performances of apes—inasmuch as they involve a transformation of process. Their difference lies in the causes which bring about this transformation. For whereas in the former cases all the data necessary for the transformation were presented simultaneously, in the cases now under discussion something new is required which can only be provided by the animal's activity itself, since no animal could from the mere inspection of the puzzle box discover the device for opening its door, whereas potentially an animal should be able to perceive a box in one corner as a tool useful for reaching a lure suspended from the centre of the ceiling.

Animals master both kinds of tasks. Historically "trial and error" experiments preceded "insight" experiments, and it is these former which clamour for a law of effect or success. For I am as fully convinced as Thorndike himself that—in these cases—the success of the action performed is responsible for its being learned. I differ from Thorndike only in the interpretation of this effect of success. For Thorndike, success, i.e., the pleasure of obtaining the goal, stamps in a previously existing "connection." In my theory success transforms a process in such a way as to give it a new "meaning," i.e., a new rôle in its total goal-directed activity. In my theory success need not be the only effect to change the trace of a unitary process. Failure may be another, punishment a third, and there is still room for many other varieties of results of actions.

THE AFTER-EFFECT OF TRACES

Thus we have discussed the three aspects of learning and can now take up our two remaining problems, the after-effect of traces in its various forms, and the arousal of a new process in thought, two problems which, as we have seen, are not unrelated to each other.

The first problem arises from the preceding discussion when we analyze the term "availability" which we have used so often with reference to traces. Availability means only that the trace, by becoming part of the field of a new process, exerts an influence upon it, the *kind* of influence exerted remaining as yet undefined. It is this influence which we are to analyze now. Our procedure must be empirical in the sense that we take up one by one a number of such influences as we know from experience, a more systematic approach being excluded by the insufficiency of our knowledge.

Acquisition of Skills. We begin with the acquisition of skills. A great amount of experimental work has been done in this field, practice curves have been obtained for a variety of different accomplishments, and their theoretical significance has been discussed. Our problem, however, will be a different one. We accept the fact of improvement by practice. We ask what this improvement can mean in terms of trace-process dynamics. Furthermore we take it for granted that the problem of achievement pertains to this field of learning as to any other. A process cannot be improved by repetition before it has happened, however primitive and crude the first occurrence of the process may appear compared to its later stages. Therefore the problem *how* the particular process occurs for the first time will also remain outside the scope of the present discussion. That new processes occur again and again during the progress of learning seems to be proved by the transitions in the learning curve from one plateau to another.

Our problem is the problem of improvement by practice, reduced to its lowest terms of a relatively simple movement. Why has repetition the effect that it does? In terms of process-trace dynamics this problem has two parts: a certain performance leaves a trace; improvement must be due to the effect of this trace. Therefore two questions arise: (1) How does the new process come into communication with the trace? (2) What effect has the trace on the new process with which it communicates? We shall defer the discussion of the first point, since it enters each and every trace function. What can we say about the second? The general nature of the effect of a trace on a process has been developed before. A trace can influence a process only if it belongs to the field in which the process takes place. We now have to discuss the specific form of this field influence in the acquisition of skill. Previously we have found that a trace field arising from a unitary temporal process exerts its influence on the continuation of this process by causing certain new part-processes to occur more easily than others (see Chapter X, p. 449), the ones favoured being those which would give good continuation and closure to the whole process. But the acquisition of skills cannot be treated as one unitary process in the same sense in which a melody must be treated as such (see p. 533), and therefore we cannot simply take over this principle from the old case. Instead we must introduce new assumptions: a first hypothesis would be that a trace as part of the field of a process exerts an influence on the process in the direction of *making it similar to the process which originally produced the trace.*

First Assumption about the Effect of a Trace. We have encountered an example of such an influence at the end of the last chapter (pp. 506 f.), the face taking the place of a chaos of lines which will ever afterwards be seen as a face. This case illustrates our hypothesis very well: a stimulus constellation which can give rise to several perceptual organizations calls out one of them only as soon as this one has occurred and left a trace. Ambiguity of the stimulus pattern with regard to the ensuing process of organization means that the actually occurring process is not caused by the stimulus forces alone; other forces, extraneous to the stimulus pattern, must have tipped the scales in favour of the actual process. A trace of a similar process, this we infer from our example, can be such a force; when it is, it has exerted the influence formulated in our first hypothesis.

The Principle of Action and Reaction Applied to the Trace-Process Relation. We shall meet with other manifestations of this influence later. Now we shall try to explain it. Must we introduce this hypothesis as a new assumption to explain a number of different effects, or is it possible to derive it from a more fundamental principle inherent in our system? We shall attempt the latter course. If a process occurs in a field, it is influenced by that field; but because of the law of action and reaction the field must also be influenced by the process. Consequently, when a trace forms part of the field of a process, it will be affected by the occurrence of the process, a possibility which we have previously discussed (see p. 524).[2] If now the trace is stable, it will resist change and will therefore determine the new process in such a way that it will not induce such a change. This is achieved when the new process is similar to the one which originally produced the trace. If this argument is right, our first hypothesis about the influence exerted by a trace on a process has been derived from a far more general principle, the principle of mutual interdependence of old trace and new process, which will help us to explain a number of other trace influences as well and which, as a matter of fact, we introduced some time ago in our explanation of the arousal of melodies (Chapter X, p. 449).

This Principle Applied to Improvement by Repetition. Now at last we can raise the question whether our first hypothesis explains the gradual acquisition of skills. And we see at once that it does not. It will explain the relative persistence of a skill, new move-

[2] Probably such effects can be very profound. At least it is possible to interpret one of Huang's results in this way. Children would falsify their memories under the stress of contradictory perceptions (pp. 79 f.).

ments being performed with a fairly high degree of perfection even after long periods of disuse, for here the new process more or less approximates the old ones. But the hypothesis does not yet explain why consecutive performances become increasingly better. The hypothesis as it stands explains recurrence of a process, but not improvement. However, with the help of the more general principle of the interaction of trace and process we can approach this problem also. Above we assumed that the trace which formed part of the field of a process was in itself stable. Under this condition it would have the effect of making the new process as similar to the original one as possible. But if the trace is not stable? Then it is under stress towards stability, as we have seen in the last chapter. And therefore its field influence will be such as to produce a process which in its turn will react on the trace so as to make it more stable. In this case, then, the trace would not favour a mere recurrence of the old process to which it owes its existence, but rather the occurrence of a more stable process. In other words such a trace would lead to improvement. The rôle of repetition for the acquisition of skills would be explained if we could apply this conclusion to this function. This would mean that we assumed the traces of the first processes to be highly unstable, an assumption which on the face of it seems very plausible. It would have two consequences, both subject to experimental testing. On the one hand a highly unstable trace has, as we have seen (Chapter XI, p. 507) a low survival value.[3] Therefore we should expect that repetition will have no effect if the single performances are spaced too far apart. This certainly seems true and is in striking contrast to the fact just mentioned that an acquired skill will not be lost after a long period of disuse. The low survival value of an unstable trace is opposed to the high survival value of a stable trace system. On the other hand an unstable trace, before it disintegrates, will tend to change in the direction of greater stability. The acquisition of skills seems to show features well compatible with such an assumption, although Hunter's excellent review of the experiments on learning contains no reference to any experimental work done to establish this point. I mean a sort of "latent" learning, the fact that the performance after an interval of rest is often better than at any previous learning period. If this effect which many people will probably confirm from their own

[3] This does not contradict the fact that under the special conditions investigated by Zeigarnik unstable ("incomplete") traces may at a certain time possess a high availability.

experience is found to be a true fact,[4] it would indicate that the traces have changed during the rest period in such a way as to produce better performances, and that means, in the terms of our theory, in the direction of greater stability. This assumption would also explain one of the best established facts of learning, viz., the advantage of distributing the repetitions over a long period of time as compared to their accumulation in a few blocks.

All this is hypothesis, but an hypothesis which really explains the acquisition of skills. No doubt it is an abstraction inasmuch as virtually no skill is so simple that it is improved by progress in one direction only. As a rule the process will have to vary in a number of different directions before it becomes perfect, and not all of these directions may be present in the first performances. In other words new *achievements,* in the sense of our definition, may occur at various stages of the learning process and thereby complicate the picture enormously. Moreover such new achievements may be made possible by previous developments of the processes. In short, on purely theoretical grounds we cannot expect the learning curve to be simple, and that the less since the learning curve represents merely one or a few manifestations of learning which in many, if not in most or all cases, reflect but a part of the actual learning achieved.

Associative Learning. THE DOCTRINE OF ASSOCIATIONISM. The next function of memory to be discussed is so-called associative learning in its various aspects. Associationism has in the course of history meant a number of different things, but since the end of the last century it has become a very definite and essentially simple doctrine which tries to explain every acquisition by experience in terms of newly formed *associations,* i.e., connections between independent units by virtue of which one of them is capable of reproducing the other. Association, in this theory, is the cause of reproduction, although formerly the term association was used indiscriminately for cause and effect, the item reproduced through association being called an association as well as the bond which was thought to have caused its reappearance. To avoid misunderstandings we shall reserve the term association for the cause, the connection established by experience, and use the term reproduction for the effect, i.e., the item produced by the bond, and the working of the bond. In this sense association in the form of the strict traditional theory means a

[4] Several persons have told me, for instance, that whereas immediately after a concert they can remember no new melodies played in the recital, they will recall a number of them after an interval of one or several days.

bond between two or more items, established by mere spatial or temporal contiguity of these items, therefore the same in kind for all items, i.e., independent of their nature. How little such a concept is compatible with the principles of physical science has been duly emphasized by Köhler in a passage which we have previously quoted (see p. 167). Nevertheless, that it was the true concept of association dominating the theorizing and experimenting of psychologists for at least fifty years is proven by the method of their experimentation. No innovation in psychology is praised more highly, no single event in the history of psychology valued beyond Ebbinghaus's invention of nonsense syllables for the investigation of memory. Now I am far from minimizing this achievement of this highly original and active psychologist who gave us a new tool with which to work experimentally on problems which before had been the domain of uncontrolled everyday observation and pure speculation. But I want to point out that Ebbinghaus's method presupposed a very definite theory of learning, viz., the theory of association as I have just presented it. Any investigation of learning must use material which is not yet learned at the time of the experiment. This is a truism. So we might begin to learn long poems or pieces of prose, and Ebbinghaus himself did just that. Why then did he also begin to learn nonsense syllables, a painful achievement with no gain to one's knowledge? The reason is simple under the associationistic assumptions: since all learning consists in the formation of associations it can best be studied with material which is entirely unassociated when learning begins. Words, which form the elements of poetry and prose, have entered into innumerable associations before the learning of the particular text begins and therefore such learning is not learning from scratch but learning partly supported, partly inhibited, by an uncontrollable mass of pre-existing associations. Only meaningless new material should therefore be used when one wants to control all effective factors. This argument, however, is conclusive only if the processes of learning meaningful and meaningless material are identical in kind, different only in degree of complexity. Only if every connection between several items is of one and the same kind, viz., association, one kind of material can be selected to study the laws operative in learning of every kind of material. Therefore the difference between the two sequences:

Pud sol dap rus mik nom and
A thing of beauty is a joy for ever,

does not lie in the kind of connection existing between the different members of each series, but only in the complexity of the associative pattern. In the second there are many associations in existence when the line is being learned, some of which need only be strengthened by the learning process, like "a thing," "of beauty," "is a," "a joy" or even "is a joy," "for ever," while the first pattern has to be built up entirely during the learning process. On the other hand, the terms of the second series must have incurred previous associations which inhibit or obstruct the forming of new ones according to the law of associative inhibition which says: if an item A has been associated with an item B it will be more difficult to associate it with an item C than if it had not been previously associated with B. Thus "a" has been connected with innumerable other words, so has "is," "for," "beauty." Since no such inhibition exists for the terms of the first series, it is not easy for association theory to explain why the second line is learned and retained so much more easily than the first, a difficulty which, as far as I know, was never explicitly mentioned by the associationists. In order to complete this side of the picture we need only add that associations are also formed between terms not following upon each other directly, e.g., between *pud* and *dap* in the first series, their strength depending not only upon the proximity of the terms but also upon their position within the series. The same is of course true of the second series, so that in each product of learning we have a complicated set of associations of various strength, in both meaningful and meaningless material. The association theory can at best ascribe to these associations, their facilitating and inhibiting effects, definite quantitative values *after* the learning effect has been established—and even that has never really been attempted—but it cannot predict before the event which will be strong, which weak; this is only another way of saying that it cannot really explain the difference between the learning of meaningless and meaningful material, if one means by explanation the deduction from previously established principles.

Association, then, has meant something much more specific than "the establishment of functional relations among psychological activities and states in the course of individual experience," a definition which Robinson (p. 7) introduces.[5] Association has meant *one kind* of functional relationship, produced by mere contiguity and independent of the properties of the terms. It is, to use a German term, entirely "sachfremd," i.e., external, adventitious, contingent.

[5] In his text, however, association has a very much more special meaning than that expressed by the above definition.

But there is still another side to associationism. In considering association as *the cause* of reproduction one considers it as a *force,* a force which starts a new process. The fact that A and B have become associated not only makes it *possible* for B to appear when A has been reinstated, it would even make it *necessary* if there were no other forces operative at the moment. Since, however, at any one moment numberless associations are operating, the association A B is only one component in the complex interplay of forces, the additive resultant of which will determine the result.

Associationism and the Würzburg School. It was here that the first reaction against associationism set in. It seemed incredible that this resultant should so often lie in the direction of an ordered and purposive sequence of ideas or train of thoughts. Although, as we have seen, it was quite impossible to predict the strength and number of the individual associations operating at a given time, it was in many cases perfectly possible to predict the results, i.e., the actual course which the train of thought will take. We recall merely the experiments on the learning of a new relation reported in Chapter XI (pp. 509 f.). How can we predict that a person instructed to name the opposite will answer "bad" to the word "good," and not "man" or "boy," or "is," or "better," or "hope," although we have not the faintest idea of the relative strength of these different associations? The clear recognition of this difficulty by Oswald Külpe gave rise to the work of the Würzburg school which about thirty years ago began to shock the psychological world and destroyed many a bond of personal allegiance and loyalty. Unfortunately the solution which this school proposed for the difficulty it had discerned was not tenable, and so it happened that its real discovery, the insufficiency of associationism, was buried together with its positive contribution. The Würzburg school found itself in the same predicament as the Graz school and shared its fate; psychologists were equally ungrateful to both. The Graz school, following up the ideas of von Ehrenfels, found that no sensation theory could explain shapes, and therefore they added to the concept of sensation, which they left untouched, the concept of a higher mental function "production" and of its product the "Gestaltqualität," the "produced idea," the "idea of extrasensory origin." Similarly the Würzburg school found the concept of association insufficient to explain the orderly and purposive nature of our thinking, and so they added to it, without modifying it, the concept of a new force, the "determining tendency," which was defined in terms of its effects, just as the process of production was by the Graz school. Both concepts were introduced to explain order, order imposed upon material which by itself lacked order; in each case a new force appeared as a *deus ex machina,* introducing a profound dualism into psychology, a dualism between blind mechanical and ordered mental forces. In short, both solutions were vitalistic, and for that reason both are equally unacceptable to us.

As a matter of fact the introduction of the determining tendency left the scheme of associationism in one sense intact. The principle of the resultant force as the strongest by mere algebraic addition was retained in the system for a long time, till Selz recognized its inadequacy.[6] The determining tendency entered this scheme solely as a new force, non-associative in origin, to be added to the multitudinous associative forces, strengthening those bonds which would lead in its direction. It was therefore only consistent with the general principle when Ach conceived the idea of bringing an association and a determining force into conflict and thereby measuring the strength of the latter by the strength of the former, which he regarded as measurable. If the combination "good fellow" has been very strongly associated, then it should occur that a person instructed to respond with the opposite replies to the "stimulus word" "good" by saying "fellow" instead of saying "bad." Ach, working not with such meaningful material but with nonsense syllables, made many experiments which he interpreted as supporting his view. We shall discuss them later when we develop a positive theory. They were mentioned here chiefly to show the nature of the Würzburg principles: the conservation of the associative *forces,* and the additive character of the combination of association and determination.

THEORY OF ROTE LEARNING. After this brief historical survey, which acquainted us with the oldest and most hallowed of all psychological theories, let us approach our problem systematically. The association principle was supposed to have universal application. In our systematic procedure we must start from a definite case, and since rote learning has played such a large part in the experimentation of the associationists, we shall choose it as our starting point. What is the effect of rote learning? In the first place: that we can, when we so desire, reproduce, i.e., recite, the material learned by heart; that we can continue the sequence when somebody else starts it, a test which in the case of series of nonsense syllables takes the form of the method of paired associates, in which one member of

[6] I shall omit Selz's contribution from this discussion, since, as I have explained elsewhere (1927 a), it does not seem to me to make a positive contribution in the right direction.

the series is repeated to the learner and he has to reproduce the next one. There are other effects of rote learning, notably that we recognize the material, an effect which will be discussed later when we discuss the problem of recognition, and besides that many more which we shall neglect, since they do not directly concern the problem of association as manifested by our material.

A DISCREPANCY BETWEEN FACT AND ASSOCIATION THEORY. Let us then say that a person has learned a series composed of twelve nonsense syllables. He encounters one of these syllables again; what will happen? According to the association theory this syllable should at once reproduce the one that followed or preceded it, unless other associations were stronger at the moment. Such other associations would have to originate in *other* data encountered simultaneously with the syllable, since the strongest association which the syllable has formed connects it with either of those two other syllables. If, therefore, other data are removed, as far as that is possible, the above result should inevitably follow. But this is not the case, as special experiments by Lewin have proved (1922, I, pp. 227 f.). Syllables which had been learned by 300 repetitions and which, if tested by the method of paired associates, would yield correct responses with short reaction times, failed to call up anything if presented under a neutral instruction, according to which the subject was to read the syllable presented in the exposure apparatus but to refrain from any *active* attempt at reproduction. This result, not derivable from the law of association as usually formulated, can mean two things in terms of our theory. Since reproduction of the following (or any other learned) syllable would mean that the trace system of the learned series had come into communication with the newly perceived syllable, forming part of the field in which this perceptual process occurred, failure to reproduce must mean either that no such communication took place or that the trace field, even when it is in communication with the process, is not capable of producing the *process* of naming, or thinking of, another syllable. Thus the fact of reproduction raises at once the problem of the communication of the new process with an old trace or trace system. Without such communication the old experience can have no possible bearing upon the new process, a point clearly discerned by Höffding (1889-90), but practically forgotten since then, until Köhler took it up again in his paper read before the International Congress of Psychology at Copenhagen in 1932.

TWO POSSIBLE EXPLANATIONS OF THIS FACT. The result of the Lewin experiment, if it could be interpreted as due to a failure of the new process to communicate with the old trace, would mean that such communication presupposed, at least in the case of nonsense syllables, a definite Ego attitude: when the subjects were instructed to name the following syllable, they could do so with great facility, whereas this syllable did not emerge when, owing to the instruction, they had no wish or attitude of reproducing. This conclusion depends, of course, on the truth of our interpretation. Fortunately Lewin's account of his experiment contains some extra evidence which makes it at least very plausible. For reproduction is not the only effect which a trace system has upon a process with which it communicates: there is the more primitive effect of recognition, which, whatever its dynamics, presupposes some such communication. Therefore, if the syllables had been recognized and yet led to no reproduction, our interpretation would be wrong; while, on the other hand, a lack of recognition accompanied by failure to reproduce, would greatly increase its probability. As a matter of fact, in Lewin's experiments the second alternative was realized; the syllables that failed to have a reproductive effect also failed to be recognized. Therefore it seems fairly safe to assume that they did not come into communication with the old traces. So our conclusion about the effect of Ego-attitudes upon such communication would be justified.

But this does not mean that the second of the two alternatives enumerated above is excluded, namely, that traces, though in communication with a present process, do not lead to reproduction. The result of Lewin's experiment, if interpreted in my way, says nothing about the effect that a trace system exerts upon a process with which it is in communication. It may or it may not be capable of enforcing reproduction by its mere communication, without any special force like an Ego-attitude. While working in the famous laboratory of the University of Würzburg as early as 1909, I made some experiments which throw some light on this question (1912). They were similar to Lewin's experiments in using practically the same instruction; they differed from them in being a modification of the old type of association experiment rather than a modification of the paired-associate memory experiments. I called out a word to my subjects, who were instructed to listen and passively wait for anything that might come to their consciousness. The results corresponded perfectly to Lewin's. The passive attitude proved to be very unstable, tending to be quickly replaced by a definite active attitude, often unknown to the subject. But before such an attitude developed my subjects were as much at sea as Lewin's:

nothing would come to their minds, and the experience of passive waiting was distinctly painful. In all these respects the two sets of experiments are in exact correspondence. But dynamically there is this difference between them: the words that my subjects were presented with were understood by them, i.e., they did communicate with older trace systems. The failure to reproduce anything in my experiments can therefore not be explained by lack of communication. Here a trace field existed, and yet its influence alone was not sufficient to start a process of reproduction, whereas reproductions of various kinds occurred with great ease as soon as "latent attitudes" had developed. The second alternative may thus be a very real one. There exist conditions under which a trace field in communication with a process is not capable of influencing this process in the sense of reproduction.

That much we can deduce from my old experiments, but no more. At least to me it would seem premature to generalize that under *no* conditions can a trace field have this effect.

THE RÔLE OF THE TRACE IN REPRODUCTION. Before we follow up the two problems raised in the preceding discussion, viz., the causes which make a process communicate with a trace and the rôle which special attitudes play in reproduction, we shall treat a third one, corresponding to the problem discussed in the section on motor skill: What is the function of a trace in those cases where reproduction occurs? We hear "to be or" and we continue "not to be"; we want to recite a poem that we have learned, and we do it; we are presented with a syllable from a previously well learned series and instructed to name the one that followed upon it, and we produce the right answer. In the last two cases our intention is without a doubt among the causes of the respective processes, the recitation and the naming of the syllable; in the first case, it is not so easy to establish the existence of a similar attitude. But in all three cases the present performance would be impossible without traces from earlier ones. Therefore we accept it as a fact that these traces are in communication with the processes, and we grant that these processes are set in motion by causes external to the traces (intentions, attitudes). Even so, the trace has a very definite influence on the process. Of what kind is this influence? Can we derive it from the general law formulated on pages 554 f., viz., that a trace will influence a process in such a way that the reactive influence exerted by the process on the trace will not diminish, but if possible increase, the latter's stability? We can, as soon as we envisage the traces as products of organization and not, as associationistic psychology was accustomed to do, as a number of separate items merely joined or coupled together by some bond. That we must treat traces as organized products of organized processes has been demonstrated in the last two chapters; it is therefore no new hypothesis introduced in order to explain reproduction.

Rote Learning a Process of Organization. We shall now apply this principle to our present case: In what sense is a series of nonsense syllables organized? We have seen in the historical introduction to this section that this material was chosen just because it seemed to fit the associationistic assumptions: a number of unconnected items. And judged by *accomplishment* the learning of such material seemed good proof of these assumptions. But accomplishment of so crude a kind gives us no knowledge of the processes which made it possible, a point stressed sufficiently in our previous discussions. Variation of experimental procedure has instead produced ample proof that the *performance* which leads to the learning of a nonsense series is a process of organization. Thus it is impossible to learn a series of ten nonsense syllables without some rhythmization; as a rule these series are learned in trochaic rhythm, so that they become organized into five pairs which form real parts of the whole series, just as each syllable of a pair is a real part of it. This formation of pairs is a fact of true organization, and not explicable in terms of mere association. A purely associationistic explanation of this fact would have to explain the formation of pairs like this: the members of a pair are more closely associated with each other than either of them with its other neighbour; i.e., the associations (all in a forward direction) between an odd and an even member are stronger than those between an even and an odd one. For example, in a series: *a b/ c d/ e f/*, *c* is more strongly associated with *d* than with *b*, or than *d* with *e*. That this explanation of the pair character is wrong has been proved by very ingenious and elaborate experiments by Witasek, posthumously published by Auguste Fischer. Only one of the many experiments will be reported here.

Witasek's Experiments. On one day the subject learned four preliminary series of ten nonsense syllables, symbolized thus:

$$I_1 I_2 \quad I_3 I_4 \quad I_5 I_6 \quad I_7 I_8 \quad I_9 I_{10}$$

$$II_1 II_2 \ \ldots\ldots\ \ II_9 II_{10}$$

$$III_1 III_2 \ \ldots\ldots\ \ III_9 III_{10}$$

$$IV_1 IV_2 \ \ldots\ldots\ \ IV_9 IV_{10}$$

Here the Roman figures refer to the number of the series, the Arabic ones to the syllables within the series. Learning was regarded as completed when the subjects were able to recite the series at the rate of seven seconds per series. One hour later they had to learn three test series of the following kind:

$$A:\ x\,I_3\ I_4\,II_5\ II_6\,III_7\ III_8\,IV_9\ IV_{10}\,x$$

$$B:\ x\,II_2\ II_3\,III_4\ III_5\,IV_6\ IV_7\,I_8\ I_9\,x$$

$$C:\ xx\ IV_3\,IV_4\ \ I_5\,I_6\ \ II_7\,II_8\ \ III_9\,III_{10}$$

That is: each of these new series A, B, and C was composed of eight syllables learned in one of the first four series and of two new ones, symbolized by x. To understand the principle according to which these series were built we glance back at the first four series and consider a feature not yet discussed. Since all these series were learnd in trochaic rhythm they were articulated into five pairs. Now, on the associationistic assumption, a pair is distinguished from a non-pair by the greater strength of the associative bond that exists between its members. Thus the strength of association between two successive members of a series must vary periodically, being stronger when an odd member precedes the even than when an even precedes the odd. Thus the first syllable is more strongly associated with the second than the second with the third, the third more strongly with the fourth than the fourth with the fifth, and so on. I have symbolized this by connecting two successive syllables in the schema by loops, two loops indicating a stronger association than one. The same symbolism has been employed for the three critical series A, B, and C, but this time not to designate the strength of the associations to be created by the learning of these new series, but that of the associations taken over into the new series from the old ones. Thus one sees that both series A and C contain four strong associations built up by the learning of the four original series, while series B contains only four old weak associations. Therefore, if group formation were nothing but association, series A and C should be learned with equal ease, more easily than B. That the other points of difference between these three series do not, according to the association principle, favour A more than the others has been shown in an elaborate discussion by Witasek.

Each subject had twelve sittings, i.e., they learned twelve sets of four preliminary and three critical series. The result contradicted the expectation derived from the associationistic premise: in order of difficulty the three series ranked: A > B ⪢ C, i.e., C was by far the easiest, and the slight difference between A and B was in favour of B. For a full discussion of this result the reader must again turn to the original. Its main bearing, however, is clear: group formation is not association, i.e., a bond between individual items which can vary only in the dimension of strength, but organization, through which the two members of a pair have become a real unit, separated from the next unit. For in C, the series most easily learned, the pairs were retained *as pairs;* in A, the series most difficult to learn, the same number of strong associations was preserved as in C, but now it was to be no longer an association of members of one pair, but an association between the last member of a preceding and the first of a succeeding pair; in B finally the weak associations of this inter-pair character were maintained. I.e., association in these experiments counts not as association *per se* but through the function which the association has in the organization of the series. This means, of course, that the term "association" is no longer appropriate, since the *kind* of connection takes on the decisive rôle, a characteristic for which the association theory has no place.

To explain the results of Witasek's experiments concretely is impossible because of two possibilities between which we cannot decide: (a) it is possible that a trace system in which the syllables k and l are members of a pair obstructs the formation of a new organization in which they belong to different pairs, k being the second member of the preceding and l the first of the succeeding; or (b) it is possible that the k l trace is brought into play only if the new process has the same organization, but not if it is of the type of series A, i.e., i k, l m.

However, for our purposes it is not necessary to decide between the two alternatives, since both prove that a *learned* series is an *organized* series and that therefore the traces must be organized too.

Interaction of Organized Trace and Process and the Law of Reproduction. And now we can take up our question as to the function of a trace system in the reproduction of material learned by heart. We said it could be derived from our general principle of the dynamic relation between trace and process, viz., that the former will influence the latter so that by interaction it does not lose stability (see p. 563). If a whole series has been learned, then its trace system forms an articulated unit. When the subject begins to recite the series, his process must be in communication with this trace system. If, then, the first syllable has been recited, the part of the trace corresponding to this syllable has been in communication with a process while the rest has not, so that, if the process should stop, the whole trace system would have been changed by the fact that to one part of it something had happened and to the other not. If the trace is stable it will resist such change and it can do so by inducing the continuation of the process until all members have been in communication with a new process; i.e., the trace will exert a force on the field in which the process occurs so as to make the process "complete." To explain reproduction we do not need an assumption of special associative bonds; rather the possibility of reproduction follows from the fact of organization and the general principle of the interaction between trace and process. And the traditional law of association should be replaced by the following formulation: if a process communicates with a part of a trace system, the *whole* trace system will exert a force on the process in the direction of making it as complete as it was when it created this trace system.

That this formulation is indeed compatible with the facts is easily proved. I can adduce as witnesses Müller and Pilzecker, whose work is one of the finest of pure associationistic literature. Nobody could accuse G. E. Müller of a bias in favour of gestalt theory.

Müller and Pilzecker's *Initial Reproductive Tendency* as Supporting Our Theory. Müller and Pilzecker write: "If one says to an educated German the word 'Eisenhammer,' then most probably he will recall the unitary word complex 'Der Gang nach dem Eisenhammer,'[7] and many other examples could be given for similar occurrences. Experiences of this kind seem to warrant the following conclusion: if a series of successive ideas, once or several times repeated, form a unitary complex of ideas, then each constituent of this complex, and particularly its terminal member, when it recurs in consciousness, has the tendency to reproduce first the initial member and then the others in their proper sequence. We shall designate this reproductive tendency, at first directed towards the initial member of the complex, as the *initial reproductive tendency*" (p. 199).

Two things have to be distinguished in this quotation, the fact and the interpretation of the fact. The fact is the re-instatement of the whole complex by one of its parts; the interpretation culminates in the term *initial reproductive tendency,* which dissolves this fact into an associative relation between two isolated members. True

[7] "Der Gang nach dem Eisenhammer" is a well-known ballad by Schiller. English equivalents might be: "The Ancient Mariner" will call up "The Rime of the Ancient Mariner," "Galuppi": "A Toccata of Galuppi's," "Dreadful Night": "The City of Dreadful Night."

enough, the two authors leave it an open question whether the tendency aroused by the part is directed only towards the initial member, which in its turn reproduces the next and so forth, or whether it is directed immediately towards the reproduction of the whole complex. But characteristically they discuss this alternation only in a footnote, while the above quotation with the introduction of the new term occurs in the text. And by coining and employing this term they tacitly accept the first interpretation, whereas to an unbiassed observer the second is undoubtedly the more plausible one. A glance at the English examples given in the last footnote will make this clear: it is not the definite or indefinite article—in each case the "first term of the complex"—which is being directly reproduced, but the main word which completes the meaning. But then the initial reproductive tendency, whose efficacy Müller and Pilzecker have proved by special experiments with nonsense syllables, confirms our statement of the law of reproduction: a part of a trace tends to establish the whole process that gave rise to the whole trace.

The Quantitative Aspect of the Law of Reproduction. The use of the word "tends" in this last formulation was intentional; it does not mean to emasculate the statement, nor has it a purely statistical significance; instead it is to indicate the quantitative aspect of this law: the force exerted by the trace (see our first formulation on p. 567) may vary in strength, and so may other forces which at the same time influence the process. Our law is then a law not about effects, but about causes; and the quantitative aspect implied in our last formulation has to be amplified. The force which the trace field exerts upon the new process will depend on many conditions, among which the *degree* and *kind* of communication must be very important, although at the moment we can say nothing about them. Another condition, however, is inherent in the trace itself: since the influence which the trace exerts on the process is intrinsically related to the stability of the trace, its force must be a direct function of this stability: *ceteris paribus,* the greater the stability of the whole trace, the more strongly will a part process be influenced by the trace in the direction of completion.

Stability of a Trace. Contiguity as One of Many Factors of Organization. Meaningless and Meaningful Material. Stability of a whole trace means that in this unit each part is held in its place by strong forces which resist a displacement. The stability of a trace must therefore be a function of its dynamic structure. The "better" this structure, the more will the whole be a real unit and consequently the parts dependent on each other and their function in this whole. We have studied unit formation in earlier chapters and can apply the knowledge gained there to our present problem. There we encountered proximity as a strong factor, the same factor which appeared in associationism as contiguity. We now understand its meaning. Contiguity plays its part in reproduction to the degree to which it has unified the contiguous parts. Thus, although each syllable in a series of nonsense syllables is contiguous to two others it will reproduce one of them more easily than another, viz., the one that belongs to the same pair. For unit formation depends upon a number of factors other than mere contiguity. Parts which "fit" each other, which jointly form a "good curve," are more strongly unified than such as have no intrinsic relation and are linked by mere proximity. Such "good continuation" distinguishes a meaningful text from a nonsense series; therefore the process corresponding to the apprehension of the meaningful material must be better organized than that corresponding to a nonsense series, and hence the trace of the former must be more stable than the trace of the latter. This greater stability will endow the former trace with a "greater reproductive power"; if one of its parts is in communication with a process, the whole trace will exert a stronger influence on that process than if a part of a nonsense-trace communicates with a process. For in the former case the process finds in the stability of the trace greater resistance to its proceeding in a different way than it does in the latter. It is a common experience that we can recall meaningful material better than meaningless, an experience which was long ago quantitatively confirmed by Bühler, whose experiments at the same time indicate that recall does not go from part to part, but from part to whole. The difference between meaningful and meaningless material is, therefore, not a difference in number and strength of associations, as associationism assumed (see pp. 556 ff.), but a difference in kind of organization. Just as there is a practically infinite number of shapes, so there is an equally great number of "ideational" organizations, different from each other in kind, complexity, and stability. Once more: mere contiguity, qua contiguity, has no effect. It enters the causal series only through its effect on organization. Even there it is not enough. We have seen that series of nonsense syllables can be learned only if they are read in a definite rhythm, i.e., when they are being organized by an extraneous factor. On the other hand, von Restorff's experiments have shown that under other conditions meaningless material can be learned fairly easily and without this extraneous influence. But in her experiments again proximity (contiguity) was not the only factor, but proximity of similars in a surrounding of differents. Here the unifying principle was the gradient between the "isolated" and the "repeated" material (cf. Chapter XI, pp. 485 f.). In discussing her experiments we distinguished between two possible explanations of the difficulty involved in learning a series of nonsense syllables, the one based on its "monotony," the other on its "nonsense" character. Von Restorff's experiments emphasized the first factor, which heretofore had been neglected in favour of the second. But it would be a misinterpretation of her results to think that the other factor played no rôle at all. We have just discussed the greater stability which a trace must possess when it derives from a meaningful rather than from a meaningless process. But what is true of the stability of the trace is also true of the process of organization itself which builds the trace. Meaningful material is more easily organized than meaningless, although it may be difficult to transform (more or less) meaningless material into (more or less) meaningful material, as when we gradually come to understand a mathematical proof.

Summary: Arbitrary Connections Replaced by Dynamic Organizations. Summarizing, we can say that we have so far examined one aspect of the concept of association: the arbitrary character of the associative connection. We have seen that the organization of arbitrarily joined items in one whole is only an extreme case in a whole class of cases, and that even in this case mere contiguity is not a sufficient factor. The connection: *pud-sol* is certainly not the archetype of all connections or, rather, organizations. Instead there are numberless possibilities of organization in which the members of the whole are held together by *intrinsic* relations, which in our theory must be regarded as *dynamic* relations of the nervous processes.

Does This Lead to "Psychologismus"? Psychology and Logic. Such a theory seems to imply an extreme *Psychologismus,* i.e., the view that all logical, *subsistent,* relations can be explained by psychological or even physiological *existing* relations. This view, which had gained ground at the turn of the century, was violently attacked by some of our best philosophers, notably Edmund Husserl, who claimed to have refuted it once and for all. But his argument rested on the assumption, implicit or explicit, in all "psychologistic" theories, that psychological relations were merely factual or external. A "psychologism" based on this assumption has indeed been refuted by Husserl and other philosophers. But this refutation does not affect our psychologism—if our theory can rightly be given this name—since in our theory psychological and physiological, or rather psychophysical, processes are organized according to intrinsic or internal relations. This point can only be alluded to. It means that in our theory psychology and logic, existence and subsistence, even, to some extent, reality and truth, no longer belong to entirely different realms or universes of discourse between which no intelligible relationship exists. It is here, if anywhere, that psychology will have to prove the integrative function that we assigned to it in the first chapter.

Association as a Force. Lewin. It is now time to consider the other aspect of association, according to which it is a *force* which by itself causes reproduction (see p. 559). Against this side of the old concept Lewin has levelled a most energetic and well supported attack (1926). He summarizes his conclusions in the following words:

> "The experimental investigation of habit formation (association) has shown that the couplings created by habit never supply as such the motor of a mental event; such an interpretation is erroneous also if one sees the essential side of habit—and practice—processes not in the formation of piecewise associations, but in the transformation and creation of definite activity-wholes. Rather in all cases certain mental *energies,* originating as a rule in a pressure of will or needs, i.e., mental systems *under stress,* are the necessary conditions of mental events" (p. 311).

Lewin rightly distinguishes, in this quotation, between couplings, on the one hand, and forces and energies on the other. "Mere connections," he says, "are never 'causes' of events in whatever form they may exist" (pp. 312-3), and he applies this distinction with equal force to old atomistic associationism and to a gestalt interpretation of the connections. The application to atomistic associations is easy. Lewin himself uses the analogy of the train where all carriages are coupled together, but move, not because of the couplings, necessary though they are, but because of the steam power of the locomotive. Indeed, the concept of association being primarily a concept to explain *connections,* it is difficult to see how it can at the same time fulfil the function of a propelling force and a reservoir of energy. The mere fact that the concept was endowed with this double function (of connecting and propelling) is no defence against Lewin's criticism, for associationism has never shown how the same substratum of association could function in this double manner. But Lewin goes further than that; he shows that the "strength of an association," if measured by the result it *can* produce under definite instructions or attitudes, may be quite different from the "strength of association" if measured by what it *must* do under *any* instruction; or rather that only the former can be measured and therefore defined, whereas the latter may in many cases be zero. In other words: in the terms of the association theory, the definition of association as a bond has sense, whereas its definition as a "motor" has none.

Our Theory Escapes Lewin's Criticism. It Supplies (a) Forces. But, as we have seen, Lewin levels the same criticism also against a non-associationistic theory, which "considers not a chainlike coupling of members but the integration of the parts in the whole as the 'cause' of the event" (p. 311), because, as he adds in a footnote, such an hypothesis does not use the concept of tensions in a dynamic system. It is immaterial to examine how justified he was when he wrote his unusually significant and important article. Instead we shall see whether his criticism is applicable to the theory developed in the preceding pages. We have, on purpose, left this question in abeyance, discussing merely what kind of influence a trace must exert on a process, no matter how such a process was started. But the answer to our question treated the trace as a dynamic system under tension, a tension which would favour one kind of process and obstruct other kinds. Therefore it is no longer obvious that Lewin's arguments affect our hypothesis as they did the association theory. If the trace as an organized system under stress exerts a force upon a process it is no longer evident why it should not also be able to start a process, why, in other words, the revival of a part of a larger whole, if in communication with the whole trace, should not of and by itself, through its relation to the trace, lead to reproduction of the whole, why *under all conditions* another, external, force should be necessary. As far as the forces are concerned, "automatic" or "spontaneous" reproduction, i.e., reproduction without the "intention to reproduce," should be perfectly possible.

(b) Energies. But there remains the energy aspect. To quote again from Lewin: "In order for a process to occur, *energy capable of doing work* must be set free. *Hence for every mental event the question must be raised as to the origin of the effective energies*" (p. 313). Every system under stress contains energy capable of doing work, and therefore the needs and quasi-needs (intentions, resolves) which Lewin introduces as "motors" of events are well equipped to play that rôle. Since in our theory trace systems are also systems under stress it might seem as though they also might be thought of as supplying the energy for the process. Such an assumption would, however, run into great difficulties if it considered the trace systems as such as the store of energy. For, since reproduction is possible in an unlimited number of single occasions, the store of energy in the trace system would have to be practically unlimited also, and that is an assumption too improbable to be admitted.

How else then can we account for the energy consumed in the process? To answer this question we must make explicit an implicit feature of Lewin's theory. We have seen that in his system the cause of my writing a letter lies in a need or quasi-need to do so, i.e., in a system under stress which ultimately supplies the energy for this action. The word "ultimately" was used on purpose, for the acts of opening a drawer to get the necessary stationery, of unscrewing the fountain pen, of moving the chair to the right place, and finally of tracing the words on paper consume disproportionately more energy than is stored in the need-system; it is the energy stored in our muscles which is being liberated and directed by this system. The energy relation between the system which acts as "motor" of the activity and the executed actions is thus a very indirect one. The original energy achieves the result by liberating and steering this energy, even in Lewin's theory.

With this knowledge let us return to spontaneous reproduction. A part of a larger whole process is rearoused and communicates with a trace system. Then, according to our hypothesis, the whole trace system is put under new pressure, because of the fact that only one of its parts is in communication with a process, a stress which can be relieved by the reinstatement of the whole process. Is it then an illegitimate assumption that the energy of this pressure liberates other energy stored in the brain field to keep the process going? It seems to me no more so than the assumption implicit in Lewin's theory that the wish to write a letter succeeds in liberating energy stored in the muscles. Perhaps an even simpler assumption is possible: the energy put in the trace system by the tension might go directly into the new process. Both assumptions escape the difficulty inherent in the assumption of a trace as an inexhaustible store of energy. For in both the energy is supplied to the trace system by its communication with a process which in its turn was caused by forces outside the trace system, e.g., in perception. Thus it seems as though spontaneous reproduction were perfectly possible within the framework of our theory. This, of course, is not tantamount to saying that spontaneous reproduction, i.e., reproduction determined by no outside forces, is the normal or even the most frequent case. It would still be possible even if it never occurred in reality. That it does occur occasionally seems to me, however, very probable when I think of the first example given on page 563 ("to be or . . .") or those in the footnote on page 567.

OUR THEORY AND THE EXPERIMENTAL WORK. However, we cannot conclude this argument without a consideration of Lewin's experimental work. Is it compatible with our theory or not?

ACH'S ATTEMPT TO MEASURE THE STRENGTH OF A VOLUNTARY ACT. In order to cast a very summary glance at the experimental work we have to go back to Ach's experiments published in 1910. For after all, however much one may disagree with his theoretical conclusions, Ach was the first to treat the question of the dynamic side of association experimentally. His setting was that of the Würzburg school of which he was one of the first members. Thus he accepted the traditional concept of association with its undiscriminated double aspect of bond and force, and at the same time introduced the "determining tendency" as a new force which by algebraic addition with the associative forces would determine the actual mental event. In his experiments he tried to prove the principle of summation of these forces. Supposing an item *a* is associated with an item *b*, then it will reproduce this item more promptly if, simultaneously with this association, a determining tendency exists that by itself would arouse *b* than when a determining tendency is operative that would lead to item *c*. And conversely, a determining tendency leading from *a* to *b* will be more effective if it is supported by an association *a-b* than when it is in conflict with an association *a-c*. In the case of conflict, either a retardation of the reproduction should take place, or, if the associative force were stronger than the "determining" one, then the subject should give a *wrong* response; otherwise expressed, his habit should overcome his will. Thus the strength of the determining tendency originating in an act of will can be measured by the association which is just strong enough to overcome it.

His method was simple and ingenious. The subjects learned three series of eight nonsense syllables, one normal, one in which the second member of a pair was always the "inverted" first member, like *rol-lor,* and one where the second member rhymed with the first, like *zup-tup*. After each of these series had been learned on seven successive days, each having been repeated eighty times, the four odd syllables of each series mixed with four unknown syllables were presented for reproduction according to the method of paired associates. On the following days the subjects started by reading the three series another ten times, and were then tested by different methods: on the tenth day the instruction was the same as on the seventh, i.e., to reproduce another syllable after being shown one in the exposure apparatus. On the eighth and twelfth days, however, they were told to respond to the stimulus syllable by inverting, and on the ninth and eleventh days, by rhyming it. We can divide the test syllables into four groups: *o* the syllables taken from the ordinary series, *i* those from the series in which the members of a pair were in the relation of inversion, *r* those from the third series in which the members of a pair rhymed, and *n* the new syllables. On different days these syllables were under the influence of different tasks: reproducing, inverting, and rhyming respectively. This must lead to algebraic summation of associative and determining tendency. When inverting is the task, the *i* syllables are subjected to two forces which have the same direction; for if the pair *rol-lor* has been learned, then on the basis of association *lor* should be reproduced by *rol,* and equally should it be produced from *rol* by the mere determining tendency to invert. Contrariwise both the *o* and the *r* syllables are under the same instruction exposed to conflicting forces. For the syllable *zup,* associated with *tup,* would on the basis of this association reproduce the latter, whereas the task demands the reply *puz;* and similarly the syllable *dur* should reproduce, on an associative basis, say, the syllable *tik* with which it had been learned, and not the syllable *rud* demanded by the determining tendency.

The same is true of the instruction to rhyme; only the *r* and the *i* syllables have changed their places, the former now being favoured, the latter, together with the *o* syllables, being handicapped.

It is harder to say how Ach interprets the dynamics of the instruction to reproduce. But it seems that he considers it, somewhat inconsistently, as the case where the associative tendency finds neither support nor resistance. With this interpretation the dynamic situation for each of the three kinds of syllables under the three different instructions may be represented by Table 29, + meaning the direction of the determining tendency, and — that the associative tendency has a different direction, 0 that one of the tendencies does not exist (the first symbol will refer always to the determining, the second to the associative, force).

TABLE 29

syllables	task: reprod.	task: invert	task: rhyme
o	0 +	+ −	+ −
i	0 +	+ +	+ −
r	0 +	+ −	+ +

Therefore, the syllable demanded by the instruction should be most promptly supplied in the two + + cases, next in the three 0 + ones, and least in the four + — ones; in the latter, errors should be likely to occur. The *n* syllables are omitted from this discussion, since they contribute nothing conclusive either way.

The actual reaction times, taken from Ach's table, are contained in Table 30, the figures representing the median of all reactions in thousandths of a second.

TABLE 30
(from Ach)

syllables	task: reprod.	task: invert	task: rhyme
o	881	841	1132
i	767	664	895
r	871	804	777

To some extent this table confirms our expectations: the highest figure occurs with a + — constellation, the lowest with a + + one. But there are a number of discrepancies, which will appear when we look at the rank order of the different constellations.

1. 664 + +
2. 767 0 +
3. 777 + +
4. 804 + −
5. 841 + −
6. 871 0 +
7. 881 0 +
8. 895 + −
9. 1132 + −

The most striking facts are the relatively short reaction times in Nos. 2, 4, and 5, and all three have something to do with inverting. No. 2, the second shortest of all, concerns the reproduction of inverted syllables, Nos. 4 and 5 the inversion of *r* and *o* syllables. Also the *n* syllables, so far excluded from our discussion, have significantly lower reaction times for "inverting" than for "reproducing" and rhyming.

A last way of looking at the figures of our table is to average the values for the + +, the 0 +, and the + − cases.[8]

TABLE 31

Constellation	+ +	0 +	+ −
Average reaction time	745	1090	1059

This survey confirms the expectations only inasmuch as the + + constellation has the shortest reaction times, but the two others, whose difference is probably insignificant, are in contradiction with Ach's assumption.

The quantitative analysis of the reaction times (and this holds for Ach's other subjects as well as for the one from whose results our tables are taken), although giving some indication of the expected results, fails to confirm the theory, thereby showing that factors must have been at work which are not included in Ach's theory. We mention only the fact that the pairs of the *i* series were more strongly associated than those of the two others, and that, as the subjects reported, they were easier to learn. It is characteristic of the period in which Ach worked that, although he particularly stresses this point, he does not see its incompatibility with strict associationistic principles. For according to these the material properties of the terms associated should have no bearing on the strength of the association between them. The fact that they have, therefore,

[8] I have averaged not the medians but the averages, contained in Ach's but not in my table. The rank order of these averages is different from that of the medians, above, but contains as many discrepancies.

invalidates these principles: it proves again that organization has taken place and that within the range of organization possible for nonsense syllables the symmetry of a syllable and its "mirror image" is particularly stable.

The most significant among these quantitative results, the shortening of the reaction times if the "homogeneous" task is substituted for the mere reproduction, and the lengthening of it when the heterogeneous task takes its place, is clearly realized even in this model case, only for the task of inverting and not for that of rhyming. In other experiments even this regularity disappears, so that we cannot accept the figures as proofs of Ach's theory.

On the other hand the qualitative results add some evidence in favour of Ach's assumption. With the two heterogeneous activities of inverting and rhyming a great number of errors occurred, namely twelve out of a possible twenty for rhyming, and seven out of a possible twenty for inverting. In these cases not the syllable demanded by the instruction was named but the one closely associated with the stimulus syllable. Habit has been stronger than will, if Ach's interpretation is right. Again we must add, however, that no other subject showed so many wrong reactions as this one, that in several cases they failed to appear at all. I am using this statistical argument only to point out that evidently Ach's conditions are not compulsory and that therefore other factors than those he discriminated and sought to control may have played an important rôle.

LEWIN'S WORK. We can now pass to Lewin's work, for he succeeded where Ach failed: he could create conditions which would produce wrong reactions or at least strong retardations of reaction time, and such as would lead to neither the one nor the other. Before he achieved this he had repeated Ach's experiment with a greatly simplified method. A number of ordinary (*o*) series of nonsense syllables of varying length were learned during sixteen days with a total of 270 repetitions. Thereupon 70 new syllables (*n* syllables), arranged in five series of twelve and one of ten, were repeated six times in such a way that each syllable changed its place at each repetition so that it would not become associated with any special one. Finally the activity of inverting was practised with a number of different syllables. Then in the critical experiments in which the subject had to respond by inverting the presented syllables, *o* and *n* syllables were presented in alternation. Under this instruction the *o* syllables would fall under the scheme $+\,—$, the *n* syllables under the $+\,0$; i.e., the latter should yield shorter reaction times, the former, owing to the great number of repetitions, some wrong responses. Neither of these effects appeared, the reaction times were equal within the limits of error and no false reactions occurred, with one single exception which occurred at the end.

This result, clearly as it contradicts the expectation, is not new. If one goes through Ach's tables and compares the reaction time of *o* and *n* syllables with inverting (and rhyming) one finds cases in which they are equal (5), cases in which the *n* syllables have the shorter reaction times (3), and even one case where the *o* syllables are favoured. On the other hand we saw that in Ach's experiments wrong reactions occurred. As a matter of fact only *one* such wrong reaction occurred in Ach's experiments with an *o* syllable and the task of inverting, five in all with *o* syllables and the task of rhyming, and altogether these wrong reactions were not frequent in Ach's experiments.[9]

The results so far seem unclear, although they certainly do not confirm the underlying assumptions. A conflict between association and determination does not regularly appear. We saw before that the opposite result, mutual support of these two factors, was not regularly present in Ach's experiments, and it failed to appear at all in Lewin's experiment performed with an interesting modification of Ach's technique. In these experiments associations were not formed by presenting series of syllables to be read and learned, but by presenting syllables to which the subjects had to respond by naming a new syllable which could be produced from the presented ones by changing the first consonant in a prescribed manner. For instance, if the syllable began with *d* they had to pronounce a syllable beginning with *g* but otherwise equal, e.g., presented syllable *dak*, response *gak*. Since the traditional law of association establishes only the conditions that two items must have occurred in contiguity (and with sufficient frequency), this method is as good as the other. With this method one can obtain + + and + — cases in the test, and no difference in the reaction times appeared, nor any wrong reactions.

Thus Lewin's results are in strict contradiction to those of Ach and to the assumptions which guided this author. In order to explain the contradiction Lewin introduced an entirely new theory. We know already that he denies that an association can be the "motor" of any activity. The motor must be something else, a mental act, intention, or "set." And thus he concludes that wrong reactions

[9] I am referring to his experiments according to Procedure I, high numbers of repetitions, which alone are comparable to Lewin's experiments.

occur only where a wrong set is operative, retardation, only where two sets are in conflict. To the proof of this assumption he devotes a number of highly ingenious experiments which can be simplified so as to be performed in the classroom. The underlying idea is that the same result may be accomplished by two different activities, and more easily by the one than by the other, and that the subject will sooner or later choose the easier activity even if it is not the one required by the instruction. This will lead to no mistake as long as the original condition is fulfilled, viz., that the wrong performance leads to the right result. If, however, this wrong activity is exercised on material where it does *not* produce the correct result, then either the result will be wrong, or a conflict will occur between two activities, with a resultant retardation. These conclusions were amply confirmed.

The procedure was as follows: Eight syllables were "associated" with other syllables by the method last described. That is to say, four of them had to be responded to by another syllable in which the hard initial consonant was to be replaced by a soft one and *vice versa* (*r* syllables), example *tak-dak,* while the four others had to be inverted (*i*-syllables). Each syllable was presented thirty-two times, a comparatively small number if compared with the high number of repetitions in the previous series. A very important aspect is the mode of presentation. At first all four *r*-syllables were presented, each syllable being repeated before the next was named, e.g.:

stimulus	response
dak	*tak*
dak	*tak*
ged	*ked*
ged	*ked*

This whole procedure was repeated, and then the same syllables were repeated twice more in simple alternation without successive repetition. Then the *i* syllables were subjected to the same procedure. Then came more repetitions of the first and the second kind of material, until both had the required 32. After the completion of the learning the testing took place. Again the subjects were presented with syllables, their task being to respond by changing the *vowel.* First 20 *n* (new) syllables were called out, then an *r* syllable, five more *n* syllables, then an *i* syllable, six *n* syllables, another *r* syllable, and one more *n* syllable. I.e., the three critical syllables which had been practised before were interspersed in a great number of neutral syllables, with the result that *no* wrong reaction occurred and that the average reaction time of those critical syllables was exactly the same as the average time of the *n* syllables. Thus, this first test only confirmed the previous result. But now a new test was added: the instruction was hard-soft rhyming, and the first four syllables were the four *r* syllables with which this activity had been practised before; they were followed by two syllables taken from these same *r* syllables, then came the *i* syllable of the first test, and then the two other *r* syllables. The result was that the reaction time of the *i* syllable was 144% (880σ) longer than the average of the *r* syllables. The same *i* syllable, which in the first test had not led to any retardation, produced a very large one in this. The experiment finished with a last test in which the task was to invert and in which the procedure was the same as in the preceding, except that the two *r* syllables used in the first test were interspersed in the midst of *i* syllables. One of them led to a wrong reaction, the other to a retardation of 74% (480σ).

Since the same syllables show retardation and wrong reaction in one kind of test but not in another, the cause of these effects cannot be the association which should have shown up in either of them, both conforming to the type + —. The true cause is easy to find. In the two last tests the first six syllables offered for the particular activity, rhyming and inverting, had been learned in conjunction with a rhymed and inverted syllable respectively. There are therefore two ways of fulfilling the task of rhyming an *r* syllable: either really to rhyme it, or to do with it what has been done before, i.e., to reproduce the following syllable. Similarly, when we are asked to add 8 + 4 we answer 12 without a new process of addition by mere reproduction. Just so the subjects after rhyming one or two *r* syllables would no longer really rhyme them but *reproduce.* The method of original presentation for purposes of learning, double presentation of each syllable, had been chosen because it would tend to favour this mode of procedure. There exists, then, a *set* to *reproduce* which is as much a set as the set to rhyme, and this set, if applied to an inappropriate syllable (*i* syllable for rhyming, and *r* syllable for inverting), must lead to wrong reactions, or if this is checked, to a considerable retardation. When on the other hand, as in the first test, a number of neutral syllables are given for the execution of a task, then there is only one way of doing it, and reproduction cannot take its place. Consequently no set to reproduce develops and the *r* and *i* syllables are just as easily and quickly changed in the right way as the *n* syllables.

This explanation invalidates one of Ach's assumptions which we have listed in our table on page 576 as 0 +, the assumption, namely, that reproduction is the *mere* effect of association without any special set.

THE RELATION OF LEWIN'S WORK TO OUR THEORY. However, our main question remains as yet unanswered: Are Lewin's results compatible with our theory? Do they prove that an association, or rather an organized trace system, exerts no force on the new process? As far as I can see, and I have Professor Lewin's assent to this opinion, they do not. For the same explanation which we gave to his experiments with a perfectly passive attitude (see p. 561) is equally applicable here. It is not proven that in the cases where no retardation or wrong reaction occurred the old traces were in communication with the new process. But if they were not, then they could not, of course, exert any influence upon it. If this is the true explanation of Lewin's results, they are perfectly compatible with our own theory. Thereby their significance is not in the least diminished. Instead of bearing on the effect exercised by a trace upon a process they bear on the opposite relationship, the effect produced by a process on the trace system. For they prove that, in terms of the association theory, the re-arousal of an *a* does not necessarily carry with it a tendency towards the re-arousal of *b*, which had previously been associated with *a*, because the re-arousal of *a* does not necessarily communicate with the *a b* trace. In other words, even in terms of its own theory the law of association was incomplete. The recurrence of an *a* can arouse a tendency for *b* to appear only when *a* establishes a communication with the old *a b* trace system.

Lewin's experiments prove more than this, revealing as they do a very powerful factor which determines this communication. However, before we follow this lead we shall briefly discuss the fact itself. It seems self-evident, and yet it has gained no recognition in associationistic psychology although it was clearly pointed out and vigorously emphasized by Höffding in 1889. Höffding argued like this: I see an apple and am reminded of paradise. Now, the apple that I am seeing at present was never together with a picture of paradise, but a picture of an apple, different from the present one, may have been contained in a picture of paradise, or a mere idea of an apple may have been together with an idea of paradise. However this may be, the present apple, so Höffding argued, must first come into connection with the memory trace of the old apple, because only this can lead to the idea of paradise.

The "Law of Substitution" (or "Assimilation"). This interpretation was not accepted by psychologists, who at the time were completely under the sway of associationism, because it implied the efficacy of similarity for the evocation of the trace by the new process. They preferred to base their theory on the law of contiguity alone. And so they introduced another law, the law of substitution, to explain the same fact. This law says: if an association between *a* and *b* has been formed, then not only *a* will be able to reproduce *b*, but also any *a′* which is similar to *a*, the strength of the reproductive tendency aroused by *a′* varying with the degree of similarity between *a′* and *a* (Müller and Pilzecker). In America this law has been called the law of assimilation—not a good name, since the term assimilation had been used much earlier by Wundt for a very different phenomenon (see Chapter III, p. 103)—and appears as a real law in the recent presentation of associationism by Robinson. It seems to me, however, that this law *names* what it considers to be a fact without explaining it. It would indeed be an explanation if one assumed, as Höffding did, that the trace *a* can be re-aroused by a process *a′*, different from, but similar to *a*, and that therefore *a′* can reproduce *b*. But without this assumption, which the law of substitution was intended to make unnecessary, this law is unconnected with the main body of associationism, if one means by associationism an explanatory theory and not a mere collection of purely empirical laws.

But even as such an empirical law the law of substitution is false, as follows directly from Lewin's experiments, for he has proved even more than Höffding claimed. To apply Lewin's results to Höffding's example we may say: if we have seen an apple next to a vase and see the same apple again, then there need arise no tendency towards the reproduction of the vase. This reproduction will take place only when the special conditions of the case ensure that the new perception communicates with the old trace. The same is true *a fortiori* for the case where the apple that we see now is different from the apple that we saw lying by the vase, so that the law of substitution contains within itself the still unsolved problem: When does a process communicate with a trace?

The Rôle of Attitudes or Sets in Reproduction. To this problem Lewin's experiments contribute an answer of high significance: they prove that such communication may be created by a "set," attitude, intention, or otherwise expressed that forces starting within an Ego-system can be powerful factors in bringing about communication between a process and a trace both of which belong to the environmental field. We had come to the same conclusion before, at the end of the eleventh chapter, when we discussed the attempt to recall a name (p. 525), and at the beginning of this, when we discussed another of Lewin's experiments. Thus Lewin's results demand that kind of Ego-environment hypothesis which, starting from entirely different premises, we have introduced in Chapter VIII (p. 333), an hypothesis by which Ego and environment are in dynamic intercourse both in the process of actual present organization and in the accumulation of traces of such organizations.

Before we follow up this idea and discuss the problem of the communication more thoroughly, we must add a few words about the relation of Lewin's work to our theory and a section about other types of associative learning.

Although our theory implies that communication of trace and process, by producing tensions in the trace, is apt to create a force between trace and process in the sense of reproduction, it does not mean, as pointed out before, that such spontaneous reproduction must inevitably follow. In the first place, reproduction would be truly spontaneous only if the process had formed its trace without the co-operation of a set or attitude. This possibility we shall have to assume, as will be shown later. But even when communication takes place, the tension created in the trace system cannot be accepted as explaining the whole process of reproduction as it occurs in memory experiments. The fact that the subject actually pronounces the reproduced items is indeed more than can be derived from our hypothesis. Whether he does or not, must depend upon forces extraneous to those between trace and process, i.e., upon attitudes, intentions, sets. And if one includes these aspects of reproduction, then Lewin's claim that association (or the existence and participation of an organized trace) can never be the motor of any mental activity is perfectly true.

We must, however, go even further than that. Continually, old large trace systems are in communication with present part processes, and yet, in any controlled activity, reproductions that lead away from the goal of that activity occur very rarely, even in the form of mere "knowledge" or "thinking about." Köhler (1929, pp. 335 ff.) has insisted on this point sufficiently for us to pass it over with these few words. But even this does not contradict our theory. For as we know, a controlled activity means an activity under the rule of strong forces, forces partly external and partly internal to the organization of the process and the trace which it is building up (see our discussion in Chapter IX, pp. 418 f.). Compared to these forces the tensions arising in the trace will often be negligible.

OTHER TYPES OF "ASSOCIATIVE LEARNING." The question may even be legitimately raised whether such tensions in a whole-trace will arise under all conditions when a part process communicates with a part of it. We have so far treated reproduction as though it were the only effect that a whole-trace could exert upon a new process. But this is far from the truth. And we can choose another type of so-called associative learning to discover a very different effect. The method of nonsense syllables was the contribution of an earlier epoch in psychology—German psychology—to the investigation of learning. Two other methods have since then been introduced and have gradually surpassed the old in the scope of their application, viz., the method of the conditioned reflex, invented in Russia, and the method of the maze, developed in America. Both methods share with the nonsense syllable method the aspect of complete arbitrariness of the items to be connected. The conditional sitmulus can be selected at random, and similarly the structure of the maze with its different blind alleys and its true path is entirely at the discretion of the experimenter. Nothing in the situation itself demands, say, a bell to be connected with feeding, or the building of the maze according to any one of the principles employed in the different investigations, just as little as the syllable *zut* demands that the syllable *pid* follow upon it. We shall not treat the conditioned reflex experiments, because by their very construction they cannot make any direct contribution to our problem. Moreover, the theory of the conditioned reflex has been very searchingly discussed during the last few years, notably by Tolman and Humphrey, so that a new discussion would not advance us very much further.

Maze Experiments. The maze experiments, on the other hand, have, in the hands of ingenious experimenters, acquired a new meaning which is relevant to our present discussion. In the ordinary maze experiment the animal learns the maze in the attempt to reach the food contained in the food box. The progress of learning consists in the animal's obtaining its reward more and more quickly and with fewer and fewer errors, i.e., by entering fewer and fewer blind alleys. Learning here is defined by behaviour continuously approaching an optimal type, it is the steady improvement of one and the same accomplishment, in that sense again similar to the learning of series of nonsense syllables. One can, however, alter the procedure in such a way that during the first part of the "learning period" the accomplishment of the animal is different from that of the second.

Will then the practice in the first accomplishment aid the second one?

"Latent Learning." The best and simplest way would probably be one suggested to me once by Dr. Mintz: put the animal into a maze and let it stay there for, say, a couple of hours without rewarding it. Repeat this a number of times and then introduce food in the food box. Compare the behaviour of such animals with that of a control group which has been trained in the same maze by the usual method, i.e., by having food in the food box from the first day of training. As far as I know this experiment has not yet been performed, but experiments by Blodgett and by Tolman and Honzik, briefly referred to in an earlier part of this chapter (p. 547), are similar enough to allow a prediction of what would happen if it were carried out. The last two authors put rats into a maze and took them out, without feeding them, as soon as they reached the exit box, feeding not taking place till two hours later, in their living-cages. After this had been done for ten days, food was introduced on the eleventh. "On the twelfth day they exhibited an enormous drop in both errors and times" (Tolman, p. 52); as a matter of fact their error curve dropped on that day below that of a normal control group which had been running this maze for the same number of days with food in the exit box, whereas on the preceding day the control group had made far fewer errors. To express the result in this way is, of course, not correct. For the term error has meaning only for the animal that wants to get quickly to the food box, i.e., for the control group and the test group after the eleventh day. Before this day an entry of a blind alley was in no sense an error, except for the experimenter who wants to tabulate the results. This experiment proves that the activity of exploring the maze with a great number of "errors" is at least as advantageous for the desired effect, the quick and errorless reaching of the food box, as the activity of running for that food box. But in the former the difference between the pre-critical and the critical activities is much greater than in the latter; in the former the trace of the older activities has the effect *not* of reproducing, with modifications, these activities, but of giving rise to *new* activities. It is therefore highly probable that the experiment suggested by Dr. Mintz would also have a positive result: living in the maze would help the rats to find the food box quickly as soon as they became motivated to run for it.

"Latent Learning" as an Example of a Trace Influence That Is Not Reproduction. Thus we have come across a striking example

of a trace-effect which is *not* reproduction. The trace formed by the non-rewarded runs in the maze becomes a more and more articulated system which forms part of the field in which the later motivated activity takes place, and directs it according to field structure and motivation. It seems quite unnecessary to assume that the rat will be impelled, in its run for food, to choose a path that leads in a wrong direction simply because it had chosen it in its non- (or differently) motivated activity.

THE GENERAL FIELD-INFLUENCE EXERTED BY A TRACE UPON A PROCESS. So this experiment brings us back to the discussion interrupted a while ago. And we find now that a part process in communication with a trace which is part of a larger trace system need not be affected by this trace at all in the sense of reproduction corresponding to the whole trace. The communication may have altogether different effects. It might seem that this conclusion contradicted the theory which we took such great pains to develop, viz., that such communication would set up tensions within the total trace which would exert a force towards reproduction. But this contradiction disappears as soon as we consider that the effect of the communication upon the trace must depend upon the nature of the trace. In the case under discussion the trace system influencing the test runs may be not that of the previous run, but that of the maze pattern which, as previously mentioned (p. 547), arose out of the other traces. Furthermore not all traces can be so constituted that asymmetrical communication changes their stability and thereby gives rise to stresses. Only those where this is the case can cause spontaneous reproduction, and since probably they are in the minority, spontaneous reproduction should, according to our theory, occur still more rarely than would follow from our earlier discussion. And therefore Lewin's criticism of this concept becomes the more significant.

To say which traces are of the one kind, which of the other, would require a much better knowledge of traces than we possess today. The main value of my hypotheses, if they have any, seems to me to lie more in their heuristic than in their explanatory character. They pose problems, problems which an associationistic psychology could never have raised. The only indication of an answer to our question seems to me this: traces resulting from rote learning are particularly apt to become endowed with tension through communication with part processes and thereby to be capable of initiating spontaneous reproduction. It is plausible to connect this with the fact that they form more or less isolated, self-sufficient systems, whereas most other traces must be connected with innumerable other trace systems.

But the discussion of the Tolman-Honzik maze experiment has given us an even more important insight. A trace system may exert influences other than reproduction on the continuation of a process. The influence studied in this experiment was one upon the animal's activity. We can describe it best by saying that the trace developed during its non-rewarded runs influenced its activity in the food-motivated runs in a manner similar to that in which a maze which the animal could *perceive* in all or many of its details would. If the animal sees or feels that an alley is blocked at one end it will turn back; if it sees that another alley leads to the lure it will enter it. The Tolman-Honzik experiment and our everyday experience demonstrate that the trace can have a similar effect. What the animal has developed during its "latent learning" is a trace of the maze; this trace, being in communication with the present activity, regulates it more or less as the perception of the maze would. Just so, when I want a book I leave my chair and turn to the book-case at the side of the room which at the moment is outside my perceptual field. The trace field of the whole room in which I am staying is in communication with my present activity and thereby directs it in such a way that orderly action, started by needs or intentions, becomes possible. Again, dynamically it makes no difference whether the required book stands on my desk within the field of perception or in the book-case at the side.

Why This Theory Is Not Associationistic. But is this not association? Let us see what this claim would mean. In writing this chapter I was reminded of an experiment on "latent learning." This had become associated with Tolman's book, because I had first read it there. Therefore the idea of the experiment reproduces the idea of the book. This in its turn is associated with the shelf on which I have put it, and therefore the idea of the bookshelf arises. And now? The idea of the bookshelf is associated with many other ideas, e.g., with that of all my cases containing reprints; are they or any other associated ideas reproduced? Not at all. What happens is that I rise from my chair and fetch the book. Has Tolman's book been associated with this activity? If not, why, on purely associationistic principles, do I rise? In this presentation of the associationistic explanation I have disregarded the fact that spontaneous reproduction, on which this whole explanation rests, is a very rare occurrence. Even so, the explanation fails to explain what it set out to. Granted then that my final action requires some other kind of explanation, what of the preceding events? Why does the idea of Tolman's book reproduce the idea of the bookcase and not that of the many seminar evenings on which I discussed it, or that of my review of it, which by "frequency" and emotional intensity should be favoured? Surely it is not chance that at this moment the bookshelf association proved to be the strongest while at other moments entirely different ones would be dominant, occasions at which I would never think of the place of the book, but of its contents, or its author, or what not. Certainly I could think of neither of these unless the "Tolman-trace" were connected with all those other traces. But neither is the fact of the connection enough, nor has the connection been proved to be of the type of association. In short, if one calls the explanation of my activity which I gave above an associationistic one, one shirks the issue. Association has unwittingly assumed a meaning which makes it practically synonymous with experience. And a theory based on experience, a *genetic* theory, is for that very reason a desirable theory. Therefore the great attachment to associationism. But association is far from being synonymous with experience. It is *one* way of coping with experience, *one* conception to treat experience scientifically. Therefore a criticism of associationism, however negative it may be, is not a rejection of a genetic theory. There are other, and I believe *better,* ways of treating experience than the concept of association.

A Reference to Older Experiments on Memory. In many respects the preceding discussion of associative learning was incomplete. Its omission of a reference to most of the results reached by the older experiments is due to the fact that their theoretical meaning is, to say the least, highly ambiguous. Take the facts expressed in Jost's law: two series of nonsense syllables, A and B, of which A has been learned some time before B and with more repetitions, will rank differently according to the method used in testing them. By the method of paired associates B may be the one better retained, whereas by the saving method A may appear superior. The traditional explanation has been a one-factor explanation, in agreement with the traditional theory which knows only one variable: the strength of association. It says that the *average* strength of association is greater in A than in B, and therefore it can be relearned more easily, while the individual number of associations which are supraliminal, i.e., which are strong enough to effect reproduction, is greater in B, accounting for its superiority in the method of paired associates. But such a simple explanation overlooks the dynamics of the situation. There are three problems involved: the effect of the trace on the process once it is in communication with it—this is the equivalent in our terms to the old theory—the case of communication between the present process and the trace, and, thirdly, the effect of new repetitions on the existing trace systems. It seems to me very unlikely that the facts can find their explanation in terms of the first problem alone, but since we lack experimental evidence to decide this point, I shall omit these and numerous other effects.

But our discussion of associative learning was incomplete also because it left the second problem just mentioned unanswered, although we encountered it again and again. It is not, however, a problem specific of associative learning. It was equally obvious in our discussion of the acquisition of skills, and it is of no less importance for the problem of recognition. Therefore, before treating it we shall turn to this new achievement of memory.

CHAPTER XIII

LEARNING AND OTHER MEMORY FUNCTIONS II

Recognition and the Problem of Communication Between Process and Trace. Theories of Recognition and Their Problems. The Causes of Communication Between Process and Trace. The Law of Similarity. Other Laws. The Arousal of a New Process. Thinking. The Relation of Logic and Psychology. Problem Solving. Two Steps. M. R. Harrower's Experiments. How Is the Solution of a Problem Found? "Insight." Organization in Perception and Thought Compared. Experimental Studies. The Original Reorganization. The Law of Effect. Our Picture of Behaviour. Intelligence. Different Types of Reorganization

RECOGNITION AND THE PROBLEM OF COMMUNICATION BETWEEN PROCESS AND TRACE

Unfortunately it is not easy to define what we mean by recognition. I recognize a pencil as a pencil, and my special pencil as *my* pencil; but in a sense this latter effect will occur only if I see it among others and not when I take it out of my pocket. A similar example is given by Maccurdy: "If I meet one of my students[1] in London I recognize him; if I see the same man in my lecture room in Cambridge I do not recognize him, although I know he is there" (p. 113).

We must then distinguish first of all "class" recognition and individual recognition, and, secondly, explicit and implicit recognition, the explicit being characteristic of Maccurdy's meeting his student in London, the implicit of his meeting him in the lecture room. For it seems to me not correct to say that in this last case no recognition takes place. For if I, or Maccurdy, were asked whether we knew this or that student in our class we should unhesitatingly answer "yes," and this answer does not presuppose that the question has *changed* the perception of the student; my affirmative answer is the direct outcome of the perception, even though it lacked that tone of familiarity which it would have in a different context (e.g., in London).

Still, we are dealing with different cases, and the theory of recognition finds itself continually hampered by that difficulty. How the difference between class- and individual recognition makes it impos-

[1] I have substituted the word "students" for Maccurdy's word "class" in order to avoid unnecessary ambiguity in my text.

sible unambiguously to evaluate her own quantitative results has been pointed out by von Restorff.

Theories of Recognition and Their Problems. There was a time when recognition was a major problem in psychology. Katzaroff published a paper on the subject in 1911 in which he enumerated and discussed fourteen different theories. One fundamental fact stands out for every theory of recognition: an object A cannot be recognized unless some object A′ had occurred previously. In the terms of any theory except that of Wheeler—whose application to recognition I can understand even less than its application to recall—this must mean that a present process is under some influence of a trace of A′. The problem is: Of what kind is this influence and what produces it, i.e., why, in our terminology, does the process communicate with the trace A′? In 1906 Schumann, surveying the experimental work on the psychology of reading, said: "Today the assumption is made fairly universally that in the act of recognition the images of former perceptions of the same object are being re-excited, fuse with the sensations and give to the perceptual process its 'quality of familiarity'" (p. 170). Recognition is, in this view, explained by assimilation, and inasmuch as we have rejected the assimilation hypothesis (Chapter III, p. 103) we shall not accept this explanation of recognition. Nevertheless I find Bartlett's judgment of this hypothesis entirely too harsh when he says: It "is a striking example of a fruitless hypothesis, and can never be either proved or disproved" (p. 192). For apart from its specific form this hypothesis claims a connection between a process occurring now and a system of traces left behind by earlier processes, and this claim, though, like all our physiological hypotheses, not amenable to direct proof, finds a number of facts to substantiate it, facts which would remain unexplained without some such hypothesis. Schumann himself points to the fact that a word of 25 letters tachistoscopically exposed can be seen clearly and distinctly in all its parts, and that furthermore this clearly perceived word may be more or less different from the actually exposed one, whereas of 25 unconnected letters at best a small fraction will be so perceived. Of course I agree with Bartlett, if he applies his criticism only to the hypothesis of fusion of sensations and images, but even there I must plead for Schumann that at the time of his report no other possibility of a connection between a process and a trace had been envisaged.

The Theory of Katzaroff and Claparède. That in recognition the process is under the influence of a trace is, as I said before, the minimum that any theory of recognition has to assume. That this minimum is not enough was the claim of Katzaroff, which was vigorously defended by Claparède (1911). Claparède produced cases where indubitably a connection of trace and process had occurred and where nevertheless recognition had failed to appear. The bulk of his material is taken from post-hypnotic suggestion and from the Korsakoff syndrome, characterized by an extreme memory defect. He points out the discrepancy manifest in Korsakoff patients between their achievements in recognition and voluntary recall on the one hand, and their orientation in the hospital on the other: whereas the former may be completely absent, the latter may be normal. Thus a woman who was perfectly well oriented in the hospital, found her way to the lavatories, bathrooms, etc., would not recognize her nurse, who took care of her for six months. If the nurse asked her whether she knew her she replied: "Non, madame, a qui ai-je l'honneur de parler?" (Claparède, p. 84.) I have reproduced this quotation in order to show what lack of recognition means, and how different it is from the case of the student in the lecture room which we discussed previously. In terms of that discussion the answer of Claparède's patients proves a lack of individual recognition, not of class recognition. As a matter of fact, as Maccurdy, whose own observations fully confirm those of Claparède, points out, the nurse is not only recognized as a woman, but as a woman to whom respect is due. Claparède has made experiments with these patients; a particularly neat one is reproduced by Maccurdy. I omit it here and give instead an ingenious experiment by Maccurdy himself: "I would give the patient my full name and address. Within a few minutes this was totally 'forgotten.' Later on, I would present the patient with a list of ten Christian names, another of ten surnames, another of street numbers, and another of street names. From this he would be asked to guess which one was mine. To my surprise, the guesses were nearly as accurate as would be the conscious memory for such data of normal subjects. But the response remained to the subject a mere guess, it was associated with no feeling of me-ness; on no occasion did the patient think that he had the slightest reason for picking one name rather than another from the list" (p. 121). The striking point in this experiment, as in those by Claparède, is that the new process, the "guessing," must have been in communication with the trace left by the information given before the experiment. This is proved by the degree of correctness of the choice. And yet, although the process was in communication with the trace, it lacked all recognition, the correct choices were made without conviction, they appeared as pure guesses.

Therefore mere communication cannot be enough, some other factor must be added. This other factor is found by Katzaroff and Claparède, with whose interpretation Maccurdy more or less agrees, in the "feeling of me-ness." In Katzaroff's words: "One may therefore assume that the feeling of familiarity (*sentiment de familier*), *déjà vu,* which accompanies a repeated sensation results from the fact that this sensation, when it passed through our consciousness for the first time, became associated with the very feeling of our 'Ego' (*s'est associée au sentiment lui-même de notre 'moi'*) and was, so to speak, enveloped by it" (p. 78).

Today it may seem surprising that this theory has found so little support. Bartlett, who distinguishes four theories of recognition, does not even mention it. But we must not forget that at the time the theory was proposed, experimental psychology had no place for the Ego. Thus in the book which I published in 1912 I refused to accept Claparède's explanation, whereas now, when the Ego has a prominent place in the psychological system here presented, I recognize its value and admire the insight of its author. Many theorists had acknowledged the "feeling of familiarity," the *"Bekanntheits-Qualität"* of Höffding, but they had been satisfied with a discussion whether this quality was an emotional or an intellectual element of experience, without an acknowledgment of the fact that the "familiar" is "familiar to *me,*" i.e., that recognizing involves an object-Ego relationship.

This Theory and Our Ego-hypothesis. Our theory of the Ego, as it was developed in the preceding chapters, allows us to accept Claparède's theory, freeing it from those aspects which are the outcome of the period at which he worked, and to incorporate it without any new hypothesis into our own system. In the eighth chapter we saw how the necessary assumption of a permanent Ego system involves the assumption of an environment system from which this Ego system remains segregated. In Chapters X and XI we have developed this hypothesis from the point of view of a trace theory, and now we can reap the harvest. I believe that it strengthens the status of our theory that it was developed from facts different from those which are now to be explained by it. It became necessary on the grounds of a general theory of organization, and now it provides an explanation of recognition and voluntary recall.

In our theory the trace retained the dynamics of the process in a latent form. We also know that our environmental field does not consist of a number of "dead" or "indifferent" things, but that these things possess dynamic characters, such as physiognomic, functional, and demand characters. All these characters imply an object-Ego relationship, i.e., an interplay of forces between the Ego and the environmental objects. Therefore, the trace of an object is, as a rule, part of a larger trace of which the object is but one sub-system, while a part of the Ego is another, these two sub-systems being connected by forces corresponding to the forces obtaining in the process of perception. Communication of the trace with a new object-process means, therefore, at least potentially, communication of this whole trace with the new process. And according to Claparède's theory, recognition can take place only when the *whole* trace becomes involved and not merely the object sub-system.

This is the translation of Claparède's theory into our own, as will be seen more clearly still when we envisage Claparède's theory in its most general aspects. "One must distinguish between two sorts of connections: those which establish themselves *eventually between ideas,* and those which establish themselves *between the ideas and that which constitutes the Ego,* the personality. In the case of purely passive or reflex association of ideas the first kind of connections will function alone; in the case of voluntary recall or of recognition, where the Ego is involved, the second kind would play its part" (Claparède, p. 86). In our terms, communication with a part of a trace system may bring into play either such other parts of the system as do not include the Ego, or those which belong to the Ego also. The effect on the present process must be different in the two cases.

The case is similar to that of the command of the executive. The same distinction between intra-Ego-, Ego-environment- and intra-environmental forces that proved so fruitful there, finds its application here. The forces within the trace which affect the process now occurring may be of any of the three kinds. The first has not been mentioned by Claparède, but the two others correspond closely to his distinction.

This theory allows certain deductions about the conditions under which recognition is more or less likely to occur. Since it depends upon the participation of the Ego-part in the particular trace systems, the structure of this system will be of great importance. The closer the dynamic intercourse between the Ego and the object part, the more likely, *ceteris paribus,* will recognition be. Now in the structure of the behavioural environment there are things close to and remote from the Ego and even some that have practically no Ego-connection. According to the theory, and to all appearances in conformity with the facts, the former are better recognized than the latter. In many cases the Ego-object relationship will be, at least partly, due to the interests and attitudes of the Ego. Thus whatever has interested us, attracted our attention, is relatively easily recognized. "The things we deny ever having done, in the face of ample testimony from honest observers, are acts performed 'absent-mindedly,' automatically. Automatic behaviour has no me-ness attached to it." Thus Maccurdy (p. 124).

THE QUALITY OF FAMILIARITY. Can we explain also why the positive impression of familiarity fails to appear with objects which are too well known? When we formulate the question in this way we have to remember that even well-known objects may carry that quality of familiarity if they appear in a new environment; we recall Maccurdy's student. This fact gives us the clue for our explanation. When we see the well-known object in its normal environment, then our attitude towards it is also, as a rule, the normal one. Therefore, the process which communicates with the trace is not simply the process of perceiving the object but the process of perceiving this object which, corresponding to the prevailing attitude, is in a definite relation to the Ego. This new process will at once communicate with the whole Ego-object trace; conversely, when the object is encountered in a new environment with a different Ego-attitude, then the communication takes place between object process and object trace, and the effect of this communication of a part trace with a part process will be the one derived in our theory of reproduction: the whole trace will be put under tension. We derived from this tension the possibility of spontaneous reproduction, and indeed recognition is very often accompanied by spontaneous reproduction. But we are now forced to the conclusion that this stress, if it involves the Ego-object pattern of the trace, must also account for the quality of familiarity in recognition. On the other hand, we see the justification of including as true cases of recognition also those where a known object appears without this quality. For we had to assume that in these cases a communication between process and trace occurred, a communication, however, of the kind that produced no stresses in the trace. And when we compare this case with the one *without* recognition, e.g., Claparède's Korsakoff patient, we see indeed that the line of cleavage runs between *these* two, and not between the first two cases (i.e., student in London and in the lecture room).

Our theory also accounts for the fact that the quality of familiarity can be more or less impressive. It must explain the impressiveness (or intensity) of the quality of familiarity by the amount of stress set up in the object-Ego trace, and it is a direct consequence from the theory that this stress can continuously vary in intensity.

In applying this hypothesis one must not forget that our formulation was greatly oversimplified. In order to find the principle of the underlying dynamics it isolated one single object with *one* Ego relationship. In reality much more complex conditions will obtain. But in order to understand these complexities one must first have grasped the principle of a simple, even though fictitious, case.

The question of what kind the influence exerted by a trace or a process in recognition is has been answered only in part. We have said more about the traces which exert the influence than about the actual influence itself. The reason is obvious. We know the influence only through direct experience—and I do not see how any observation of the behaviour of animals can reveal it, for the behaviour of the Korsakoff patient in his normal environment does not look different from that of a normal person; the fact that it is behaviour without recognition and voluntary recall is not amenable to this kind of observation—but we do not know anything about the dynamic connection between trace and process except what we have to assume in order to explain the facts of direct experience or those interpreted with the help of direct experience. All we can say, therefore, at the present moment is that a process that communicates with a trace must be different from one that does not, and that the *kind* of trace it communicates with will also determine the nature of this influence.

The Causes of Communication Between Process and Trace. And now we can at last turn to the problem so often deferred, viz., the problem of the causes of the communication between process and trace. Thus we shall now complete the discussion begun in Chapter X (pp. 461 ff.), and again we have to select between two ways of approaching this problem; we might either survey all the known facts and try to derive as many special laws from them as possible, or we might analyze the communication and its effects as such, try to derive from each analysis a general law, and then fill in as many special cases as we can find. I choose the second way, because the empirical data are very scant, and apart from as yet unpublished experiments by Köhler and von Restorff, they have not been collected for the purpose of solving our problem.

The General Principle. Let us then consider the event in its broadest aspect. A process is aroused—for simplicity's sake we assume a perceptual process caused by sensory stimulation; this process occurs at the tip of a "trace column" (see p. 447); it may communicate with practically any one of the innumerable trace systems. Since the process will be affected by this communication, the choice which it makes among the existing traces will determine its own future. We have encountered similar conditions before, and we have found that under these conditions the choice must depend upon its influence on the future of the process. Our description of the circular perceptive-motor process given in Chapter IX (pp. 373 f.) can be translated into these terms. The field F_0 which starts the movement selects such movements as determine its own future in such a way that the subsequent fields F_1, F_2, . . . are progressively under less stress. It is therefore no new hypothesis if we apply this general principle to the problem of the selection of a trace by a process: this selection must have something to do with the nature of the process, it must further one kind of development of this process rather than others. Let us call the kind of development which is thus being furthered the stability of the process, just to have a convenient name. The actual choice will then depend upon this stability. Those traces will communicate with the process which will give it the particular stability it needs. When we say that in this way our problem has become a problem of organization we say nothing new, but with this formulation we connect our problem with others, the solution of which has been previously indicated. Again, in this aspect also, memory appears not as an entirely new function with completely new laws, but as a special case of a very general function.

The Law of Similarity. One of the first laws of perceptual organization which we encountered was the law of similarity. If we could apply this law to our present problem it would mean that a process would exert a dynamic influence on a trace which had been built up by a similar process so as to produce communication with it. In our previous discussion in Chapter X we demonstrated the necessity of such a law and saw that similarity must mean similarity of patterns. This law of similarity has also been recognized, if we discount the different terminology resulting from a different theoretical foundation, by many psychologists in their theory of recognition. I recall Höffding, Schumann, and Semon.[2] And indeed it would be impossible to explain recognition and a great amount of so-called associative reproduction without such a law. However, we must not

[2] I refrain from giving a survey of Semon's theory and from discussing how far it agrees with the one here presented and how far it is different. Such a discussion would unnecessarily break up the course of our discussion without making any positive contribution. I must add, however, that this omission is not due to a lack of appreciation of Semon's great achievement.

forget that similarity is not absolute similarity, not similarity *in vacuo*. On the one hand, when we first introduced a similarity law of organization we formulated it as a similarity-proximity law. Two simultaneous similar processes will interact the more the closer they are together. Inasmuch as this law applies to our problem it means that *ceteris paribus* a similar trace will have a better chance to be chosen by a present process when it is recent, i.e., near the tip of the trace column, than when it is old. It is important to stress the condition *ceteris paribus,* since other factors of selection, which we shall discuss presently, may overcome the handicap of age.

On the other hand similarity has in this connection to be subjected to the same criticism that von Restorff applied to her concepts of repeated and isolated material (see Chapter XI, p. 485). If a number of similar processes occur in close succession in such a way that their communication with the trace of any of the previous ones does not contribute to their stability, then they will soon cease to produce such communication, and therefore a new similar process which would profit by communication with the trace system will also fail to select it. When instead a process A is followed by a number of different processes, B, B′, B″ . . . A′, then A′ will be much more likely to communicate with the trace of A. This has been proved by the unpublished experiments by Köhler and von Restorff which I previously mentioned, and on which Köhler gave a brief report at the International Congress at Copenhagen in 1932. In our discussion of Restorff's argument, which was concerned with the aggregation of traces, we saw how this definition of similarity has its exact counterpart in perception, and thus presents a general feature of organization. Therefore the same law found valid for the relation between process and trace automatically makes this relation one of organization.

The Relation Between the Law of Similarity and the General Principle. But we cannot be satisfied with this discussion of the law of similarity, since we started out with a much more general law according to which communication between process and trace was determined by the stability of the former. We must therefore examine the relation of this general law and the special law of similarity. This investigation will be handicapped by the fact that we have not properly defined the term stability. Thus we could easily fall into the trap of a teleological explanation, looking at the *result* of communication and using this result as a cause of the process. To say: a certain process occurs because it is biologically useful, would be the kind of explanation we have to guard against. For the biological advantage of a process is an effect which has to be explained by the process, but the former cannot be used to explain the latter. A process must find its explanation in the dynamics of the system within which it occurs; the concept of biological advantage, on the other hand, does not belong to dynamics at all. And therefore teleological explanations in terms of biological advantage have no place in gestalt theory.

How, then, can we connect the general law of stability with the special law of similarity? Let us turn back to the first effect exerted by a trace on a process which we discussed, viz., the acquisition of skills, and let us consider an example previously introduced, that of the Southerner on the ice-covered streets in the North. We saw how the improvement of his skill in crossing these streets is due to the interaction between trace and process. And the cause of the communication must be in this case, as in the case of recognition, the similarity between trace and process. But, bearing in mind our theory of this improvement, we can look at it from a different point of view. We explained the improvement by the fact that the original process, and therefore the trace left by it, was not stable, and that communication resulted in processes of greater stability. That is, we assumed the fact of communication and derived a specific change of the process from it. We can now look at the same total event differently and connect not only the change of the process with its communication with the trace, but also the latter with the former; i.e., we can say: the particular trace was selected because communication with it would lead to an improved process. At the same time, as we have seen, the selected trace derived from a process similar to the one now occurring, so that similarity and stability have become connected in our theory. Similarity is one way by which greater stability can be reached.

The case of motor skills was particularly suitable for our argument, because the increased stability of the process had been previously derived and did not have to be assumed merely for the sake of establishing a connection between stability and similarity. In the case of recognition we are not in such a favourable position, because we have not yet deduced that recognition stabilizes the process, which we must claim if we want to interpret the relation between stability and similarity in the same manner. And yet some stabilizing effect must occur in recognition if our theory is right. That the kind of stability must be different in the two cases, recognition and improvement of skill, is obvious. In the former its main aspect cannot be a change in the internal organization of the process itself—

although such an effect will frequently accompany recognition—rather must the greater stability of the new process, which it achieves by recognition, be due to its becoming related with previously existing trace fields. At the end of Chapter XI (p. 526 f.) we have tried to show how a trace can gain stability by communication with other traces. A trace from a process which communicated with other traces will itself be in communication with them. And thus a "recognized" process will have a more stable trace than a similar process without such communication. Because of the constant dynamic relation between a process and its own trace, which we developed in the tenth chapter, we may well include this trace effect of the "recognized" process among the aspects of its greater stability.

However, the preceding reflections raise no other claim than to have demonstrated the possibility of connecting our special law of trace selection with the general one for the case of recognition. They have pointed out dynamical possibilities, but it must be left to future research to find out whether realities correspond to them.

Similarity as It Enters the Law. In applying the law of similarity to the selection of a trace by a process one has to exercise great care. One must bear in mind that similarity must exist between, and therefore be defined in terms of, the process and the trace; hence similarity or partial identity between the two sets of *stimuli* which gave rise to the formation of the trace and the process now occurring is *not* an adequate criterion for the application of the law. And therefore any formulation like the following one is essentially wrong: If an organism has reacted in a certain way to the stimulus complex A B C D E F, it will later respond in the same way to the recurrence of a part of this complex, say B C D. This formulation presupposes that the second B C D communicates through similarity with the first which occurred within the total complex A B C D E F. This is, however, totally spurious as a general assumption. There are cases where this communication will occur, but there are others, and if we think in terms of stimuli, probably incomparably more, where it does not. The reason is obvious. We know that the response to a stimulus complex is not the sum of all responses to its individual components, but an organized pattern in which each part depends upon the organization of the whole. Chapters IV and V contain many examples of this fact. Therefore it will happen only *under special conditions* that the process aroused by the stimulus complex B C D is in any way dynamically similar to the part B C D in the process aroused by A B C D E F. Often enough it will not even be a proper part of it, i.e., in the process aroused by the whole complex there will be nothing corresponding to the process aroused by the partial complex. Then, of course, the latter will not be able to select the former.

GOTTSCHALDT'S EXPERIMENTS EXPLAINED. Of the truth of this deduction there is abundant proof. The reader will at once think of Gottschaldt's experiments, which were arranged according to the pattern of our argument, except that the temporal sequence of whole- and part-stimulus was transposed. The *a* figures (see p. 155) can be described as stimulus complexes B C D, the *b* figures as complexes A B C D E F. Practice with the former had not the slightest influence upon their recognition in the latter. Naturally, since the process aroused by B C D was quite different from the part process aroused by B C D in the total complex A B C D E F. Thus we can now understand *what* is proved by Gottschaldt's experiments: he interprets them as a proof that in the field which he investigated experience produces no forces but only systemic conditions, or, otherwise expressed, that in his field of research no automatic or spontaneous effects of experience occur. And he correlates his results with Lewin's formulation that association is never a moving force (1929, pp. 80 ff.). But the same criticism which we levelled against Lewin's formulation (see p. 582) holds with regard to Gottschaldt's interpretation. A trace can exert a force on a process only if it is in communication with it. We explained Lewin's results as proving that such communication did not occur under conditions in which it should according to the traditional association theory. And the same interpretation explains Gottschaldt's results. The *a* figures could not influence the perception of the *b* figures, because the latter did not spontaneously communicate with the traces of the former. One can call this an absence of an automatic effect of experience, but then one must be clear that the effect which fails to appear lies not in an influence of a trace upon a process, but in the opposite relation from process to trace. In the old theory, with very few exceptions, these two relations were not distinguished, and therefore, in attacking the old theory, both Lewin and Gottschaldt failed to make that distinction themselves, thereby imparting to their own theories a bias which obscured the real significance of their results. We learn from Gottschaldt's experiments, as from Lewin's, the proper use of the law of similarity for the selection of trace by process.

That comparatively slight changes in the new stimulating situation can often result in dissimilarity between process and trace such that no communication ensues has been demonstrated by Köhler, who thereby explains the results of Shepard and Fogelsonger and of Frings (1929, pp. 315 f.), which in their turn disproved the traditional association theory.

THE TRACES CONSIDERED FROM THIS POINT OF VIEW. Similarity, if it is to effect communication between process and trace, must be similarity between process and trace. This was the theme of our last sections, but only one side of this relationship was treated in them. We showed what conditions a process must fulfil in order to be similar to a trace. But the other side is equally important: the trace too must fulfil conditions in order to be similar to a process. Communication will not only fail to appear when the new process is different from the one which aroused the trace—the case we have just discussed—but also when the trace has changed so as to be no longer sufficiently similar to a process equal to that which originally produced it. We have studied changes which occur in traces because of stresses within themselves or interaction with other traces. Such changes can easily destroy that degree of similarity which is necessary for communication. Experimentally this has appeared chiefly in the case of aggregation. We remember that in those experiments by Lewin in which he presented the subjects with syllables from very well learned series and asked them to wait passively for what other ideas might come to their consciousness (see p. 561), these syllables were not even recognized by the subjects. We saw further in our discussion of von Restorff's experiments that recognition was affected in the same way, if not to the same extent, as recall by the conditions of isolation and repetition, the latter impeding, the former favouring it. In these cases we are fairly safe in assuming that no communication took place between process and trace and that this failure was due to the condition of the trace.

RECOGNITION AND RECALL. This argument leads to a new question with regard to the relation of recognition and recall. We have found cases where recognition is followed by recall, others where neither of them took place, and finally others where, as in the Korsakoff syndrome, no recognition ensued, while other effects of traces on the process were manifest. But there are also cases where not only does recognition fail to be followed by recall—a possibility which we have already discussed—but where despite recognition recall is, at least at first, *impossible*. The discussion of an example will best show us the problem involved here. I come across the beginning of a poem which I recognize as one I have learned before. I try to recall it, but I am only partly successful at my first attempt; a number of words fail to appear. However, after a few more trials I can recite it without gap or mistake.

This example is interesting for two reasons: in the beginning there is communication between trace and process (the hearing or reading of the first line), as proved by my recognition, without the possibility of complete recall. Afterwards this possibility has been re-established. What does this signify for the theory of traces? We must assume that at the time of recognition the whole-trace of the process had lost so much articulation as no longer to be able to effect a correct process of reproduction. This change of the whole-trace was not sufficient to prevent the process from "finding" the trace, because the part process, corresponding to the first line, is a sufficiently independent part so as not to be seriously affected by the degeneration of the rest of the trace. My first efforts to recall, partly successful as they are, bring about the arousal of a process, my faulty recitation, in communication with the degenerated trace. As we know, in our theory, such communication between trace and process has effects on the trace, in the sense of making it more stable. Therefore, if we assume that our efforts have "improved" the trace, we introduce no new hypothesis: this new effect follows from the general laws which we have previously derived.

Altogether recall is an achievement of higher grade than recognition. This fact is too well known to require proof. I mention only that our vocabulary, in our mother tongue and even more in a foreign one, is considerably larger for understanding than for speaking. Now this greater facility of recognition may be due to either, or both, of two causes. It may be that the conditions of communication are more readily fulfilled under the circumstances of recognition, or it may be that a condition of the trace which suffices for this achievement is insufficient for the other. The first possibility will be discussed a little later. The second seems highly plausible also. A trace which has lost its articulation to a greater or smaller degree will be less "destabilized," put under less stress, by communication with a partial process than a well articulated one, i.e., it will have less reproductive power, while on the other hand it may have preserved enough of its general structure to be arousable by a similar process and thereby lead to recognition.

Other Laws. The formulation of our general law, and the interpretation of the selection of a trace by a process as a process of organization, make it unlikely that similarity is the only factor to determine this dynamic interplay. As a matter of fact we have already introduced, in connection with similarity, the factors of proximity and isolation. But there are other laws of organization, notably those of good continuation and closure. Do these factors also play a part in our problem? I believe that thinking cannot be understood without giving an affirmative answer to this question.

THE LAW OF CONTRAST. The older empirical psychologists, before the era of experimental psychology, had included a law of contrast among their laws of association, which, as we have pointed out previously, meant for them reproduction as well as association proper. Some of these early psychologists were shrewd observers, and therefore there is a presumption in favour of the belief that the law of contrast was based on the observation of true facts, even though the law did not adequately explain them. It does happen that our thoughts turn from a concept to its opposite, often under conditions when the assumption that a previous strong association exists and is responsible for the reproduction is neither proven nor probable. If we accept it as a fact that in a train of thought an idea may evoke its opposite, or, to put it better, that a thought process may move from one item to its opposite, without the existence of a trace in which the two opposites have become organized together, then we should have to say that such a process, in order to run its proper course, in other words, in order to achieve stability, will communicate with a trace which was aroused by the "opposite" process. The law of association by contrast could be a valid one: for it would mean that the selection of the trace with which the process of the moment was to communicate was governed by the relationship of contrast or opposition, whenever the intrinsic course of the process demanded such a communication.

Three Possible Interpretations. The theoretical situation is, however, complicated. There exist at least three different possibilities to explain the reproduction of opposites, as represented by the following three schemata.

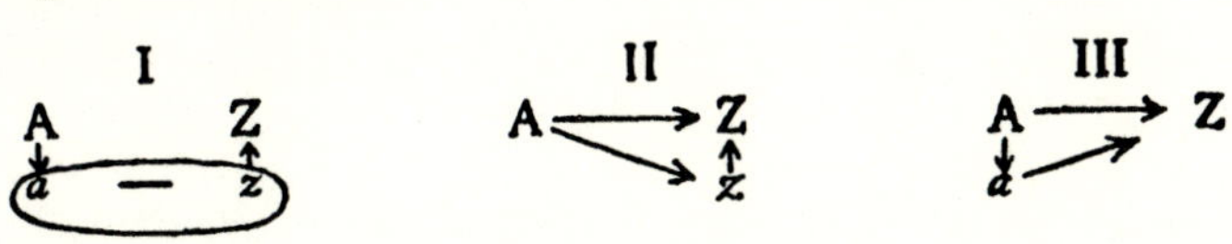

In these schemata the capital letters signify processes, the small letters corresponding traces. Schema I is the traditional associationistic interpretation, amplified so as to contain the trace-process communication, and to be applicable to a gestalt interpretation of association. The process, having reached stage A, communicates with the trace system (*a*—*z*) (*z* being the opposite of *a*), and under the influence of this trace field the process continues to Z. Such processes are perfectly possible.

The second schema represents our interpretation of the law of contrast. The process at stage A, directed towards its opposite, communicates directly with trace *z*—it may also communicate with *a*, but no $(a - z)$ trace system exists—and this communication, together with the direction of the process at A, leads it towards Z. The first two cases have one feature in common: the effect of communication between A and *z* (either directly as in II, or mediated by *a* as in I) produces Z, i.e., the effect which in these two hypotheses the trace exerts on the process is to turn it into a process similar to the one which produced the trace. This is the first effect of traces which we have studied. But we have found that the effect of a trace on a process may be different in kind. This possibility is utilized in Schema III. Here, as in I, A communicates with trace *a* (by similarity); as in II, *a* is not part of an $(a - z)$ system, but, in contrast to I and II, communication of A with *a,* together with the directedness of A, leads to Z; i. e., this hypothesis assumes that the effect of communication between a trace and a similar process may be the continuation of the process in *the sense of contrast.* This hypothesis, then, would interpret the law of association by contrast differently from the second.

A Fourth Possibility. Before we discuss the plausibility of these hypotheses we must introduce a fourth possibility.

IV

$$A \rightarrow Z$$

In this case the progression from A to Z occurs without the influence of trace fields—certainly trace fields must have been in communication with A, but they are not responsible for Z, and are therefore not contained in the schema. In this case Z is determined, or even "created," by the fact that it fulfils the condition of being the opposite of A; otherwise it is completely unknown, no trace exists of such a process, since it never occurred before.

What we mean may be exemplified by the following instance: the simple algebraic formula $(a + b)\ (a - b) = a^2 - b^2$ has done signal service; e.g., it makes it possible to divide $(a^2 - b^2)$ by $(a + b)$ and by $(a - b)$. No such possibility exists for the sum of the two squares $a^2 + b^2$. I wish, some fictitious mathematician might have said, that numbers had properties so as to give a similar formula for the sum of two squares. What kind of number must they be? Here the new numbers are determined just by the function they have to fulfil, and this determination would lead to the discovery, or invention, of complex numbers, even if the mathematician had not previously come across them. For $(a + bi)\ (a - bi) = a^2 + b^2$. The process would never end with Z, for the Z would, by communication with trace systems, be developed until it had been connected with other parts of one's knowledge. Nevertheless, for the first occurrence of Z no specific trace system is responsible.

If we accept Schema IV, we have no reason to reject Schema III. Although this weakens the argument in favour of Schema II, since in most observed cases either schema will fit the facts equally well, as far as we know them, I believe that this case has as good right to be considered as the others. In each actual occurrence there is influence from process to trace (selection) and from trace to process (field influence). And so far everything speaks in favour of the assumption that the laws which govern these two influences are the same, even though the evidence at hand is still very slight.

We have discussed the law of contrast because it seems to exemplify the working of other laws than similarity in the process-trace communication. When we introduced this topic (on p. 605) we referred to the more general laws of good continuation and closure. Contrast should be considered as a special case of these other two factors, selected chiefly for historical reasons, the law of contrast being one of the oldest laws of association. Of course our discussion of contrast applies equally to other relations possible under the laws of closure and good continuation. When we discuss thought processes we shall take up this thread again.

ATTITUDES AS INFLUENCING COMMUNICATION. We now turn to a different factor of great power in producing communication, the factor which was proved so abundantly in Lewin's and Gottschaldt's experiments, I mean the "set" or attitude of the Ego. If, as we did, we interpret the practical non-existence of spontaneous reproduction in Lewin's experiments as due to a lack of communication between process and trace, then we must also explain the fact that reproduction occurred easily under the proper attitude as due, at least in part, to a direct effect of attitude on communication. Attitude may have done more than that, but it certainly must have done that. And similarly the effect of attitude in Gottschaldt's experiments must have been to put a process in communication with traces which, without such an attitude, they could not "find."

This conclusion seems inevitable. But it raises the question *how* attitudes can have such effects. No final answer to this question can be given, but the following considerations are intended to show what definite possibilities our system contains for indicating the outline of an answer. We have, in our theory of recognition, made use of the fact, integral to our whole theory, that the total field, both as actual process and as trace column, is organized into Ego and environment, the two sub-systems being dynamically dependent parts of the whole systems. This same circumstance will help us also in our present problem. Let us again begin with an example. One day we see a number of figures, and among them +. On the next day we see a number of other figures, and among them 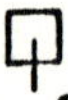. In a neutral attitude, or an attitude of remembering as many of the new figures as possible (or a number of other attitudes), we shall see this figure as a square with a vertical line bisecting its lower side. But if, in looking at these figures, we were told that they were similar to figures shown on the first day and that we should try to discover for each new figure the figure of the preceding day to which it was similar, then with great probability we should see the figure as a cross with three added lines; i.e., under the first kind of attitude the new figure was not in communication with the traces of the old one, under the second it was. And we have to explain why. In order to do this we have to examine the dynamic meaning of the second attitude. What happens in the total field when I am "set" to find something old in something new? Since I understand the task, since I know that I am to look for figures which were shown to me yesterday, a communication must exist between my Ego as it is now and some experiences it had yesterday. The field in which any process is to happen now comprises already the large trace system of yesterday's figures, since the "present" Ego is in communication with it. Therefore, when a new figure is presented, it does not have to create this communication. All it has to do is to select within this large system the particular member with which it will most intimately communicate.

Let us, for a moment, simplify our case. Let only *one* figure be shown on each day, + on the first, 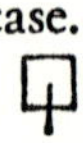 on the second. Then, when the search attitude exists on the second day, the 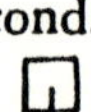 pattern will be impressed on the retinae and will give rise to a process in a field which comprises the trace of +. Then the process started by the  pattern will be profoundly changed by the trace. As a matter of fact, a true search attitude does much more than establish the communication between trace and process, it determines the new process not only through such communication but also by prescribing what the result of the communication is to be: the new process is to be organized in terms of the trace. For many purposes it would be highly interesting to produce conditions where the attitude had *only* the effect of incorporating a trace within the field of a process without determining the process directly at the same time. However, for our present problem the example discussed will suffice, since it was constructed in conformity with actual experiments (Gottschaldt). It shows that attitude is not enough to produce such communication. If the figure were 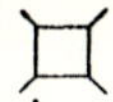 instead of 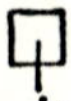 it would not communicate with the trace of + even though it occurred in a large field which includes that trace. Furthermore if the figure were 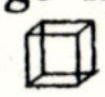 instead of +, communication would be more difficult. That is to say, even when we investigate the influence of attitude, we have to retain certain conditions inherent in the relation between process and trace which are to communicate.

The attitude, then, becomes effective by creating a trace field. It seems to me the main advantage of our theory is that it provides a possibility for this effect. We must remember the trace column with its preservation of the Ego-environment organization, and we must also remember the continuity of the Ego, which gives a special kind of structure to the Ego part of the column. Inasmuch as the Ego is, as a rule, more or less in the centre of its environment, we can picture the Ego part of the trace column as its core and the environmental part as a shaft, keeping in mind that core and shaft support each other. We know that the shaft is full of strains and stresses which produce aggregation and other unifications of traces at various levels. But we also know that the core, despite its great internal complexity, has, as a whole, a much stronger unity than the shaft as a whole. If then an attitude arises, what will happen? To follow up our example: if I want to link up figures shown to me now with figures presented yesterday, what is my attitude, and how does it become effective? In the first place this attitude has the character of a quasi-need, it corresponds to a tension in the Ego part at the tip of the column. This tension can be relieved only through that part of the trace column which contains yesterday's figures, since a linking up of today's with yesterday's is possible only if these traces influence the new process. In other words, the attitude requires the creation of a field which includes these particular traces. Now, in directing our attention to a particular event that occurred in the past, we link up our present Ego with this particular part of the past Ego; our present Ego continues that particular past Ego and continues it dynamically. In looking at the new figures I am the one who looked at the old figures, in a much more definite sense than I am the one who went to a concert last night. My concert Ego is but indirectly connected with my "psychologically experimenting Ego," but my Ego experimenting today is directly connected with my Ego doing so yesterday. The great complexity of the Ego, which we have previously discussed (Chapter VIII, pp. 334 ff.), accounts for these facts. Now, dynamic continuation means dynamic intercourse, so that the attitude towards the figures presented yesterday can make their traces part of the field, because, through the general attitude of psychologizing, the Ego of yesterday's experiments, with that of ever so many other occasions, was already in communication with the present Ego. That the attitude will have an effect not only on the core but also on the shaft, i.e., not only on the old Ego but also on special objects in the environment of the old Ego, is not hard to explain. For Ego and object are again dynamically related, and in cases like those now discussed this dynamic relation is close and strong. We *looked at* the pictures yesterday; they aroused interest, curiosity, ambition, or some other attitude, in our past. Thus the *total* trace of that event must contain a strong Ego-object connection. Therefore when the object part of the trace is needed for dynamical reasons (attitude, set, desire) and the Ego part is already in communication, the field will easily be extended so as to embrace the object trace.

Let us compare with this case the other where without any attitude whatever the + figure which was seen on the first day will recur on the second. To assume that its recognition can take place without any participation of attitudes would mean that a process at the tip of the *shaft* can directly communicate with a trace further down, across layers of other traces. That recognition will occur only when the Ego also becomes involved we have already discussed. But in the case now under discussion the process would first find a trace in the shaft, and the shaft-trace thus aroused would involve the core-trace with which it had formed a larger unit. Thus, on the grounds of our hypothesis, spontaneous recognition, recognition without a corresponding attitude, should be much more difficult than recognition under a corresponding attitude.

It is significant that recent investigators have gone so far as to doubt the occurrence of spontaneous recognition. Thus Lewin finds the existence of a "tendency to identify" necessary for the arousal of the qualities of familiarity and unfamiliarity in recognition (1922, II, p. 114), and Bartlett maintains that "Recognizing is possible if the orientation or attitude which marked an original perception is carried over to re-presentation" (p. 193) and claims that "recognition depends upon the coincident arousal of two different functions: (1) a specific sensory reaction, and (2) an attitude, or orientation, which we cannot ascribe to any localized physiological apparatus, but which has to be treated as belonging to 'the whole' subject, or organism, reacting" (p. 191).

It is possible to interpret both Lewin and Bartlett as asserting that communication between process and trace as an event entirely within the shaft of the trace column does not occur.[3] Whether such a claim is true or not, experiments will have to decide. Personally I do not believe it. Again I hold that dynamic relations within the shaft, i.e., within the environmental field, and between core and shaft, may be effective, and not only dynamic relations within the core, the Ego system. Despite this belief, which, as I just said, will have to be tested by experiments, I recognize the enormous importance of attitudinal factors. As I envisage the problem, the alternative, either spontaneous recognition or recognition always mediated by attitude, does not exist. That intra-shaft forces are necessary even where an attitude made communication possible, we have seen above. Thus a frank acceptance of the effectiveness of all the forces that may come into play seems the safest position to adopt before new experimental evidence is adduced.

In ascribing an effect on the process trace communication to attitudes we have not only discussed the rôle they play in recognition but implicitly also a part which they can play in reproduction. It was, as a matter of fact, by experiments on reproduction that Lewin proved the efficacy of attitudes. Inasmuch as this influence on reproduction is the same as on recognition it is to be explained in our theory in the same way. Again we are in good agreement with

[3] I shall not stress the point whether this interpretation is absolutely correct. Probably both authors did not, when they wrote the quoted sentences, envisage the process of recognition as concretely as we are doing it here. Particularly Bartlett could say that he meant only that some attitudinal factor entered the process of recognition at some stage, and that it enters also in our theory through the environment-Ego relationship. This interpretation of Bartlett's is not incompatible with the rest of his theory, according to which an object to be recognized must at its first presentation have been in dynamical relation to the Ego, not only *heard* but *listened to,* and similarly in other sensory realms. The point that has not become quite clear to me in Bartlett's presentation is, however, whether he applies this condition to the previous occasion only or also to the new one when recognition takes place.

Bartlett: "A new incoming impulse must become not merely a cue setting up a series of reactions all carried out in a fixed temporal order, but a stimulus which enables us to go direct to that portion of the organized setting of past responses which is most relevant to the needs of the moment. There is one way in which an organism could learn how to do this. It may be the only way. At any rate, it is the way that has been discovered and it is continually used. An organism has somehow to acquire the capacity to turn round upon its own 'schemata' and to construct them afresh" (p. 206). In the first of the sentences quoted Bartlett formulates our problem of communication, in the last he solves it by an act of the Ego. I shall not harp on the differences between Bartlett's and my approach, I shall only point out that a theory of the trace column as developed in this book makes this "turning round of the organism upon its own schemata" possible. In Bartlett's theory the organism has to *acquire* this capacity *somehow,* in our theory it follows from the assumption of the dynamical structure of the trace column and the dynamics of the present process. Perhaps it would be more correct to say that it would follow if our knowledge of these dynamic structures were more concrete and detailed than it is. For I know perfectly well that the description of the effect which I gave a few pages ago is far from being complete or adequate. But admitting all this I have to contend that my theory, developed as a theory of field organization, provides for the "turning round" which is needed for the explanation of recall, whereas in Bartlett's theory it appears without previous preparation merely to overcome the difficulty presented by the facts of reproduction.

That our theory, on the other hand, is in accord with Bartlett's most general conclusions is evident. Bartlett maintains that "Remembering is not the re-excitation of innumerable fixed lifeless and fragmentary traces. It is an imaginative reconstruction, or construction . . ." (p. 213). Our field theory of traces, including the effect of attitudes, is a concrete hypothesis which tries to explain this "constructiveness" of memory.[4]

ANOTHER RÔLE OF ATTITUDE IN REPRODUCTION. However, the rôle of attitude in reproduction is not exhausted by bringing about the required communications, it can also determine what the *effect* of such communication will be. I recall merely our discussion of the "naming of opposites" (pp. 509 f.) to indicate what I mean. This effect, however, has not been explained yet. We may well grant that

[4] In my book of 1912 I have already indicated a standpoint which in this respect is similar enough to Bartlett's to deserve a mention here (p. 279).

through the "core" the present may come in contact with traces of the past, but we do not yet know how such contact can determine the present process in the *specific* form defined by the task. How can we, to start with a definite instance, exert an attitude of "opposition" on an incoming idea so that we continue the idea by its opposite? How does the mind become possessed of this faculty?

Gestalt Dispositions. We came across this problem at the end of Chapter XI (p. 510), when we discussed certain properties of traces. And indeed, the problem of the voluntary arousal of attitude must be a memory problem. For how shall I search for an opposite unless I know what opposite means, and how can I know it unless "oppositeness" had first happened to me without an "opposition-attitude"? In other words, it seems necessary to assume certain traces, traces of dynamic relations, of definite progressions, in order to understand how such progressions can be initiated at will. Dallenbach's experiment, reported on page 509, corroborates this deduction. Before the boy could name the opposite to "good" he had to have experienced "good—bad" in opposition. This experience has left a trace, which can become effective not only, not even chiefly, in the recognition or recall of this specific occasion, viz., "good—bad" in opposition, but, to use Spearman's terminology, in "educing the correlate" of the opposition relation for any new term. A voluntary attitude, therefore, presupposes that the *specific* dynamical aspect of that attitude must have occurred previously in a non-attitudinal form, and that in the attitude the trace of this former occurrence becomes effective.

What is true of the attitude of "opposition" is equally true of any other attitude, therefore also of that of "reproducing" which in so many cases is necessary for the occurrence of reproduction. But if this is so, the reproduction must have occurred previous to the existence of an attitude of reproducing, since the latter becomes possible only through the former. Therefore spontaneous reproduction has to be assumed to explain "intended" reproduction.

In a former publication (1925) I made use of the concept of gestalt disposition, referred to on page 514, to explain these facts. Although this concept lacks concreteness, as I pointed out before, it expresses the fact which we have just derived, viz., that specific sets or attitudes, voluntarily aroused, mean dynamically the inclusion of older trace systems in the field of the present process, an inclusion which is produced by the Ego system. Therefore, a complete understanding of the voluntary determination of processes presupposes an intimate knowledge of the Ego system and its relation to traces in the environmental system I must leave the matter at that. Here lies a vast field practically unexplored by the psychologist, and the exploration of it ought to yield results of the highest significance for our understanding of mental activity.

I shall also forbear to treat extensively a serious problem which has given rise to much psychological and philosophical discussion, viz., the problem of the "temporal reference" of ideas or images. I believe that this problem can as yet find no final solution, but that our general framework of "core" and "shaft" contains the elements which will make such a solution possible.

THE AROUSAL OF A NEW PROCESS. THINKING

Instead I shall now take up the last problem of this chapter, the arousal of new processes. It follows naturally upon our discussion of attitudes, since we saw that attitudes require traces of certain processes. How then are these processes started, or produced, or created? How do thoughts originate, how do thought processes run their course?

The Relation of Logic and Psychology. Perhaps in no field will the specific quality of gestalt psychology become so manifest and its integrative function so important as in this. On the one hand, a thought process is a natural event; on the other, it is rational, meaningful, significant, faulty, or irrelevant. To traditional psychologists, and to the bulk of philosophers, it appeared evident that, viewed as natural events, there is no difference between true and false thoughts. Philosophers who wanted to retain an objective difference between truth and error were therefore forced into a sphere different from nature to account for this difference. We have touched on this problem before (pp. 570 f.) and have shown how from the point of view of an isomorphistic gestalt theory it gains an entirely new aspect. A true solution is different from a false one not only in terms of logic, not in a realm of mere *subsistence*, but this difference must, if our fundamental views are right, be duplicated in the realm of natural *existence*, i.e., dynamically there must be a difference between true and false solutions. This view has been clearly expressed by Duncker (1926, p. 694).

Thought processes as meaningful natural events reveal the basic conceptions of gestalt theory more than any other events, because in good thought processes the rôle of the contingent or arbitrary has been reduced to a minimum. In perception the stimulus distribution on the sense surface is an unavoidable element of contingency. In pure thought processes this is lacking, the contingent factors that may influence them being merely in the trace column. Therefore these processes can give us the deepest insight into gestalt dynamics, the most compulsive proof of the truth of gestalt principles. It is to be hoped that Wertheimer will before long publish the results of the work which he did in this field for many years. But before this work is available, I prefer to treat thought within the framework so far erected, i.e., as a process within the system with its vast and complex store of traces—relying on the published work, small in bulk as it is.

Problem Solving. Two Steps. A new process can occur in various ways, as we have discussed on pages 549 ff. Frequently the situation is a problem situation; at first the problem cannot be solved, later on it can. The transformation which takes place in such cases implies as a rule that trace systems at first out of communication with the present process are brought into communication with it (see p. 550, and Duncker, p. 705). The solution then involves two steps: the achievement of a communication with the proper trace systems and the proper effect of this communication upon the process.

Let me illustrate this by a joke. A asks B: "What did Noah say when he heard the rain patter on the roof?" B does not know the answer, and therefore A has to give it himself: " 'Ark"! A little later B puts the same question to C, and when C does not know the answer he supplies it by saying: "Listen." In this case B, who does not solve the problem spontaneously, fails even to get it when A tells it to him. The word " 'ark" is properly understood, i.e., the present perceptive process communicates with the trace of the word, or rather the significance of it, but this trace fails to exert the proper influence on the process. Instead of communicating first with the trace of the flood situation it stays within its own sphere and therefore fails to elicit the double meaning, with the result that in trying to repeat the joke B makes a fool of himself. B might have failed to understand the joke for another reason, viz., if the word " 'ark" in the context of Noah and the flood had failed to communicate with the trace of the "listening" complex. Thus our joke exemplifies the two processes distinguished above. These two effects, though different from each other, will, as a rule, not be mutually independent, since, as we have seen, the choice of a trace system is influenced by the effect which it can exert upon a process. As a matter of fact, in many cases the *effect* which the communication can produce seems to be the main reason which we can adduce for the communication. I borrow an example from Claparède's highly suggestive recent essay (1934): "Somebody proposes to a friend to go with him on a trip to Spain, and receives the answer: 'I should like to very much, but I have not got the money'" (p. 35). Here the fact that the idea of Spain communicates with the trace system of the person's financial affairs is clearly connected with the fact that such communication can settle the problem aroused by the question. The trace system, then, appears to be directly under the influence of stresses in the present process distribution, a proposition which goes beyond our previous deduction that communication depends upon stresses in the Ego system (see pp. 607 f.).

M. R. Harrower's Experiments. To this, as to many other problems relevant in this connection, the work of M. R. Harrower has made a valuable contribution.

The Completion of Jokes. In one set of experiments she read to her subjects a number of uncompleted jokes and asked them to complete them. I give an example. The joke as read: "A young lady called on Rubinstein, the pianist, who condescended to listen to her playing. 'What do you think I should do now,' she inquired when she had finished. Rubinstein: '. . . . .'" The answers as classified by Harrower:

"Go to Germany to learn."	"Leave off."	"Raise cabbages."
"Learn to play."	"Give up."	"Get married."

In all these groups, the answers imply the effect of memory traces, in the first, e.g., the memory that Germany is a country with many excellent conservatories. In each case the particular trace selected makes a solution, i.e., a completion, possible. But in the last group the problem is solved in a more specific way; it turns the incomplete part into a real *joke,* i.e., the *form* or *shape* of the thought process, not only its content, becomes effective in the choice.

The rôle of the form of the thought process appeared particularly clearly where two "joke" solutions were possible and about equally good. Example: The Prisoner in Court: "But, your worship, I wasn't going 50 miles an hour, nor 40, nor 30. . . ." The Judge: ". . . . ." Answers:

"Well, you'll be going backwards soon."	"No, I suppose you were going 60 miles an hour."
"You won't be going at all soon."	"No, you were going faster."

In both sets of answers the trace system selected by the presented part, viz., the knowledge of the car's propulsion, becomes effective for the answer. But *within* this system a selection occurs according to the direction which the joke takes in the mind of the listener. In the first group of answers the process is continued, 50—40—30 . . . 0 or even $< 0 =$ reverse (positive type); in the second the process is reversed, 50—40—30 . . . 60 (negative type).

THE REALITY OF THE JOKE PATTERN IN THE TRACE. This joke pattern is a very real affair; it is retained in the trace and may be selected by a new process, thereby determining its completion. This was proved by special experiments of Harrower's. She constructed two jokes similar in structure to the Judge joke but different in content; one was given the "positive," the other the "negative" ending. One of these jokes was the last of a number of jokes read to the subjects; it was followed by the Judge joke which the subjects were asked to finish. Eight subjects heard the positive, seven the negative joke. The following table shows in percentages how the subjects completed the Judge joke when no joke of a similar structure had preceded and when the joke with the positive and that with the negative completion had been presented first.

TABLE 32

(from Harrower, p. 80)

(n = number of subjects)
(F = failure to complete)

Neutral n = 17			+ influence n = 8			— influence n = 7		
+	—	F	+	—	F	+	—	F
35.4	35.4	29.2	100	0	0	0	100	0

This result was confirmed under conditions which even more than the last exclude an explanation in terms of attitude. The subjects' task was to repeat as accurately as they could what was being read to them, accurately not only as regards content and formulation, but also as regards the experimenter's tone of voice. They were then read four finished jokes, each of which was repeated by the subject. The third of these was the joke which served in the last experiment to induce a "positive" completion. After the fourth joke, i.e., not immediately succeeding this inducing joke, the incomplete Judge joke was read, and the series ended with another complete joke.

None of the eleven subjects behaved with regard to the critical, the Judge, joke, as they did with regard to the others; they finished it either spontaneously or after having asked whether they should do so, and *all* of them gave it a completion corresponding to the inducing joke. Since without the preceding inducer the Judge joke had been completed as often in the positive as the negative direction and had yielded an appreciable number of failures, the 100% results of this and the last experiments prove that the trace of the old joke must have been in communication with the new one. The cause of communication can only have been the structural similarity, and the tension set up by the incompleteness of the new joke.

RECALL OF JOKES. FACTORS OF AVAILABILITY. The last experiment has shown that this effect can take place also when the selected trace is not the most recent one. But of course, whether the stress in the field—be it an Ego-environment or a pure environment stress as in the last experiment[5]—will succeed in selecting the proper trace, proper for the resolution of the tension, must depend upon the availability of the particular trace (see pp. 525 f., and 546 f.). Two experimental series of Harrower's deal with this problem, availability being tested by recall. In one series sixteen jokes, alternately finished and unfinished, were consecutively read to 25 subjects in all. Immediately afterwards the subjects had to write down the jokes they remembered. Five of these 25 were asked for a second recall three weeks later. The following table contains the results in percentages:

TABLE 33

(from Harrower, p. 97)

(n = number of subjects)

	unfinished remembered	finished remembered	P
immediate recall n = 25	48.5	29	1.67
recall after 3 weeks n = 5	45	26.2	1.71

We can express our results in terms of the P quotients which we introduced in the discussion of Zeigarnik's work, viz., $\frac{\text{number of unfinished remembered}}{\text{number of finished remembered}} = P$, and then we see that the

[5] We use the word "environment" here in the broad sense in which it is synonymous with the non-Ego part of the field, i.e., in our case with the joke qua incompleted structure.

two P quotients are nearly as great as those obtained by Zeigarnik for the difference between incomplete and completed tasks (see p. 335). Since under the conditions of the experiment no subject completed the unfinished jokes spontaneously the results prove that the traces of unfinished jokes are more readily available than those of the finished ones.

In another series sixteen jokes were read to twelve subjects. Of these eight were incomplete and had to be finished by the subjects themselves, four were finished, and the remaining four were also finished but were accompanied by the presentation of a proper diagram.

This needs a word of explanation. In special experiments Harrower had shown that it is possible to diagrammatize jokes, i.e., to draw simple figures which picture the "shape" of the jokes, and that subjects can select the "proper" diagram of a joke out of a number of different diagrams. For example, three figures were chosen correctly by fifteen subjects in 100%, 73%, and 73% of the cases under conditions where chance would have decreed 25%.

We can now return to the experiment: One week after the presentation of these sixteen jokes the subjects were tested for recall, eleven of the twelve were retested after another three weeks, five of them again after another ten days and still again after another three weeks. The results are perfectly clear. The finished jokes are recalled the least, those finished with diagrams most frequently; the unfinished self-completed ones fall between them, though they are much nearer to the best remembered. The following table, calculated from Harrower's tables, summarizes the results in quotients similar to the P quotients.

TABLE 34

(from Harrower, p. 93)

	unfinished self-completed / finished	finished & diagram / finished
After 1 week, n = 12	2.1	2.9
After 4 weeks, n = 11	2.5	4.0
All four recalls combined, n = 5	7.1	10.5

The high numbers in the last row are due to the fact that these five subjects recalled from the beginning only a very small number of finished jokes; at the same time the *number* of recalled jokes varied extraordinarily little during the four recall periods, although different jokes might be recalled at different times. Another way of presenting the same results is to list the total number remembered in each category—halving the number of the unfinished ones, since they were twice as frequent as the others. Then we get:

TABLE 35

finished	unfinished	finished & diagram
16	48.5	69.5

The total possible for each group is 132.

A further analysis of the data revealed some other significant results. Some of the unfinished jokes which the subjects were to complete were not actually completed, and of these a great number were remembered, relatively almost as many as of the finished diagram jokes. Again some of the unfinished jokes were badly completed. They were either forgotten altogether or remembered without the poor completion, only 25% of them being recalled in the completed form, almost 10% less than the average of all unfinished jokes.

TABLE 36[6]

(from Harrower, pp. 98-99)

	$\frac{\text{unfinished}}{\text{finished}}$	$\frac{\text{arbitrary diagram}}{\text{finished}}$	$\frac{\text{proper diagram}}{\text{finished}}$
Immediate recall n = 10	2.22	1.28	2.7
After 10 days n = 5	5.0	1.0	6.0
After 7 weeks n = 5	4.0	0	12.0

In order to understand the effect produced by the presentation of the diagram and to confirm the other results a last series was undertaken with ten new subjects, twelve jokes being used, divided into four groups of three. These were: the normal finished jokes, jokes left completely unfinished, jokes with a proper diagram, and jokes

[6] After seven weeks both the finished and the arbitrary diagram jokes were practically forgotten. None of the latter were recalled, and only one of the former, and that in a changed form so that in Harrower's table it is assigned the value .5. Therefore the two high quotients of the last line.

accompanied by an arbitrary diagram. If the mere fact that *some* figure was shown simultaneously with the presentation of the joke was responsible for the high recall value of the diagram jokes, then the last two groups should be equally well recalled. All subjects were tested immediately after the presentation of the series, five after ten days, and the other five after seven weeks. In Table 36 (p. 620), we present the results again in the form of ratios, always putting in the denominator the number of the finished jokes recalled. Or adding up all recalls at the three different test periods we get:

TABLE 37

finished	arbitrary diagram	unfinished	proper diagram
11.5	13.5	32	42.5

The result is obvious. The arbitrary diagrams have no effect whatever on recall, whereas the proper diagrams again occupy the first position. Moreover, the finished and the arbitrary diagram jokes are much more affected by the passage of time than the two other groups. After ten days these are recalled as well as immediately after presentation, whereas the two other groups taken together have dwindled from 20.5 recalls to 4! After seven weeks, when these last two have virtually disappeared, the proper-diagram jokes have increased their superiority over the unfinished ones; however, the number of cases is not sufficient to make this result absolutely reliable.

AVAILABILITY AND "GOODNESS" OF TRACE. Now to the interpretation. Are we justified in explaining the results in terms of availability of traces? This question necessitates a new discussion of the term availability. In discriminating between the deterioration and the availability of a trace we had assumed that traces of equal "goodness" might possess a different degree of availability. Thereby we might have given the impression that goodness of trace and availability were entirely independent of each other. In reality, however, the goodness of a trace seems to be one of the factors that determine its availability, though by no means the only one. In the experiments just described a trace might be good enough to produce recall—they were probably all good enough to produce recognition—and yet not be available, or not as available as other traces. The first contention is proved by a fact already mentioned, viz., that recall at successive periods does not always yield the same jokes. Some jokes which appeared on the first day may not ppear on the second, but return on the third or fourth, and contrariwise jokes which are repeated on a later occasion may have failed to be named on the first.[7] The second contention is proved by the fact, corresponding to a fact observed by Zeigarnik, that in the actual recall the unfinished jokes tended to precede the finished ones. It also happened that a subject reported having recalled a finished joke only because of a previously recalled unfinished one ("An unfinished joke about a dog led her to wonder if there were any more animal jokes, etc."). Thus the superiority of the recall of certain groups over others proves that their traces were more available. If we take the ordinary finished jokes as the norm, the self-completed, incomplete, and proper-diagram jokes leave traces of increasingly greater availability. The common factor in these three types is, as Harrower has shown in a detailed discussion, that in them, as compared with the normal case, the structure of the joke was enhanced, a structure which keeps the parts of the joke well articulated. Such articulation requires forces, and therefore the traces of the better-recalled jokes are under higher stress than the others.

But this explanation necessarily implies the conclusion which we have just derived, viz., that deterioration of a trace involves a loss in availability. For deterioration means a loss in structure. The trace becomes more and more "colloidal" and thereby loses in internal stress, which in its turn is one of the factors on which availability depends. At the end of the eleventh chapter we discussed the greater survival value of more highly organized traces compared to more chaotic ones. We find now a close correlation between survival value and availability.

EMBEDDEDNESS. Two other of Harrower's experiments deal with the problem of availability of traces. In the first the variable was the kind of connection established between the required trace and other traces; in the second the variable was the kind of organization of a large articulated trace system. Both will be briefly described. In the first the answer to incomplete jokes which the subjects could not finish was contained in two different kinds of texts which the subjects read either after or before they were presented with tne jokes. The one kind of material was connected prose, the other a number of meaningful, but totally unconnected, sentences. There were altogether 32 subjects, one half of whom read the connected

[7] The same fact appeared in experiments performed by Cree Warden (p. 200), to be briefly discussed later.

prose, the other half the loose sentences. Only in one case did the connected prose help in finding the answer (and this when the conditions were most favourable, the subjects being given the reading matter before the jokes, and being told that "perhaps this will help you in the next experiment"). On the other hand, the loose sentences provided the solution in sixteen cases, of which only six occurred under the most favourable conditions. Therefore we see: a trace strongly "embedded" in a trace system is less available for a new process than a trace loosely embedded. These experiments confirmed at the same time the influence of the subjects' attitude on the availability of the traces. Thus we see that the unconnected sentences proved vastly superior to the former, and that the more so, the more the instruction of the subjects implied that the non-joke material contained the required solutions. But the fact that attitudes played an important part by no means invalidates our other conclusion. Even if, owing to the attitude, the observer is directed towards the trace system of the reading matter, the participation of a specific part of that large trace system in the process of solution must be determined by the intrinsic properties of trace and process.

TABLE 38

(from Harrower, p. 105)

n = 32
Number of recalls

	I	S	O
absolute	11.5	87.5	84.5
in % of all answers given	6.3	47.7	46.0

RELATION BETWEEN PROCESS AND TRACE. In the second experiments, performed with a number of variations with a total of 54 subjects, twelve pairs of proverbs were read to the subjects, and were immediately afterwards tested for recall by the method of paired associates, the experimenter reading aloud the first member of the pair, the subject having to write down the second. The twelve pairs were divided into three equal groups:

(1) The two proverbs in a pair had no connection with each other; *indifferent* (I).

(2) The two members of the pair were similar in meaning, though not in content (example: "In for a penny, in for a pound"—"As well be killed for a sheep as a lamb"): *similar* (S).

(3) The second member had a meaning opposite to that of the first (example: "Out of sight, out o mind"—"Absence makes the heart grow fonder"): *opposite* (O).

Table 38 on page 623 gives the results of the normal procedure, three different series of proverbs being used.

There is no significant difference between the S and O groups, but both are vastly superior to the I groups. This group remained inferior, though to a diminished degree, when the proverbs belonging to it were read twice or even three times, while the proverbs of the two other groups received as before only one reading; and also when the I proverbs were particularly familiar and the S and O rather rare. I give absolute figures for these three constellations:

TABLE 39

(from Harrower, p. 106)

Number of Recalls

	I	S	O
I proverbs read twice, n = 14	19	41.5	43
I proverbs read 3 times, n = 14	21	42.5	47
I proverbs extremely familiar, n = 4	3.5	12	13.5

These clear-cut results confirm the theory of reproduction which we have previously developed (see pp. 566 ff.). In these experiments communication between process and a previous trace was insured; in all cases there was the same attitude, the same desire of the subjects to reproduce. But those traces which were organic subsystems of a larger trace system were far superior to those which were more indifferently related parts, in making the other part of the trace system (which was not directly aroused by the new process) available for the continuation of the process, i.e., for recall. The forces aroused in the well-organized whole trace system by the communication of one of its parts with a new process were stronger in the one case than in the other. Therefore, the trace of the second member was more available in the S and O groups than in the I group, even when under other conditions, because of their greater familiarity, the latter would be more available than the former. The reality of a "purely logical" relation has again been proved in the dynamic interplay between process and trace which occurs in recall. Again we find intrinsic, meaningful, rational factors of organization effective. This same fact came out in experiments by Cree Warden in which the memory for pairs of words was tested in immediate and delayed recall. The words paired with each other stood in one of five different relationships to each other—there was nothing, however, that corresponded to Harrower's "indifferent pairs"—and significant differences between the recall value of these relationships were found.

How Is the Solution of a Problem Found? This discussion has dealt with certain conditions which pertain to the arousal of a new process. But the main problem of the psychology of thinking is: How does a problem find its solution, how does the stress set up by a question contrive to create those conditions which will make the answer possible? We have previously (pp. 615 f.) given a first answer to this question, inasmuch as it concerns the communication with old traces. But this answer was very unsatisfactory: an explanation of an event by its effects. Even though we shall not be able to go much beyond this unsatisfactory stage, we shall now discuss the problem in a much wider frame.

This Problem a Problem of All Behaviour. The problem of the arousal of a new process is not in all cases a problem of traces. Indeed the case where such traces play an important rôle, frequently though it may be realized, is but a special case of a much larger problem: a need arises which cannot be satisfied in the normal way; how does the organism manage to satisfy it? The question thus formulated gives us a lead as to its answer. Since it will be very hard to draw a border-line between "normal" and "non-normal" satisfaction, an analysis of a normal case might provide us with a clue for the solution of our question. Such normal cases are involved in all behaviour. I want a drink, I walk to the refrigerator, take a bottle of beer, open it, pour the beer into a glass, and raise the glass to my mouth. Without a doubt much in this behaviour series is learned. But the question is *how*. Does every one of the numerous single movements included in this action arise from mere random trial and error? When I *know* that a bottle of beer is on the ice, will I then, before I have learned to fetch it, have to go through a random series of movements before I come to the refrigerator? Certainly not. The knowledge of the location of the beer and the wish to obtain it are sufficient to cause the *adequate* movements directly, without chance trials. But how, this is our question, can the "knowledge" innervate the musculature? Here is a need, and this need contrives to produce such muscle innervations as will satisfy it. The reflex arc theory tried to give an answer to this question in terms of pre-established anatomical structures, i.e., neurone connections. In Chapter VIII we have rejected this theory, replacing it by a dynamic theory which, however, is to a certain degree open to the same objection which we have raised to our theory of the arousal of new thought processes: it explains an event by its consequences. We saw that such movements as would increase the total tension in the system are excluded, and that the dynamic situation demands such movements as will decrease the tensions. This explanation is perfectly good as far as it goes, but it is incomplete inasmuch as it leaves the actual dynamics in the dark; it does not show how the organism manages to find those movements which will lead to a relief of the tensions which cause the movements. In a very few cases only, notably in those of certain eye movements, we were able to go further and point out the operative forces. However, theoretically, there is no difference between eye movement and such movements of the whole body as are executed in order, say, to quench our thirst. And yet, in the latter case we have much less insight into the actual forces at work that determine every step.

AN EXAMPLE OF A NEW MOTOR PERFORMANCE. This argument becomes more impressive when we consider cases where the motor performance, though completely automatic or spontaneous, is entirely *new,* albeit the only one that could achieve the required result. A particularly striking case is fully reported by von Allesch, who vouches for the accuracy of his description. During the war he was on a patrol in the Alps. He had to make a descent from a rocky crag by means of a chimney whose upper mouth gaped about ten metres under and far to the side of his position. Having climbed down on a rope he found himself hanging in the air and several metres to the left of the chimney, with no more rope for a further descent which would have landed him on a ledge by which he had hoped to reach the chimney. He determined to reach the opening by swinging on the rope. In doing this the rope slipped from his feet, and his hands were not able to support his weight. "The situation was extremely critical. No emotions arose, instead suddenly the clearly formulated thought, 'This is the end.' The next moment the author realized (and this point is absolutely certain in his observation) that he had taken hold of the rope with his teeth. Thereupon followed another formulated thought: 'That cannot last long either.' In the next moment his feet waving in the air had caught hold of a projecting piece of a slab [and thus he succeeded in saving himself and reaching the chimney]. The important point in the process is, that this action, *not* belonging to the technique of mountain climbing, never previously considered, and of course never previously practised, the only one which could save me, arose spontaneously without any conscious deliberation. The event regulated itself" (pp. 148-49). Here was a real problem, a problem which we might put as a question to test a subject's intelligence: "What would you do under those conditions?" And the solution was *not* produced by an act of thought, but at a time when the rational part of the organism had concluded that no solution was possible—"This is the end." The stress between Ego and surrounding field succeeded in finding *that* movement which alone could relieve it.

Reorganization and Its Causes. Such a statement is unsatisfactory because it says nothing about the *how* of this success. Therefore one can understand the attraction of empiristic explanations. An explanation by previous experience would at least supply one link to fill the gap between cause and effect. But we have argued against the validity of empiristic explanations too often to be satisfied with such an easy escape. The explanation must lie in the dynamic structure of the psychophysical field itself. We must try to find out how needs, tensions, act on the motor system of the organism, what properties of the system under tension and of the motor system are responsible for the communication between them. Expressed in conceptual language we can describe the critical event in von Allesch's adventure like this: the mouth *changes its function,* from an organ of speech or food intake to an organ of clasp; a reorganization has taken place within the executive part of the Ego system. We know the fact of this reorganization and we know its ultimate cause, the urgency of the moment. But we do not yet know its immediate causes.

In this respect the solutions of thought problems are identical with von Allesch's case. The solution very often presupposes a reorganization of which the ultimate but not the immediate causes are known. To find these immediate causes is perhaps the fundamental problem of thinking, and of learning in its achievement aspect, for the arousal of each new process offers the same difficulty.

This problem has been clearly recognized by recent workers in this field, Wertheimer, Duncker, Maier, Claparède. The last author particularly emphasizes this problem again and again and confesses that his own investigation has failed to give an answer to this question. Being aware that the psychology of thinking is in this respect no worse off than other parts of psychology,[8] we shall the better appreciate any contributions which the study of thought processes has made to our general problem.

"INSIGHT." One frequently finds it stated that the achievement of gestalt theory in the field of thought psychology is the introduction of the concept, or term, "insight." Such a statement is true or false according to the view which one takes with regard to the rôle which insight is supposed to play in gestalt theory. It was introduced in Köhler's ape book in order to establish the reality of one type of behaviour, its irreducibility to another type. Insight, as the direct utilization of the relevant parts of a situation, was contrasted with blind trial and error, and it was shown that the latter was not the type manifested by anthropoids under certain conditions. In Köhler's book insight did not appear as an explanatory principle. It was established as a fact containing a *new* problem. At the same time the new problem pointed towards new solutions. Insightful behaviour does not occur, as I tried to prove in "The Growth of the Mind," by processes travelling along predetermined pathways. Instead it presupposes processes of organization and reorganization. What remained unknown was the exact cause of these processes of organization. Perhaps many misunderstandings might have been avoided had this gap in the theory, this defect in our knowledge, been more strongly emphasized by me. The general principle was clearly stated: "The situation forces the animal to act in a certain way, although the animal possesses no pre-established special devices for the act" (Koffka, 1925 a, p. 135). But the question, "How is this possible?" could only be answered in rather general terms. We shall therefore have to examine what such general answers can mean for a concrete causal theory. But once more: the term insight does not supply this answer, insight is *not* a force which creates solutions in a mystical way.[9]

AN ANALYSIS OF A TRAIN OF THOUGHT. Before we cast a glance on the experimental work performed in our field it will be expedient to analyze a train of thought which might easily occur. A person, familiar with the first elements of algebra only, finds himself faced with the problem of discovering the length of the sides of a rectangle whose area is known to be b sq. m. and one of whose sides to be a metres longer than the other. His familiarity with algebra will make it easy for him to formulate the data of this

[8] It is significant that Claparède also points out the similarity between thought and movement with regard to their dynamics (p. 147).

[9] This is made very clear by R. M. Ogden (1932, pp. 350-55).

problem. The area of a rectangle is equal to the products of its sides. Therefore, if the length of the shorter side be called x, $b = x\ (x + a)$, or $x^2 + ax = b$. Our fictitious person has not learned to solve quadratic equations. What is he to do, apart from giving up and asking somebody else? At first no step seems possible. All he did in solving linear equations was to separate the unknown and the known quantities, and that has already been done. The equation is as simple as it can be, but how is it to be solved? He might resort to mental trial and error! What does that mean? Mere random fumbling with this equation? Thus he might write:

$$x^2 + ax = b$$
$$100\,x^2 + 100\,ax = 100\,b$$
or
$$x^2 + ax + 35 = b + 35$$
or
$$x^4 + 2\,ax^3 + a^2x^2 = b^2$$
or
$$x^2 - b = ax$$

or an infinite number of other equally true equations. But would he? Unless there were some reason in his mind for doing it, he certainly would not. But trial and error might mean: fall back on vaguely remembered procedures practised with other tasks. But there is nothing in his previous experience he can fall back upon in this vague manner. Trial and error may then mean that he gets a "hunch" from the data themselves and tries this "hunch" out. This would no longer be random activity, but activity determined by the nature of the task and in so far insightful. He might, for instance, write $x^2 = b - ax$ because he sees that he can extract the square root from x^2, only to find that now he has no longer only known quantities on the right side. So he returns to the old form $x^2 + ax = b$. But the idea persists: find an expression which is a square. He knows the formula $(a + b)^2 = a^2 + 2\,ab + b^2$, but so far this potential knowledge has not become actual. If this knowledge enters the present situation what will happen? Supposing the person had read the left side again and again, and one of these readings had recalled that old formula. Has he thereby found the solution? By no means: the mere fact that the old formula is recalled is not sufficient; it is necessary that its recall combine with the present equation in a certain way. The mere recall might indeed lead to its rejection: "Oh, no, that is no good; in this formula a square is expressed by three terms, whereas on the left side of my equation I have only two; therefore the formula does not help me. Try something else." And then the recall of the old formula would have prevented the solution. But if the formula makes the person see the left side as "two terms of a possible three," then indeed he has made a large step towards the solution. Thus he may formulate:

$$x^2 + ax + ? \sim a^2 + 2ab + b^2$$

$$x^2 \sim a^2 \qquad ax \sim 2ab \qquad \therefore ? \sim \left(\frac{a}{2}\right)^2$$

$$x \sim a \qquad a \sim 2b$$

$$\frac{a}{2} \sim b$$

where ~ stands for "corresponds to."

Therefore he writes: $x^2 + ax + \left(\frac{a}{2}\right)^2 = b + \left(\frac{a}{2}\right)^2$ and sees that this transformation leads to the required solution, because he has now a square on the left side of the equation and only known quantities on the right.

The example is very simple. Only two real steps are necessary: he must see that the left side is to be a square and that it is not "enough of a square," to use Duncker's terminology. Probably the second step would be impossible without previous knowledge of the old formula. But this knowledge alone is insufficient. In the first place it must become available at the present moment, in the second place it must influence the data in a specific manner. The first of these effects need not be so accidental as we described it in our analysis. The idea that the left side should be a square might of itself recall the knowledge that a square may be expressed in more than one term, and thereby the formula. If this is the case, then the process is more directed than in our first analysis, and the chance of the old formula's failing to help is greatly diminished. Instead the old formula will easily lead to the idea: "left side an incomplete square; complete it!" And this determines at once the effect that the knowledge of the formula exerts on the present datum. It might even happen that the idea "left side should be a square" leads directly to the addition of $\left(\frac{a}{2}\right)^2$ without an explicit recall of the formula. In this case the trace of the old formula would have come into communication with the present process but instead of leading to recall would at once have led to the correct process. In this case, one single step would have led to insight, whereas the other possibilities would have required two or more steps for its development, although each step in itself would have been a case of partial insight. Therefore insightful behaviour is not necessarily a behaviour in which the full solution occurs at once. Criticisms of the term insight based on this assumption are therefore spurious.

THE FORCES OF ORGANIZATION. Our example is indeed one in which "the animal is forced by the situation to act in a special way although it possesses no special devices for the particular act." And we can see, up to a certain point, *why* it is forced. The occurrence of the square of the unknown enforces the idea of the operation of extracting a square root; the other fact that the unknown also appears in the first power leads to the apprehension of the left side as an incomplete square, and this, with the help of previous knowledge, to the proper transformation of the equation. The whole process stays, as it were, inside the boundaries set by the data of the problem. If the solution is found, *intrinsic* relations must have acted as dynamic relations. If one wants to deny this consequence one has to defend either of two positions: either one has to reject the claim that the process was guided by intrinsic relations and explain it by the workings of blind mechanisms (as has been the tendency of experimental psychology for a long time) or one has to introduce a new factor, a mind, which is able to grasp intrinsic relations and utilize such understanding in its interaction with the body. This alternative would lead to a vitalistic or spiritualistic dualism which we, in full agreement with the vast majority of psychologists, have refused to accept. The first alternative is incompatible with the facts. The three recent investigators, Duncker, Maier, and Claparède, are unanimous about this point. Intrinsic relationships enter every true problem solution. But then our former conclusion is unavoidable: the dynamics of the process are determined by the intrinsic properties of the data. Expressed in this way, the proposition is not new to us; it was the theme on which our whole treatment of perceptual organization played. What seems so startling in the application of this proposition to thought processes is that the *kind* of intrinsic properties which are to be considered as dynamically effective seem to exclude such a consideration. How can a purely logical relation exert a real force on a real process in a nervous system? Homogeneity and inhomogeneity of stimulation as intrinsic properties of areas could well be treated as the origin of forces, but how can the idea "incomplete square, complete it," be so considered? And yet, even here we possess a good analogy in perceptual organization: the principle of closure. Just as a perceived circle will, as a psychophysical process, "tend" towards completion, so will $x^2 + ax$, once it is seen as an incomplete square, tend to be completed.

Organization in Perception and Thought Compared. Although I do not wish to claim that every thought relation has a counterpart in a perceptual relation, yet the similarity between the two fields is closer than is generally recognized. It was to bring out this fact that Harrower first introduced her joke diagrams (see above, p. 619). She also draws attention to language which frequently enough uses spatial or dynamical terms to describe properties of thought, as "a balanced sentence," and she quotes Titchener, a witness least likely to be considered biassed in favour of this view, who describes his understanding of a text as accomplished by a visual schema (Harrower, p. 58).

If we take this argument seriously, we have made a decisive step in our answer to the problem as to the immediate causes which produce the reorganization in thought processes. In our attempt to answer concretely the question why things look as they do, we have enumerated a number of principles of organization, i.e., we have discovered a number of intrinsic properties of psychophysical processes that determine which of them will become unified, which segregated, the mode and shape of this unification, and so forth. Similarly, in answering the question: Why do we think as we do? Why are thoughts what they are? we have to find intrinsic properties of psychophysical thought processes which account for their organization. Each of the two problems has its particular advantages and disadvantages. The perceptual problem keeps us closer to the actual physiological events than the thought problem where physiological hypotheses are speculative to a much greater degree even than in the field of perception. On the other hand, the "purer" thought processes are, the more they will reveal the efficacy of properties which are apt to be obscured in perception because of the contingent stimulus distribution.

At the present time problems in perception and in thinking will, therefore, probably have to be investigated at "different levels." Answers which must satisfy our curiosity on the level of thought will have to be much more concrete on the level of perception. But if our argument is correct, this difference in level is a difference in our knowledge of things and not a difference in the things themselves. In either field we have to find intrinsic properties which explain field organization, and though at the moment we may often enough be able to express these properties of thought processes only in logical terms we ought to feel convinced that to these logical terms there correspond psychophysical realities, just as we assume that in perception psychophysical realities correspond to qualitative properties of the perceived objects.

INTRASYSTEMIC FACTORS. The discovery of such properties, however, does not finish our work. In the discussion of our algebraic example we have pointed out such properties, and yet the solution will not be reached by every person, and those who find it will not all find it in the same way. Therefore the knowledge of these properties alone is not sufficient to derive the result. A law knows no exceptions or individual differences. If individual differences remain unexplained, our law is not yet complete. To give a simple example from physics: the trajectory of a thrown ball can be derived from the force of gravity and the initial velocity (its magnitude and direction) of the ball (disregarding the "twist" imparted to the ball, the air resistance, and the wind). No two actual trajectories will be alike; though as a rule they will be parabolas, they may also be straight lines, namely, when the ball is thrown straight up. But each individual trajectory is predictable from the law, provided we know the initial velocity and the constant of gravitation at the place where the ball is thrown. The law is that the ball will fall with constant acceleration, the intrinsic properties the masses of earth and ball.

To account, then, for the individual differences of thought processes we have to know a great deal more than the intrinsic properties so far discussed. In our example a 3-term expression is needed instead of the given 2-term one. The fact that the situation demands the extraction of a square root is the prominent intrinsic property of the situation. But whether this property will be able to transform the *complete* 2-term expression $x^2 + ax$ into an incomplete 3-term expression $x^2 + ax + ?$ depends partly on the firmness of the 2-term structure. And this in its turn depends, without a doubt, on the anatomico-physiological constitution of the nervous system, even though we know as yet nothing at all about the particular aspects of this constitution which account for such differences.

Our ignorance about the physiological side of the person's constitution need not, however, prevent us from finding out psychological characteristics. We can recall differences in the Ego structure which we discussed in Chapter VIII (p. 342), to show the kind of differences we mean. Thus in one person a process distribution will be more isolated and more rigid than in another, so that an organization once produced will be harder to change. Such a person would, e.g., have greater difficulty in transforming the $x^2 + ax$ into

$x^2 + ax + ?$, and at the same time the first expression would be much less likely to communicate with the trace system of the formula $(a+b)^2 = a^2 + 2ab + b^2$. One could deduce a number of characteristics inherent in the thought processes of different persons from such differences in their psychological make-up.

But our main problem remains to study the intrinsic character of the processes which will, under favourable circumstances, result in proper reorganization, i.e., lead to the required solutions.

Experimental Studies. To study this problem one has to put subjects into problematical situations and observe their behaviour. Such observation can be greatly facilitated by a method suggested by Claparède in 1917 and employed in his last investigation as well as by Duncker. The subjects are instructed to "think aloud," i.e., to formulate every idea that occurs to them during their attempts to find the solution.

In such studies the choice of the problem is of paramount importance, just as the choice of the figures was decisive in the experiments on the change of traces (Wulf and his successors, Chapter XI, p. 496); for the forces in the field which regulate the behaviour are determined by the problem. Different problems are therefore liable to reveal different forces, different intrinsic properties of objects, perceptual or imagined, which become dynamically effective. If, in the following lines, we attempt to distinguish between various kinds of problems, we do not intend to give an exhaustive classification.

THREE DIFFERENT TYPES OF PROBLEMS. A first type of problem is exemplified by our algebraical example. Here the data themselves contain everything that is needed for the process of solution. One might object to this statement that the formula $(a+b)^2$ must be known beforehand. Even so, the conditions for this piece of knowledge to be reproduced are potentially inherent in the datum. Of course the datum must be apprehended as a question, not as a statement, but when we speak of datum we mean always the *process* to which the objective (geographical) datum gives rise.

Duncker has largely used problems of this type, and Wertheimer has discussed several falling under this group. In genuine solutions the intrinsic properties of the data are operative; the solution occurs uninfluenced by external factors, external, that is, to the situation of the data themselves.

A second kind of problem are the jokes which were to be completed in Harrower's experiments and most of the tasks set by Claparède, which consisted in finding a legend for a cartoon or connecting two phases of a picture story by events which might have happened between them. In two senses the solution has, in these cases, to go beyond the data. A joke, a cartoon, refers to situations of everyday life. To treat them adequately a more or less specific knowledge of the events concerned is necessary. But over and above this, a joke is a joke, and therefore the completion of the unfinished structure has to conform to this general "atmosphere" (Claparède). If this "atmosphere" failed to appear or to influence the solution, then such completions would be made as are exemplified in the first group of answers reproduced on page 616. As pure answers they are perfectly correct; Rubinstein might have said so; but they fail to complete the unfinished structure so as to make it a joke.

In this group of problems the solution depends upon many more factors than in the first, although here too, as Harrower has shown, various degrees of ambiguity are possible. And clearly: the more the solution depends on internal factors, the less ambiguous it will be. Again both much and little ambiguity have their respective advantages: the first chiefly by demonstrating a great number of different processes that will occur, the second by a clearer definition of a few essential factors. At the present moment, even though I may have a personal preference, I can see no good reason why one type of problem should be used to the exclusion of another.

A third type of problem is that used so successfully by Köhler and modified and put to various uses by later workers. As a rule the physical (geographical) situation contains everything that is necessary for the solution. But the togetherness of the different elements is in itself contingent. This fact distinguishes it from the first group, where the togetherness itself was necessary. To exemplify: the problem of reaching a lure that is not directly accessible does not imply that a stick *must* be at hand. If it happens to be there, it is a fortunate circumstance. But in the equation $x^2 + ax = b$ a part of a square cannot help appearing on the left side.

This difference is likely to appear in the dynamics of the solution. One might argue: the task is complete without the presence of a stick; the solution is: I must have something to extend my arm, and for this conclusion the presence of a stick is not necessary. It is indeed perfectly possible that a solution could be reached in this way and that thereupon the person or animal proceeded to search for or fabricate a stick. But chimpanzees would never have solved the problem in this way, as proven by the fact that even *after* they have used a stick once or twice they will not for some time employ one which is not visible simultaneously with the lure (Köhler).

With this difference between the third and first groups another one is closely connected. In the first group the question, and therefore the principle of its solution, lies entirely within the datum, i.e., the environmental part of the field, whereas in the third the problem arises from a relation between Ego and environment. As long as the ape is not hungry, there is nothing in his behavioural situation that would cause him to use a stick in order to get a banana. But the equation $x^2 + ax = b$ is always a question, even if the person who understands this equation refuses to worry about and solve it. The result of this difference is that the problems of the third group require, if not to a higher degree, then in a different manner, forces between Ego and environment. To say that problems of the first kind are quite independent of Ego forces is obviously wrong. As we just stated, one might refuse to worry about their solution and then, as a rule, they will remain unsolved. We know from the testimony of great thinkers that in order to solve difficult problems they persevered in concentrating on them. But this concentration is effective only inasmuch as it supplies the problematical external situation with sufficient energy to make reorganization possible. The reorganization itself must, if it is to be right, depend upon the properties of the field alone and not upon any field-Ego relationship. In the third group the Ego is one of the parts of the problem itself, and therefore Ego-properties as well as object-properties must become effective in the final reorganization of the field.

The distinctions which I have drawn between different kinds of problems is an idealized abstraction. No problem is in reality quite free from Ego forces. It is at least very doubtful whether a problem of an entirely objective nature will solve itself if we refuse to deal with it seriously. If such cases could be established they would be ideal cases in which the working of intrinsic environmental [10] properties would be manifested in the purest form. But they will be exceptions. On the other hand no real solution is independent of intrinsic field properties, and therefore also the experiments of the third group reveal their dynamical effects.

EXPERIENCE AND ITS RÔLE IN THE SOLUTION. The recent investigators have by their experimental procedures and theoretical considerations contributed a great deal to the foregoing analysis. They are all

[10] "Environmental" is here again used in the sense: not belonging to the Ego. See footnote, page 618.

agreed that a problem is equivalent to a system under stress, and that the mere recourse to experience is quite insufficient to explain problem solutions. Maier (1930) has even gone so far as to provide his subjects with the experiences necessary for the solution. But of 37 subjects only one (=2.7%) found the solution, and he was one of a group of 28 which had been told that these experiences were to be applied in the solution of the real problem. On the other hand eight out of twenty-two subjects (=36.4%) who had been given a "directional" hint in addition to these experiences were successful. Harrower's experiments reported on pages 622 f. can be interpreted in the same way. The existence of knowledge—having read the required solutions in a different context—is not sufficient for its utilization. In her experiments such knowledge was only utilized once out of 18 possible cases when no hint as to its possible usefulness was given.

These results are not astonishing after our analysis. The *existence* of utilizable traces is not sufficient for the solution; the utilizable trace must be utilized, and this utilization is often the chief part of the solution. This point was well brought out in Wertheimer's example (1920) of the lawyer who looks for a paper belonging to case A, the files of which have been carefully preserved, whereas the files of other cases, B, C, . . . have been destroyed. The solution comes when the lawyer "remembers" that the paper he is looking for belonged *also* to case B. *Now* he knows actually that it has been destroyed; before, he knew it "potentially," but this knowledge was useless for the present occasion. The paper could not recall the fact of its having been destroyed before it had been recognized as belonging to case B.

In this case the actualization of potential knowledge follows immediately upon the reorganization of the principal item in the field, and here the difficulty lies not in the former but in the latter. Probably, wherever the problem is difficult, some reorganization must occur before the utilizable material is utilized, but the first step will not always lead to the second as quickly as in Wertheimer's example. Everything depends upon the relation between the reorganized item and the potentially available material.

AVAILABILITY OF TRACES AND PERCEPTUAL DATA COMPARED. Whether this material is a trace or a part of the perceptual field makes no essential difference. We cannot even say that under all conditions it is easier to make a perceptual object available than a trace, availability depending, as we have seen, on too many factors. One of these is clearly envisaged by Maier (1931 a, pp. 343-4) and has, for memory material, been proved by Harrower, for perceptual material in much simpler tasks by Heiss (reported by Volkelt, pp. 129 f.): the object potentially available may be so strong a part of a larger object or be possessed of a functional character so different from the one needed that it will not yield to the pressure in the field. Now this difficulty may be greater for a perceptual object than for an object present merely in the form of a trace. It might, for instance, be necessary to use a pair of pliers as a weight. A person who sees the pliers before him may because of their very definite functional character be prevented from using them—just as one of Köhler's apes, perfectly familiar with the use of a box, failed to utilize one on which another animal was seated (1927, p. 178 f.; see also Koffka, 1928, p. 215)—whereas if the person had faced the problem: what object likely to be around could I possibly use as a weight, he might more easily have hit upon a pair of pliers.

The presence of an object with a very definite functional character may also prevent the proper reorganization. When I know that I can use only the things now at my disposal, and there is no other heavy object except a pair of pliers, then its presence might prevent the reorganization of the problem as one which required a weight. On the other hand, as we have pointed out before (stick experiment), the perceptual presence can be of enormous importance.

"FITTINGNESS." If we treat the problem of the utilization of material in the same way, whether the material is actually or only "memorially" (trace) present, we can deduce new principles of interaction between process and trace. In an experiment by Lipmann and Bogen (p. 28) a child has four different sticks at its disposal for pushing a ball lying behind bars (see Fig. 111).

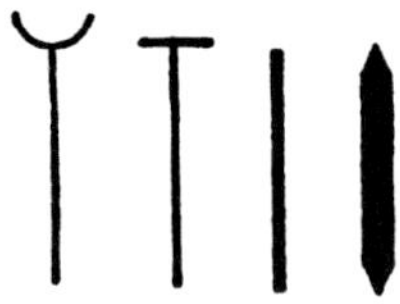
1 2 3 4

Fig. 111

Clearly, 1 is the best, 4 the worst. If then the child selects the proper stick this selection is due to intrinsic characters of the objects; the tool "fits" the ball, and this fittingness acts as a principle of selection.

Since all problem solutions can be said to consist in finding the *fitting* part which will relieve the existing stress, a law of fittingness would be the most universal law to explain thinking, and with it the arousal of new processes. Such a law would be a generalization of the laws of good continuation and closure. In establishing such a law one must, however, be careful lest one explain an event by the event, i.e., one has to define "fittingness" concretely in such a way that it can become dynamically operative. What is the nature and the seat of the forces which draw an element, originally absent from a situation, into this situation? Before such a task is accomplished, the law is not yet a true law but only a demand for finding a law. However, even as such it has its value, for it refuses an explanation of "fitting" events in terms of extraneous factors which have nothing to do with their fittingness, an explanation which derives the intelligible from the merely contingent. This was implicitly or avowedly the aim of empiricism and positivism, and therefore a law of fittingness is another manifestation of the anti-empiristic[11] and anti-positivistic attitude of gestalt theory.

Nevertheless, the claim that there should be a law of fittingness is not the proof that there is one. In order to establish such a proof it would be necessary to show what particular properties of physiological processes make them "fit" and make them attract each other. As regards the laws of good continuation and closure in spatial organization, which, as we just said, can be regarded as special cases of a more general law of fittingness, we attempted to give the beginning of such a proof by considerations of systemic equilibrium. In an organization which conforms to these two laws the forces must be better balanced than in others. Even such a proposition, however, could be proved only in a few very simple cases, the main burden of our proof being empirical. But a proposition like the one just formulated makes it possible to *understand* the empirical evidence. If now we try to generalize and establish our law of fittingness we are in a less favourable position. True enough, when the solution of a problem has been found, the forces are better balanced than they were before, the problem stress has been relieved, but, as we have pointed out before, the sequence of events that leads to this final state is not thereby explained. In spatial organization the general conditions are such that only a few organizations are possible under a given stimulus distribution, and the one which fulfils the conditions of the laws of good continuation and closure is among them. Thus we discussed the problem, why, in a given case, articulation a b c/d e results, and not a b/c d e? (See Chapter IV, pp. 164 f.) But when we deal with problems of thought the very condition which made the treatment of spatial organization so

[11] It will not be necessary to point out that an anti-empiristic attitude does not mean the denial of the enormous value of experience. Not *that* it makes use of experience causes our objection to empiricism, but *how* it makes use of it.

comparatively simple is mostly lacking. The question here is often a b c x, where x, the unknown, is not necessarily present, and if present *not* in connection with a b c but with e f g.

With these last remarks we have connected our present problem with an earlier discussion (see pp. 625 f.). Our law of fittingness would be an answer to the question: Why do we think as we do? (See p. 632.) And we shall have to be satisfied if we establish its validity on a "higher" level than that of the laws of spatial organization (see p. 632).

UTILIZING FACTORS OF ORGANIZATION TO PRODUCE ERROR. Such proof requires a number of different steps. The laws of spatial organization were derived from experiments in which several organizations were *a priori* possible, but only one or a few actually realized or even realizable, thus revealing the operative factors. A similar procedure would be extremely useful in the field of thinking. We ought to create conditions where dynamically the true solution is not the only possible one but where false solutions are favoured by the distribution of the forces at work. The beginnings of such a procedure have been indicated by Harrower. I quote: "We may tell a subject this:—'swimming under a bridge there came two ducks in front of two ducks, two ducks behind two ducks, and two ducks in the middle' asking him how many there were in all. The first spontaneous answer is 6, with the formation

o o
o o.
o o

For the concept of 'twoness' implies a pair of ducks, and a pair would be spatially equidistant from the observer, since pairedness implies[12] equality. Again, it is as if three such pairs are seen; for each mentioned spatial position ('in front of,' 'behind,' and 'in between') 'demands' a pair of ducks to fill it.

"The correct solution is *four* ducks, swimming in single file. This organization, however, has properties which are against its ever being seen as the required one. For if we are thinking in terms of 'pairs,' the 'single file' aspect will not even be considered" (p. 112).

Here the question is put in such a way that the forces must produce a wrong organization (provided the person asked is not closely familiar with swimming ducks). To the forces enumerated by Harrower I may add that in the false solution the pairs remain constant for each specified relation, whereas in the true solution

[12] The meaning and the importance of implication as a psychological concept has been amply and adequately discussed by Claparède (pp. 101 ff.).

the pairs themselves are variable, a factor which in itself favours the former tremendously with regard to the latter.

A systematic employment of this method should reveal a number of factors which determine organization in thought processes. Experiments which provoke false thinking should prove as fruitful for our understanding of thought processes as the study of optical illusions has proved for perceived shape, and some modern methods (Jaensch, 1921, pp. 170 f., G. Heider, pp. 37 ff.) for the theory of so-called colour constancy.[13]

THE COMBINATION OF OPERATIVE FORCES. TWO DIFFERENT POSSIBILITIES. If such experiments have given us insight into a number of concrete factors of organization, then there arises a new problem as to their combination. Either they might act independently of each other, in a summative manner, or they might themselves be organized into a meaningful whole. When Duncker says: "A problem solution is due to insight inasmuch as its relevant traits are immediately determined by those traits of the problem situation which they satisfy" (p. 701), he disregards this distinction. And yet, as Wertheimer never tires of emphasizing, it is quite fundamental. *Full* insight is distinguished from partial insight by this very difference. In full insight the different traits of the situation that determine its relevant features and thereby the solution form themselves a *coherent* system and are not independent of each other. To exemplify again with an example from elementary algebra. A person who transforms the equation $x^2 + ax + b = 0$ first into $x^2 + ax = -b$, because he wants to separate the known and the unknown variables, then takes the next step which makes the left side a square, $x^2 + ax + \left(\frac{a}{2}\right)^2 = \left(\frac{a}{2}\right)^2 - b$ does not have the same insight as a person who sees that the second step is compatible with the principle of separation of unknown and known, since it leads to $x + \frac{a}{2} = \pm\sqrt{\left(\frac{a}{2}\right)^2 - b}$, where the separation is as easy as in the original equation. Unless he sees that $x^2 + ax$ can be made into the square of a sum of an unknown and a known quantity, the coherence of the solution is partly obscured and the result, although it follows necessarily, contains an element of surprise, that is, the final solution is not entirely free of stress.

FITTINGNESS AND ARTICULATION. Solutions can be, and often are, reached without full insight, i.e., without complete organization of

[13] Maier (1930, pp. 141 f.) discusses two examples which can be utilized from this point of view.

all the determining factors, but a *complete* solution requires such complete organization. This conclusion leads to very important consequences for the relation of psychology on the one side, and logic and epistemology on the other, consequences which we cannot discuss here. Instead I shall refer to a particular aspect which reveals a difficulty intrinsic in all thought. We just said (p. 636) that no problem is entirely free from Ego stresses. The fact that "we" concentrate on a problem shows that the Ego is needed to hold the problem in the actual behavioural environment. On the other hand the problem may be of such a kind that the organized pattern of forces which are to determine its solution does not contain the Ego at all. Therefore, in such cases, the Ego has to be in dynamic intercourse with a process, supply it with energy, and yet *not* determine how this energy is to be organized. When we envisage the situation thus we understand why our wishes so easily influence our thought. The dynamic situation as we have just described it almost demands such an effect. To give an example: I am trying to verify a special hypothesis; naturally it would please me if I could find in my store of knowledge such items as would confirm it, particularly if this special hypothesis were closely linked up with my general theory. My trace system contains a number of relevant facts; it is exposed to the forces of the "hypothesis" and, almost unavoidably, also to the Ego forces originating in a wish to see the hypothesis confirmed. Therefore it is not surprising that such facts as fulfil both conditions emerge more readily than those that fulfil only the first.

We turn back to the investigation of the law of fittingness. We return to the example of the four sticks taken from Lipmann and Bogen (p. 638). Except by chance, the selection of the proper stick can take place only if the shape of ball and sticks are clearly perceived. Otherwise expressed, fittingness applies to the behavioural and not to the geographical data. Fittingness thus presupposes a definite organization of the total field. In a badly articulated field fittingness will be differently determined from what it is in a well articulated field. Our stick example shows that improved articulation results in improved selection, for the less clear the difference between the sticks, the less likely is a correct choice to be deliberately made.

However, the relation between field articulation and fittingness is not so simple as it would appear if we considered just this one example. Not only the degree, but also the *kind* of articulation enters this relation. Thus in the duck example the articulation into three pairs is very clear indeed, and by its clearness makes the true solution so difficult.

THE ORIGINAL REORGANIZATION. In such cases, as in many if not most others, a reorganization of the field has to take place as the first step in the thought process. This reorganization has been investigated and described by Duncker and Maier. Duncker speaks of the "functional value" of a situation ("lure *too high*," "stick *too short*," etc.); Maier says that "we see the difficulty to lie at some particular point" (1930, p. 137); different subjects may choose different points in one and the same objective task, thereby producing different solutions of at least partially different behavioural tasks. Thus in the problem of tying together two strings suspended from the ceiling at such a distance that the subject, holding one in his hands, could not reach the other, four possibilities existed and were realized, each leading to a special solution:

"(1) How to make one cord stay in the centre while the other cord is reached . . .

"(2) What to do to make the cords long enough to bridge the gap . . .

"(3) What can be done to extend the reach . . .

"(4) As the one cord cannot be reached while holding the other, one cord must in some way be made to move toward the other" (1931, p. 190). What "fits" one of these organizations will not fit the others. In the first a chair to tie one string to will be fitting, in the second a piece of cord lying around, in the third a stick, and in the fourth a weight.

Since "fittingness," however, is a relation between at least two things, it is not only the problem which must be organized in a special way so as to make something fit it, there must also be objects which can fit the problem so organized. Since these objects need not be perceptually present, this imposes a certain condition on traces if they are to fit into the problem. They also must be organized, and organized in special ways. And often the form of the problem will influence the organization of the objects; i.e., an object will *become* the kind that fits, because it is exposed to the stress of the problem. Thus, when one of Köhler's apes broke a branch from a tree to use it for pulling in bananas, a "branch" had become a "stick"; a behavioural object had been so reorganized as to fit the problem. This reorganization, of course, presupposed that the object had certain properties which made this reorganization possible. But when we remember how difficult it is to utilize knowledge (Maier and Harrower) we recognize the real achievement of this animal. We can liken the animal to Maier's subjects who had been told everything that was necessary for the solution of their problems or to Harrower's who had read the solution of their incomplete jokes in a different context. Just as they are acquainted with the necessary material, so the ape knows branches as long, rigid objects. In each case the utilization of this knowledge for a new problem is the decisive step. Again such reorganizations may happen with objects not perceptually present. When one of Köhler's apes ran into her sleeping room and fetched a blanket to use as a stick, she utilized an object which was "present" only through recall. This raises the question whether the stress of the present problem can directly produce a reorganization of the trace system, a question which I dare not answer.[14]

THE LAW OF EFFECT. But one cause of such reorganization deserves special mention because of its intrinsic interest and the rôle which it has played in the discussion of the laws of learning. Supposing that in the Lipmann-Bogen stick experiment the child selected the sticks at random and happened in a later trial to use the best stick for the first time. Then the manipulation of the ball will be easier, and the experience of this greater ease may bring about the required articulation: the fittingness of this stick will be recognized as well as its difference from the others. In other words: the result of an activity, taken in the broadest sense, may reorganize the conditions which were responsible for this act. This is the law of effect and the interpretation we have given of the rôle of success in learning in Chapter XII (p. 540).

According to it the "effect" can have the required backward result only if the action performed and the environment in which it is performed are behaviourally unified, and the result will vary directly with the degree of this unification. An act therefore which is objectively successful but which uses an object not included in the relevant behavioural situation should remain without consequences,[15] a conclusion confirmed by an observation of the McDougalls, father and son. A rat engaged in opening a latch which was locked by another latch succeeded in this task by accidentally pressing the second latch by a random movement of the hind paw; 173 such trials did not perfect this action, and when this particular latch was set tighter so that the random movement did not turn it the rat

[14] I recall again Huang's experiment mentioned in Chapter XII, p. 554 n.

[15] In a different context we have derived the same conclusion at the beginning of the twelfth chapter (pp. 537 f.).

was completely baffled, and concentrated all its efforts on the first latch (p. 166).

The result of success will vary according to the conditions. It may lead to full insight or to a very partial understanding, sufficient only to make the response more adequate than it was before.

Thorndike, whose unfailing and ingenious attempts to prove the validity of a law of effect or success must command the admiration of every psychologist, saw that such a law was a necessity for every trial and error theory of learning. His proof, being independent of such a theory, seemed to lend strong support to it. This connection, however, disappears in our theory. The unity of act and environment, which we found a necessary supposition of this law, excludes pure trial and error, i.e., behaviour entirely at random, completely uninfluenced by features of the environment.

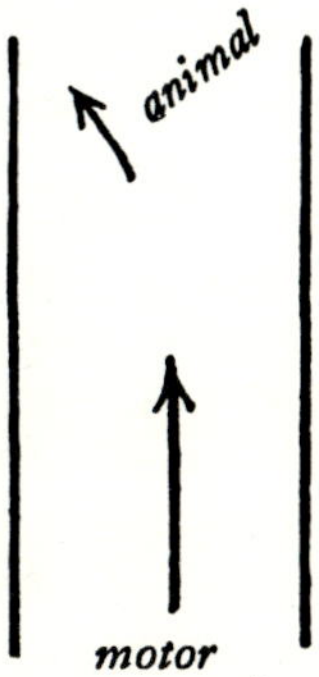

Fig. 112

I am convinced that the law of effect is responsible for a great many reorganizations, i.e., for a great deal of learning, both in men and in animals. In order to fill in a gap left open in Chapter IX (p. 372) I will discuss one special example. In that chapter I explained as an effect of experience the fact that animals often escape an approaching motor car by running to the side, although the field forces alone should drive them along in advance of the moving vehicle. How can an animal have learned this? My conjecture is that the animal did it the first time "accidentally," i.e., that the conditions were such that the direction of the force of the approaching car became effective only with one of its components. If, for instance, the animal was walking across the road in the direction indicated in this sketch, then we can consider the direction of the animal's body as a constraining condition which allows only that component of the force of the approaching car to become effective which coincides with it. Such an accidental success may, however, lead to a reconstruction of the field, such that in the future the proper reaction will follow directly and independently of the position of the animal. This case is of special interest because it shows that a reorganization of the field can change the direction of the operative forces, a conclusion very important for our understanding of the detour when the initial path lies geometrically in the direction directly opposite to the attracting goal.

OUR PICTURE OF BEHAVIOUR

If now we look back on the picture we have sketched of mental dynamics and of behaviour in general, we find that this picture represents a continuous sequence of organizations and reorganizations. New events happen practically every moment, events new by virtue of their organization. These new organizations are brought about by the forces arising through the relation between the organism and the environment and through field forces originating in the trace system. The function of the latter is, in our picture, primarily that of making new appropriate organizations possible, and not that of repeating what was experienced or done previously. Thus we are in full agreement with Bartlett, who says: "In fact, if we consider evidence rather than presupposition, remembering appears to be far more decisively an affair of construction rather than one of mere reproduction" (p. 205).

The preceding chapters have attempted to show that such a formulation is very much more than purely verbal, that "organization" has a very definite and concrete meaning, and that it follows very definite laws.

Intelligence. In conclusion we add only a few words: the behaviour of an organism, resulting as it does from psychophysical organization, is determined by the kind of this organization. Comparative psychology is therefore the study of the different kinds of organizations of which organisms are capable. This problem has two aspects, closely related to each other. In the first place, there arises the question of generic, specific, and individual differences. What is it that distinguishes the behaviour of insects from that of vertebrates, of rodents from that of primates, of anthropoids from that of humans, of one individual from that of another? Thus the question of intelligence arises, which will have to find its answer in terms of internal organic conditions which make certain organizations possible. Each organization has many apsects: stability, rigidity, complexity, degree of articulation and so forth. For different organizations different characteristics may be of dominant importance. Therefore it seems probable that there is not one kind of intelligence, but different kinds according to the particular organizations especially favoured. This does not mean, however, that we must necessarily distinguish different intelligences according to the *field* or material in which they become operative, but rather according to the kind of organizations that are being produced. To distinguish a motor, a practical, and a theoretical intelligence seems to me therefore much less warranted than, let us say, a geometrical and an arithmetical, a "quick" and a "slow," a "poetic" or a "mathematical" one.

Different Types of Reorganization. The solution of this problem introduces the second aspect of the general problem of comparative psychology just mentioned, viz., a systematic survey of the different kinds of organizations and reorganizations that are possible. I shall refrain from elaborating this point. I have enumerated and discussed a number of such forces in a previous book (1928), and R. M. Ogden has treated this aspect very systematically (1926, pp. 239 ff.).

CHAPTER XIV

SOCIETY AND PERSONALITY

The Incompleteness of the Preceding Discussion. The Main Problem. The Sociological and the Psychological Group. The Reality of the Sociological Group. The Reality of the Psychological Group. The "We." Formulation of the Problem. The Psychological and the Sociological Groups Connected by a Circular Process. The Formation of Psychological Groups. The Nature of Psychological Groups. Unification and Segregation. Stability. Articulation. The Results of Group Formation. Products of Civilization. Civilization as a Framework. Personality

THE INCOMPLETENESS OF THE PRECEDING DISCUSSION

Let us suppose that in the preceding chapters we had completely solved all the problems discussed. Should we then possess a full knowledge of behaviour? We need only raise this question to see that we have hardly approached behaviour as it really occurs. For we are members of a society, and our behaviour is determined by this fact to a degree which psychologists have only begun to realize. Therefore, without understanding the social factors of behaviour we cannot hope to understand behaviour. We must know the dynamics of the social factors and the results they produce.

The study of a science implies, as we have seen, the discovery of the laws which govern the phenomena investigated and of the conditions under which these laws operate and produce the concrete effects. So far we have neglected that most important set of conditions which we call the social conditions. If we disregard them, then our programme of developing a psychology that can explain the facts of civilization cannot be carried out.

Therefore we devote this last chapter to a brief survey of the main problems of social psychology. This subject is so vast that volumes larger than this can be written about it. Therefore our treatment will have to be sketchy, confining itself in the main to the drawing of outlines without filling them in with material.

THE MAIN PROBLEM

The Sociological and the Psychological Group. An important distinction is necessary for the formulation of our main problem: When we speak of a group—and I shall use this word instead of the more specific one "society" to designate any collections of organisms—we may mean two different things, viz., in our old terminology, a geographical or a behavioural group. I shall in the future call the former the sociological group, since the science of sociology has such groups as its subject matter, and the latter the psychological one. In what sense do these groups exist?

The Reality of the Sociological Group. Let us begin with the sociological group, and let us consider one composed of *n* members. What do we mean when we call these *n* persons a group? One answer would be that this term is nothing but a convenient name for the *n* members considered together, but that no reality corresponded to this concept over and above the reality of the members. This answer would, therefore, deny the existence of a group in the strict sense. Now it is surely true that there exists no $(n + 1)$th member, called the group, apart from the *n* members which compose it. Any group concept that implies, in however subtle a manner, such an interpretation will be rejected by us at the outset. But is this tantamount to rejecting the reality of a group? Let us remember our treatment of melodies. We saw that and how they are real, and yet the same argument that we just raised against the reality of the group was long ago raised against the reality of melodies: "a melody cannot be real, because if it consists of *n* tones, there is no $(n + 1)$th tone."

Melodies are behavioural events, and we are now discussing not the reality of the behavioural or psychological, but that of the sociological, group. And therefore it might seem as though we could not apply the melody argument to the group. But this would be a wrong impression, since we know that gestalten are not restricted to the mental or behavioural realm.

A group, then, may be a reality even though it need not be a new item added to the number of individuals which compose it. That certain groups *are* realities we have indicated in a much earlier part of the book (Chapter II, p. 58), where we showed very briefly that certain modes of behaviour are typical of individuals as members of groups and not of isolated persons. Similarly Bartlett proves the reality of sociological groups by giving detailed descriptions of "reactions which are *specific* to groups, found in them, and *not found outside them*" (p. 241). A sociological group, then, has existence, in the sense in which a gestalt has existence, and since the criterion we have used for the reality of the group is at the same time a criterion of its gestalt character, we must infer that a group is a gestalt. Such a statement, however, means very little unless we know what kind of a gestalt it is.

Two Gestalt Characteristics of Sociological Groups. In this respect groups have a number of very definite characteristics, they are gestalten of a very particular kind. I shall only mention two closely related particularities. In the first place the "strength" of the gestalt may differ over an enormously wide range. The strength of the gestalt character is defined by Köhler by the degree of interdependence of the parts. The stronger the gestalt, the more will each of its parts depend on all the others, and the more will this dependence affect every aspect of the parts. From this point of view practically all of the groups with which we are familiar are relatively weak, but groups in other cultures are much stronger. The difference which Becker calls that of the sacred and the secular society is a good illustration. The stronger the group, the more not only will the behaviour, but the entire status, of its members depend upon their relation to the other members. Thus, in primitive societies, loss of connection with the group may bring about the isolated member's death. To stay nearer home, we may compare the village with the city to exemplify differences in gestalt strength of groups. The strongest groups that we encounter are probably teams in games like football.

The fact that groups may have a very low degree of gestalt coherence derives from the second peculiarity that I want to point out. The group is composed of individuals, and the existence of individuals, although largely group-determined, is not exclusively so. To produce children, to rear and educate them, all these are socially determined activities; but much as we may wish to have children of a certain kind, it is not in our power to realize this wish. Again social factors enter to mould the characters of the young independently of our desires, but there remains an element that is no longer social. And though we cannot measure or evaluate the magnitude of this non-social element, we have to recognize it. Individuals are different from each other apart from social influences, and since the individuals, by composing the group, determine to some extent its nature, there remains a non-social element in groups. What this means will become clearer when we compare groups with other and stronger gestalten like melodies. In the composer's mind the tones do not exist prior to or independently of the melody. Here the melody, the whole, entirely determines its own members. The fact that the members of groups are not thus completely determined by the group is the same as saying that the group is not of the strongest gestalt type possible. This characteristic becomes especially important the less natural, the more artificial, the groups are. If a number of individuals join to form a club or a society, then the character of the members is already established, and the particular characteristic which such a new group assumes will to a large extent depend upon these characters of its members.

The Reality of the Psychological Group. The "We." And now we turn to the behavioural group. In what sense does it exist? Here the answer is easier. The reality of the psychological group finds its expression in the pronoun *"we."* "We" means not simply a plurality of persons which includes myself, it means in its most proper sense a unified plurality of which I and the others are true members. Otherwise expressed: when one says: "*We* do this," then one means not that the persons included in the "we" are doing this each for himself and independently of the others, but that we do it jointly. The speaker experiences himself as part of a group, and his actions as belonging to this group. Of course, the word "we" can also have the other meaning. "We have assembled here because we were all born on the same day." The two we's in this sentence are not quite identical. Only the second is a purely summative plural, while the first would carry at least the beginning of a true "group-we."

Here the question might be raised whether the "we," when it is used in the non-summative sense, is equivalent to an expression of a psychological group. It seems, at least at first, to be advisable to treat the "we" as more general than the psychological group; for the "we" applies to a great variety of personal relationships not all of which are groups of the same kind. Thus the "we" of bridge players may pertain to all four players or to a pair of partners; similarly a football player might use the word either to designate both teams or only his own. Similarly, I might say, of Mr. X and me, that we had a discussion on gestalt psychology, and this particular event might be the only one in which I should include him and myself under this term. It is clear that the two partners or the members of a football team form a psychological group of a different kind, if not in a different sense, from that formed by all players. And the group of the last example is entirely of that second kind. In all these cases, however, the word "we" refers to a reality. It is never a mere abbreviation of "they and I," or "he and I." For the I to which it refers is dependent upon the "we." In other words, the plurality to which the word "we" refers is not composed of a number of members which would be identical in all possible pluralities, but codetermines its own members. I feel differently, my behavioural Ego is more or less different, when I address a strange audience, when I speak in a dining club of which I am an old member, and when I walk in an academic procession.

Details of this relationship will be discussed later; here it only serves to prove the reality of the "we."

Formulation of the Problem. Having established the reality of both the sociological and the psychological groups, we can now formulate our main problem: What is the relation between them? In general outline the answer to this question is obvious: a sociological group presupposes a psychological one. For the sociological group differs from a mere collection of individual persons in that the behaviour of these persons, and the accomplishments to which it gives rise, depend upon the behaviour of the other persons. Now the behaviour of another person as a geographical event can influence my behaviour only in the same way in which any geographical event can influence my behaviour, i.e., by determining my *behavioural* environment (see Chapter II). This general proposition does not contain any statement about the particular kind of behavioural environment that would account for the formation of sociological groups. But we can see that, although "we-experiences" are not the only ones that contribute to group behaviour, they are a *conditio sine qua non* for the formation of groups. The mere presence in my behavioural field of other human beings will not lead to social behaviour. If a person or a group of persons is in my way, I shall make a detour in order to get what I want, just as I would if an inanimate object obstructed my path. My behaviour might be as little social in the first case as in the second.

Such arguments may even seem pedantic in view of the fact that we experience a "we," a belonging to a psychological group; therefore it seems natural to connect the geographical, or sociological, groups with the psychological ones.

Granted then that sociological groups arise through the mediation of psychological ones, the concrete nature of this dynamic connection becomes a problem, which again must first be stated in broad outline. Given a sociological group g composed of *n* members, it must owe its origin to the existence and interaction of *n* psychological groups G_n, and the interaction of these G_n becomes the fundamental problem. How do events within behavioural fields, the G_n, lead to the establishment of a geographical reality, the g?

The Psychological and the Sociological Groups Connected by a Circular Process. We have in various places discussed similar problems on a simpler level (see Chapter VIII, pp. 311 f., and Chapter IX, pp. 373 f.). Thus we saw in our discussion of movement how behavioural events gave rise to geographical ones by a circular process. If we apply this principle to our present problem we find the following situation: in the field of k, who is a member of the n who form the group, there exists a psychological group, a "we," and this part of the field is, for some reason or other, under stress. Then movement, behaviour, will be started in such a way that it leads to a new field which is under less stress than the original field. Although this general statement is obviously true, it is far too vague to characterize the ensuing behaviour sufficiently. What more can we then say about it? K's behaviour will affect the fields of the other persons in the group, a—j and l—n, changing the stresses of their behavioural fields and thereby leading them to act. Their action similarly will change k's field. It was the function of k's action to reduce the pressure in his own field. Therefore his action will fulfil this function only if the actions of a—j and l—n, to which it gives rise, lead to such a reduction of stress in k's field. The relation between the action arising from stress in a field and the result of this action on the stress of the field is therefore much more indirect than in the case of the eye-movements, mediated by other fields and their stresses. But for all this difference there remains a fundamental similarity: no new law is needed, only the application of the old law to a vastly more complex set of conditions.

Of course all members of the group have an equal right to be considered as k; i.e., in group behaviour we have an interplay, mediated by action, of n different behavioural fields, which may, and often does, produce organized behaviour, organized as well in each individual person as in the whole, sociological, group. Our principle explains, indeed, true sociological behaviour by deriving it from psychological behaviour; g has been explained by the interaction of the G_n.

I am prepared to assert that the problem of social psychology consists in filling in this general frame. In the rest of this chapter I shall discuss only a few points within this frame. They will fall under the following headings: (1) How do psychological groups become organized? (2) What are their main characteristics? (3) What are the results of social activity and how do they influence such activity?

As we have seen so often during the course of this book, different problems distinguished in a certain field are in reality interdependent. The same is true of the last three questions, none of which can be answered entirely without reference to the others.

THE FORMATION OF PSYCHOLOGICAL GROUPS

Nevertheless, we can start with the first problem and inquire into the formation of psychological groups. These groups, being parts of behavioural fields, must arise through processes of field organization. They are different from such group organizations as we have previously studied (point groups, line groups, etc.) in the fact that they include the Ego. Although this fact need not deter us from trying to apply our laws of organization to such instances, since we have met with a sufficient number of occasions in which the Ego is to be treated like other field objects, it is of extreme significance for the Ego. The Ego, being part of a group, will have characteristics due to this membership, a topic which we shall take up in the context of our third problem. Now we must try to discover forces which are responsible for behavioural group-formation.

The Law of Similarity. We begin with an extremely simple case, not because it is the most significant or typical one, but because it will clarify the problem in the easiest way. When we enter a room, we see the people in it as a group, separate from all the other objects, and more or less independent of their spatial distribution. This organization is, at least in part, reducible to the law of equality or similarity; thus far it offers no new problem. And as long as the matter remains there, this group formation is not the one we are now interested in. At first, on entering the room, we do not belong to the group. A little later, however, we may. What has produced this new group, containing not only the other people but also ourselves? Does it seem far-fetched to apply the same law to the formation of this new group which was found operative in the formation of the first? I believe not. Though surely not the only factor, the similarity between ourselves and the others seems definitely to contribute to this new organization. Thus one feels distinctly out of place when one is in evening dress while none of the others are, even when no social mistake is involved on either side.

Similarity and Physiognomic Characters. I will admit, however, that the factor of equality is not the strongest force in group formations. But it will lead us directly to other and more important ones as soon as we begin to analyze the equality or similarity itself. Why is my Ego, which is given only to a small extent in visual terms, similar to other persons, who are predominantly given in such terms? The answer must be that my Ego must be similar to other persons with respect to characters which, though they *may* be carried by visual characteristics, need not be so carried. We have encountered these characters before (Chapter VIII, pp. 359 f., and Chapter IX, p. 407), when we called them physiognomic characters. We saw that through these characters particularly strong Ego-object forces are aroused; therefore it is not a new step when we now connect group formation in general, and similarity in particular, with them. For something that we know as characteristics of our Ego appears also in those parts of the field which we call human beings, and to a lesser degree in animals. We perceive, through vision and audition, *persons,* i.e., objects endowed with the same kind of spontaneity that we possess, with purpose and hesitation, with joy and sadness, courage, ambition, and so on; and we experience ourselves also as persons. If, then, equality is an active factor in group formation, it must be equality of physiognomic character. Thus a sophisticated person will fall in easily with other sophisticated or even blasé ones, and will readily develop in his field a psychological group to which they and he belong; conversely, a direct and simple person will not easily find himself a part of a "we" if he is thrown in with a number of sophisticated people. Similarly, to be sad tends to exclude one from a gay group. That physiognomic similarity can lead to group formation is evidenced by certain mixed swarms of birds composed of different species with different life habits. Stresemann (quoted by Katz, 1926, p. 466) believes that he has found the causes of this group formation. "The little birds which come into proximity to an impressive and usually noisy swarm are attracted by it; they hurl themselves into the living maelstrom and are not easily able to extricate themselves from it."

The Origin of Physiognomic Characters. How We Perceive "The Other Person's Mind." But the dynamic characters play a far greater rôle than that of merely determining the boundaries of psychological groups; they are also largely responsible for the group structure and group behaviour. Therefore our next step must be to answer the question raised in Chapter IX (p. 407), how persons as behavioural objects possess physiognomic characters, or, more popularly expressed, how we perceive the other person's mind. I can confine myself to a brief treatment, since Köhler has discussed this problem very fully in the seventh chapter of his "Gestalt Psychology." I forbear to refute the two most widely held theories according to which we understand the other person's emotions by an inference based on analogy or by association. Both theories have been amply disproved by Köhler and C. D. Broad. The latter author therefore concludes: "Hence only two alternatives seem to be left. Either (1) there are certain cognitive situations which actually contain other minds or certain of their states as objective constituents; or (2) the visual appearance of certain bodily forms, movements, gestures, and modifications, has for us an *unacquired* meaning" (p. 327). It is interesting to see how Broad deals with these two possibilities. Although he gives dominance to the second, he is disinclined to reject the first completely. But the first is even less acceptable than the two rejected traditional theories, because it implies a theory of perception which to me at least appears mystical. For it would negate the difference between a behavioural and a geographical world. If somebody else's mind could be given to me directly, it would be simultaneously and identically the same object in my behavioural and in the geographical world. The second possibility, on the other hand, is another way of acknowledging the existence of physiognomic characters. Therefore everything depends upon the elaboration of this second possibility, i.e., on the answer to the question how persons as behavioural objects can possess physiognomic characters, physiognomic characters moreover which have cognitive value, which coincide with essential aspects of the other person as a geographical object. Broad's answer is this: "We must suppose that the innate constitution of human beings (and probably of other gregarious animals) is such that, when one sees any body which *in fact* resembles his own closely enough, he instinctively believes it to be animated by a mind like his own" (p. 330). This, of course, is highly unsatisfactory. It is not true that one believes the other body to be animated by a mind *like one's own*. Köhler has stressed this point: ". . . sometimes I understand others as being highly different from me. The characteristic manliness of Douglas Fairbanks is something which impresses me very much, though, unfortunately, I shall never be able to achieve it myself" (1929, p. 237). But apart from this inadequacy Broad's explanation is no explanation in a true sense. All it does is to invoke man's innate constitution, his instincts. This explanation is of the type of the famous *vis dormitiva,* and therefore resolves itself into a renaming of the problem which it pretends to solve. If we take it seriously, we have to apply it to concrete cases. How does it deal with questions like these: Why does *this* face appear to me sad, that gesture resigned, this voice exultant? Have we for each such experience a special kind of constitution, a separate instinct? And how does each special occasion contrive to appeal to a particular part of the constitution or to arouse a special instinctive faculty? Since a theory like Broad's must leave all such questions unanswered, it gives no real solution of the problem.

How, then, can forms, movements, gestures, have an unacquired meaning? This question does not strike us as particularly new or startling, for we have encountered a number of properties which behavioural objects possess directly (apart from the sense qualities). A line may be curved or broken, a figure symmetrical or out of shape, a tone in a melody flat or sharp, to name only a few instances. Behavioural objects possess these properties because of the organizations to which they owe their existence. We have also, in a special discussion, added the physiognomic characters to the list of such properties of behavioural objects, indicating that for them it is as a rule more difficult to point out the details of the underlying organization. Yet it is possible to produce clumsy or graceful objects in anybody's behavioural world without confronting him with other persons. A good draughtsman can produce graceful lines, clumsy figures, gay and melancholy patterns. This is still easier when we employ temporal arts. Indeed, very few objects of our behavioural worlds are so charged with emotion as good music is. Another example would be puppets, puppets which need to bear very little geometrical resemblance to human beings and yet are capable of carrying a wealth of emotional characters. The best examples for our argument are perhaps certain trick films after the pattern of Mickey Mouse, for here there is objectively neither motion nor emotion, but a mere sequence of strange drawings. But this sequence gives rise to objects in the behavioural world of the observers which move, and are agile or clumsy, exuberant or dejected, and so forth. The merit of this example lies in the fact that here all these characters are *only* in the behavioural objects and entirely absent in the geographical ones. The "meanings" which those forms and motions possess for us are therefore most clearly aspects or results of the psychophysical organizations produced by the stimuli.

But why are these "meanings" physiognomic, why do they convey emotions or other mental characteristics? This is a good question, if it is intended to signify only why objects have *physiognomic* characters, like sad and gay, and so forth. But it becomes at once misleading if it stresses the word "mental" or opposes it to "bodily" or physical. For many, if not most, words which we apply to subjective experience are equally well used for objective experience. Köhler, from whom this argument is taken, adduces a number of examples borrowed from Klages: "a *bitter* feeling," "a *soft* mood," "*sweet* love," etc. Therefore, what we have to explain is not the *mental* nature of these properties, but their *quality*. Why bitter and not sweet, calm and not excited, black and not bright!

In order to solve this problem we turn to a different class of cases, those where the physiognomic character is, more or less, veridical. I see an irritable person, and the person really is irritable; I meet my friend in the morning and find him depressed, although he tries to conceal it; I am shocked by the meanness of that face, and in truth a mean soul dwells behind that ugly mask. Such cases will lead us further, because here the geographical object possesses certain characteristics which are due to its intrinsic nature and which in some way or other become operative in proximal stimulation. Thus the movements of an irritated or a depressed person will be causally connected with his state of mind, and will on the other hand provide proximal stimuli for other persons who observe him. Thus a situation arises with two main relations: let us call the irritated or depressed person A, his friend who observes him B. Then the first relation is inherent in A, viz., that between his mood and his movements; and the second between these movements as possible stimuli for B and B's perception of A and his mood. That the mood or emotion of A influences A's actions is obvious. Action springs from stresses within Ego systems, and emotions bear, as we have explained in Chapter IX, a close relation to these Ego stresses. Even so, the dynamic relation between the two might be of different kinds. Emotion might cause or influence action by mere release; in this case the form of action would be independent of the emotion which released these actions, depending only on the "motor-mechanisms" thus brought into play. But all along in our discussion of action we have found the concept of release quite inadequate to deal with the facts; everywhere we found actions not only released, but also guided or steered by forces residing in the total field. Therefore we shall have to consider this possibility in our present problem. If an emotional stress steers action, then the ensuing movements will, to some extent, mirror the emotions; characteristics of overt behaviour will map characteristics of the field in which this behaviour is started. The slow dragging movements of the depressed, the jerky, discontinuous movements of the irritable, correspond indeed to the leaden state of depression or the disrupted state of irritability. The one, viz., the overt side, is as much depression or irritability as the other, the conscious side. Therefore it is meaningful to say that *real* behaviour, as defined in Chapter II (pp. 39 f.), is emotional.

And now we turn to our second relation, that between A's overt behaviour and B's perception of A. On B's sense organs, notably his eyes and ears, there is a proximal stimulation, determined by the shape and the actions of A. This stimulation gives rise to the spatio-temporal organization of A in B's behavioural field. It maps A's movements on B's retinae, his speech on his ear drums. Our total situation now looks like this:

$$E_A \sim M_A \sim R_B \rightarrow ?$$

E_A is A's emotion or mood, M_A his overt movements, R_B the image produced by these on B's retinae (and also the vibration pattern set up in his ears), $\sim$ stands for "maps." E_A is mapped by M_A and this in turn by R_B which determines the perception of A by B. However, there is a difference between the two kinds of mappings: R_B maps M_A *geometrically,* i.e., point by point according to the laws of perspective, and therefore R_B is not a *dynamical* map, as we discovered when we discussed the nature of the retinal image in Chapter III (p. 75); there we confined our discussion to the spatial picture, but it is easy to see that the same argument applies to the temporal picture which is important in our present context. Temporally also R_B is a mosaic of stimulations, for what happens at any one moment in R_B does *not* depend upon what happened *there* at the immediately preceding moment, but on the light rays which happen to strike the retina at the moment. On the other hand M_A maps E_A *dynamically.* Now we know that the *result* of R_B is a dynamic organization in B's psychophysical field, the relation of which to R_B we have studied in general terms in Chapter III and in detail in Chapters IV and V. There we saw that often this organization maps the distant stimulus better than the proximal one. If this were true in our case, if A_B, A as he is perceived by B, were a more or less true map of M_A, then we could understand how B becomes aware of A's emotion without association or inference by analogy. The behavioural object is a dynamic map of the distant stimulus object when and inasmuch as the proximal stimulus distribution possesses such geometrical characteristics as will produce a psychophysical organization similar to the one of the distant stimulus object. Thus I see the ashtray on my desk as a separate thing because the stimulus distribution is discontinuous along its boundary lines and therefore produces a segregated object of a particular shape in my behavioural environment. When we apply this argument to the M_A–R_B–A_B relationship we see that in many cases R_B will, as a geometrical map of M_A, have such characteristics as will produce an A_B dynamically similar to M_A. Thus a raising of A's voice will produce a temporal stimulus pattern in which each sound is followed by a louder one, and this stimulus pattern will give rise to the experience of a crescendo. Similarly A's jerky movements will result in a jerky spatio-temporal stimulus distribution on B's retinae and these in turn to B's experience of a jerky movement.

Thus to some extent A_B must be a dynamical map of M_A, but the question remains how much of M_A will A_B map. The crescendo of A's voice or his total behaviour may be the expression of his rising excitement, the jerkiness of his movements may express his irritability. So far we have only shown that A_B will possess the character of crescendo or jerkiness. But our real problem was to explain that A_B is excited or irritable. The difficulty seems to lie in the transition from crescendo to excitement or from jerkiness to irritability. But this difficulty is more apparent than real. Experienced crescendo and jerkiness are thoroughly dynamic events, and their dynamic aspect is but inadequately described by the terms crescendo and jerkiness, which may be interpreted geometrically. If we try to find words by which to describe the dynamic side of these experiences we are driven to use such terms as excitement or irritability. This is the reason why, as we mentioned previously (p. 657), we use the same adjectives to describe "mental" and "physical" events. It seems a false rationalization to assume that originally a crescendo is experienced simply as a change of intensity and is only later endowed with the character of excitement. This view has already been rejected at the end of Chapter VIII (p. 360), where we claimed that the more primitive a behavioural world is, the more physiognomic it is. Therefore we may assume that excitement is of the warp and woof of a crescendo experience, so that a crescendo A_B *is* an excited A_B.

Therefore our main problem has been solved in general terms. To work out the details we have to consider a number of points. The words which we have so far used in order to describe spatio-temporal patterns of R_B were very general. There are many kinds of crescendo and of jerkiness. Language fails to do justice to the variety of such patterns, which, qua patterns, are all different from each other. As different patterns they will owe their origin to different M_A and hence to different E_A, and conversely they will give rise to different A_B. Furthermore, the A_B depends not only on the R_B but also on the constitution of the nervous system of B. Thus what to one individual may appear as a grossly impertinent behaviour may to another seem nothing more than the awkward expression of shyness and modesty. The same (or a very similar) R produces a cruder organization of A in one observer (K) than in the other (L), just as in a concert a musical person receives more highly organized impressions than a less musical one (i.e., $A_K \neq A_L$).

Thus the more general the emotion expressed is, the more will the individual expressions be similar to each other and the more widely will such expressions be understood. Thus Katz summarizes the work done on the vocal expression of birds by saying that these expressions are the less understood the greater the difference between the species of birds, but that certain sounds, like those expressing fright, seem to be similar to a great variety of species and to be understood by them. The warning cries of certain pewits are even understood by the mammals with which these birds live in community.

We must also not forget that each behaviour takes place in a field, and that therefore the A_B will depend upon the field in which it takes place. This field is of course a field of B's, and that means that B's understanding of A will depend on the field in which he sees him acting. Thus A's behaviour may entirely change its aspect to B, when B notices the presence of another person whom at first he had not noticed, because A's behaviour appears now in dynamic relation to this other person. This point is of great importance; for behaviour is directed towards an object, living or dead, and if this object fails to be included in the observer's behavioural field, he will often get a wrong impression of the actions and gestures with which he is confronted. A case of particular significance is that in which the person's actions are directed towards the observer himself.

Before we conclude this discussion we must recall the fact that of our first three examples we have neglected the third, the mean face. It is different from the two others inasmuch as the organization involved may be purely spatial; we may perceive the meanness also in a portrait or a photograph. Without going into the theory of this case I will only mention that the face at any one moment is, as it were, a cross section of a motion, one frame taken out of a motion picture sequence, and that it bears the marks of being a part and the outcome of motion. This fact has been symbolized in "The Picture of Dorian Gray."

Group Formation as Due to Other Factors Besides Similarity. We can now return to the problem of behavioural group formation. The factor of similarity served well to introduce the general principle, to demonstrate forces in the field which pull the Ego towards other human beings. This factor would be effective even if *per se* each individual were "complete"; otherwise expressed similarity would lead to group formation even if the Ego in whose field no similars existed were free from stress; the stress towards group formation which arises from mere similarity is, to use an old terminology, a pure environmental-Ego stress, with the specification that the particular objects between which the stress exists are the Ego and his fellow creatures.

INCOMPLETENESS OF THE EGO. Now the most natural of all groups, the family, does not originate in this way. The helpless baby is not "complete," it depends for the satisfaction of its needs on the actions of others, and the first intimate relationship in a person's life is to those who administer to his needs. Conversely, having to administer, having to help the pitiably helpless, is another and not less strong force to produce group connection, to which is added the paternal relationship: flesh of my flesh. Parents are also no longer "complete" without their children.

But is any human being "complete" in isolation or would he be if he had grown to adulthood without ever coming into contact with his fellow creatures? We feel convinced that he would not. On the one hand he will want a mate, on the other comrades.

MC DOUGALL'S THEORY. This survey shows that the Ego itself must contain stresses which can be relieved only by its inclusion in various kinds of (behavioural) groups. And thus we seem to have reduced the causes of group formation to a theory of instinct. Indeed, when we look through McDougall's latest list of instincts, or, as he calls them now, propensities, we find all the needs we have just enumerated listed as such. Thus the need which attaches the infant to his parents or nurses corresponds to McDougall's 9th and 11th propensities, viz., submissive and appeal propensities, the need that binds the parents to their children to his sixth, protective or parental propensity; then, of course, he lists the sex propensity ("to court and mate," No. 3), and the gregarious propensity, No. 7 (1933, pp. 97 f.).

This parallelism reveals a fundamental reason for the adoption of an instinct theory. Behaviour, human and animal, cannot be described or explained without the assumption that the Ego is a seat of stresses which require particular kinds of reliefs. Furthermore, it makes no difference whether one uses the more general and neutral term "Ego-stress" or the more specific and controversial one "instinct." The real problem is what one means by either of these terms, what rôle they are to play in the theoretical system. Now we have criticized McDougall's concept before (Chapter IX, pp. 403 f.), and the criticism presented there applies as well to his use of the term with regard to our present problem. Also in his new book McDougall treats the instinct, or rather propensity, as a permanent innate disposition which may become "excited" and then "generates an active *tendency*, a *striving*, an *impulse*, or *drive* towards some goal" (p. 118). And it is at this point that my way of looking at the facts—acknowledged as much by me as by him—differs from McDougall's. I give another quotation. He speaks of a boy who has two abilities which he has never used. "Then one day he is among a group of boys who begin to 'show off' under the stimulus of fair spectators; his *latent propensity*[1] to shine, to excel . . . is roused by way of his perception of the situation" (p. 68). Passages like these seem to me to indicate that all propensities are permanent entities which may pass from the latent to the effective stage by excitation, and thus, since a number of the propensities are distinctly social in character, social behaviour is reduced to individual capacities. Now we have seen that individual characteristics of group members are determinants of the groups, but McDougall's theory goes far beyond such a statement. As long as we treat psychological groups we remain within the fields of individual persons. McDougall explains psychological group behaviour by dispositions which produce processes according to their own nature; the (behavioural) environment has no other function than to "excite" these dispositions. To this we oppose the view: the total field, and more particularly its relevant parts, set up the stresses in the Ego which determine behaviour according to the properties of the whole field. If we claimed that the Ego was "incomplete" without a number of social relationships we meant that the Ego, which itself is a product of organization, is an incomplete organization, a structure under stress, unless the total field fulfils certain conditions, viz., that it contains objects with definite dynamic characters. Thus McDougall's propensities are for us not ultimate explanatory concepts, but gross descriptions of certain main types of behaviour which it is the task of social psychology to explain. Propensities are formulated questions but not solutions.

That the difference between our theory and that of McDougall is more than terminological follows from the manner in which either theory treats the relation between behaviour and its underlying causes, as we have just demonstrated. But this point is so important that it needs a further elaboration. With some exaggeration, necessary to make the theoretical distinction as sharp as possible, one might say: for McDougall the Ego with its propensities and the environment which excites these propensities are independent en-

[1] Italics mine.

tities; in our theory they develop together and in close interaction by a process of field organization. Just as the behavioural environment depends upon the Ego which it surrounds, so the Ego depends upon the environment by which it is surrounded. In this relation of interdependence certain parts of the behavioural environment, our fellow creatures, play a particular rôle, and that because between them and the Ego certain forces can arise which alone can organize the Ego completely. Social behaviour, therefore, is not the result of "social propensities" within the Ego, but the result of field organizations of special kinds.[2]

Just because social behaviour results, in our theory, from field organization, it seems more fruitful for the progress of the theory to concentrate less on fundamental factors, which can at best be analyzed from fictitious cases, than on actual group behaviour, which shows field organization at work. We became, each of us, members of many groups for purely "social reasons," quite apart from an instinct or a propensity of gregariousness. We move to a new town and thereby become a part of the social life of that town, sociologically and psychologically. What happens in our behavioural social field under such circumstances? In answering this question we turn to the second of our main questions—the nature of the psychological groups—drawing only one more conclusion before we leave our first topic. If the behavioural Ego is incomplete in isolation, then the real, or geographical, organism is also incomplete as an individual. For the presence of fellow creatures in the behavioural environment presupposes the presence of real persons in the geographical environment. Intercourse in the behavioural social field is mediated, as we saw before, through a sociological field. Neither psychologically nor biologically is the isolated individual a complete part of nature.

THE NATURE OF PSYCHOLOGICAL GROUPS

If, now, we turn to our second question, we shall do well to free ourselves from the restriction to psychological groups which we have so far observed. We shall include in our discussion properties of groups to which we ourselves do not belong. This is legitimate since we have established the principle that sociological group properties are mediated by psychological ones. Therefore it is permissible to use the former as indications of the latter.

[2] A relevant discussion of kindred problems is contained in an earlier book by Bartlett (1923) and in my review of this book, particularly pp. 284 ff.

Unification and Segregation. In investigating the nature of groups we shall utilize our knowledge of other products of organization. The first of these which we met was unification and segregation along a boundary line. This is easily applicable to social groups, psychological and sociological. Groups are more or less closed, with more or less defined boundary lines. Consequently, the more closed they are, the more difficult it is to introduce new members into them. This has been confirmed by Köhler, whose chimpanzees nearly killed a new animal when it was introduced to their group, and by similar observations of the poultry yard (Schjelderup-Ebbe). Furthermore, if a member of a group drops out, the group very quickly closes again; the absent member will be missed much less by the group than the group by him, a fact which Köhler observed again in his chimpanzees.

Exclusion from a group may profoundly affect the Ego of the excluded member. We have mentioned before (p. 650) that in primitive societies it may lead to his death. But in our society also exclusion may have the gravest results. Schulte has developed a very ingenious theory of paranoia from this case of group dynamics: a particularly close group cohesion is demanded by the situation, and special circumstances, either within the personality of a certain member or more or less adventitious, prevent this member from yielding to this stress. The result may then be a total reorganization of the social field: "we," meaning "I within the group," changes into "I *and* they," "I *opposed* to the group," whereby the whole Ego-field relationship, and thereby the whole structure of the Ego, may be profoundly altered.

Stability. Connected with the closedness of the group is its stability or conservativeness. It seems that the degree of closure and of resistance to innovations vary directly with each other. Thus the rural group is more conservative than the city group. The more primitive a group is, the stronger its closure and the greater its conservativeness. In isolated primitive groups change is resisted most vehemently. Nevertheless, through contact with other peoples, new elements of culture may be introduced. Changes resulting from such innovations, as psychological events, have been studied by Bartlett with great success. His main conclusion is "that the imported elements change, both in the direction of existing culture and along the general line of development of the receptive group" (1932, p. 275).

Articulation. Closure, as a property belonging to the whole and, not to the parts, presupposes interaction between the parts. And we find generally that actions of parts of the group have reverberations all over the group, depending in kind or extent on the kind of action and the status of the agents. Perhaps the most interesting effect of this interaction is the articulation of the group. Hardly any group which has a more than temporary existence is entirely homogeneous. All articulation within an organized unit depends upon the relative properties of its parts, just as its segregation from the rest of the field depended upon a gradient.

Leader, Follower, Comrade. Thus in a group in which one member is much more intelligent or efficient than the rest, this member will have a unique position, often as the *leader*. On the other hand, a member deviating in the other extreme will be the "scapegoat"—again I may refer to Köhler's chimpanzees. This seems a trite statement, but I believe that the apparent triteness derives only from the fact of its intrinsic truth. That A, the most efficient member, is the leader does not mean only that all others try to do as he does because he does it best, but that they submit to his leadership with the result that what he does is best because he does it. The authority of the leader is much more than the acknowledgment of his superiority in special tasks. If A is the leader, the others are followers; the relation of each of the other members to A involves a special relation of these members to each other. The case, though much more complex, is of the same nature as that of repeated and isolated material investigated by von Restorff. And as there the isolated material acquired properties by being isolated, so the leader will acquire properties by the mere fact of being a leader. We shall give an amusing example of this when we discuss the articulation of some animal groups (p. 669). Here we only point out that such effects follow in a general way from our theory. To be the leader of a group means that the leader's psychological group is different from that of the followers in a fundamental respect, and therefore his Ego must be different too as a consequence of the first difference. If we say the leader looks down upon his followers, the followers look up to the leader and are on the same level with each other, we have expressed what Bartlett (1922) called the three fundamental tendencies that determine social relationship, viz., assertion, submission, and primitive comradeship (pp. 36 f.). It is clear that any individual might experience either of these according to the group of which he is a member and the position which he holds in it.

Mental Nearness. In an unusually fine article Dodge has recently introduced a new concept, "mental nearness," which must not be confused with Bartlett's primitive comradeship. "Nearness of minds is a fundamental frame of community between one person and others" (p. 235). Mental nearness is an aspect of what we have called "we-ness" and applies to the leader-follower relationships as well as to the follower-follower ones. It must be a direct function of the connectedness of the Ego and the other person. The leadership relationship may, of course, influence it by the particular kind of relation it is. But the leader may be as much the utterly beloved master as the admired but feared ruler.

Leadership and "Isolation." In our argument leadership was derived from inhomogeneity or isolation of one member of the group. In many respects our argument needs to be made more complete. In the first place we selected a particular kind of property, efficiency, for isolation, and no doubt it is a very important one. But it seems to me a true problem of social psychology to find out whether and how isolation as such (in the sense defined by von Restorff) is responsible for leadership, or whether the isolation must concern particular characteristics. May the wittiest person be the leader as well as the strongest one or the most beautiful? Very clearly the weakest, the most stupid and the slackest will not, i.e., isolation must be in the upward and not in the downward direction; but is the dimension in which the up and down exists of paramount importance, or is it not? Such questions lead at once to concrete problems; they can be answered only by the study of particular groups, and the answer may easily depend upon the kind of group studied.

Allied to this question is the other: Is leadership the only characteristic which can emerge from up-grade isolation? On purely theoretical grounds we have to infer that it is not; rather, when the degree of isolation becomes too great, the isolated member will lose its connection with the group, tend to become segregated; and this conclusion seems well in accord with the facts of everyday life and even with such little experimental work as has been done. Thus Leta Hollingworth concludes that "too much intelligence tends to disqualify a child (or an adult) for popular leadership," a fact which she ascribes to isolation.

But even when the outstanding person remains within the group, is it sufficient to characterize him as leader? May this term not be a class term comprising a number of different types? May it not even be that the outstanding person is *not* the leader in the ordinary sense of the word? Groups are far too complex structures, and my knowledge of the subject is far too limited, to make any attempt at answering these questions advisable.

Further, we have simplified the situation by assuming that *one* individual stands out from all the others who, compared with him, are all relatively similar to each other. In reality conditions will hardly ever be so simple. What then will happen when more than one inhomogeneity occurs in a group?

Leadership and Behaviour. A last point I want to make is this. Here is a sociological group with a leader A. Let us consider the psychological groups of A and some other member K. In the first, G_A, the Ego will be on top, whereas in the second a "he" will have this position. It is clear that each of these behavioural fields must determine, first, the behaviour of the person whose field it is, and then the behaviour of the others. Being at the top of one's behavioural group *implies* that certain actions be committed and others omitted, the former those that will *keep* the Ego on top, the latter those that will lower it. What kind of actions these will be in a particular case must, of course, depend upon the particular group and the particular kind of leadership. They will be different for the tyrant and for the beloved master. "Noblesse oblige" is the motto of a fine kind of leadership, and if a nobleman acts without heeding his obligations he acts not as a leader but in despite of his leadership, under the impulsion of different forces.

The same is true of the behaviour of K, one of the followers. If he submits to the leader, he does not display the action of an instinct or a propensity of submissiveness, but acts again in conformity with his behavioural field and in such a way that its structure be preserved or strengthened.

From this starting point one can enter thousands of avenues and investigate the dynamics of the rebel, the sceptic, the grumbler, the envious, the fanatic—both leader and follower—and so forth. And one may also try to find the origin of morality in the dynamics of group behaviour. Such an attempt should not, however, be confused with those modern tendencies which, by deriving morals from sociological factors, deprive them of any independent status and make them the result of blind and mechanical social forces. What in earlier chapters (pp. 570, 614) was said about the relation of psychology and logic applies, *mutatis mutandis,* to the relation of psychology to ethics.

Complex Groups—Articulation. Animal Groups. the pecking list. We return to the problem of group articulation itself. Our example of a homogeneous group with only one outstanding member is at best rarely realized. Consequently group articulation will be much more complex. In animal groups, this leads to an intricate system of dominances, which is the rule for birds, of which Schjelderup-Ebbe has observed more than fifty kinds; it seems typical of groups of mammals also (Katz, 1926). Birds living together determine individually their relation of dominance and submission, which, once established, tends to remain constant for a long period of time if not forever. The decision falls either in actual battle or in the course of a challenge in which one partner shows greater courage than the other. The symptoms of dominance are that the superior will peck at the inferior, most frequently during feeding time, while the inferior accepts the blows; concomitantly the superior "struts," the inferior "cringes." The factors which determine dominance are not altogether clear. One of the most powerful ones is naturally physical strength, but it is by no means the only one, as evidenced by the fact that the "pecking list" is very seldom a simple list, in which the first member of a group of n hens pecks at $n-1$, the second at $n-2$, and so forth, until the nth pecks at no one and is being pecked at by everyone. A typical irregularity is the triangle: A superior to B, B to C, and C to A.

I have briefly referred to these facts because they seem to be facts of social psychology and not facts of the psychology of birds. This will be demonstrated in various ways. First we apply our gestalt principles of group formation to birds. We deduced above that to be a leader involves a definite kind of Ego and behaviour, different from that of the followers. A continually corroborated observation of Schjelderup-Ebbe's verifies this deduction for bird societies. If one compares the behaviour of the bird at the top of the pecking list, the despot, with that of one very far down, the second or third from the last, then one finds the latter much more cruel to the few others over whom he lords it than the former in his treatment of all members. As soon as one removes from the group all members above the penultimate, his behaviour becomes milder and may even become very friendly, much to the surprise of the other bird (1924). It is not difficult to find analogies to this in human societies, and therefore one side of such behaviour must be primarily the effect of the social groupings, and not of individual characteristics.

THE ORIGIN OF THE PECKING LIST. THE UPWARDS TENDENCY OF THE EGO. Have we any sort of explanation for the existence of the "pecking list" itself? Otherwise expressed: Can we derive the fact that any two birds must establish their relative dominance when they meet, from general principles of group dynamics? Because of the close interconnection between group and Ego the following remarks are offered with some reserve and in full knowledge that they must in many ways be inadequate.

From the preceding discussion we know that behavioural groups are, as a rule, not homogeneous. The I and the various you's do not have the same rank. On the other hand, we have seen that there are many factors operative to give to the Ego a central position in his field, make him unique. The Ego, merely by being an Ego, possesses therefore properties of leadership, or at least a strong tendency towards leadership. Piaget's description of the egocentric behaviour of young children seems to tally well with such a view. Now, often enough, the social group is not such that it will brook the leadership of a particular person. For his behavioural field this means that his domineering behaviour will lead to very unexpected results; instead of preserving or strengthening the organization of his psychological group, his behaviour will weaken or even disrupt it. Therefore, unless he allows himself to be ejected from the group, he will have to change his behaviour in such a way that a well organized group results. This he can do only by being less despotic, and the resulting organization, not only of the sociological but also of his psychological group, will be one in which he is the leader no longer. If this description gives an approximate, though entirely schematic, picture of the true state of affairs, then we should infer that in all behavioural groups there is a force which propels the Ego upwards, a force of paramount importance for group dynamics.

Experimental Evidence. Can we accept the existence of such a force as an established fact? One might think of the data on which psychoanalytic and related theories are based, and indeed such facts could be utilized for proving our thesis. However, we forbear to include such material in our discussion and confine our argument to more strictly experimental work. The investigation most closely related to our problem is that by Hoppe on success and failure, briefly referred to in Chapter IX (p. 414). His subjects were presented with difficult tasks which, as a rule, they could not accomplish before a considerable amount of practice. Each trial was therefore, objectively speaking, either a success or a failure, and the former did not occur at the beginning of the practice series. But this description of the objective distribution of success and failure is *not* at the same time a description of the subjective experience of success and failure. For very soon the subject substitutes, at least temporarily, for the task given him, an easier one, a task in which success is liable to occur very soon. Otherwise expressed, the subject, instead of aspiring to accomplish what is demanded of him, lowers his standards; to use Hoppe's terminology: he establishes a *level of aspiration* which may fall far short of the accomplishment demanded by the experimenter. Thus, if the task is to hit the bull's eye of a target every time, the subject may at first substitute the task: hit the target, then hit ring 50, then 75, and only then 100, i.e., bull's eye. This level of aspiration, and not the real task, determines the experiences of success and failure, and these in their turn determine the level of aspiration, the former tending to raise, the latter to lower it. However, if the task is either too high above or too far below the aspiration level, neither failure nor success is experienced. We do not feel failures because we cannot prove a certain difficult mathematical proposition (unless we are mathematicians, so that the task belongs to our level of aspiration), nor do we experience success because we can carry out the task of fetching a book from a shelf. This fact in itself argues for a close relation between experienced success and failure on the one hand and the Ego of the agent on the other. Success "heightens," failure "lowers," our Ego, i.e., the opinion we have of ourselves. This effect explains the changes of the level of aspiration, if we assume that the Ego is always under a force which propels it "upwards" (see p. 670). For, in order that success can occur, the level of aspiration must be kept sufficiently low to make success sufficiently frequent. The question then arises why this level is ever raised as it is, by one or more successes. And this question can be answered only in terms of social factors. If the level of aspiration is low, it means that the Ego is low within his group. Thus the lowering of the level of aspiration leads to two conflicting effects: on the one hand, by facilitating success it satisfies the condition that the Ego be raised, while on the other it lowers the *Ego level* by being relatively low. The level of aspiration is therefore always very delicately balanced between two opposing forces, one which tends to lower, and one which tends to raise it. And both these forces originate in the relation between the Ego and the group. These conclusions were amply supported by the behaviour of the subjects, who would often explain their failures by objective reasons, blaming the quality of the instruments put at their disposal, and doubting the skill of the experimenter. The fact previously mentioned, viz., that tasks too far above or below the aspiration level do not lead to experiences of failure or success is explained by the same principle, since in the first case failure does not lower, in the second success does not raise, the Ego level. Thus Hoppe's results confirm our assumption of the upward tendency of the Ego, an hypothesis which is expressly introduced by this author (p. 35).

Another argument in favour of the same assumption can be derived from the interesting investigation by W. Wolff. In his main experiments, the results of which were corroborated by evidence obtained with different materials, a subject had to judge the character of a person from a voice which he heard in a gramophone. A number of persons had been made to speak the sentence, "Good day, I am curious whether these experiments will yield any results" [3] into a recording machine, and when later on a person had to judge character from a number of these voices, his own was as a rule among them. Now out of fourteen such cases twelve did not recognize their own voice—a result which probably finds its explanation in facts external to the main problem. These twelve subjects, then, and a few others (sixteen in all,[4] p. 279) judged their own voice in the same way as they judged the others, and yet, if one compares their judgments of themselves with the average of the judgments which others gave about them, one finds a number of significant differences. In the first place the judgments about their own voices were as a rule considerably more detailed than those about other people's voices, despite the fact that the subjects did not recognize their own voices; they also betray a deeper insight into the character of the speaker. In the second place the self-appraisals (unwitting ones to be sure) are always more affective than the average of the appraisals by others, and in the majority of cases more positive. Of the sixteen cases investigated only one does not conform to this rule, and in this case the appraisal by other observers had an enormous scatter, some judges having a high, others a low, opinion of his character. Of the remaining fifteen cases, twelve are more positive than the average, five indeed are the best of all judgments, and five more fall within the first third. The explanation of this result is that "the judge reacts to his own unrecognized voice exactly as in ordinary life he reacts to his Self: without recognizing his own voice he judges it as though he had done so" (p. 290). This hypothesis was proved by special experiments which I omit. It means, however, that the Ego is striving to be as high up on the ladder as possible. This is not only proved by the cases, embracing the more normal or better adjusted persons, who judge themselves better than they are judged by others, but also by the small group whose self-appraisal deviates in the opposite direction: for their behaviour is a result of a tension between their very high ideal and their conscious-

[3] In reality, of course, this sentence was in German.

[4] I cannot find out how the author arrived at the two different figures, twelve and sixteen. The following discussion, however, is based on the greater number.

ness of insufficiency with regard to that ideal. Just because they strive for so high a goal they are dissatisfied with their present achievements.

A third line of support comes from an as yet unpublished investigation by Dr. Dembo which, in continuation of the work previously discussed, she carried out in my laboratory. Again she provided conditions for the arousal of anger; the subjects had to perform very easy but perfectly nonsensical tasks, like scattering a box of paper clips over the floor and then collecting all the clips again in the box, possibly repeating this action, and similar ones, several times. The principal purpose of this investigation was, however, a study of the social forces in the arousal of anger, a problem on which her first work had already thrown some light, inasmuch as the relation between the subject and the experimenter appeared to be one of the determining factors. Consequently, in this new study this relation was varied. In one group of experiments the subject was alone in the room, finding her tasks on slips of paper which she took one by one from a pile; the experimenter, needless to say, observed her from the next room through a carefully concealed chink in the wall. In other groups of experiments the experimenter was in the same room with the subject, varying her behaviour from pure passive observation to actual quarrelling. For our purposes it is sufficient to compare Group I with a group in which the experimenter interfered with the work of the subjects. In both situations anger occurred; but when the subject is alone her anger is freely expressed, it leaves no after-effect once the experiment is over, and it is not directed against the experimenter. In all three points the anger of the person disturbed by the experimenter is different. Expressions of anger are absent, not because there is no anger, but because of an extraordinarily strong self-control demanded and brought about by the social situation. As a matter of fact the anger was much stronger in these experiments than in the former ones, as evidenced by the duration of the after-effects. As a rule the subjects are unable to record their introspections at the end of the experiment, a task which offered no difficulty to the subjects of the first group. It sometimes took weeks or even months before the subjects could speak about these experiments and relate their experiences, which often consisted of desires for revenge to be wreaked on the experimenter. For in this group the anger is primarily directed against this personal cause of all the trouble.

I think it is fair to interpret the enormous influence exerted on the strength, direction, after-effect, and expression of the affect as due to the Ego-alter dynamics, the pressure under which the Ego of the subject is put just by its *sub*ordination under the will and whim of the experimenter. This stress points clearly to the existence of a force which raises the Ego and is therefore diametrically opposed to the stress of this particular social situation. Dr. Dembo's experiments contain far more material relevant for a social dynamics, but I refrain from giving any more detail since the author has not yet found the time to write up her results in a systematic form.

THE RESULTS OF GROUP FORMATION

Products of Civilization. We can now turn to our third and last question: What are the results of group formation, and how do such results influence future behaviour? Truly, we have already discussed some of the more or less temporary results, but now we turn to more permanent ones, those results which *par excellence* may be called products of group- or social activity. I am, of course, thinking of our customs and modes, our fashions and conventions, which are palpable only in the actual behaviour types in which they reveal themselves, and of those more "solid" products like buildings, books, works of arts, and the objects of our daily use. In short, the aggregate of the products of social activity is what we call civilization. Such products, originating in social activity, determine future social activity, just as a trace originating in a psychophysical process determines future psychophysical processes. It would be a tempting task to apply the questions which we have raised about traces to the products of social activity, but the treatment of these questions, apart from being entirely beyond the capacity of the author, would require a separate book.

Civilization as a Framework. Instead we confine ourselves to a few remarks. Products of civilization are not fortuitously connected with the social group which produced them, but are always to some extent *intrinsically* connected with the dynamic characteristics of these groups, however much purely adventitious factors (like the availability of certain materials and not of others) may determine certain aspects of these products. Secondly, these products, being social in their origin, will be misunderstood and misinterpreted if considered as individual actions. Products remain and influence behaviour even when such behaviour types as produced these products no longer occur. "We may legitimately speak of customs, traditions, institutions, technical secrets, formulated and unformulated ideals and numerous other facts which are literally properties of groups, as the direct determinants of social action . . . in actual fact they constantly constrain human action as directly as anything ever can do" (Bartlett, p. 254).

We can very well say that such products of civilization form a framework—the term is also used by Bartlett—in which practically all behaviour takes place, just as all spatial localization takes place in and depends upon a spatial framework. Thus actions and attitudes which appear on the surface to be entirely individual are found on closer inspection to be determined by social frames.

Examples. This point has been very convincingly proved for food aversions by Julian Hirsch. If one asks a person why he will not touch addled eggs, one will get the answer: "Because they are disgusting," and yet putrid eggs are a delicacy for the natives of Bruni; if, to explain this difference of taste, one wants to fall back on individual differences between those natives and ourselves, one has only to envisage another example: the orthodox Jew who has a violent aversion to pork is apt to explain it by the dirty habits of live pigs, whereas the Gentiles and the freethinking Jews have no dislike of pork, although they know as much about the conditions of pigsties. On such facts Hirsch bases his conclusion: "The avoidance of certain foods is not caused by aversion to the foods, but the aversion is caused by the avoidance." He then proves for a great number of cases the social origin of the avoidance. Today this origin has been forgotten, yet avoidance and averison persist as effects of the social framework.

A very general and lucid discussion of the effects of social frameworks is given by Sapir, who draws on many different fields of social activity. Since I have so far neglected language, perhaps the greatest and most powerful product of civilization, I will choose some of Sapir's linguistic examples. "So powerfully, indeed, are we in the grip of our phonetic habits that it becomes one of the most delicate and difficult tasks of the linguistic student to discover what is the true configuration of sounds in languages alien to his own. This means that the average person unconsciously interprets the phonetic material of other languages in terms imposed upon him by the habits of his own language. Thus, the naïve Frenchman confounds the two sounds 's' of 'sick' and 'th' of 'thick' in a single pattern point—not because he is really unable to hear the difference, but because the setting up of such a difference disturbs his feeling for the necessary configuration of linguistic sounds" (p. 136). In a somewhat different terminology we should say: the Frenchman, because of his linguistic framework, *hears* the "s" and the "th" as two variants of one and the same sound, whereas within the framework of English they are as different sounds as "s" and "t." Just so, for the Englishman, the *i* sound in cockney "lydy" is heard as a variant of the *a* sound in lady, whereas for the foreigner who has learned English and arrives in London for the first time, these are two different sounds, with the result that he does not even understand the word "lydy." And a last example from Sapir: "From a purely objective standpoint the difference between the k of 'kill' and the k of 'skill' is as easily definable as the, to us, major difference between the k of 'kill' and the g of 'gill' (of a fish). In some languages the g sound of 'gill' would be looked upon, or rather would be intuitively interpreted, as a comparatively unimportant or individual divergence from a sound typically represented by the k of 'skill,' while the k of 'kill,' with its greater strength of articulation and its audible breath release, would constitute an utterly distinct phonetic entity" (p. 134).

Our total social framework is composed of a great number of special parts, which find their expression in language, customs, traditions, laws, modes of thought, styles of artistic creation, fashions, and so forth. Even such a casual enumeration will make it clear that some of these parts are more stable than others, although none are quite immutable. At the same time, they are all interdependent, although the degree of interdependence between any two may vary considerably and not even be constant during the history of development. Here are problems which connect the work of the psychologist with that of the linguist, the sociologist, the historian.

Personality. While we shall not pursue these problems we shall take up a last consequence of our theory of psychological and sociological groups. We have already seen how the Ego, as part of a We, must depend for its nature upon the kind of We to which it belongs and upon the place which it occupies within it. But at that point of our discussion we had not yet included the products of civilization, the social framework. And yet, the social framework is of paramount importance for the development of the Ego. When we speak of personality we think as a rule of the Ego within its culture, i.e., determined by its social framework. Development of personality by education has for centuries consisted chiefly in making the young acquainted with the masterpieces of the past. School and college curricula were predominantly, if not entirely, based on the classics and on mathematics, thus introducing the students into an old framework of culture. I do not pretend to speak with any authority when I confess that to me these old ideas of education do not appear so bad or antiquated as they are sometimes made out today, even though I would not deny that the mere rigid continuation of a particular system is apt to lead to petrification.

Be that as it may, the educated or cultured person lives in a framework that owes its existence to continued social creativeness and not simply to the inert transmission of such social products as those characteristics of behaviour which are common to the educated and the non-educated, of which the food aversions were given as an example in our previous discussion.

The problem of personality is one of the intrinsically greatest problems of all psychology. Nowhere is it easier to miss the point, and to run either into the Scylla of blind statistical investigation of traits, or the Charybdis of ultimately unscientific abstract discussion. It is easy to comprehend why men of culture and knowledge who were interested in the study of personality turned away with contempt from work done on this problem by experimental psychology and claimed that no "explanatory" psychology could ever master this problem, and that only a psychology different in essence, an "understanding" psychology, would be equipped to deal with it. We discussed this dilemma in the first chapter and refused to accept it. Our reason lies in our general principle: if psychology reveals organization, i.e., intrinsic connections of properties, and if this holds for personality as well as for the other fields we have studied, then indeed psychology should reveal personality in all its richness and significance by its general methods.

Is Personality a Gestalt? The question, therefore, can be formulated: Is personality a gestalt, and if so, what kind of gestalt is it? These are concrete questions which can be investigated by scientific methods. What would it mean if personality were not a gestalt? That its different behaviour units or traits were independent of each other and could be united in any combination. If, on the other hand, personality is a gestalt, then there would be interdependence between its various manifestations, and a great number of combinations of traits would be excluded.

If we remain in the realm of experimentally established facts, we have to confine our purview to a relatively small number of relationships, to those, namely, between character- or personality-traits and physiognomic characters. The last year has seen the publication of a highly important book on expressive movements by Allport and Vernon, at the end of which the authors formulate the following conclusion, based on a vast material of experimental results: "The evidence indicates clearly that the expressive movements of personality are not specific and unrelated; on the contrary they form coherent, if perplexing patterns. . . . From our results it appears that a man's gestures and handwriting both reflect an essentially stable and constant individual style. His expressive activities seem not to be dissociated and unrelated to one another, but rather to be organized and well-patterned. Furthermore, the evidence indicates that there is congruence between expressive movement and the attitudes, traits, values, and other dispositions of the 'inner' personality" (pp. 247-8). And this conclusion is not reached lightly, but after a thorough discussion of other findings and theories as well as of their own results.

I shall mention only one other piece of experimental work, since Allport and Vernon's book gives an excellent survey of the literature; this is an investigation from the University of Berlin by Arnheim. He asked his subjects to match different aspects or expressions of persons—for example, handwritings, with known personalities (Leonardo, Michelangelo, Raphael), or portraits with handwritings; again portraits of men with quotations from their writings or descriptions of certain modes of behaviour (like drinking habits). The number of correct matches was always greater than chance would have decreed and often considerably greater, and many errors were "good" errors, inasmuch as the matching was not at fault but the understanding of one of the terms—thus in the experiments with the great painters very few confusions between Michelangelo and Raphael occurred. There were in all 779 matches, and of these only 36 were co-ordinations of Michelangelo's writing to Raphael or Raphael's to Michelangelo, whereas the correct co-ordinations for Michelangelo, Raphael, and Leonardo were 221, 192, and 175.

Results like these, just like the good agreement in the judgments of Wolff's subjects (in the experiments described above), can be looked at from two different points of view. On the one hand they prove that physiognomic judgments are possible, fairly uniform, and much oftener correct than can be expected from mere chance. On the other hand they confirm Allport and Vernon's conclusion; for these judgments could not be correct as often as they are if *any* combination of traits were equally possible. If the handwriting of Michelangelo did not possess some characteristics which were *indicative* of the person as he was known to the judges, how could they have acquitted themselves so well! Thus physiognomic experiments lend a weighty support to the view that personality is a gestalt.

WHAT KIND OF GESTALT IS PERSONALITY? The other question, what kind of a gestalt it is, is much more difficult to answer, if one wants to stay within the frame of the theory developed in these pages. Such an answer would have to consider all the different sub-systems of the Ego, the richness and complexity of which we have discussed in the eighth chapter; the way in which these sub-systems are organized, their relative degrees of dominance, their mutual communication, and their relative "depth." By this we mean their surface-centre localization, or their connection with the Self, the very core of the Ego. Furthermore the "openness" or "closedness" of the whole Ego would have to be investigated, i.e., its relation to the surrounding field, and particularly to the social field. The dynamic intercourse between Ego and environment must depend to a large extent upon the nature of the Ego itself. And in this investigation the products of civilization must be included. Which of them have most profoundly influenced the Ego, which of its sub-systems have been chiefly affected, and how strong has this influence been?

Present-day psychology has rediscovered the importance of the problem of personality without which no psychology is complete, and many writers have made valuable contributions to it; among them William Stern and McDougall must be specially mentioned. I shall, however, forbear to report their views, since I could contribute nothing over and above the questions which I have just formulated. Gestalt theory has been rather consistent in its development. It has studied the fundamental laws of psychology first under the most simple conditions, in rather elementary problems of perception; it has then included more and more complex sets of conditions, turning to memory, thinking, and acting. It has started to approach those conditions under which personality itself enters the investigation. But since this is but the barest beginning it seems wiser to bide our time. And thus this section is unduly brief not because I underrate the importance of the problem of personality, but because I have too high a regard for it to treat it less consistently than any other part.

CHAPTER XV

CONCLUSION

A Retrospect. The Theoretical Setting. The Meaning of "Gestalt." The Integration Achieved. Positivism and Gestalt Theory

When one comes to the end of a long journey one likes to compare what one has done with the plan one drew up before starting. And so it seems appropriate, after we have traversed the land of psychology, to glance back on our programme and see how much of it we have carried out, and to recapitulate the main stages of our journey. We developed two programmes, one, in the first chapter, very general in scope, the other, at the end of the second chapter, more concrete and limited. We have followed the directions of the second programme. How much of the first have we carried out in so doing?

A RETROSPECT

Let us briefly recall our steps. The province of the world which we mapped out for our investigation was the province of behaviour in all its forms and aspects. Behaviour, we found, is always behaviour in an environment. This proposition led to the fundamental distinction between the geographical and the behavioural environments and thus to the problem of the relation between them. This problem was made tractable in a non-dualistic theory by the introduction of the psychophysical field with its field properties. The relation between the geographical environment and the psychophysical field, and thereby the behavioural environment, was complicated by the fundamental distinction of distant and proximal stimuli. Although only the latter are in direct causal connection with the psychophysical field and thereby with behaviour, behaviour is, as a rule, adapted not only to the behavioural, but also to the geographical environment, the world of the distant stimuli. A theory of the relation between the psychophysical field and the proximal stimuli had therefore to be checked by the test of whether it represented the relation between behavioural and geographical environment correctly.

The first question that was asked was the fundamental question of perception: Why do things look as they do? The discussion of this question led to a rejection of a number of psychological theories, deeply ingrained in our modes of thinking, even if not made explicit, and introduced us to the concept of organization. Perceptual organization was then studied, revealing an amazingly intricate interplay of forces and at the same time a lawfulness that knows no exception. We tried to understand why we perceive space and things within it, why these, behavioural, things have the properties they have, like unity, shape, size, colour, why they can move or appear at rest.

We then proceeded to show how the perceptual field can instigate movements of our limbs, how it can influence behaviour. This new problem required no new general principle to be added to the principles of organization previously developed, but a mere expansion and application of these principles to the new problems.

But the discussion of this problem led us of necessity a long step further. Whereas we had started from the proposition that behaviour requires an environment in which it takes place we were now forced to accept the other proposition that behaviour requires an Ego which behaves. Thus the Ego had to be introduced, and the introduction of the Ego again required no new principle, no factor extraneous to the system so far developed. Rather did the principles of organization supply a method by which the Ego, which had defied most psychological systems, could be consistently treated. To the organization of the Ego we then turned our attention, trying to probe into its enormous complexity and the influence it exerts on the field. Attempting to confine ourselves to experimentally established facts, we could not even hope to do justice to this problem in all its richness and significance, having to be satisfied with laying the foundation of a more complete future understanding.

Only then did we include the continuity of behaviour in our discussion, the continuity whose basis we call memory. And again the power of our originally introduced principles became manifest. Memory did not appear as a new entity or function, but as the result and the determiner of organized processes. We built a trace hypothesis, in which traces are endowed with dynamic properties from which their function is deducible. Several functions of memory were discussed in detail supplied by experimental work. Learning, that category of psychology which has continually gained in importance, was theoretically analyzed, a task that involved a criticism of the famous doctrine of associationism. The necessity of including the Ego in the theory of memory functions was demonstrated, particularly in our discussion of recognition, and finally an attempt was made to sketch the dynamics of that process we call thinking, an attempt that again could be based upon the laws of organization.

In a last chapter we applied our principles to the problems that arise from the social intercourse of animals and men, our chief purpose being to formulate the problems of social psychology in such a way that they link up with all other psychological problems. Again the concepts of the psychophysical field, consisting of Ego and environment, and the laws of field organization and field reorganization through action proved to be capable of dealing with this new problem. As a matter of fact only in this context could the theory of the Ego be further developed, since only as a member of a group does an individual develop his personality.

THE THEORETICAL SETTING

Thus we can say that we have studied psychology in a theoretically consistent manner. We have not divided behaviour or mind into so-and-so-many different functions or elements, each to be studied in isolation. Instead we have followed the principles of organization as they become manifest under diverse conditions, starting from the simplest and proceeding to those of higher and higher complexity. At the same time the results of organization became increasingly more complex, richer and more significant. All our facts have been presented in a theoretical setting, and our selection of facts was largely determined by their value for the theory. Many facts of equal interest had to be omitted, many even that might have been used in the development of the theory as well as those we reported. This was necessary in order to keep some sort of balance between the various chapters and to confine the book within manageable limits.

THE MEANING OF "GESTALT"

But what of the concept of gestalt from which this book derives its name? We have not used the word in this summary directly, but it is implied in our term "organization." The word gestalt "has the meaning of a concrete individual and characteristic entity, existing as something detached and having a shape or form as one of its attributes" (Köhler, 1929, p. 192). A gestalt is therefore a product of organization, organization the process that leads to a gestalt. But as a definition this determination would not be enough unless one implied the nature of organization, as it was expressed in the law of prägnanz, unless one remembered that organization as a category is diametrically opposed to mere juxtaposition or random distribution. In the process of organization, "what happens to a part of the whole, is determined by intrinsic laws inherent in this whole" (Wertheimer, 1925, p. 7). On the basis of this definition we can call the process of organization no less "*gestaltet*" than the products of organization, and in this wider connotation the term has been used in the title of this book and all along by gestalt psychologists. It carried in its connotation the *chaos–kosmos* alternative; to say that a process, or the product of a process, is a gestalt means that it cannot be explained by mere chaos, the mere blind combination of essentially unconnected causes; but that its essence is the reason of its existence, to use metaphysical language for an idea which has been presented so many times in this book in notions as free from metaphysics as any science can be.

THE INTEGRATION ACHIEVED

Has this book carried out the broader programme announced in the first chapter? If the reader turns back to the last words of Chapter I which contain what I conceive to be the ideal of psychology, he will see how little the book has done to realize this ideal. But he may discern that it has made an effort to approach it. For it has attempted to give explanations of the most complex events, those which create civilization, in terms which are also applicable to the simplest events, the motions of electrons and protons in a simple atom, without in the least destroying the difference between the two kinds of events. Again I am tempted to quote Browning:

Say not "a small event!" Why "small"?
Costs it more pain that this, ye call
A "great event," should come to pass,
Than that? Untwine me from the mass
Of deeds which make up life, one deed
Power shall fall short in or exceed!

There are great events as well as small in which power may fall short or exceed, for a calm view of the universe cannot share the optimism of Pippa. But there are perfect small events, like the wonderful stability and symmetry of a crystal, and perfect great events, like the heroic simplicity of Captain Scott. If we understood scientifically the second event as well as we do the first, it would thereby lose not a particle of its grandeur or beauty. It would be a great and beautiful action, even if nobody knew about it, just as the crystal would have its perfect symmetry if there were no eyes to see, no minds to understand it. I shall not pursue this line of argument any further, since it would take me much further into metaphysics than I am prepared to go. But this much had to be said, lest my attempt at integration might be misunderstood to mean the very opposite of what it intends: an equalization of all events, one appearing as blind and meaningless as the others.

To become more concrete: Has our psychology contributed to the integration of nature, life, and mind? That it has attempted to do so must, I believe, be affirmed. The judgment whether it has been successful must depend upon the ultimate truth or adequacy of the gestalt concept. For this concept cuts across this division of realms of existence, being applicable in each of them. Köhler's demonstration of physical gestalten laid the foundation for a new unification of nature and life; there is no reason to postulate new factors of order specific of life, if order pervades inorganic nature. Wertheimer's and Köhler's principle of isomorphism integrated mind with nature and life. This principle has proved eminently fruitful for experimental research, because it gives definite directions to physiological hypotheses, which in their turn lead to new psychological experiments. This, I believe, has been amply demonstrated in the course of the book. But at the same time this principle has implications of great philosophical significance. It leads us back to an argument which we have just dropped. If a thought process that leads to a new logically valid insight has its isomorphic counterpart in physiological events, does it thereby lose its logical stringency and become just a mechanical process of nature, or does not the physiological process, by being isomorphic to the thought, have to be regarded as sharing the thought's intrinsic necessity? Our attempt at integration has claimed the latter, thereby incorporating the category of significance within our system. That at this point the development of the theory will have to overcome great difficulties is perfectly obvious to me. At the same time it should be recognized that a beginning has been made to face these difficulties and to conquer them.

POSITIVISM AND GESTALT THEORY

If there is any polemical spirit in this book, it is directed not against persons but against a strong cultural force in our present civilization for which I have chosen the name positivism. If positivism can be regarded as an integrative philosophy, its integration rests on the dogma that all events are equally unintelligible, irrational, meaningless, purely factual. Such an integration is, however, to my way of thinking, identical with a complete disintegration.

Being convinced that such a view is utterly inadequate in face of the facts, I had to attack it, and that the more since its hold over our generation is strong. It makes a difference to one's life whether one is a thorough positivist or not. I believe that a truly integrative philosophy will lead to a better life than a purely destructive one. But the scientist dare not be swayed by such considerations. His only standard is truth.

I am as convinced as any reader that each one of the many special hypotheses advanced in this book is in need of further verification; I am doubtful about the future fate of many of them. But this attitude towards particular hypotheses must not be confused with the general principle, which is independent of special applications. Gestalt theory would not be refuted if its hypotheses of perceived motion were proved to be false. The truth of the gestalt principle will have to be tested by the course that science takes in the future. But I should not have written this book based upon a non-positivistic theory, were it not my deep scientific conviction that truth demands such a philosophy.

BIBLIOGRAPHY

A. Aall, 1913, Ein neues Gedächtnisgesetz? Zts. f. Psych. *66*, pp. 1-50
N. Ach, 1910, Über den Willensakt und das Temperament. Göttingen
—— 1930, Über die Gefügigkeitsqualität. Ber. üb. d. XII Kongr. f. exp. Psychol. 1929, Jena, pp. 45-52
A. Ackermann, 1924, Farbenschwelle und Feldstruktur. Psych. Forsch. *5*, pp. 44-84
G. J. von Allesch, 1931, Zur nichteuklidischen Struktur des phänomenalen Raumes (Versuche an Lemur mongoz mongoz L.). Jena
Gordon Allport, 1930, Change and Decay in the Visual Memory Image. Brit. J. of Psych. *21*, pp. 138-148
G. W. Allport and P. E. Vernon, 1933, Studies in Expressive Movement. New York
R. P. Angier, 1927, The Conflict Theory of Emotion. Amer. J. of Psych. *39*, pp. 390-401
R. Arnheim, 1928, Experimentell-psychologische Untersuchungen zum Ausdrucksproblem. Psych. Forsch. *11*, pp. 2-119
P. Bahnsen, 1928, Eine Untersuchung über Symmetrie und Asymmetrie bei visuellen Wahrnehmungen. Zts. f. Psych. *108*, pp. 129-154
H. Banister, 1929, Hearing I. In "The Foundations of Experimental Psychology," ed. by C. Murchison. Worcester, Mass., pp. 273-312
F. C. Bartlett, 1923, Psychology and Primitive Culture. Cambridge
—— 1932, Remembering. A Study in Experimental and Social Psychology. Cambridge
S. H. Bartley, 1933, Gross Differential Activity of the Dog's Cortex as Revealed by Action Currents. Univ. of Kansas Stud. in Psych. *1*, Psych. Mon. *44*, No. 1, pp. 30-56
E. Becher, 1911, Gehirn und Seele. Heidelberg
Howard Becker, 1932, Säkularisationsprozesse. Kölner Vierteljschrft. f. Soziol. *10*, pp. 283-294
W. Benary, 1924, Beobachtungen zu einem Experiment über Helligkeitskontrast. Psych. Forsch. *5*, pp. 131-142
I. M. Bentley, 1899, The Memory Image and Its Qualitative Fidelity. Am. J. of Psych. *11*
I. M. Bentley, *see also* W. H. Mikesell
V. Benussi, 1913, Psychologie der Zeitauffassung. Heidelberg
—— 1916, Versuche zur Analyse taktil erweckter Scheinbewegungen. Arch. f. d. ges. Psych. *36*, pp. 59-135
C. Berger, 1932, Zum Problem der Sehschärfe. Berlin dissertation
G. Berkeley, 1709, An Essay towards a New Theory of Vision. In "The

Works of George Berkeley, D.D., former Bishop of Cloyne," Vol. I, Oxford, 1901

F. Beyrl, 1926, Über die Grössenauffassung bei Kindern. Zts. f. Psych. *100*, pp. 344-371

G. Birenbaum, 1930, Das Vergessen einer Vornahme. Isolierte seelische Systeme und dynamische Gesamtbereiche. Psych. Forsch. *13*, pp. 218-284

H. Bogen, *see* O. Lipmann

J. Borak, 1922, Über die Empfindlichkeit für Gewichtsunterschiede bei abnehmender Reizstärke. Psych. Forsch. *1*, pp. 374-389

E. G. Boring, 1930, A New Ambiguous Figure. Am. J. of Psych. *42*, pp. 444-445

—— 1933, The Physical Dimensions of Consciousness. New York, London

C. D. Broad, 1925, The Mind and Its Place in Nature. London, New York

J. F. Brown, 1928, Über gesehene Geschwindigkeiten. Psych. Forsch. *10*, pp. 84-101

—— 1931, The Visual Perception of Velocity. Psych. Forsch. *14*, pp. 199-232

—— 1931 a, On Time Perception in Visual Movement Fields. Ibid., pp. 233-248

—— 1931 b, The Thresholds for Visual Movement. Ibid., pp. 249-268

E. Brunswik, 1929, Zur Entwicklung der Albedowahrnehmung. Zts. f. Psych. *109*, pp. 40-115

—— 1933, Untersuchungen über Wahrnehmungsgegenstände, see Brunswik 1933 a, Eissler, Holaday, and Klimpfinger

—— 1933 a, Die Zugänglichkeit von Gegenständen für die Wahrnehmung. Arch. f. d. ges. Psych. *88*, pp. 377-418

K. Bühler, 1908, Über Gedankenerinnerungen. Arch. f. d. ges. Psych. *12*, pp. 24 ff.

—— 1913, Die Gestaltwahrnehmungen. Stuttgart

—— 1922, Handbuch der Psychologie. I. Teil. Die Struktur der Wahrnehmungen. 1. Heft. Die Erscheinungsweisen der Farben. Jena

—— 1924, Die geistige Entwicklung der Kindes, 4. Aufl. Jena. (1st ed. 1918)

W. Burzlaff, 1931, Methodologische Beiträge zum Problem der Farbenkonstanz. Zts. f. Psych. *119*, pp. 177-235

M. W. Calkins, 1910, A First Book in Psychology. New York

H. Cantril and W. A. Hunt, 1932, Emotional Effects Produced by the Injection of Adrenalin. Am. J. of Psych. *44*, pp. 300-307

H. A. Carr, 1925, Psychology, A Study of Mental Activity. New York

P. Cermak und K. Koffka, 1922, Untersuchungen über Bewegungs- und Verschmelzungsphänomene. Psych. Forsch. *1*, pp. 66-129

E. Claparède, 1911, Récognition et Moïïté. Arch. de Psych. *11*

—— 1925, Does the Will Express the Entire Personality? In "Problems of Personality, Studies in Honour of Dr. Morton Prince." London, pp. 39-43

E. CLAPARÈDE, 1934, La Genèse de l'Hypothèse. Arch. de Psych. *24*, pp. 1-154

A. DAHL, 1928, Über den Einfluss des Schlafens auf das Wiedererkennen. Psych. Forsch. *11*, pp. 290-301

K. M. DALLENBACH, 1926, A Note on the Immediacy of Understanding a Relation. Psych. Forsch. *7*, pp. 268-269

K. M. DALLENBACH, *see also* J. P. Guilford, J. G. Jenkins, and G. Kreezer

C. W. DARROW, *see* E. S. Robinson

T. DEMBO, 1931, Der Ärger als dynamisches Problem. Psych. Forsch. *15*, pp. 1-144

H. R. DESILVA, 1928, Kinematographic Movement of Parallel Lines. J. Gener. Psych. *1*, pp. 550-577

R. DODGE, 1933, Mental Nearness. J. of Abn. and Soc. Psych. *28*, pp. 233-244

H. DRIESCH, 1925, The Crisis in Psychology. Princeton, N. J.

K. DUNCKER, 1926, A Qualitative (Experimental and Theoretical) Study of Productive Thinking (Solving of Comprehensible Problems). Ped. Sem. *33*, pp. 642-708

—— 1929, Über induzierte Bewegung. Psych. Forsch. *12*, pp. 180-259

K. DUNLAP, 1928, A Revision of the Fundamental Laws of Habit Formation. Science *67*, pp. 360-362

M. EBERHARDT, 1922, Über die phänomenale Höhe und Stärke von Teiltönen. Psych. Forsch. *2*, pp. 346-367

—— 1924, Untersuchungen über Farbschwellen und Farbenkontrast. Psych. Forsch. *5*, pp. 85-130

A. S. EDDINGTON, 1928, The Nature of the Physical World. Cambridge, New York

K. EISSLER, 1933, Die Gestaltkonstanz der Sehdinge bei Variation der Objekte und ihrer Einwirkungsweise auf den Wahrnehmenden. Arch. f. d. ges. Psych. *88*, pp. 487-550

N. FEINBERG, 1926, Experimentelle Untersuchungen über die Wahrnehmung im Gebiet des blinden Flecks. Psych. Forsch. *7*, pp. 16-43

J. C. FLÜGEL, 1930, The Psychology of Clothes. London

H. M. FOGELSONGER, *see* G. F. Shepard

H. FRANK, 1923, Über die Beeinflussung von Nachbildern durch die Gestalteigenschaften der Projektionsfläche. Psych. Forsch. *4*, pp. 33-37

—— 1926, Untersuchungen über Sehgrössenkonstanz bei Kindern. Psych. Forsch. *7*, pp. 137-145

—— 1928, Die Sehgrössenkonstanz bei Kindern. Psych. Forsch. *10*, pp. 102-106

—— 1930, Über den Einfluss inadäquater Konvergenz und Akkommodation auf die Sehgrösse, Psych. Forsch. *13*, pp. 135-144

E. FREEMAN, 1931, Untersuchungen über das indirekte Sehen (Speziell

zur Analyse des Aubert-Foersterschen Phänomens) Psych. Forsch. *14*, pp. 332-365
M. von Frey, 1923, Über Wandlung der Empfindung bei formal verschiedener Reizung einer Art von Sinnesnerven. Psych. Forsch. *3*, pp. 209-218
G. Frings, 1914, Über den Einfluss der Komplexbildung auf die effektuelle und generative Hemmung. Arch. f. d. ges. Psych. *30*, pp. 415-479
W. Fuchs, 1920, Untersuchungen über das Sehen der Hemianopiker und Hemiamblyopiker. I: Verlagerungserscheinungen. Zts. f. Psych. *84*, pp. 67-169
—— 1921, Untersuchungen über das Sehen der Hemianopiker und Hemiamblyopiker. II: Die totalisierende Gestaltauffassung. Zts. f. Psych. *86*, pp. 1-143
—— 1922, Eine Pseudofovea bei Hemianopikern. Psych. Forsch. *1*, pp. 157-186
—— 1923, Experimentelle Untersuchungen über das simultane Hintereinander auf derselben Sehrichtung. Zts. f. Psych. *91*, pp. 145-235
—— 1923a, Experimentelle Untersuchungen über die Änderung von Farben unter dem Einfluss von Gestalten. Zts. f. Psych. *92*, pp. 249-325
A. Galli, 1932, Über mittels verschiedener Sinnesreize erweckte Wahrnehmung von Scheinbewegung. Arch. f. d. ges. Psych. *85*, pp. 137-180
A. Gelb, 1914, Versuche auf dem Gebiet der Zeit- und Raumanschauung. Ber. üb. d. VI. Kongr. f. exp. Psych. in Göttingen. Leipzig, pp. 36-42
—— 1920, Über den Wegfall der Wahrnehmung von "Oberflächenfarben." Zts. f. Psych. *84*, pp. 193-257
—— 1921, Grundfragen der Wahrnehmungspsychologie. Ber. üb. d. VII. Kongr. f. exp. Psych. Jena, 1922, pp. 114-116
—— 1930, Die Farbenkonstanz der Sehdinge. In "Handbuch d. norm. und pathol. Physiologie," her. von Bethe u.a. *12*, 1, pp. 594-678
—— 1932, Die Erscheinungen des Simultankontrasts und der Eindruck der Feldbeleuchtung. Zts. f. Psych. *127*, pp. 42-59
A. Gelb und K. Goldstein, 1920, Zur Psychologie des optischen Wahrnehmungs- und Erkennungsvorgangs. In "Psychologische Analysen hirnpathologischer Fälle," her. von Gelb und Goldstein, I, Leipzig, pp. 1-142. Also in Zts. f. d. ges. Neurol. und Psychiatrie *41*
A. Gelb und R. Granit, 1923, Die Bedeutung von "Figur" und "Grund" für die Farbenschwelle. Zts. f. Psych. *93*, pp. 83-118
J. J. Gibson, 1929, The Reproduction of Visually Perceived Forms. J. Exper. Psych., *12*, pp. 1-39
K. Goldstein, 1925, Das Symptom, seine Entstehung und Bedeutung für unsere Auffassung vom Bau und von der Funktion des Nervensystems. Arch. f. Psychiatr. und Nervenkrankht. *76*, pp. 84-108

K. Goldstein, 1927, Die Lokalisation in der Grosshirnrinde. In "Handb. d. normalen und patholog. Physiologie," her. von Bethe u.a. *10*, pp. 600-842

K. Goldstein, *see also* A. Gelb

K. Gottschaldt, 1926, Über den Einfluss der Erfahrung auf die Wahrnehmung von Figuren. I. Psych. Forsch. *8*, pp. 261-317

—— 1929, Über den Einfluss der Erfahrung auf die Wahrnehmung von Figuren. II. Psych. Forsch. *12*, pp. 1-87

W. Götz, 1926, Experimentelle Untersuchungen zum Problem der Sehgrössenkonstanz beim Haushuhn. Zts. f. Psych. *99*, pp. 247-260

C. H. Graham, 1929, Area, Color, and Brightness Difference in a Reversible Configuration. J. Gener. Psych. *2*, pp. 470-481

A. R. Granit, 1921, A Study on the Perception of Form. Brit. J. of Psych. *12*, pp. 223-247

—— 1924, Die Bedeutung von Figur und Grund für bei unveränderter Schwarz-Induktion bestimmte Helligkeitsschwellen. Skand. Arch. f. Physiol., pp. 43-57

A. R. Granit, *see also* A. Gelb

J. P. Guilford and K. M. Dallenbach, 1928, A Study of the Autokinetic Sensation. Amer. J. Psych. *40*, pp. 83-91

M. R. Harrower, 1929, Some Experiments on the Nature of γ Movement. Psych. Forsch. *13*, pp. 55-63

—— 1932, Organization in Higher Mental Processes. Psych. Forsch. *17*, pp. 56-120

—— to be published shortly in Brit. J. of Psych., Some Factors Determining Figure-Ground Articulation

M. R. Harrower, *see also* K. Koffka

H. G. Hartgenbusch, 1927, Gestalt Psychology in Sport. Psyche, No. 27, pp. 41-52. Originally published as: Beobachtungen und Bemerkungen zur Psychologie des Sports. Psych. Forsch. *7*, pp. 386-397

L. Hartmann, 1923, Neue Verschmelzungsprobleme. Psych. Forsch. *3*, pp. 319-396

V. Hazlitt, 1926, Ability, A Psychological Study. London

H. Head, 1920, Studies in Neurology, 2 vols. London

—— 1926, Aphasia and Kindred Disorders of Speech. 2 vols. Cambridge

F. Heider, 1927, Ding und Medium. Symposion *1*, pp. 109-157. Also separately published as "Sonderdruck des Symposion." Heft 7

G. M. Heider, 1933, New Studies in Transparency, Form and Colour. Psych. Forsch. *17*, pp. 13-56

R. Heine, 1914, Über Wiedererkennen und rückwirkende Hemmung. Zts. f. Psych. *68*, pp. 161-237

H. von Helmholtz, 1866, Physiologische Optik (3rd ed., 3 vols., 1909-1911). Hamburg und Leipzig

H. Helson, 1929, The Effects of Direct Stimulation of the Blind Spot. Amer. J. Psych. *41*, pp. 345-397

H. Helson and S. King, 1931, The *TAU* Effect: an Example of Psychological Relativity. J. Exper. Psych. *14*, pp. 202-217

L. Hempstead, 1900, The Perception of Visual Form. Amer. J. Psych. *12*, pp. 185-192

E. Hering, 1868, Die Lehre vom binokularen Sehen (1. Lieferung). Leipzig

—— 1870, Über das Gedächtnis als eine allgemeine Funktion der organisierten Materie. Wien

—— 1879, Der Raumsinn und die Bewegungen des Auges. In "Hermanns Handb. d. Physiol." *3*, pp. 343-601

—— 1920, Grundzüge der Lehre vom Lichtsinn. Berlin. (The first instalment appeared in 1905)

M. Hertz, 1929, Das optische Gestaltproblem und der Tierversuch. Verhandl. d. deutsch. Zoolog. Ges. 1929, pp. 23-49

F. Hillebrand, 1922, Zur Theorie der stroboskopischen Bewegungen, Zts. f. Psych. *89*, pp. 209-272; *90*, pp. 1-66

J. Hirsch, 1922, Über traditionellen Speiseabscheu. Zts. f. Psych. *88*, pp. 337-371

H. Höffding, 1889, 1890, Über Wiedererkennen, Assoziation und psychische Aktivität. Vierteljschr. f. wissensch. Philosophie *13*, pp. 420 ff.; *14*, pp. 27 f.

B. E. Holaday, 1933, Die Grössenkonstanz der Sehdinge bei Variation der inneren und äusseren Wahrnehmungsbedingungen. Arch. f. d. ges. Psych. *88*, pp. 419-486

H. L. Hollingworth, 1909, The Inadequacy of Movement. Arch. of Psych. No. *13*

—— 1910, The Central Tendency of Judgment. J. of Philos., Psych., and Sci. Meth. *7*, also in "Experimental Studies in Judgment," Arch. of Psych. No. *29*, 1913, pp. 44-52

Leta Hollingworth, 1931, Special Gifts and Special Deficiencies. In "Handbook of Child Psych.," ed. by C. Murchison, Worcester, Mass., pp. 627-642

F. Hoppe, 1931, Erfolg und Misserfolg. Psych. Forsch. *14*, pp. 1-62

E. M. von Hornbostel, 1922, Über optische Inversion. Psych. Forsch. *1*, pp. 130-156

—— 1923, Beobachtungen über ein- und zweiohriges Hören. Psych. Forsch. *4*, pp. 64-114

—— 1930, Das räumliche Hören. In "Handb. d. norm. und pathol. Physiol.," her. von Bethe u.a. *11*, pp. 602-618

E. M. von Hornbostel und M. Wertheimer, 1920, Über die Wahrnehmung der Schallrichtung. Berliner Ber. *20*, pp. 388-396

I Huang, 1931, Children's Explanations of Strange Phenomena. Psych. Forsch. *14*, pp. 63-180

G. Humphrey, 1933, The Nature of Learning in Relation to the Living System. London, New York

W. A. Hunt, *see* H. Cantril

W. S. Hunter, 1929, Experimental Studies of Learning. In "Foundations of Experimental Psychology," ed. by C. Murchison, Worcester, Mass., pp. 564-627

E. Husserl, 1900, Logische Untersuchungen I. Halle a. S.

M. H. Jacobs, 1933, Über den Einfluss des phänomenalen Abstands auf die Unterschiedsschwelle für Helligkeiten. Psych. Forsch. *18*, pp. 98-142

E. R. Jaensch, 1909, Zur Analyse der Gesichtswahrnehmungen. Erg. Bd. *4* d. Zts. f. Psych.

—— 1911, Über die Wahrnehmung des Raumes. Erg. Bd. *6* d. Zts. f. Psych.

—— 1914, Über Grundfragen der Farbenpsychologie. Ber. üb. d. VI. Kong. f. exp. Psych. in Göttingen. Leipzig, pp. 45-56

—— 1920, Einige allgemeinere Fragen der Psychologie und Biologie des Denkens, erläutert an der Lehre vom Vergleich. Arb. z. Psych. und Philos. her. von E. R. Jaensch, No. 1, pp. 1-31

—— 1921, Über den Farbenkontrast und die sogen. Berücksichtigung der Beleuchtung. Zts. f. Sinnesphysiol. *52*, pp. 165-180

E. R. Jaensch und E. A. Müller, 1920, Über die Wahrnehmung farbloser Helligkeiten und den Helligkeitskontrast. Zts. f. Psych. *83*, pp. 266-341

J. G. Jenkins, 1930, Perceptual Determinants in Plain Designs. J. Exp. Psych. *13*, pp. 24-46

J. G. Jenkins and K. Dallenbach, 1924, Obliviscence During Sleep and Waking. Amer. J. Psych. *35*, pp. 605-612

J. R. Kantor, 1922, The Psychology of Reflex Action. Amer. J. Psych. *33*, pp. 481-510

L. Kardos, 1934, Ding und Schatten. Erg. Bd. *23* d. Zts. f. Psych.

T. von Kármán, 1916, Das Gedächtnis der Materie. Die Naturwiss. *4*, pp. 489-494

A. Karsten, 1928, Psychische Sättigung. Psych. Forsch. *10*, pp. 142-254

D. Katz, 1911, Die Erscheinungsweisen der Farben und ihre Beeinflussung durch die individuelle Erfahrung. Erg. Bd. 7 d. Zts. f. Psych.

—— 1926, Sozialpsychologie der Vögel. Ergeb. d. Biologie I, pp. 447-478

—— 1929, 2. Sammelreferat über Arbeiten aus dem Gebiet der Farbenwahrnehmung. Psych. Forsch. *12*, pp. 260-278

—— 1930, Der Aufbau der Farbwelt. Erg. Bd. 7 d. Zts. f. Psych., 2. Aufl.

D. Katzaroff, 1911, Contribution à l'étude de la récognition. Arch. de Psych. *11*

F. Kenkel, 1913, Untersuchungen über den Zusammenhang zwischen Erscheinungsgrösse und Erscheinungsbewegung bei einigen sogenannten optischen Täuschungen. Zts. f. Psych. *67*, pp. 358-449

S. King, *see* H. Helson

S. Klimpfinger, 1933, Über den Einfluss von intentioneller Einstellung und Übung auf die Gestaltkonstanz. Arch. f. d. ges. Psych. *88*, pp. 551-598

S. Klimpfinger, 1933 a, Die Entwicklung der Gestaltkonstanz vom Kind zum Erwachsenen. Ibid., pp. 599-628

H. Klüver, 1929, Contemporary German Psychology. A Supplement in G. Murphy: Historical Introduction to Modern Psychology. London, New York

K. Koffka, 1909, Experimentaluntersuchungen zur Lehre vom Rhythmus. Zts. f. Psych. *52*, pp. 1-109

—— 1912, Zur Analyse der Vorstellungen und ihrer Gesetze. Leipzig

—— 1915, Zur Grundlegung der Wahrnehmungspsychologie. Eine Auseinandersetzung mit V. Benussi. Zts. f. Psych. *73*, pp. 11-90

—— 1919, Über den Einfluss der Erfahrung auf die Wahrnehmung. Die Naturwiss. *7*, pp. 597-605

—— 1922, Perception, an Introduction to the Gestalt-Theorie. Psych. Bull. *19*, pp. 531-585

—— 1922 a, Über den Linke'schen Kreisbogenversuch. Psych. Forsch. *2*, pp. 148-153

—— 1922 b, Die Prävalenz der Kontur. Ibid., pp. 147-148

—— 1923, Zur Theorie der Erlebniswahrnehmung. Ann. d. Philos. *3*, pp. 375-399

—— 1923 a, Über Feldbegrenzung und Felderfüllung. Psych. Forsch. *4*, pp. 176-203

—— 1923 b, Über die Messung der Grösse von Nachbildern. Psych. Forsch. *3*, pp. 219-230

—— 1923 c, Über die Untersuchungen an den sogenannten optischen Anschauungsbildern. Psych. Forsch. *3*, pp. 124-167

—— 1924, Introspection and the Method of Psychology. Brit. J. Psych. *15*, pp. 149-161

—— 1925, Psychologie. In "Lehrbuch der Philosophie," her. von M. Dessoir. Berlin, pp. 497-603

—— 1925 a, Mental Development. In "Psychologies of 1925," ed. by C. Murchison, Worcester, Mass., pp. 129-143. Also in Ped. Sem. *32*, pp. 659-673

—— 1926, Psychologie der Wahrnehmung. VIIIth Internat. Congr. of Psych. held at Groningen. Proceedings and Papers. Groningen, pp. 159-165

—— 1926 a, Review of Bartlett, 1923. Psych. Forsch. *7*, pp. 283-287

—— 1927, On the Structure of the Unconscious. In "The Unconscious, a Symposium," ed. by E. Dummer. New York, pp. 43-68

—— 1927 a, Bemerkungen zur Denk-Psychologie. Psych. Forsch. *9*, pp. 163-183

—— 1928, The Growth of the Mind, 2nd ed. (1st ed. 1925, 1st German ed. 1921). London, New York

—— 1930, Some Problems of Space Perception. In "Psychologies of 1930," ed. by C. Murchison, Worcester, Mass., pp. 161-187

—— 1931, Die Wahrnehmung von Bewegung. In "Handb. d. norm. und pathol. Physiol.," her. von Bethe u.a. *12*, *2*, pp. 1166-1214

K. Koffka, 1931 a, Psychologie der optischen Wahrnehmung. Ibid., pp. 1215-1271

—— 1931 b, Gestalt. Encyclopaedia of the Social Sciences. New York

—— 1932, Les notions d'héréditaire et d'acquis en psychologie. J. d. Psych. *29*, pp. 5-19

—— 1932 a, Some Remarks on the Theory of Colour Constancy. Psych. Forsch. *16*, pp. 329-354

—— 1932 b, A New Theory of Brightness Constancy; a Contribution to a General Theory of Vision. Report of a Joint Discussion on Vision by the Physical and Optical Societies. Published by the Physical Society. Cambridge, pp. 182-188

—— 1933, Review of Tolman, 1932. Psych. Bull. *30*, pp. 440-451

—— 1935, On Problems of Colour Perception. Acta Psychologica *1*, pp. 129-134

K. Koffka and M. R. Harrower, 1931, Colour and Organization. I. Psych. Forsch. *15*, pp. 145-192; II. Ibid., pp. 193-275

K. Koffka and A. Mintz, 1931, On the Influence of Transformation and Contrast on Colour- and Brightness-Thresholds. Psych. Forsch. *14*, pp. 183-198

K. Koffka, *see also* P. Cermak

W. Köhler, 1913, Über unbemerkte Empfindungen und Urteilstäuschungen. Zts. f. Psych. *66*, pp. 51-80

—— 1915, Optische Untersuchungen am Schimpansen und am Haushuhn. Berliner Abhandlg., Jhg. 1915, phys.-math. Kl. Nr. 3

—— 1917, Die Farben der Sehdinge beim Schimpansen und beim Haushuhn. Zts. f. Psych. *77*, pp. 248-255

—— 1918, Nachweis einfacher Strukturfunktionen beim Schimpansen und beim Haushuhn. Berliner Abhandlg. 1918

—— 1920, Die physischen Gestalten in Ruhe und im stationären Zustand. Braunschweig

—— 1923, Zur Theorie des Sukzessivvergleichs und der Zeitfehler. Psych. Forsch. *4*, pp. 115-175

—— 1923 a, Zur Theorie der stroboskopischen Bewegung. Psych. Forsch. *3*, pp. 397-406

—— 1923 b, Tonpsychologie. In "Handb. d. Neurol. d. Ohres," her. von Alexander und Marburg. Berlin und Wien, pp. 419-464

—— 1924, Gestaltprobleme und Anfänge einer Gestalttheorie. Jahresber. üb. d. ges. Physiol. 1922, pp. 512-539

—— 1925, An Aspect of Gestalt Psychology. In "Psychologies of 1925," ed. by C. Murchison. Worcester, Mass., pp. 163-198

—— 1925 a, Komplextheorie und Gestalttheorie. Antwort auf G. E. Müllers Schrift gleichen Namens. Psych. Forsch. *6*, pp. 358-416

—— 1927, The Mentality of Apes. 2nd ed. London, New York (1st German ed. 1917)

—— 1927 a, Zum Problem der Regulation. Wilh. Roux' Arch. f. Ent-

wicklungsmechanik *112* (Festschrift für Hans Driesch. II), pp. 315-332
W. Köhler, 1929, Gestalt Psychology. New York, London
—— 1930, Some Tasks of Gestalt Psychology. In "Psychologies of 1930," ed. by C. Murchison. Worcester, Mass., pp. 143-160
—— 1933, Zur Psychophysik des Vergleichs und des Raumes. Psych. Forsch. *18*, pp. 343-360
H. Kopfermann, 1930, Psychologische Untersuchungen über die Wirkung zweidimensionaler Darstellungen körperlicher Gebilde. Psych. Forsch. *13*, pp. 293-364
A. Korte, 1915, Kinematoskopische Untersuchungen. Zts. f. Psych. *72*, pp. 194-296
G. Kreezer and K. M. Dallenbach, 1929, Learning the Relation of Opposition. Amer. J. Psych. *41*, pp. 432-441
J. von Kries, 1901, Über die materiellen Grundlagen der Bewusstseinserscheinungen. Tübingen und Leipzig
O. Kroh, 1921, Über Farbenkonstanz und Farbentransformation. Zts. f. Sinnesphysiol. *52*, pp. 113-186
E. G. Lammer, 1906, Thurwieserspitze. In "Empor," Leipzig. Also in G. E. Lammer's book "Jungborn," 2nd ed. München, 1923, pp. 64-77
K. S. Lashley, 1929, Brain Mechanisms and Intelligence. Chicago
—— 1929 a, Nervous Mechanisms in Learning. In "The Foundations of Experimental Psychology," ed. by C. Murchison. Worcester, Mass., pp. 524-563
O. Lauenstein, 1933, Ansatz zu einer physiologischen Theorie des Vergleichs und der Zeitfehler. Psych. Forsch. *17*, pp. 130-177
—— 1934, Bemerkungen zur Sehgrössenkonstanz. Psych. Forsch. *19*, pp. 191-192
K. Lewin, 1917, Kriegslandschaft. Zts. angew. Psych. *12*, pp. 440-447
—— 1922, Das Problem der Willensmessung und der Assoziation. I. Psych. Forsch. *1*, pp. 191-302; II. Ibid. *2*, pp. 65-140
—— 1922 a, Der Begriff der Genese in Physik, Biologie und Entwicklungsgeschichte. Berlin
—— 1926, Vorbemerkungen über die psychischen Kräfte und Energien und über die Struktur der Seele. Psych. Forsch. *7*, pp. 294-329
—— 1926 a, Vorsatz, Wille und Bedürfnis. Ibid., pp. 330-385.
—— 1931, Environmental Forces in Child Behavior and Development. In "Handbook of Child Psychology," ed. by C. Murchison. Worcester, Mass., pp. 94-127
K. Lewin und K. Sakuma, 1925, Die Sehrichtung monokularer und binokularer Objekte bei Bewegung und das Zustandekommen des Tiefeneffekts. Psych. Forsch. *6*, pp. 298-357
S. Liebmann, 1927, Über das Verhalten farbiger Formen bei Helligkeitsgleichheit von Figur und Grund. Psych. Forsch. *9*, pp. 300-353
E. Lindemann, 1922, Experimentelle Untersuchungen über das Entstehen und Vergehen von Gestalten. Psych. Forsch. *2*, pp. 5-60

J. Lindworsky, 1922, Umrisskizze zu einer theoretischen Psychologie. Zts. f. Psych. *89*, pp. 313-357
O. Lipmann und H. Bogen, 1923, Naive Physik. Leipzig
B. Löwenfeld, 1927, Systematisches Studium der Reaktionen der Säuglinge auf Klänge und Geräusche. Zts. f. Psych. *104*, pp. 62-96
J. T. MacCurdy, 1928, Common Principles in Psychology and Physiology. Cambridge
W. McDougall, 1923, Outline of Psychology. New York, London
—— 1930, The Hormic Psychology. In "Psychologies of 1930," ed. by C. Murchison. Worcester, Mass., pp. 1-36
—— 1933, The Energies of Men. New York
W. McDougall and K. McDougall, 1927, Notes on Instinct and Intelligence in Rats and Cats. J. Comp. Psych. *7*, pp. 145-176
E. Mach, 1865, Über die Wirkung der räumlichen Verteilung des Lichtreizes auf die Netzhaut. Wiener Ber. *52*
—— 1885, Die Analyse der Empfindungen (5th ed. 1906). Jena
R. B. MacLeod, 1932, An Experimental Investigation of Brightness Constancy. Arch. of Psych. No. *135*, pp. 1-102
N. R. F. Maier, 1930, Reasoning in Humans. I. On Direction. J. Comp. Psych. *10*, pp. 115-143
—— 1931, Reasoning in Humans. II. The Solution of a Problem and Its Appearance in Consciousness. J. Comp. Psych. *12*, pp. 181-194
—— 1931 a, Reasoning and Learning. Psych. Rev. *38*, pp. 332-346
W. Metzger, 1926, Über Vorstufen der Verschmelzung von Figurenreihen, die vor dem ruhenden Auge vorüberziehen. Psych. Forsch. *8*, pp. 114-221
—— 1930, Optische Untersuchungen am Ganzfeld. II. Zur Phänomenologie des homogenen Ganzfelds. Psych. Forsch. *13*, pp. 6-29
—— 1931, Gestalt und Kontrast. Psych. Forsch. *15*, pp. 374-386
—— 1934, Beobachtungen über phänomenale Identität. Psych. Forsch. *19*, pp. 1-60
W. H. Mikesell and M. Bentley, 1930, Configuration and Brightness Contrast. J. Exp. Psych. *13*, pp. 1-23
A. Mintz, *see* K. Koffka
E. A. Müller, *see* E. R. Jaensch
G. E. Müller, 1896, Zur Psychophysik der Gesichtsempfindungen. Zts. f. Psych. *10*
—— 1913, Zur Analyse der Gedächtnistätigkeit und des Vorstellungsverlaufs. III. Erg. Bd. *8* d. Zts. f. Psych.
—— 1916, Über das Aubert'sche Phänomen. Zts. f. Sinnesphysiol. *49*, pp. 109-244
—— 1917, Zur Analyse der Gedächtnistätigkeit und des Vorstellungsverlaufs. II. Erg. Bd. *9* d. Zts. f. Psych.
—— 1923, Komplextheorie und Gestalttheorie. Ein Beitrag zur Wahrnehmungspsychologie. Göttingen

G. E. Müller, 1930, Über die Farbenempfindungen. Psychophysische Untersuchungen. 2 vols. Erg. Bd. *17* und *18* d. Zts. f. Psych

G. E. Müller und A. Pilzecker, 1900, Experimentelle Beiträge zur Lehre vom Gedächtnis. Erg. Bd. *1* d. Zts. f. Psych.

E. B. Newman, 1934, Versuche über das Gamma-Phänomen. Psych. Forsch. *19*, pp. 102-121

A. Noll, 1926, Versuche über Nachbilder. Psych. Forsch. *8*, pp. 3-27

R. M. Ogden, 1926, Psychology and Education. New York

—— 1932, Insight. Amer. J. Psych. *44*, pp. 350-355

E. Oppenheimer, 1934, Optische Versuche über Ruhe und Bewegung. Psych. Forsch. *20*, pp. 1-46

M. Ovsiankina, 1928, Die Wiederaufnahme unterbrochener Handlungen. Psych. Forsch. *11*, pp. 302-379

F. T. Perkins, 1932, Symmetry in Visual Recall. Amer. J. Psych. *44*, pp. 473-490

—— 1933, A Study of Cerebral Action Currents in the Dog under Sound Stimulation. Univ. of Kansas Stud. in Psych. *1*. Psych. Mon. *44*, No. 1, pp. 1-29

F. T. Perkins, *see also* R. H. Wheeler

J. Piaget, 1923, The Language and Thought of the Child. London, New York. 1926. (The first date is that of the original French edition.)

—— 1924, Judgment and Reasoning in the Child. London, New York. 1928

—— 1926, The Child's Conception of the World. London, New York. 1929

—— 1927, The Child's Conception of Physical Causality. London, New York. 1930.

A. Pilzecker, *see* G. E. Müller

C. C. Pratt, 1933, Time Error in Psychophysical Judgments. Amer. J. of Psych. *45*, pp. 292-297

H. von Restorff, 1933, Über die Wirkung von Bereichsbildung im Spurenfeld. Psych. Forsch. *18*, pp. 299-342

G. Révész, 1923, Experiments on Animal Space Perception. VIIth Internat. Congr. of Psych. held at Oxford. Proceedings and Papers. Cambridge, 1924, pp. 29-56

E. S. Robinson, 1932, Association Theory To-Day. New York, London

E. S. Robinson and C. W. Darrow, 1924, Effect of Length of Lists upon Memory for Numbers. Amer. J. Psych. *35*, pp. 235-243

C. O. Roelofs, *see* H. G. van der Waals

H. Rothschild, 1923, Über den Einfluss der Gestalt auf das negative Nachbild ruhender visueller Figuren. Graefes Arch. f. Ophthalm. *112*, pp. 1-28

E. Rubin, 1915, Synsoplevede Figurer. Studier i psykologisk Analyse. Kóbenhavn og Kristiania. (German ed. 1921, Visuell wahrgenommene Figuren.)

E. Rubin, 1927, Visuell wahrgenommene wirkliche Bewegung. Zts. f. Psych. *103*, pp. 384-392
—— 1934, Bemerkungen veranlasst durch eine von W. Wolff aufgestellte Kontrastbedingung. Psych. Forsch. *19*, pp. 187-190
H. Sakuma, *see* K. Lewin
E. Sapir, 1927, The Unconscious Patterning of Behaviour in Society. In "The Unconscious, a Symposium," ed. by E. Dummer. New York, pp. 114-142
M. Scheerer, 1931, Die Lehre von der Gestalt. Berlin und Leipzig
T. Schjelderup-Ebbe, 1922, Beiträge zur Sozialpsychologie des Haushuhns. Zts. f. Psych. *88*, pp. 225-252
—— 1923, Weitere Beiträge zur Sozial-und Individualpsychologie des Haushuhns. Ibid., *92*, pp. 60-87
—— 1924, Zur Sozialpsychologie der Vögel. Ibid., *95*, pp. 36-84
M. Scheler, 1923, Wesen und Formen der Sympathie. Bonn
—— 1928, Die Stellung des Menschen im Kosmos. Darmstadt
P. von Schiller, 1933, Stroboskopische Alternativversuche. Psych. Forsch. *17*, pp. 179-214
W. Scholz, 1924, Experimentelle Untersuchungen über die phänomenale Grösse von Raumstrecken, die durch Sukzessiv-Darbietung zweier Reize begrenzt werden. Psych. Forsch. *5*, pp. 219-272
W. Schriever, 1925, Experimentelle Studien über stereoskopisches Sehen. Zts. f. Psych. *96*, pp. 113-170
H. Schulte, 1924, Versuch einer Theorie der paranoischen Eigenbeziehung und Wahnbildung. Psych. Forsch. *5*, pp. 1-23
F. Schumann, 1907, Psychologie des Lesens. Ber. üb. d. II. Kongr. f. exp. Psych. in Würzburg. Leipzig, pp. 153-183
E. Schur, 1926, Mondtäuschung und Sehgrössenkonstanz. Psych. Forsch. *7*, pp. 44-80
O. Selz, 1913, Über die Gesetze des geordneten Denkverlaufs. I. Bonn
—— 1922, Über die Gesetze des geordneten Denkverlaufs. II. Bonn
R. Semon, 1921, The Mneme. London, New York
G. F. Shepard and H. M. Fogelsonger, 1913, Studies in Association and Inhibition. Psych. Rev. *20*, pp. 290-311
A. Sinemus, 1932, Untersuchungen über "Beleuchtung" und "Körperfarbe" bei Mikropsie. Zts. f. Psych. *125*, pp. 1-37
K. Steinig, 1929, Zur Frage der Wahrnehmung von Zwischenstadien bei stroboskopisch dargebotenen Bewegungen. Zts. f. Psych. *109*, pp. 291-336
A. Stern, 1926, Die Wahrnehmung von Bewegung in der Gegend des blinden Flecks. Psych. Forsch. *7*, pp. 1-15
G. F. Stout, 1909, Analytic Psychology. 2 vols. London
—— 1913, A Manual of Psychology. 3rd ed. London
C. Stumpf, 1883, Tonpsychologie. I. Leipzig
—— 1890, Tonpsychologie. II. Leipzig

J. Ternus, 1926, Experimentelle Untersuchungen über phänomenale Identität. Psych. Forsch. *7*, pp. 81-136
E. Thelin, 1927, Perception of Relative Visual Motion. J. Exp. Psych. *10*, pp. 321-349
E. L. Thorndike, 1931, Human Learning. New York
R. H. Thouless, 1923, Some Observations on Contrast Effects in Graded Discs. Brit. J. Psych. *13*, pp. 301-307.
—— 1928, The Psychology of Climbing. The Rucksack Club Journal *6*, pp. 155-165
—— 1931, Phenomenal Regression to the Real Object. I, Brit. J. Psych. *21*, pp. 339-359
—— 1931 a, Phenomenal Regression to the Real Object. II. Ibid. *22*, pp. 1-30
—— 1932, Individual Differences in Phenomenal Regression. Ibid. *22*, pp. 216-241
—— 1934, The General Principle Underlying Effects Attributed to the So-called Phenomenal Constancy Tendency. Psych. Forsch. *19*, pp. 300-310
E. B. Titchener, 1910, A Text-Book of Psychology. New York
—— 1911, A Note of the Consciousness of Self. Amer. J. Psych. *22*, pp. 540-552
E. C. Tolman, 1932, Purposive Behavior in Animals and Men. New York
B. Tudor-Hart, 1928, Studies in Transparency, Form and Colour. Psych. Forsch. *10*, pp. 255-298
P. E. Vernon, *see* G. W. Allport
P. Vogel, 1931, Über die Bedingungen des optokinetischen Schwindels. Pflüg. Arch. *228*, pp. 510-530
H. Volkelt, 1926, Fortschritte der experimentellen Kinderpsychologie. Ber. üb. d. IX. Kongr. f. exp. Psych. Jena, pp. 81-135
H. G. van der Waals und C. O. Roelofs, 1930, 1930 a, Optische Scheinbewegung. Zts. f. Psych. *114*, pp. 241-288; *115*, pp. 91-193
—— 1933, Über das Sehen von Bewegung. Zts. f. Psych. *128*, pp. 314-354
Cree Warden, 1933, A Study in the Recall of Perceived Relations. Univ. of Kansas Stud. in Psych. *1*. Psych. Mon. *44*, No. 1, pp. 195-206
J. B. Watson, 1925, Experimental Studies on the Growth of the Emotions. In "Psychologies of 1925," ed. by C. Murchison. Worcester, Mass., pp. 37-57
H. Werner, 1926, Einführung in die Entwicklungspsychologie. Leipzig
M. Wertheimer, 1912, Experimentelle Studien über das Sehen von Bewegung. Zts. f. Psych. *61*, pp. 161-265
—— 1920, Über Schlussprozess im produktiven Denken. In "Drei Abhandlungen zur Gestalttheorie." Erlangen, 1925, pp. 164-184. (First published separately.)

M. Wertheimer, 1923, Untersuchungen zur Lehre von der Gestalt. II. Psych. Forsch. *4*, pp. 301-350

—— 1925, Über Gestalttheorie. Symposion, *1*, pp. 1-24. Also separately published as "Sonderdrucke des Symposion," Heft 1

—— 1928, Gestaltpsychologische Forschung. In "Einführung in die neuere Psychologie," her. von E. Saupe. Osterwieck a. H., pp. 46-53

—— 1933, Zu dem Problem der Unterscheidung von Einzelinhalt und Teil. Zts. f. Psych. *129*, pp. 353-357

M. Wertheimer, *see also* E. M. von Hornbostel

R. H. Wheeler, 1929, The Science of Psychology. New York

R. H. Wheeler and F. T. Perkins, 1932, Principles of Mental Development. New York

A. N. Whitehead, 1926, Science and the Modern World. New York, London

S. Witasek, 1910, Psychologie der Raumwahrnehmung des Auges. Heidelberg

—— 1918, Assoziation und Gestalteinprägung. Zts. f. Psych. *79*, pp. 161-210

E. Wohlfahrt, 1928, Der Auffassungsvorgang an kleinen Gestalten. Ein Beitrag zur Psychologie des Vorgestalterlebnisses. Neue Psych. Stud. *4*, pp. 347-414

Werner Wolff, 1932, Selbstbeurteilung und Fremdbeurteilung im wissentlichen und unwissentlichen Versuch. Psych. Forsch. *16*, pp. 251-328

Wilhelm Wolff, 1933, Über die kontrasterregende Wirkung der transformierten Farben. Psych. Forsch. *18*, pp. 90-97

R. S. Woodworth, 1929, Psychology. Rev. ed. New York

F. Wulf, 1922, Über die Veränderung von Vorstellungen (Gedächtnis und Gestalt). Psych. Forsch. *1*, pp. 333-389

W. Wundt, 1903, Grundzüge der physiologischen Psychologie, 5. Aufl. 3 vols. Leipzig

J. G. Yoshioka, 1930, Size Preference of Wild Rats. J. Genet. Psych. *37*, pp. 159-162

—— 1930 a, Size Preference of Albino Rats. Ibid., pp. 427-430

—— 1932, A Further Note on Size Preference of Albino Rats. Ibid., *41*, pp. 489-492

B. Zeigarnik, 1927, Über das Behalten von erledigten und unerledigten Handlungen. Psych. Forsch. *9*, pp. 1-85

INDEX

Aall, A., 336, 521-522
Absolute impression, 476
Accommodation, 74, 82, 83, 114, 119, 123, 124, 172, 173, 237, 238, 238 n., 311-313, 316, 317, 342-344
Accomplishment, 37, 38, 414, 456, 457, 482, 501, 523, 544, 553, 564, 585, 586
Ach, N., 394, 395, 560, 574, 575, 576, 577, 577 n., 578, 579, 579 n., 582
Achievement, *see* Problem of achievement
Ackermann, A., 253
Acquired, 548, 549
Action, 310, 331, 333, 334, 342-345, 354, 356, 364, 366, 367, 384, 389, 391-393, 402, 405, 413, 419, 421, 653, 658, 668, 679, 682; automatic, 417; controlled, 418, 584; field, 345, 418, 419; involuntary, 416, 418, 420; voluntary, 416-420
Action and reaction, 554
Action at a distance, 41, 42
Adaptation, 81, 96, 113, 241
Adapted behaviour, 68, 76, 122, 179, 361, 368, 369, 373, 375, 376, 423, 536, 680
Adequacy of behavioural world, 375, 376; *see also* Cognition
Adrenalin, 415
Aesthetics, 347, 348, 350, 351
Affective transformation, 500
After-images, 141, 143, 144, 171, 172, 198, 199, 199 n., 211, 212, 222, 223, 318
Albedo, 112, 243, 245, 249, 251, 257 n., 260
Algebraic, addition of tendencies, 574, 575
Allesch, G. J. von, 279, 626, 627
Allport, G., 493, 494, 495, 495 n., 496, 497, 498, 498 n., 499, 502, 677, 678
Ambiguous figures, 83, 183-186, 190 f., 362, 554
Ambiguous motion patterns, 300, 303
Ambition, 341, 610
Anger, 403, 407-410, 414, 673
Angier, R. P., 410 n.
Anisotropy of space, 275-279; tridimensional, 276-278
Anthropomorphism, 30, 39, 66
Apollinian philosophy, 416, 417
Appearance, 33, 35
Appurtenance, 246-248, 260, 260 n., 283; *see also* Belongingness
A priorism, 305, 549
Arbitrariness, 570, 585, 614
Arnheim, R., 678
Arousal of (specific) new process, 541, 542, 547, 548, 552, 586, 615, 625, 626, 638; *see also* First performance and Problem of achievement
Articulation, 116, 119, 150, 171-174, 186, 193, 194, 197, 201, 203, 205, 206, 208, 209, 235, 291, 311, 314, 324, 346, 363, 376, 389, 390, 449, 508, 509, 526, 544, 566, 587, 604, 622, 639, 641, 642, 644, 646, 665, 666, 668
Assertion, 405, 666
Assimilation hypothesis (Wundt), 103, 104, 105, 393, 463 n., 583, 592
Association, 19, 167 n., 542, 543, 548, 556-561, 564-566, 570, 572, 575, 577, 579, 581, 582, 584, 588, 589, 602, 604, 607, 655, 659; as a force, 559, 560, 571, 572, 574, 575, 579; law of, 561, 567, 579, 582; strength of, 558, 560, 565, 566, 569, 572, 574, 577, 583, 589; experiment, 562
Associationism, 372, 381, 542-544, 556-561, 563-565, 569, 571, 572, 582, 583, 587, 589, 602, 681
Associative bond, 542, 543, 556, 557, 564, 566, 567, 570, 572, 574; purely existential or external, 542, 543, 558
Associative connection, *see* Associative bond
Associative learning, 530, 556, 585, 589, 590
Asymmetry of contour, *see* Contour
Atmosphere, 201
Atomic theory, 57
Attention, 102, 113, 204, 206, 210, 319, 343, 358, 386, 387, 394, 395, 400, 500, 516, 596, 609; involuntary, 358, 395; voluntary, 358, 395; conditions of, 358, 359
Attitudes, 102, 148, 149, 157, 173, 197, 204, 206, 235, 236, 301, 303, 313, 319, 343, 353, 368, 392, 394-398, 400, 508, 521, 522, 561, 562, 572, 583, 584, 596, 607-613, 617, 624; passive, 561, 562, 582

Attraction, 165, 166, 273, 286, 287, 315, 316, 357, 439, 639
Attractiveness, 353, 355, 356, 392
Attributes, 73, 358
Aubert phenomenon, 215 n.
Aubert-Foerster phenomenon, 276, 278
Audition, 200, 201
Authority, 666
Auto-kinetic movements, 213
Automatic action, 417
Automatic reproduction, *see* Reproduction automatic
Autonomous changes (of traces), 498-501, 503-505, 519, 524
Availability of traces, 337, 522, 523, 525-527, 546, 547, 552, 555 n., 618, 619, 621-624, 630, 637, 638
Availability of perceptual data, 637, 638

Bahnsen, P., 195, 196
Balance, *see* Equilibrium
Banister, H., 220 n.
Barriers, 391, 408-411, 414
Bartlett, F. C., 506, 517, 518, 519, 520, 592, 594, 611, 611 n., 612, 612 n., 646, 649, 664 n., 665, 666, 675
Bartley, S. H., 61
Becher, E., 460
Becker, H., 650
Behaviour, 25, 27, 29, 31-40, 42, 46, 48, 49, 51, 56, 66-68, 120, 122, 201, 208, 306-308, 310, 311, 317, 330, 354, 355, 361, 362, 365, 366, 368, 372-375, 392, 393, 404, 421, 422, 457, 509, 519, 540, 541, 544, 551, 585, 586, 625, 646, 648, 650, 652, 653, 661-663, 668, 669, 674, 675, 680-682; adapted, *see* Adapted behaviour; apparent, 40, 41; phenomenal, 40, 41, 51, 382; real, 39-42, 382, 658; *see also* Group behaviour, Molar behaviour, Molecular behaviour, Knowledge of behaviour, Results of behaviour
Behavioural environment, 27-52, 55, 61, 63, 65, 70, 75, 76, 79, 122, 175, 179, 180, 193, 197, 200, 208, 210, 214, 218, 317, 319, 321, 322, 331, 333, 346-348, 350, 352, 353, 355, 356, 360, 369, 373, 375-377, 379, 381, 383, 384, 392-395, 398, 422, 431, 496, 595, 642, 652, 663, 664, 680, 682; ontological status of, 46 f.
Behavioural field, 44, 46, 48, 51-53, 85, 122, 316, 394, 444, 446, 653, 654, 659, 661, 670; insufficiency of, 46
Behavioural world, 323, 360, 384, 656, 657
Behaviourism, 26, 28, 35-38, 66, 333
Behind, 322, 390
Belongingness, 137, 246, 252, 518; *see also* Appurtenance
Benary, W., 136, 137, 138, 246, 260
Bentley, J. M., 136, 470
Benussi, V., 134, 136, 149, 298
Berger, C., 205 n., 206
Bergson, H., 424
Berkeley, G., 115, 163
Beyrl, F., 92, 238, 239, 240, 305 n.
Binnen-Kontrast, 133
Binocular parallax, 160-163, 208, 235
Binocular rivalry, 189, 190, 193
Birds, 655, 661, 668, 669
Birenbaum, G., 420
Black-white series, 252
Blind sequences, 16, 310, 311, 382, 383, 474, 684
Blind spot, 144, 144 n., 145, 146, 192, 206, 510
Blocking, 411, 413
Blodgett, H. C., 586
Blooming, buzzing confusion, 67
Bogen, H., 638, 642, 644
Bohr, N., 57, 57 n.
Boltzmann, L., 428
Borak, J., 465, 466
Boring, E. G., 298, 343
Boundary, 147, 148, 507, 665; of Ego, 320-322, 325, 331, 421; of groups, 655, 665; as characteristic of things, 71, 177, 304
Box stacking, 536, 537
Brain, 11, 117, 317, 373, 378, 381, 429, 440, 442, 452, 478, 509, 518; injuries, 117, 276, 454, 455, 514, 517, 546; localization, 54
Bridge, 482, 484
Brightness, 81, 132, 169, 171, 190 n., 243, 244, 247, 248, 253, 258, 260, 263, 263 n., 264, 277, 290, 291, 301, 304; *see also* Brightness constancy
Broad, C. D., 655, 656
Brown, J. F., 94, 276, 281, 282, 288, 289, 290, 291, 292, 293, 294 n., 295, 295 n., 296, 297, 298, 378
Browning, R., 8, 683
Brunswik, E., 226, 226 n., 227, 235, 238, 239, 242
Bühler, K., 129, 132, 153, 256, 312, 313, 569
Burzlaff, W., 239, 240

Calkins, M. W., 319
Camouflage, 77, 376
Cannon, W. B., 415, 416 n.
Cantril, H., 415
Carr, H. A., 539

Carroll, L., 180
Causal connection *vs.* factual sequence, 20
Causality, 22, 72, 378-381
Central tendency of judgment, 474-476
Centre of retina, 146, 201-208, 212, 311, 313, 315
Cermak, P., 281, 293, 295, 296
Chaotic processes, 409, 507, 523, 524, 544
Chance, 308, 332, 589
Circular process, 373 f., 598, 652, 653; in social behaviour, 652, 653
Circular relation between process and trace, 542
Chickens, 88, 89, 346, 355, 356
Chimpanzees, 88, 89, 359, 394, 508, 530, 536 f., 551, 552, 635, 643, 644, 665, 666
Chladni figures, 458
Civilization, 307-310, 361, 417, 422, 648, 674, 675, 683
Clang analysis, 394, 398
Claparède, E., 419, 494, 495, 503, 592, 593, 594, 595, 596, 616, 627, 628 n., 631, 634, 635, 640 n.
Classes, 349-351, 476, 502
Clearness, 204, 206, 237, 277, 278, 358, 642
Closure, 151, 164, 167, 168, 171, 340, 449, 450, 464, 545, 553, 605, 607, 631, 638, 639, 665
Clothes, 320, 517
Cognition, 68, 76, 78, 180, 227, 279, 280, 361, 362, 368, 376, 377, 379-382, 403, 421, 656; *see also* Veridicalness
Cohesion, 126, 135, 136, 150, 253, 277, 449, 488, 523, 524, 665
Coincidence point, 128, 253
Colour, 116 n., 117, 118, 120-122, 135, 136, 146, 163, 169, 171, 178-181, 186-189, 202, 205, 206, 219, 248, 255, 256, 260, 263, 265, 301, 303, 357, 359, 363, 497, 498, 681; hard, 127, 128, 171, 188, 189, 205, 264, 362; soft, 127, 128, 171, 188, 189, 205; concentration of, 117-119
Colour mixture, 262
Colour sense, 270; *see also* Constancy of colour
Coloured shadows, 258, 259
Combination zone, 270, 273
Communication between Ego and field, 409, 420, 679
Communication between different Ego-systems, 342, 679
Communication between sensory and motor system, 316, 373, 627
Communication of traces with processes, 461, 464, 523, 524, 527, 553, 561-563, 566-569, 573, 582-584, 587, 588, 590-607, 609, 611, 612, 615, 618, 624, 625, 630, 634; with other traces, 501-504, 508, 519, 522-524, 572, 588, 601, 603, 622
Comparison, 239, 240, 466, 467, 476, 477; simultaneous, 466; successive, 451, 452, 465, 466, 481, 497
Completion, 533; of figures, 141, 143, 146, 505, 632; of ground, 192; of jokes, 616-620; of process, 567, 568, 632; of tasks, 335, 336, 338, 340, 341, 508, 619
Complexity of the Ego, 333, 334, 338, 342, 366, 609, 610
Comrade, 666
Conation, 361, 521, 526
Concave, 192, 199
Concentration of reacting molecules, 441, 442, 444, 445, 467, 473, 479
Concepts, 454 n., 476
Conditioned reflex, 542, 585
Conditions of a process, 100, 102, 104, 138, 198, 200, 206, 210, 217, 227, 311, 337, 384, 412, 458, 459, 503, 548, 625; external, 100, 117, 227, 236, 348, 535; internal, 100, 102, 105, 117, 227, 236, 270, 348, 535; momentary, 100, 102, 392; permanent, 100, 270
Conduct and science, 7, 8
Cones, 201, 208, 285, 286
Conflict, 408, 408 n., 419
Connection between members of a whole, 557, 558, 571
Connections of neurones, 310, 312, 313, 369, 370, 552, 626
Connectionism, 371, 544
Consciousness, 10, 11, 25, 35, 36, 39, 51, 55, 56, 62, 65, 68, 193, 330-333, 360, 382, 383, 395, 401, 402, 423, 432, 433, 435, 436, 442, 444, 446, 525; as epiphenomenon, 65; of animals, 65; stream of, 332
Conservation, 308-310, 316, 369, 382
Conservative nature of behavioural things, 83
Constancy of framework, 222, 386
Constancy as characteristic of things, 72, 210, 224, 279, 304, 305
Constancy phenomena, 90, 210, 211 ff., 239, 240, 260, 305; *see also* Perceptual constancies, Superconstancy, and Unique cases in constancy phenomena; colour constancy, 34, 106, 224, 225, 227, 237-241, 254-260, 263, 265, 304,

641; intensity constancy, 240 n.; shape constancy, 222-240, 243, 244, 250, 255, 265, 273, 304; size constancy, 34, 87-95, 106, 222-230, 235-244, 255, 256, 273, 277, 278, 304; weight constancy, 240 n.; whiteness (brightness) constancy, 81, 89, 112, 227, 238-257, 259 n., 304; constancy of animals and children, 88 ff., 224, 239, 240; development of constancy, 227, 238-240; measure of constancy, 226, 227, 234, 234 n., 238, 242
Constancy hypothesis, 86, 87, 89, 95, 97, 104, 105, 115, 180, 224, 393, 448 n.
Constraining conditions, 99, 100, 102, 391, 602
Constructiveness of memory, 612
Contiguity, 149, 482, 542, 557, 558, 568-570, 583; association by, 542, 543, 558, 579
Contour, 197, 199, 216, 314; asymmetry of, 151, 181, 184, 497; double-sided function of, 182, 183; one-sided function of, 181-184, 197, 199, 208, 209, 216
Contour figures, 150, 151, 181
Contraction of distance in stroboscopic motion, 287, 315 n.
Contrast, 133, 134, 136, 137, 170, 186, 188, 241, 245, 245 n., 249, 250, 258-260, 260 n., 477 n.; internal, 133; as absolute, 134, 245, 245 n.; association by, 542, 605, 606; law of, 605-607
Controlled action, *see* Action controlled
Convergence, 123, 124, 237, 238, 269, 311, 314-317, 342
Convex, 192, 199
Co-operation between traces and stimuli, 432, 450, 523
Co-ordinated duo, *see* Duo organization
Co-ordination of the eyes, 315
Correspondence between phenomenal and real things, 305, 377-380
Corresponding points, 266-271, 273, 314, 315
Couplings, 571
Cratylus, 70
Crescendo, 659, 660
Criteria of depth, *see* Depth criteria
Critical fusion frequency, 129-132, 184, 187
Culture, 19, 676, 677
Cumulative disposition, 432, 433, 435, 436, 438, 451
Curie, P., 108, 109
Customs, 409, 674, 676
Cycloid, 284, 377
Dahl, A., 492
Dallenbach, K. M., 213, 341, 491, 492, 509, 613
Darrow, C. W., 491
Dead things, 70
Deep sensibility, 121, 390
Demand characters, 345, 346, 355-360, 363, 364, 382, 391-393, 408, 595
Dembo, T., 407, 408 f., 408 n., 410, 412, 673, 674
Demon-mask experiment, 359
Density of energy, 189, 193, 194
Depth perception, 160, 162, 163, 212, 269, 270, 272, 273
Depth criteria, 163, 266, 273, 274; *see also* Depth factors; combination of depth criteria, 266, 273, 274
Depth factors, 229, 235, 273
Depth value, 212
Descartes, R., 12
DeSilva, H. R., 291
Desire, 102, 325, 327, 368, 521, 535, 610, 624
Despot, 669, 670
Determination, 325
Determining tendency, 559, 560, 574, 575, 579; strength of, 574
Development, 308, 309, 332; mental, 332, 542; of constancy, 227, 238-240; of Ego, 529; of figures, 396-398
Difference limen, 465, 477, 480, 481
Dimensions of stimuli, 115, 116
Dionysian philosophy, 416, 417
Direct experience, 35, 36, 39, 51, 61, 64, 67, 73, 597
Direction of energy, 99, 100; *see also* Steering
Direction, temporal, 439, 445
Direction as a determinant of constancy of size, 94, 211, 236
Directions, main of space, 191, 215, 216, 218, 224, 231, 255, 275
Discipline of science, 9
Discontinuity of stimulation, 125, 129, 147, 148, 151, 152, 173, 439; *see also* Inhomogeneity of stimulation
Discrimination, 279, 444
Discrimination experiments, 189, 205, 279
Discriminanda, 34 n.; capacities, 34 n.
Disparate points, 267-269, 271-273
Disparity, *see* Retinal disparity
Displeasure, 19
Displacement, 281-284, 287-290, 385, 387
Distance, 122, 123, 211, 212, 229, 230, 236, 243, 244, 277-279, 294, 296, 301,

480, 481; normal, 236; in the brain, 478, 479; *see also* Signs of distance
Distant stimulus, *see* Stimuli, distant
Distribution of quantities, 14
Distribution of process, 138, 305, 616, 633
Dodge, R., 666 f.
Dominance, 417, 668, 669, 679
Double images, 314-316
Double representation, 178 f., 181-183, 191, 192, 260-262, 264, 451
Double vectorial determination, 234
Driesch, H., 378
Drill, 547
Drive, 67, 416
Dualism, 47, 308, 436, 560, 631
Duncker, K., 281, 282, 283, 284, 285, 287, 288, 384, 386, 389, 614, 627, 630, 631, 634, 641, 643
Dunlap, K., 536 n.
Duo organization, 153, 154, 162, 178, 181; co-ordinated duo, 154, 183, 192, 196; one on top of the other, 154, 178 f., 181 f.
Duration, 297, 298, 425, 447, 452, 454 n.
Dynamic characters (properties), 43, 45, 46, 72, 304, 391, 421, 594

Ebbinghaus, H., 557
Eberhardt, M., 253, 394, 398
Eddington, A. S., 28 n., 57 n.
Education, 676, 677
Effect, *see* Transformation of processes by effect, and Success
Ego, 39-43, 47, 51, 67, 113, 114, 121, 149, 173, 175, 197, 201, 206, 217, 219, 221, 237, 280, 282, 284, 285, 304, 317, 318-334, 338, 340, 341, 344-346, 354, 355, 359-368, 371-374, 384, 387, 389, 393, 394, 402, 405, 409, 412, 414-422, 431, 446, 508, 514, 517, 520-522, 525-527, 562, 583, 594-597, 607-613, 627, 633, 651, 654, 655, 661-664, 667-674, 676, 679, 681, 682; -field (ego -object), relation or organization, 113, 121, 358, 362, 368, 373, 392, 408, 419, 421, 584, 594-597, 609, 610, 636; in trace system, 520, 522, 525, 526; experiences, 325-328; level, 671; upwards tendency of, 669-672, 674; *see also* Complexity of Ego, Localization of Ego
Ehrenfels, C. von, 559
Eidetic imagery, 212 n.
Eindringlichkeit, 113 n.
Einstein, A., 42
Eissler, K., 226, 227, 227 n., 229, 230, 231, 233, 234, 234 n., 235, 236
Elements, mental, 55, 104, 319, 360, 393, 401, 594, 682; of behaviour, 310
Embeddedness, 622, 623
Emmert, 212
Emmert's law, 212 n.
Emotion, 13, 325-327, 329, 335, 336, 340, 345, 362, 364, 368, 400-408, 410, 414-416, 527, 657-659, 661; cold, 415
Empathy, 326, 407
Emphasizing, *see* Pointing
Empirical depth criteria, 163
Empiricism, 155-160, 209, 210, 217, 218, 223, 224, 279, 305, 312, 421, 423, 519, 542, 627, 639
Enclosing and enclosed area, 192, 192 n., 202, 207, 259, 287, 311
Energy, 99, 102, 173, 174, 189, 193, 199, 199 n., 206, 237, 238, 375, 411, 412, 453, 571-573, 636, 642; direction of, 99, 573; density of, 189, 193, 194; liberation of, 99, 173, 573; release of, 375, 658
Engram, 424, 454, 493
Environment, 27, 28, 36, 40, 67, 72, 332, 646, 680, 681; *see also* Behavioural environment and Geographical environment
Environmental field, *see* Field, environmental
Epiphenomenon, 65
Episcotister, 143, 261-264
Equality, 164-167, 182, 268, 271, 301, 439, 440, 450, 453, 462-464, 654, 655; *see also* Similarity
Equilibrium, 309-311, 314, 316, 317, 331, 405, 415, 496, 498, 503, 639
Equivalent grey, 133
Error, 640, 641
Ethics, 668
Exactness of science, 9
Excitement, 339, 402, 414, 660
Executive, 342-345, 357, 363, 391, 400, 413, 526, 627; control of, 344, 354, 355, 363, 364, 366, 369, 372, 418, 575
Existence, 571, 614
Expectation, 398, 400
Experience, 33, 44, 85, 94, 100, 104, 105, 157, 160, 161, 163, 209, 210, 217, 223, 224, 280, 303, 305, 355, 356, 358, 360, 371, 372, 393, 421, 463, 474, 509, 510, 529, 556, 589, 602, 627, 629, 636, 637, 639 n., 645; experience, direct, *see* Direct experience
Experience error, 97, 98, 105, 159, 181, 209, 313

Explaining as opposed to understanding, 20, 21
External forces of organization, 138, 139, 141, 143, 145, 163, 171, 232, 449, 496
External relations, 570
Eye movements, 208, 222, 282, 304, 311-318, 373, 384-389, 626, 653; *see also* Roaming eyes

Factors of stroboscopic motion, 287, 292
Facts, 4, 5, 6, 9, 18, 55, 176
Factual connections, 55, 684
Factual sequence *vs.* causal connection, 20
Failure, 341, 670, 671
Familiarity, quality of, 550, 591, 592, 594, 596, 611
Familiarity of figures, 146, 147, 158
Familiarity of proverbs, 424
Faraday, M., 42
Fashion, 350, 674, 676
Fatigue, 100, 102, 173, 339, 339 n., 412, 413
Fear, 325, 344, 390, 402-405, 414, 415
Feeling, 11, 19
Feinberg, N., 144 n.
Fiat, 418
Field, 42, 47, 49-51, 58, 66, 67, 120, 344, 346, 353, 391, 400, 480, 510, 511, 513, 554, 567, 587, 632, 634, 637, 645, 653, 661; behavioural field, *see* Behavioural field; physiological field, *see* Physiological field; economic, 48; environmental, 69, 74, 113, 149, 178, 326, 344, 368, 421, 431, 583, 584, 594, 608, 610, 611, 636; physiological, 52, 53; psychological, 43, 46, 49, 51, 145; psychophysical, 67, 127, 198, 232, 266, 270, 317, 330, 331, 355, 356, 368, 373, 374, 376, 380, 402, 403, 435, 449, 529, 535, 537, 561, 627, 659, 680, 682; social, 664, 679; total, 149, 346, 361, 363, 368, 372, 375, 405, 409, 520, 521, 608, 642, 658, 663; trace, 448-451, 510, 511, 521, 522, 526, 528, 537, 550, 552-555, 563, 568, 587, 588, 601, 606-613; of vision, 203 (of hemianopics), 204 (reduced); of stress, 231, 353, 407, 409
Field action, *see* Action
Figural after-effect, 210
Figure (as opposed to ground), 166, 177, 183-211, 253, 269, 270, 272, 275, 275 n., 276, 283, 291, 311, 314, 472
Figuredness, degrees of, 193, 194, 200, 207, 311
Film colour, 114, 118
Firmness of separating walls, 340, 341, 409
First performance, 535, 538, 541, 553, 556
Fischer, A., 564
Fittingness, 569, 638-644
Fixation, 283, 285, 311-316, 318, 342, 343, 370, 389
Flicker, 130-132, 142, 187
Flight, 344, 366, 405
Flügel, J. C., 320
Fogelsonger, H. M., 603
Follower, 666-669
Food, 355, 356, 360, 363; aversions, 675
Force, 43, 44, 46-48, 50, 67, 72, 98, 100, 102, 117-119, 122, 127-129, 132-137, 153, 145, 147-150, 164, 165, 173, 175, 177, 184, 197-200, 231-234, 237, 266, 269, 270, 273, 274, 286, 315-321, 333, 334, 342, 344, 353, 355, 357-359, 363, 367, 371-375, 378-380, 383, 392, 395, 398, 402-414, 418-421, 439, 440, 449, 450, 467, 476, 496, 507, 508, 527, 535, 548, 560, 567, 568, 572, 574, 582-585, 595, 602, 622, 624, 626, 631, 634, 646, 658, 661, 673, 681; *see also* Attraction and Stress; of organization, 129, 138, 140, 161, 166, 206, 451, 631; *see also* External forces of organization and Internal forces of organization
Force diagrams, 391, 405
Forgetting, 420, 421, 516, 522-525, 527, 545, 548, 620, 621
Form, *see* Shape; geometrical, 138, 140; dynamic, 138
Forward acting inhibition, 481, 492, 493
Framework, 72, 177, 183-185, 201, 211-213, 215-219, 221, 222, 224, 255, 275, 282, 283, 304, 319, 348, 349, 351, 384, 386, 389-391, 674-677
Frank, H., 88, 92, 187, 198, 212, 237, 238, 238 n., 240
Freeman, E., 278
Frequency, 525, 579, 589; law of, 538-541, 551; *see also* Repetition
Frequency and normality, 221
Freshness, 100, 102
Freud, S., 331
Frey, M. von, 62
Fright, 364, 661
Frings, G., 603
Fuchs, W., 135, 146, 147, 158, 202, 203 f., 208 n., 261
Function of science, 9
Function and structure, 206, 207, 207 n., 208, 208 n., 314, 315, 375

Functional characters, 392-394, 522, 594, 638
Functionalism, 160
Fusion of double images, 273
Fusion of periodic excitations, 127, 130, 132, 142, 184 f., 296; *see also* Critical fusion frequency
Fusion of processes in motion, 285-287, 298-300, 302-304
Fusion of sensations and images, 105

Galli, A., 303
Gamma (γ) motion, 275 f.
Gaps, 497, 505
Gefügigkeitsqualität, 393 f.
Geisteswissenschaften, 18
Gelb, A., 118, 121, 122, 129, 150, 187 f., 205, 241, 245, 246, 247, 249, 250, 251, 252, 253, 276, 298, 438
General principle of action, 367
Geographical environment, 27-41, 45, 46, 48-50, 52, 61, 67, 69, 76, 78, 79, 122, 180, 309, 331, 347, 368, 369, 373, 375-377, 379, 381, 496, 533, 656, 680; *see also* Relation between geographical environment and behavioural environment
Gestalt, 22, 62, 174, 421, 496, 499, 526, 649, 650, 669, 677, 678, 682-684; strength of, 650; disposition, 514, 613; homology, 299, 300, 462; identity, 299; theory (psychology), 17, 18, 53, 66, 147, 179, 280, 403, 433, 457, 543, 549, 571, 600, 614, 628, 639, 679, 683-685
Gestaltqualität, 559
Gestures, 656, 661, 677
Ghosts, 70
Gibson, J. J., 493, 494, 495, 497, 498 n., 500, 502, 503, 504, 505
Goal-directedness, 311
Goal-objects, 391
Goethe, W. von, 143
Goldstein, K., 117, 317, 438
Good continuation, *see* Law of good continuation
Good shape, 141, 144, 151, 152, 155, 159, 171, 175, 209
Gorki, M., 383
Gottschaldt, K., 152, 155 f., 157, 158, 210, 395, 396 f., 398, 400, 602, 607, 609
Götz, W., 88, 356
Graded disks, 169 f.
Gradient in psychophysical field, 467, 476-480, 570, 666
Gradient of stimulation, 244, 245, 245 n., 246, 248-250, 252, 255, 259, 260, 264, 276, 291, 362; effective, 247, 248, 260
Graham, C. H., 191
Granit, A. R., 141, 142, 150, 187, 188, 193
Graz School, 559
Gregariousness, 662
Grin without the cat, 180, 443 n.
Ground, 166, 177, 183, 184, 186-211, 253, 256, 269, 275 n., 276, 283, 291, 311, 314, 469, 470; auditory, 201; temporal, 468, 470
Group (social), 422, 648, 649, 653, 665-667, 682; animal, 666, 668; behaviour, *see* Social behaviour; psychological, 649, 651, 652, 654, 655, 662-666, 668, 670, 671, 676; reality of psychological group, 651, 652; sociological, 649, 650, 652, 653, 664, 665, 668, 670, 676; reality of sociological group, 649, 652
Group formation, 165-167, 512, 565, 566, 654, 655, 661, 662, 669
Guilford, J. P., 213

Habit, 420, 421, 571, 574, 578; bad, 536, 536 n.; localized, 454, 456; non-localized, 454-456
Haeckel, E., 11
Handwriting, 678
Haphazard, 382
Hard colours, *see* Colours, hard
Harrower, M. R., 127, 128, 170, 171, 188 f., 190 n., 205, 249, 250, 251, 253, 276, 339, 340, 616, 617, 618, 619, 620 f., 620 n., 622, 623, 624, 625, 632, 634, 635, 637, 638, 640, 644
Hartgenbusch, H. G., 44, 45, 389
Hartmann, L., 129, 130, 131, 132, 142, 183, 184, 187, 286, 510, 511
Hazlitt, V., 172 n.
Head, H., 15, 100, 101, 102, 117, 173, 424 n., 438, 514, 515, 516, 517, 518, 519, 520
Heider, F., 74
Heider, G. M., 135, 136, 262 f., 263 n., 641
Heine, R., 492
Heiss, A., 638
Helmholtz, H. von, 170, 179, 270, 312
Helson, H., 144 n., 298
Hemianopsia, 146, 192, 202, 203
Hempstead, L., 143, 150
Heraclitus, 70, 71
Heredity, 332
Hering, E., 62, 63, 133, 137, 190, 212, 213, 214, 237, 241, 244, 245, 314, 385, 386, 429

Hertz, M., 168
Heterogeneous, *see* Tasks, heterogeneous
Hillebrand, F., 83, 386
Hirsch, J., 675
Höffding, H., 561, 582, 583, 594, 598
Holaday, B. E., 229, 230, 235, 236
Holes, 44, 45, 208-210
Hollingworth, H. L., 474, 476
Hollingworth, L., 667
Homogeneity of fields, 43, 150, 152, 281, 289, 323, 324
Homogeneity of stimulation, 110-113, 126, 141, 147, 177, 289, 434, 448, 631
Homogeneous tasks, *see* Tasks, homogeneous
Homology, gestalt, 299, 300, 462
Honzik, C. A., 586, 588
Hoppe, F., 414, 670, 671
Hormic theory, 416, 417
Hornbostel, E. M. von, 192, 208, 220, 220 n.
H-quotient, 242
Huang I, 379, 554 n., 644 n.
Hume, D., 378, 383
Humphrey, G., 308, 309, 312 n., 316, 333 n., 382, 424, 429, 441, 529, 530, 531, 532, 533, 534, 535, 536, 585
Humphrey's principle, 308, 316, 317, 332
Hunt, W. A., 415
Hunter, W. S., 491 n., 529 f., 555
Husserl, E., 570, 571
Hypnosis, 492, 527

Idealization of our youth, 522
Ideas, 332, 559, 614
Identical points, *see* Corresponding points
Identity, 285, 299, 300, 331, 332; gestalt, 299
Illumination, 169, 243, 248, 258, 277, 304
Illusion, 76, 79, 103; *see also* Optical illusion
Images, 103-105, 332, 393, 442, 592, 614
Impenetrability, 275, 305
Implication, 640, 640 n.
Impressiveness, 113, 189, 362
Improvement, 541, 553-555, 585, 600
Incompatibility, 346, 353
Incompleteness of Ego, 661-663; of figures, 327, 449; of jokes, 618-620, 622, 644; of tasks, 334-341, 525, 555 n., 619
Indifference, 353
Indifference point, 474
Individual, 650, 661
Individual differences, 30, 332, 633, 646, 675
Induction, 147, 148
Inertia, 291, 305
Infants, 88, 89
Inference by analogy, 407, 655, 659
Inherited, 100, 529, 544, 549; *see also* Innate
Inhibition, 482 n.; associative, 557, 558; *see also* Forward acting inhibition and Retroactive inhibition
Inhomogeneity of fields, 43, 44, 117, 281, 282, 324
Inhomogeneity of groups, 667, 668, 670
Inhomogeneity of stimulation, 116, 119, 120, 149, 150, 163, 169 f. (continuous change of stimulation), 262, 325, 376, 434, 447, 545, 651; *see also* Discontinuity of stimulation
Initial reproductive tendency, 567, 568
Innate, 163, 356, 403, 548, 549, 656; *see also* Inherited
Inside, 150, 151, 181, 184
Insight, 382, 383, 552, 628-631, 641; partial, 631, 641
Insistency, 113, 116, 362
Instability, 120 (of homogeneous space); 139, 143 (of very small figures), 148 (of points), 149 (do.), 389 (of framework), 390 (do.)
Instinct, 67, 355, 356, 361, 403-406, 416-418, 520, 656, 662, 668
Insufficiency of behavioural field, 46, 49 f., 52, 67
Integration (as a task of science), 10, 13, 17, 21, 174, 571, 614, 683, 684
Intrinsic relation, 569-571, 625, 631
Intellect, 8, 417
Intellectualism, 416, 417, 420
Intelligence, 13, 509, 627, 646
Intensity, 122 (distance dependent upon), 128 (and organization), 129 (do.), 134 (in contrast); low, 141-143; *see also* Constancy of intensity
Intentions, 341, 342, 354, 355, 357, 418-420, 534, 563, 572, 579, 583, 584, 588
Interaction of traces and process, *see* Trace, interaction of traces and process
Interactionism, 47
Interests, 102, 197, 313, 343, 519-521, 526, 535, 596, 610
Internal contrast, 133
Internal forces of organization, 138-145, 162, 163, 206, 232, 377, 396-398, 400, 449, 496
Interpretation hypothesis, 86-90, 94-96, 103, 105, 224; *see also* Meaning theory
Interruption of tasks, 334-338
Introspection, 73, 319

Invariants, 218, 219, 221, 224, 229, 255, 283; of colour, 255; of motion, 283, 384, 387-389; of shape, 222, 223, 233, 233 n.; of size, 222, 236; of whiteness, 244
Involuntary action, *see* Action, involuntary
Irregularity, 139, 141, 144, 159, 168, 496, 497
Irritability, 402, 658, 660
Isolated material, 483-485, 487, 488, 491, 507, 508, 545, 570, 599, 603, 605, 666
Isolation of persons, 667
Isolation of systems, 339, 341, 409, 417, 587, 633
Isomorphism, 56, 62-66, 109, 305, 324, 381-383, 402, 614, 684

Jackson, H., 424
Jacobs, M. H., 477, 480
Jaensch, E. R., 85, 86, 237, 241, 249, 250, 250 n., 254, 255, 255 n., 260, 272, 276, 277, 278, 641
James, W., 401
James-Lange theory, 179, 401, 414
Jastrow illusion, 32, 33, 90, 295, 346
Jenkins, J. G., 136 f., 341, 491, 492
Jokes, 616-623; diagrams, 619-622, 632; pattern, 617; incomplete and unfinished, *see* Incompleteness of jokes; *see also* Completion of jokes
Jost's law, 589
Judgment, 85-87
Jung, C. G., 331

Kant, I., 305, 549
Kantor, J. R., 375
Kardos, L., 234, 237, 244 n., 248, 259
Kármán, T. von, 428 n.
Karsten, A., 407, 410 f., 413
Katz, D., 234 n., 239, 241, 242, 243, 248, 249, 254, 259, 497, 500, 655, 661, 669
Katzaroff, D., 592, 593, 594
Kenkel, F., 275
King, S., 298
Kirchhoff's law, 107
Klages, L., 657
Klimpfinger, S., 226, 227, 229, 233, 235, 236, 238, 239
Klüver, H., 19 n.
Knee jerk, 310, 333
Knowledge, 454 n., 625, 630, 637, 642-644
Knowledge of behaviour, 39
Koffka, K., 22, 34 n., 59, 66 n., 73, 115, 127, 128, 137, 159, 169, 170, 171, 188 f., 190, 205, 210, 212 n., 215 n., 217, 245, 245 n., 249, 250, 251, 251 n., 253, 255, 255 n., 258, 259, 259 n., 266, 271, 281, 282, 293, 295, 296, 310, 332, 360, 437, 440 n., 458 n., 467, 474, 510, 511, 514, 518, 529, 548, 552, 560 n., 562, 563, 612 n., 613, 628, 638, 647, 664 n.
Köhler, W., 35, 39, 53, 57, 61, 62, 63, 64, 73, 77, 85, 86, 87, 88, 89, 98, 108, 109, 116, 126, 155, 159, 164, 167, 168, 168 n., 173, 174, 179 n., 186, 193, 198, 207, 237, 281, 286, 286 n., 298, 312 n., 315, 315 n., 318, 321, 322, 329, 346, 359, 361, 373, 374 n., 375, 376, 379 n., 382, 383, 388 f., 394, 395, 400, 402, 413, 441, 441 n., 446, 451 n., 458, 465, 465 n., 466, 466 n., 467, 468, 470, 473, 476, 477, 479, 480, 481, 508, 530, 536, 537, 543, 550, 551, 557, 561, 584, 597, 599, 603, 628, 635, 636, 638, 643, 650, 655, 656, 657, 665, 666, 682, 684
Kopfermann, H., 152, 153 f., 159, 162, 181, 184 f.
Korsakoff syndrome, 593, 596, 597, 603
Korte, A., 292, 293, 294, 294 n., 296
Korte's laws, 291-296
Koster phenomenon, 277
Kreezer, G., 509
Kries, J. von, 54, 55, 460, 461, 463, 464
Kroh, O., 259 n.
Külpe, O., 559

Lake Cayuga, 217, 218, 221
Lammer, E. G., 323, 327, 330
Language, 422, 454 n., 524, 534, 632, 675, 676
Lashley, K. S., 55, 454, 454 n., 455, 456, 457, 529, 530, 531, 546
Latent attitudes, 563
Latent learning, 555
Latent learning (Tolman), 547, 588
Lauenstein, O., 236, 236 n., 441 f., 441 n., 451, 452, 453, 465, 465 n., 466, 468, 469, 470, 471, 472, 473, 474, 475, 477, 478, 479, 480, 481, 501, 502, 524
Law of assimilation, *see* Law of substitution
Law of association, *see* Association, law of
Law of closure, *see* Closure
Law of contiguity, *see* Contiguity
Law of contrast, *see* Contrast, law of
Law of effect, *see* Success, law of
Law of equality, *see* Equality
Law of exercise, *see* Frequency, law of
Law of fittingness, *see* Fittingness

Law of frequency, *see* Frequency, law of
Law of good continuation, 153, 155, 159, 168, 168 n., 171, 175, 209, 302, 332, 376, 434, 437, 448-451, 464, 545, 553, 569, 605, 607, 638, 639
Law of good shape, *see* Good shape
Law of prägnanz, 110, 138, 151, 171, 174, 195, 197, 312, 682
Law of proximity, *see* Proximity
Law of recency, *see* Recency, law of
Law of reproduction, *see* Reproduction, law of
Law of similarity, *see* Similarity
Law of the simplest path, 301
Law of size, 191-193
Law of stability, *see* Stability, law of
Law of substitution, 583
Law of success, *see* Success, law of
Law of transposition (Brown), 289, 291, 297
Laws of organization, *see* Organization, laws of
Leadership, 666-670
Leakage, 341
Learning, 209, 354, 371, 372, 414, 421, 422, 455, 456, 460, 481, 482, 484, 491, 492, 505, 508, 509, 529-543, 544 (defined), 546-549, 552, 553, 555-558, 561, 564-566, 570, 581, 585, 625, 627, 644, 645, 681; curve, *see* Practice curve
Legibility experiments, 189
Lemur, 279
Letter box example, 345, 354, 357
Letter example, 333, 334, 342-344
Level, colour, 256; *see also* Neutral level and Shift of level; general, 350; space, 185 n., 285; of aspiration, 671, 672; *see also* Personal standard
Levels of science, 49, 632
Levelling, 498
Lévy-Bruhl, L., 46
Lewin, K., 44, 46, 47, 48, 266, 272, 333, 333 n., 334, 342 n., 345, 353, 354, 391, 405, 407, 414, 416, 417, 418, 419, 420, 521, 561, 562, 571, 572, 573, 574, 578, 579 f., 579 n., 582, 583, 584, 587, 602, 603, 608, 610, 611, 611 n.
Liberation of energy, 99, 173, 573; *see also* Release of energy
Liebmann, S., 126, 127
Liebmann effect, 126-128, 171, 188
Life, 10, 12, 13, 17, 22, 174, 423, 684; nature problem, 13
Lifted weights, 465, 467, 471, 476
Lindemann, E., 141, 142, 276
Lindworsky, J., 378
Line-horopter, 267 n.
Lines, 148, 150, 151
Lipmann, O., 638, 644
Living things, 70, 72
Localization, 212-214, 218, 265, 276, 298, 384, 388, 463, 675; absolute, 218; relative, 218; of Ego, 216, 217, 219, 221; of sound, 220 f., 313; of touch, 517
Local sign, 117
Local stimulation, 96, 97, 110, 170, 192, 214, 223, 227, 244, 244 n., 379; *see also* Stimuli, proximal
Locus of an excitation, 54
Logic, 570, 571, 614, 631, 632, 642, 668, 684
Löwenfeld, B., 313

Maccurdy, J. T., 207 n., 591, 591 n., 593, 594, 596
McDougall, K., 644
McDougall, W., 25, 319, 355, 356, 401, 403, 404, 405, 406, 416, 417, 419, 644, 662, 663, 679
Mach, E., 62, 63, 108, 169, 170, 171
Mach rings, 170, 171, 447
Machine, 403
MacLeod, R. B., 241
Maier, N. R. F., 627, 631, 637, 641 n., 643, 644
Main directions of space, *see* Directions
Manifest organization, *see* Organization, manifest
Manipulanda, 30, 31
Manners, 350, 409
Marañon, G., 415
Marina, A., 313
Martius, G., 91, 241
Mass reflex, 101
Materialism, 11-13, 17, 19, 64, 65, 383
Matter, 11, 12
Maximum-minimum properties, 107-109, 116, 117, 171-174, 311, 342, 549
Maxwell, C., 42
Maze experiments, 454, 539, 540, 546-548, 585, 586
Maze habits, 454-456, 548, 551
Meaning, 13, 19-21, 26, 38, 86, 96, 163, 174, 176, 307, 309-311, 382, 383, 552, 614, 625; *see also* Significance
Meaningful material, 482, 557, 558, 569, 570
Meaningless material, 522, 557, 558, 569, 570
Meaning theory, 85, 86, 88, 89, 94; *see also* Interpretation hypothesis
Measure of constancy, 226, 227, 234, 234 n., 238, 242
Measurement of will, 574

Mechanism, 21, 308, 314, 331, 404, 417, 631
Medium, 98, 99, 109
Melody, 327, 431-438, 448, 450, 460, 510, 515, 516, 516 n., 533, 553, 649; transposition of, 460, 510
Memory, 51, 241, 305, 332, 333, 335, 336, 384, 393, 420, 421, 423, 424, 428, 429, 431, 438, 452-454, 459, 460, 464, 474, 482, 486, 488, 493, 506, 513, 517, 519-521, 524, 530-532, 538, 541, 557, 590, 598, 612, 625, 679, 681; in physics, 428, 458; spatial and temporal compared, 446; functions of, 461, 462, 482, 506, 509, 681; colour, 241, 241 n.
Me-ness, feeling of, 593, 594
Mental chemistry, 124
Mental development, 332, 542
Mental elements, *see* Elements, mental
Mental nearness, 666, 667
Mental permanence, 333
Metaphysics, 18, 416, 683, 684
Metzger, W., 111, 113, 114, 116, 118, 119, 121, 122, 123, 124, 129, 296, 298, 301, 302, 303, 468
Meyer, H., 134
Micropsia, 237, 277, 278
Microstructure of stimulus, 114-117, 119, 122, 123, 125, 129
Mikesell, W. H., 136 f.
Mind, 10, 12, 13, 21, 22, 25, 47, 48, 174, 175, 423, 631, 682, 684; body problem, 13, 47, 67, 436
Mind of the other person, 361, 407, 655-659
Mintz, A., 128, 253, 477, 480, 586
Mirror world, 215, 216
Model of ourselves, 515-517, 519
Molar behaviour, 25-27, 30, 41, 52, 56, 58, 59, 65, 66, 374, 375
Molar theory of physiological processes, 56, 58, 60, 63, 64
Molecular behaviour, 25-27, 52, 65, 374, 375
Molecular theory of physiological processes, 55, 56, 63, 64
Monochromatic illumination, 257
Monotonous series, 482, 484, 491, 504, 507, 516, 570
Moon, 78, 81, 94, 95, 279, 285
Morals, 350, 409, 688
Moral sciences, 18, 26
Mosaic of stimulation, 75, 84, 97, 98, 105, 209, 659
Motion, 78, 84, 179, 219, 276, 277, 280-304, 318, 319, 370-372, 380, 381, 384, 386-389, 435, 438, 451, 510-512, 681; acoustic, 281 n., 303; induced, 282 f., 287, 318, 384, 389; intersensory, 303 f.; "real," 281, 286, 288, 295, 298; stroboscopic, 281, 286-288, 291-295, 298-301, 303, 371, 372; dual, 287; partial, 287; singular, 287; *see also* factors of; tactual, 281 n., 303; direction of, 276, 288, 510; as characteristic of things, 71, 72
Motor of events, 571-573, 579, 584, 602
Mountain railway, 217, 218, 224, 228
Movements of fusion, 315
Movements of limbs and the body, 67, 208, 217, 222, 342-344, 371, 373, 374, 384, 386, 413, 514, 515, 517, 626, 628 n., 653, 656, 658, 681
Müller, E. A., 249, 250, 250 n., 253
Müller, G. E., 62, 63, 113, 215 n., 219, 491, 500, 508, 525, 543, 567, 568, 583
Multiple response principle, 544
Multum non multa, 5, 6

Nativism, 160, 312, 316
Nature, 10, 12, 13, 16, 17, 174, 175, 423, 684
Nearness and clearness, 277, 278
Needs, 102, 325, 327, 329, 342, 344, 345, 354-358, 360, 364, 368, 382, 391, 392, 394, 395, 419, 421, 571-573, 588, 625, 627, 662
Neurones, 55, 310; *see also* Connections of neurones
Neurotic symptoms, 344
Neutral level, principle of, 255, 256, 258
Newman, E. B., 276, 276 n.
Newton, I., 41, 42, 281 n., 451
Noll, A., 212 n.
Non-noticed, 85-87, 105, 149, 398
Nonsense syllables, 481-484, 490-492, 507, 508, 543, 544, 557, 560-566, 569, 570, 574-578, 585, 589
Non-silent organization, *see* Organization, non-silent
Normal distance, 236
Normality of framework, 221, 222
Normality and frequency, 221, 222, 503
Normalizing, 498, 499, 501, 502
Not-things, 70-72, 177, 185, 186 f.
Nuclear plane, 266-269

Object-Ego relation, *see* Ego-field relation
Objections to trace hypothesis, 452-464
Objective standards, 347, 348, 351
Objects, 175, 217, 285, 324, 329, 344-347, 358, 359, 363, 373, 391, 392, 595, 610, 643, 654
Ocular system, 285

Oculomotor system, 311, 316, 370, 373, 387-389
Ogden, R. M., 628 n., 647
One-sided function of contour, *see* Contour
Oppenheimer, E., 276, 283, 290
Optical illusions, 78, 212, 275, 510, 641
Order, 13, 15-17, 22, 174, 175, 307, 309-312, 316, 355, 474, 519, 559, 560, 588, 684
Organism, 48, 308-310, 331-333, 346, 365, 368, 369, 372, 373, 401, 424, 514, 520, 530, 535, 536, 541, 548, 549, 626, 627, 646, 648, 664
Organization (general), 67, 99, 100, 105, 107, 110, 174, 176, 266, 269, 314, 317, 376, 381, 393-395, 401, 402, 417, 419, 431, 437-439, 441, 464, 496, 512, 514, 519, 520, 549, 550, 564, 567, 569, 570, 571, 578, 594, 598, 599, 601, 604, 612, 625, 628, 632, 642, 646, 647, 653, 654, 657, 663-665, 670, 677, 681, 682; *see also* Duo organization and Unum organization; ideational, 569, 632, 640-642; manifest, 357, 381-384, 402, 404, 421; *see also* non-silent; non-silent, 317, 352-354, 403; perceptual, 98, 106, 110, 211, 230, 240, 269, 296, 300, 304, 305, 318, 342, 343, 352, 360, 361, 365, 375, 398, 400, 477, 488, 513, 524, 554, 569, 584, 598, 631, 632, 681; *see also* spatial; physical, 107; sensory, *see* perceptual; silent, 317, 318, 346, 357, 381, 382, 384, 402; spatial, 117, 118, 120, 121, 125, 127, 136-155, 159, 161, 164, 165, 167, 167 n., 168, 171, 173, 179, 183, 184, 188, 190-193, 195, 196, 198-200, 205-210, 215, 216, 231, 235, 236, 253, 260-266, 271, 273, 274, 276, 311, 315, 332, 434, 438, 439, 447, 448, 453, 462, 464, 482, 486, 531, 639, 640, 658, 659; temporal, 433, 434, 437-439, 447, 659; trimensional, 159-164, 178, 200, 265, 266; of Ego systems, 342, 633; of traces, 339, 340, 449, 450 n., 453, 461, 463, 474, 488, 491, 493, 517, 519, 520, 544, 563, 564, 566, 572, 582, 584, 605, 621, 622; laws of, 158, 159, 164, 175, 177, 193, 301-303, 305, 323, 392, 421, 451, 464, 482, 488, 489, 493, 496, 545, 549, 632, 640, 654, 682
Orientation, 184, 185, 190 f., 224, 228-230, 232-235, 255, 265, 275 n., 288, 290, 304, 319; normal, 221, 224, 230, 231, 236, 255
Other person's emotions, *see* Mind of the other person
Outside, 150, 151, 181, 184
Over-estimation of the vertical, 213, 275, 276, 276 n.
Overlapping of contours, 163, 274
Ovsiankina, M., 337

Pain, 325, 327, 328, 414
Paired associates, 483, 490, 560-562, 575, 589, 623
Pairs, learning of, 564-566, 569
Paranoia, 665
Paresis of eye muscle, 386-389
Part and whole, 26, 176, 569, 601, 602, 665, 682
Pecking list, 668, 669
Perception, 78, 85, 88-90, 103, 105, 110, 148, 172, 305, 366, 393, 400, 452, 482, 486, 488, 489, 506, 507, 510, 573, 588, 599, 632, 633, 679
Perceptual constancies, 34; *see also* Constancy
Performance (or process) *vs.* accomplishment, 530, 537-540, 552, 564, 580
Perimetric test, 204, 205
Periphery of retina, 146, 201, 202, 204-208, 315
Perkins, F. J., 61, 454, 457 f., 458 n., 459, 460, 493, 494, 495, 495 n., 496, 497, 498, 499, 526
Permeability, 101, 102
Persistence through time, 332, 333, 448
Personality, 67, 331, 419, 676-679, 682
Personal standard, 341; *see also* Level of aspiration
Persons, 655, 657, 661, 667
Perspective, 79, 280
Perspective drawings, 161
Phantom limb, 517
Phenomenal regression to the real object, 225, 226, 233, 243, 250, 251
Phenomenology, 73
Philosophy, 4, 6, 11, 12, 20, 48, 378, 383, 416, 417, 423, 614, 684, 685
Phylogenetic series, 310
Physics as a molar science, 57
Physiognomic characters, 359-363, 365, 382, 392, 407, 594, 654-658, 660, 677, 678
Physiological correlates, 62, 65, 298 (of time)
Physiological field, 52, 53, 63, 69
Physiological changes in emotions, 401, 414-416
Physiological pattern, 58, 59, 316 n.
Physiological theories, 84, 97; *see also*

Molar and Molecular physiological theories
Physiology, 26, 52
Piaget, J., 46, 379, 670
Picture on the photographic plate, 74, 75, 98
Picture on the retina, 75, 98
Pilzecker, A., 491, 567, 568, 583
Pleasure, 19, 325, 327, 552
Pointing, 498-501
Points, 148-150, 394, 400, 447
Point-to-point correspondence between stimulation and the looks of things, 84, 87
Poppelreuter, W., 146
Positivism, 17, 18, 21, 22, 222, 379, 380, 383, 639, 684, 685
Posture, 389-391, 514-517
Practice, 536-538, 541, 546, 553, 571, 586; curves, 553, 556; *see also* Repetition
Prägnanz, *see* Law of prägnanz
Pratt, C. C., 470, 471, 472
Present, 424, 433-436, 448
Primary retentiveness, 432, 433, 435, 438
Primitive people, 360, 650
Principle of the neutral level, *see* Neutral level
Principle of the shift of level, *see* Shift of level
Problem of achievement, 541-544, 547, 553, 556, 627
"Problem of memory," 541
Problem solution, 461, 625, 626, 630, 631, 633, 634, 636-643
Process in extension, 59, 60, 62, 63, 97, 110, 115
Products of social activity, 653, 674-676, 679
Production (Graz School), 559
Pronouncedness, 243
Propensities, 662-664, 668
Proper perception, 347, 348, 351, 352
Proximal stimulus, *see* Stimuli, proximal
Proximity, 149, 164-167, 270, 273, 299, 301, 315, 329, 462, 464, 481, 482, 489, 493, 513, 558, 569, 570, 599, 605
Pseudofovea, 202
Psychoanalysis, 50, 51, 331, 670
Psychological group, *see* Group, psychological
Psychologismus, 570, 571
Psychology, 3, 4, 6, 10, 13, 15, 19-22, 24, 26, 27, 35, 49, 53, 174, 306, 332, 379, 570, 571, 614, 668; experimental, 18, 19; definitions of, 25; task of, 67 f.; without consciousness, 35
Pugnacity, 364-366
Pupillary reaction, 241, 310
Purpose, 522
Purposiveness, 311, 355, 404, 559
Pursuit (eye movements of), 311, 313, 314, 318
Puzzle box experiments, 548, 551, 552
Puzzle pictures, 83, 343, 352

Quadratic equation, solution of, 629, 630, 633, 634, 641
Quality, 13, 14, 21, 22, 108, 174, 175
Quantity, 13, 14, 21, 22, 108, 174, 175
Quasi-needs, 342, 355, 357, 368, 395, 411, 572, 573, 609
Quasi-stationary processes, 108
Q-quotient, 234 n., 242

Random movements and behaviour, 625, 629, 645
Rationality of science, 6
Rats, 356, 454, 455, 546, 547, 586, 587, 644
Reading, 317, 318
Reality, 33, 35
Reality of shape, 129 f., 132, 137, 138, 379
Recall, 337, 338, 340, 461, 463, 481, 484, 485, 488-492, 494, 506-508, 521, 522, 524, 525, 545, 584, 593, 594, 597, 603, 604, 612, 613, 618-621, 624, 625, 629, 630, 644; *see also* Reproduction
Recency, 525, 541, 599, 618; law of, 551
Recognition, 444, 460, 461, 463, 481, 485, 492, 494, 495, 497, 506, 515-517, 550, 561, 562, 591-598, 600-604, 608, 610, 611, 611 n., 613, 621, 681; spontaneous, 610, 611
Reduction screen, 242, 248, 256, 257, 261, 262
Reflex, 50, 55, 58, 310, 311, 313, 314, 316, 317, 355, 362, 369; tonic, 317, 369, 370, 371; arc, 310, 316, 317, 344, 626
Regulation of behaviour, 28, 31, 37, 40, 44, 369, 588, 634
Regularity, 109, 110, 167
Reification, 401, 403, 416, 424
Relation between behavioural and physiological field, 53
Relation between geographical and behavioural environment, 46, 49, 69, 78
Relation between retinal and phenomenal lines, 214-216
Relation, new, learning of, 509, 510, 513, 559, 612

Relations of stimulation, 134 (as determining contrast)
Relative properties of parts, 666; of stimuli, 219, 221, 365; of traces, 502
Relativism, 347, 351
Release of energy, 375, 658; *see also* Liberation of energy
Relief of stresses, 342-344, 366, 367, 373, 409, 411, 419, 420, 662
Religion, 8
Remembering, 336, 337, 488, 517, 637
Reorganization, 646, 647; in perception, 506, 507, 524, 643, 644; in thinking, 627, 628, 631, 634, 636-638, 643-645; of social field, 665
Repeated material, 483, 484, 487, 488, 490, 492, 524, 570, 599, 603, 666
Repetition, 396, 397, 410, 456, 508, 531-534, 536, 536 n., 537-551, 554-556, 590
Representation without colour, 178 f., 181
Reproduction, 104, 460, 463, 494, 495, 506, 513, 515, 516, 556, 560-568, 571, 573, 575, 581-584, 587, 589, 598, 605, 611-613, 624, 634; automatic (spontaneous), 572-574, 584, 587, 588, 596, 602, 607, 613; of designs, 493, 497, 501-504, 526; of opposites, 605; law of, 566-568; *see also* Recall
Repulsiveness, 353, 355, 392
Resolves, 355, 368, 572
Restless activity, 414
Restorff, H. von, 452, 453, 463 n., 481, 482, 483, 484, 485, 486, 487, 488, 489, 490, 491, 492, 501, 502, 504, 505, 507, 508, 516, 524, 526, 544, 546, 569, 570, 592, 597, 599, 603, 666, 667
Results of behaviour, 306, 307, 309
Results of social activity, *see* Products of social activity
Resumption of tasks, 337
Retained members, 484, 486
Retention, 484, 485
Retina, 139, 145, 208, 212, 214, 215, 244, 246, 312-314, 377, 387, 659, 660; *see also* Centre of retina and Periphery of retina
Retinal correspondence, 267, 268, 272; *see also* Corresponding points
Retinal disparity, 160, 212, 235, 236, 266-268, 270, 272, 274, 315; *see also* Binocular parallax and Disparate points
Retinal elements, 311
Retinal horizon, 111
Retinal image, 198, 199, 209, 217, 222-224, 235, 238, 238 n., 261, 277, 278, 288, 384, 385, 659; of an after-image, 198, 199; *see also* Picture on the retina
Retinal points, 370, 385, 386
Retroactive inhibition, 341, 481, 490-492, 505
Reversible perspective, 83
Révész, G., 32, 33, 34, 90
Rhythm, 431-434, 437, 438, 441, 508, 564, 565, 569
Rigidity, 633, 646
Rilke, R. M., 360
Roaming eyes, 313, 314
Robinson, E. S., 491, 558, 558 n., 583
Roelofs, C. O., 281, 286 n.
Rods, 201, 208
Rote learning, 543, 548, 560, 561, 564
Rothschild, H., 143 f., 198
Rubin, E., 177, 181, 183, 186, 190, 192, 195, 210, 260 n., 283, 284, 318, 377
Rutherford, E., 57, 57 n.

Sakuma, K., 266, 272
Sapir, E., 675, 676
Saturation (of activity), 410-414; range, 413, 414
Saturation (of colour), 253, 254, 497, 498
Saving method, 589
Scheerer, M., 15 n.
Scheler, M., 12, 360
Schema (Head), 515-517, 519, 520, 612
Schiller, P. von, 277, 298, 300, 301, 303
Schjelderup-Ebbe, T., 665, 668, 669
Scholz, W., 286 f., 315 n.
Schriever, W., 274
Schulte, H., 665
Schumann, F., 592, 598
Schumann tachistoscope, 130
Schur, E., 91, 94, 95
Science, 5-9, 11, 18, 20-23, 49, 307, 347, 378, 383, 648, 685; and conduct, 7; and religion, 8; function of, 9
Sea charts, 194
Search for a name, 525, 584
Seeing (two meanings), 180
Segregation, 98, 125, 126, 128, 129, 137, 147, 151, 152, 165, 171, 175, 177, 181, 191, 199, 200, 202, 208, 209, 275, 276, 285, 313, 319-321, 323-325, 328, 331, 333, 346, 348, 362, 376, 434, 437, 439, 443, 447, 449, 453, 507, 514, 545, 594, 632, 659, 665, 666, 667
Selection of facts, 8, 61, 380
Selection of co-operating retinal points,

270, 272; of process in motion, 298-302; of tool, 638, 642; of trace by process, 436, 437, 448, 450, 461-464, 513, 532, 533, 583, 598-607, 615-618
Self, 47, 319, 324, 325, 341, 342, 366, 409, 520, 672, 679; *see also* Ego
Selz, O., 560, 560 n.
Semon, R., 598, 598 n.
Sensation, 13, 19, 55, 67, 73, 85, 88-90, 96, 103-105, 124, 224, 266, 310, 318, 319, 360, 393, 394, 398, 435, 542, 543, 559, 592
Sense of colour, 365; of motion, 365; of shape, 365; of space, 365
Sense modalities and space, 303
Sense organs, 74
Sentence, 433, 434, 437
Sentiments, 368, 400
Separation of Ego and environment, 361, 363, 420
Set, 300, 303, 579-584, 607, 610, 613
Shadows, 163, 274; coloured, 258, 259
Shape, 125, 132-139, 142, 147, 148, 150, 152, 156-161, 167, 168, 170, 175, 177, 181, 183, 185, 202, 205, 206, 209, 211, 216, 219, 222, 232, 233, 235, 265, 273, 283, 301, 303, 304, 319, 357, 359, 379, 437, 438, 443, 449, 463, 559, 569, 632, 656, 659, 681; reality of, 129 f., 132, 137, 138, 379; as characteristic of things, 71, 72; *see also* Good shape and Constancy of shape
Sharpening, 498
Shell shock, 374
Shepard, G. F., 603
Sherrington, C. S., 100, 415, 416 n.
Shift of level, principle of, 255, 256, 258
Short time of exposure, 141, 142
Sign, 160, 391
Sign-gestalt, 391
Signs of distance, 160
Signals, 357, 358, 360, 382, 391
Significance, 13, 17, 19, 21, 26, 174-176, 614, 677, 684; *see also* Meaning
Silent organization, *see* Organization, silent
Similarity, 474, 481, 485, 486, 488-491, 491 n., 493, 583, 598-604, 607, 654, 655, 661, 662; association by, 542; *see also* Equality
Simplicity, 109, 110, 131, 138, 141, 142, 146, 147, 151, 157, 158, 168, 171, 185-187, 195-197, 224, 231; of maximum event, 109, 171-174, 199, 454; of minimum event, 109, 171-174, 199, 453
Simultaneity, 292
Sinemus, A., 277
Sinn, 13
Size, 77, 78, 80, 81, 84, 191, 193, 200, 211, 222, 229, 237, 265, 273, 276-279, 288, 289, 291, 303, 346, 389, 463, 497, 499, 500, 502, 681; small, 141, 143; range of, 237; *see also* Constancy of size, Law of size
Skill, acquisition of, 424, 461, 506, 510, 513, 536, 541, 545, 548, 553-556, 562, 590, 600
Sleep, 492
Soap bubble, 14, 107
Social behaviour, 414, 422, 653, 655, 664, 674, 682
Social psychology, 648, 663, 667, 669, 682
Social relations, 410
Society, 58, 422, 648; sacred and secular, 650; *see also* Groups (social)
Sociological group, *see* Group sociological
Soft colours, *see* Colours, soft
Somatic data, 324, 325
Soul, 47, 319, 332
Space (phenomenal), 119, 121, 275, 298, 303, 304, 322, 390; dynamic theory of, 119, 237; level, 185 n., 285; perception, 160, 212, 681; sensations, 215; values, 212, 213, 385-387; *see also* Tridimensional space
Space-time, 424, 530-532
Spatialization of time, 431, 446, 452
Spearman, C. E., 613
Speculative hypotheses, 464
Spinal cord, 317
Splitting up of colour, 262, 264
Spontaneous reproduction, *see* Reproduction, automatic (spontaneous)
Sport, 44
Stability, 138, 139, 143, 151, 152, 164, 167, 183, 194, 199, 207, 212, 274, 282, 304, 311, 316, 330-332, 349, 352, 368, 389, 390, 402, 503, 507-509, 526, 537, 544, 545, 554-556, 563, 566-570, 578, 587, 598-601, 604, 605, 646, 665, 676, 683; of a trace, 339, 340; law of, 598-600
Stages of motion, 292
Stationary distributions, 107-109
Steering, 316, 375, 658
Steinig, K., 301
Stepwise phenomenon, 467, 473
Stereoscope, 161, 162, 267-274
Stern, A., 144 n., 510
Stern, W., 679
Stillness, 201, 470
Stimuli, 27, 29, 33, 35, 75, 79-81, 84, 98, 115, 155, 170, 175, 204, 209, 310,

311, 313, 314, 352, 355, 359, 379, 398, 433, 434, 448, 449, 496, 549, 597, 601, 614, 632, 639, 657; distant, 80, 97, 224, 225, 228, 242, 267, 288, 373, 374, 659, 680; proximal, 80, 82-86, 89, 96-98, 100, 104-106, 114, 117, 126, 129, 208, 210, 224, 225, 228, 232, 240, 242, 244, 244 n., 246, 248, 267, 268, 288, 373, 374, 376, 377, 379, 384, 548, 658-660, 680; *see also* Local stimulation
Stimulus-response, 26, 32, 34, 50, 310, 313, 333, 334, 356, 362, 369, 370, 421
Store house (of traces), 518
Stout, G. F., 56, 358, 432, 433, 435, 436, 437, 440, 441, 448, 450, 451
Stream of consciousness, 332
Stresemann, E., 655
Stress, 270, 273, 275, 281, 342-345, 354, 374, 443, 463, 496, 497, 499, 503, 508, 522, 525, 555, 571-573, 598, 603, 609, 616, 622, 625, 637, 638, 641, 643, 644, 653, 661, 674; *see also* Field of stress and Relief of stress
Stresses, Ego, 354-356, 363, 366, 367, 412, 414, 415, 418, 527, 595, 658, 662, 663; Ego-field or object, 344, 345, 353, 355, 357, 363, 364, 382, 388, 394, 395, 398, 405, 418, 527, 595-597, 618, 627, 636, 642, 655, 662; field, 366, 373, 418, 527, 595, 618
Structuralism, 401
Structure and function, 206, 207, 207 n., 208, 208 n., 314, 315, 375
Structure of the nervous system, 100, 633
Stumpf, C., 84, 87, 394 n.
Style, 350, 676
Subconscious, 51, 52
Subliminal differences, 140
Submission, 662, 668, 669
Subsistence, 570, 571, 614
Substance, 57, 58, 72
Sub-systems, 331, 333, 338-342, 355, 366, 389, 417, 421, 431, 520, 521, 595, 638, 624, 679
Success, 414, 540, 551, 644, 645, 670, 671; law of, 544, 551, 552, 644, 645
Succession, 292
Summative, 134 (contrast as summative), 186, 188, 259 (contrast)
Superconstancy, 227, 234
Surfaces, 118, 119, 252
Surveyability, 237
Survival value of different organizations, 507, 508, 523, 524, 555, 622
Symbolic functions, 422
Symmetry, 109, 110, 139, 152, 159, 195, 196, 312, 379, 498-500, 505, 526, 578, 683
Systems of localization, 219; of reference, separation of, 284

Talbot's law, 127-129, 261
Tasks, heterogeneous, 578; homogeneous, 578
Taste, 348, 352
Teleological explanation, 599, 600
Temporal course of stimulation, 120, 216, 377
Temporal reference of ideas, 614
Temporal unity, *see* Unity, temporal
Tension, 330, 334, 337-344, 354, 355, 362, 363, 374, 402, 403, 405, 406, 410, 411, 414, 415, 463, 533, 572, 584, 585, 587, 596, 609, 626, 627, 672; persistence of, 340
Ternus, J., 298, 299, 300, 303
Thelin, E., 283
Theories, 4, 5, 9, 55
Thingness, 71, 275, 304
Things, 44, 45, 70-72, 177, 184-187, 208-211, 275, 282, 283, 304, 305, 314, 319, 353, 401, 681
Thinking, 7, 11, 341, 342, 400, 422, 527, 551, 552, 614, 625, 627, 632, 638, 640, 679, 682
Thorndike, E. L., 539, 543, 544, 551, 552, 645
Thoughts, 326, 327, 329, 342, 343, 384, 510, 559, 605, 607, 614, 626-628, 628 n., 631, 632, 639, 642, 643, 684; form or shape of processes, 616
Thouless, R. H., 171, 223, 225, 226, 226 n., 233, 234 f., 234 n., 240, 243, 251, 389, 390
Three-dimensional, *see* Tri-dimensional
Threshold, 150, 188, 193, 253, 279, 282, 291, 449, 524
Time, 296-298, 328, 331, 332, 340, 348, 350, 377, 424-427, 433, 437, 439, 479, 531, 532; filled, 298; unfilled, 298; axis, 453, 511; difference (in sound localization), 220; error, 465, 469-472, 478; negative time error, 465, 467-471, 473, 475, 476, 479; positive time error, 468-470, 473, 475, 476, 479, 480
Timidity, 364-366
Titchener, E. B., 113, 113 n., 143, 319, 358, 632
Tolman, E. C., 25, 30, 34 n., 36, 55, 56, 356 n., 364, 365, 366, 391, 529, 538, 539, 540, 541, 547, 585, 586, 588
Tonus of musculature, 45, 50

Total reaction, 532, 534; situation, 158, 159, 459, 532
Trace, 207, 339, 340, 424, 429-432, 436, 437, 440, 443-446, 451-461, 464, 465, 470-476, 479-485, 488-493, 496-510, 514-528, 529, 533, 535-538, 541, 542, 546, 548-554, 563, 564, 567-570, 572, 584, 587, 588, 592, 594-597, 601-605, 609, 610, 613, 614, 622, 624, 630, 638, 643, 674, 681; mapping processes, 443; aggregation, 230, 481, 485, 486, 488-491, 493, 505, 508, 512, 516, 519, 524, 525, 537, 544, 545, 599, 603, 609; assimilation, 453, 468, 470, 472, 475, 476, 479, 481, 502; column, 447-449, 453, 461, 477, 597, 599, 608, 609-612, 615; core and shaft of, 609-611, 614; properties, instrinsic, 474, 499, 523, 577, 623, 631, 636; stratification, 525; systems, 454, 456, 461, 462, 470, 473-476, 481, 482, 484, 488, 489, 494, 497, 501, 503-505, 511-513, 516, 517, 522, 525-528, 537, 540, 544-546, 555, 561, 564, 567, 572, 582, 584, 592, 607, 613, 615-617, 622-624, 634, 642, 644, 646; changes of, 469, 470, 472, 473, 493, 496, 498-505, 519, 522-524, 540, 556, 603; consolidation of, 544; destruction of, 468, 523, 524; deterioration of, 621, 622; effect of on process, 509, 513, 541, 547, 550, 553, 561, 562, 566, 582, 586, 587, 589, 590, 600, 606, 607, 609, 613, 630; interaction of and process, 554, 555, 563, 566, 567, 600, 624, 638; place of different from that of process, 440, 441, 444, 457, 494; *see also* Availability of trace, Communication of trace, Co-operation between trace and stimuli, Ego-field relation in trace, Selection of trace
Transfer, 414, 430, 546, 547
Transformation, 225, 232-234, 254, 259, 259 n., 260
Transformation of processes, 550, 552, 615, 631; by effect, 551, 644
Transparency, 181, 260-265
Transposition, 460, 510; *see also* Law of transposition
Trial and error, 552, 625, 629, 645
Tridimensional organization, *see* Organization, tridimensional
Tridimensional space, 106, 115, 116, 160
Tudor-Hart, B., 135, 263 f., 263 n.
Tunnel illusion (of size), 212, 222; motion, 450, 451
Two-point limen, 202

Unconscious, 51, 52, 518
Understanding, 509, 550, 551
Understanding (as opposed to explaining), 19-21, 53, 175, 332, 677
Unification, 126, 128, 132, 137, 141, 147-149, 152, 160, 162, 164, 208, 270, 285, 328, 451, 454, 481, 504, 507, 519, 545, 569, 570, 609, 632, 644, 665
Uniformity of a unit, 135, 149, 165, 171-173, 186, 197, 262, 434, 439, 447
Unique cases in constancy phenomena, 224, 225, 227, 231, 236, 255
Unit formation, 106, 125, 126, 129, 134, 147, 168, 175, 177, 434, 437, 443, 451, 463, 466, 569
Units, 514, 566; spatial, 77, 125, 169, 176, 178, 203, 204, 275, 323, 439, 443, 449, 466, 568, 569; temporal, 437, 439, 448-451, 506, 515, 533, 550, 553; trace, 443, 444
Unity, 609, 681; spatial, 84, 97, 133, 171, 197, 346, 352, 353, 361, 439, 450, 452; temporal, 287 n., 439, 446, 452, 453; of one continuous tone, 439, 446; of a temporal pair, 439-442, 446, 451, 466
Unum organization, 153, 154, 162
Upwards tendency of Ego, *see* Ego, upwards tendency of
Usefulness, 279, 280
Utilization of signs, 160, 266

Value, 17, 19, 21, 347, 351
Vectors, 337, 372, 408, 410
Velocity, 276, 282, 288-297, 303, 378, 435; and brightness, 290, 291; and orientation, 290, 291; and size, 289, 291; objective stroboscopic, 292-295; of propagation, 99
Verbalization, 501
Veridicalness of experience, 224, 225, 227, 231, 318, 380, 658; *see also* Cognition
Vernon, P. E., 677, 678
Vestibular organ, 121
Vigilance, 100, 102, 173
Visual acuity, 205, 206, 278, 438
Vitalism, 16, 17, 19, 21, 47, 308, 331, 417, 423, 460, 560, 631
Vogel, P., 390 n.
Volkelt, H., 638
Volkmann, W. F., 145, 212
Voluntarism, 420
Voluntary action, *see* Action, voluntary

Waals, H. G. van der, 281, 286 n.
Warden, C., 622 n., 625

War landscape, 44
Watson, J. B., 390
Wax tablet, 474
We, 651-653, 655, 665, 667, 676
Weber's law, 13
Werner, H., 360
Wertheimer, M., 15 n., 18, 20, 53, 54, 56, 57, 59, 61, 62, 63, 64, 66, 110, 134, 136, 138, 149, 153, 155, 164, 166, 168, 175, 179, 215, 220, 246, 260, 280, 281, 287, 292, 301, 303, 360, 361, 371, 372, 373, 381, 449, 510, 511, 512, 513, 615, 627, 634, 637, 641, 683, 684
Wheeler, R. H., 401, 414 n., 424, 454, 457, 458, 458 n., 459, 460, 518, 592
Wheels, their motion, 284, 377
Whitehead, A. N., 380
Whiteness, 80, 81, 84, 112, 116, 128, 243, 244, 246-248, 258, 260, 263 n., 277; *see also* Constancy of whiteness
Whole, 175, 462, 463
Whole and part, 26, 176, 569, 601, 602, 665, 682
Why? 383
Will, 416, 419, 421, 571, 574, 578; measurement of will, 574
Wishes, 325, 327, 334, 343, 368, 642
Witasek, S., 212, 213, 267 n., 564, 565, 566
Wittich von, 145
Wohlfahrt, E., 143
Wolff, Werner, 672, 678
Wolff, Wilhelm, 260, 260 n.
Woodworth, R. S., 160, 401, 482 n., 529 f.
Wordsworth, W., 326, 359
Works of art, 347
Wulf, F., 493, 494, 495, 496, 497, 498, 498 n., 499, 500, 501, 502, 505, 507, 634
Wundt, W., 55, 82, 85, 97, 103, 134, 583
Würzburg school, 559, 560, 574

Yoshioka, J. G., 356

Zeigarnik, B., 334 f., 336, 337 f., 339, 340, 341, 508, 522, 555 n., 618, 619, 622
Zenith-horizon illusion, 78, 94, 95, 236, 278, 279, 388
Zeno's paradox, 424, 425
Zöllner illusion, 275
Zone law, 295

Printed in the United Kingdom
by Lightning Source UK Ltd.
117068UKS00003B/16-18

9 780415 209625